AF718962

WITHDRAWN

Comparative Neurology of the Telencephalon

Comparative Neurology of the Telencephalon

Edited by
Sven O. E. Ebbesson
Catholic University of Puerto Rico
Ponce, Puerto Rico

Plenum Press · New York and London

Library of Congress Cataloging in Publication Data

Main entry under title:

Comparative neurology of the telencephalon

Includes bibliographies and index.

1. Telencephalon. 2. Vertebrates – Physiology. 3. Anatomy, Comparative. 4. Neurology. I. Ebbesson, Sven O. E. [DNLM: 1. Telencephalon. 2. Anatomy, Comparative. 3. Physiology, Comparative. QL933 C737 (P)]
QP381.C63 596'.01'88 79-12145
ISBN 0-306-40237-8

QP
381
.C63

© 1980 Plenum Press, New York
A Division of Plenum Publishing Corporation
227 West 17th Street, New York, N.Y. 10011

All rights reserved

No part of this book may be reproduced, stored in a retrieval system, or transmitted, in any form or by any means, electronic, mechanical, photocopying, microfilming, recording, or otherwise, without written permission from the Publisher

Printed in the United States of America

Dedicated to Professor Horacio Vanegas and his son, Professor Horacio Vanegas Fishbach, whose kindness and generosity will never be forgotten by those who met in Caracas to exchange views on the evolution of the telencephalon.

Contributors

LARRY BENOWITZ • Department of Psychiatry, Harvard Medical School, and Lowell Laboratories, McLean Hospital, Belmont, Massachusetts 02178

MARK R. BRAFORD, Jr. • Division of Biological Sciences, University of Michigan, Ann Arbor, Michigan 48109

ANN B. BUTLER • Department of Anatomy, Georgetown University, Washington, D.C. 20007

JAN P. C. de BRUIN • Netherlands Central Institute for Brain Research, IJdijk 28, Amsterdam, The Netherlands

SVEN O. E. EBBESSON • Department of Anatomy, Catholic University of Puerto Rico, Ponce, Puerto Rico 00731

RAYMOND CURTIS GRAEBER • Department of Military Medical Psychophysiology, Division of Neuropsychiatry, Walter Reed Army Institute of Research, Washington, D.C. 20012

MIMI HALPERN • Department of Anatomy and Program in Biological Psychology, Downstate Medical Center, Brooklyn, New York 11203

JOHN IRWIN JOHNSON, Jr. • Departments of Biophysics, Psychology, and Zoology, Michigan State University, East Lansing, Michigan 48824

JON H. KAAS • Department of Psychology, Vanderbilt University, Nashville, Tennessee 37240

EARL KICLITER • Department of Anatomy and Laboratory of Neurobiology, Division of Biological Sciences, University of Puerto Rico School of Medicine, San Juan, Puerto Rico 00901

RICHARD A. LENDE • Deceased. Department of Neurophysiology, University of Wisconsin, Madison, Wisconsin 53706

R. GLENN NORTHCUTT • Division of Biological Sciences, University of Michigan, Ann Arbor, Michigan 48109

ELLENGENE PETERSON • Department of Anatomy, The University of Chicago, Chicago, Illinois 60637. *Present address:* School of Anatomy, The University of New South Wales, Kensington, New South Wales, Australia 2033

MICHAEL B. PRITZ • University Hospitals, University of Michigan Medical Center, Ann Arbor, Michigan 48109

GEORGE ERIC SAVAGE • Department of Zoology and Comparative Physiology, Queen Mary College, University of London, London E1 4NS, England

DOLORES M. SCHROEDER • Medical Sciences Program, Indiana University School of Medicine, Bloomington, Indiana 47401

HORACIO VANEGAS • Centro de Biofísica y Bioquímica, Instituto Venezolano de Investigaciones Científicas (IVIC), Caracas, Venezuela

WALLY WELKER • Department of Neurophysiology, University of Wisconsin, Madison, Wisconsin 53706

Foreword

When a young graduate student sat before Percival Bailey in 1960 and spoke of his longstanding interest in zoology and his recent interest in the nervous system, he asked the then Director of the Illinois Neuropsychiatric Institute if there was support in the scientific establishment for research in evolutionary comparative neurology. Bailey patted his abdomen with both hands and thought for a moment. Finally he said: "Young man, there is no place for people like you." The graduate student was crestfallen.

To a large extent what Bailey said is still true. The greater part of research in neurobiology is directed toward answering a single broad question. How do brains in general, and the human brain in particular, work? This is a legitimate and important question. It is not, however, the only question worth answering. This overweening emphasis on function, especially in regard to the human nervous system, is a result of the origins of neurology in the clinic. The professional school, site of most such research, has been remarkably well-insulated from many of the major concerns of biology.

The telencephalon has figured prominently in concepts relating to the intellectual superiority of man over the beasts. As a consequence, a great many studies have been made of the structural organization, physiological properties, and behavioral role of the cerebral hemispheres of mammalian brains. Less attention has been devoted to the telencephalon of nonmammalian vertebrates. This relative neglect was partially a result of the widespread notion that the forebrain of most nonmammalian vertebrate groups was exclusively concerned with olfaction, a sensory system with somewhat less appeal to human-oriented investigators.

As a result of pioneering experimental studies in the late 1960s and early 1970s it is now well known that there are strong organizational similarities in the forebrains of amniotes. Also, olfaction apparently does *not* dominate the forebrain of birds, reptiles, amphibians, and fishes. These findings have raised many questions. If portions of the telencephalon of nonmammalian vertebrates are "wired up" in a manner similar to the neocortex of mammals, do these cell populations perform the same functions as does neocortex? If they do, what then is the significance of the laminar organization found in mammals? If they do not, then how is the laminar organization involved in this difference in function? What were the selection pressures involved in the evolution of neocortex? Where did this neocortex first appear in vertebrate history? It is important also to remember that a frog brain is not designed to be an intermediate brain between that of a fish and that of a man. It is designed to regulate the physiological functions and behavior of a frog living in an environment that challenges the animal to survive as a frog. The frog brain is interesting from that point of view in addition to whatever it may tell us about the brain of man.

The participants in the conference which produced this book were charged with the task of assessing what we have learned about the vertebrate telencephalon since the appearance of that burst of research activity in the 1960s which continues to this day. How well they have accomplished this task must be judged by the reader. It is nevertheless encouraging to this former graduate student that there are now more neurobiologists interested in zoology and the nervous system than there were when Percival Bailey momentarily shattered his hopes. This conference was a witness to that fact. To Bailey's everlasting credit, he did not recommend the abandonment of interest in evolutionary comparative neurology. On the contrary, he suggested that a place for this interest had to be made.

C. B. G. Campbell

Preface

The fascination of comparative neurology can be compared to the fascination experienced by those who engage in a search for their individual roots through means of genealogical studies. During a period of almost 100 years, comparative neurologists have been examining animals selected from almost all vertebrate groups in order to understand how brains evolved. The search for an understanding of the neocortical evolution has particularly captivated neurologists because they believed this would lead to a better understanding of the essence of man.

The insights obtained from most neurological studies have always been highly dependent on the technology available. As new techniques for studying brain structures became available, and were applied, more meaningful interpretations were made of the highly varied and confounding brain organizations. About 20 years ago, the development of better methods for tracing neuronal pathways revolutionalized a field of exploration that had been dormant for several decades. As a result, a great number of new neuronal pathways have been traced in a broad spectrum of vertebrates. The technological breakthroughs were especially important to those researchers studying the telencephalon. All at once a completely new insight was provided into the evolution of the mammalian cerebral cortex. These data have been complemented with new exciting physiological and behavioral studies.

Recent evidence indicates that the so-called neocortex was probably formed not by an invasion of neuronal systems from caudal levels, as previously thought, but rather by differentiation and proliferation of systems already present in the brains of the earliest vertebrates. The data, at this point in time, are far from complete and provide no real insight into which selective pressures resulted in specific morphological features, although that is no doubt coming.

This book provides a review of some of the most recent data on the telencephalic structure and function in the major vertebrate groups. The focus is on the sensory systems because a great deal of factual information is already available. Other regions, such as the amygdala and the hippocampus, are not dealt with extensively because these systems, in nonmammalian vertebrates, are still not well understood and there is a scarcity of valid data.

One of the most stimulating messages that one receives, as he reads through the pages of this book, is that almost unlimited opportunities exist in comparative neurology for gaining a more complete understanding of how brains work and how each structure evolved.

The Editor

Contents

3 New Observations on the Organization and Evolution of the Telencephalon of Actinopterygian Fishes

R. GLENN NORTHCUTT and MARK R. BRAFORD, Jr.

4 The Telencephalon of Teleosts

DOLORES M. SCHROEDER

5 Projections of the Teleostean Telencephalon

HORACIO VANEGAS and SVEN O. E. EBBESSON

6 The Fish Telencephalon and Its Relation to Learning

GEORGE ERIC SAVAGE

7 Telencephalon and Behavior in Teleost Fish: A Neuroethological Approach

JAN P. C. de BRUIN

8 Organization of the Amphibian Telencephalon

R. GLENN NORTHCUTT and EARL KICLITER

9 The Telencephalon of Snakes

MIMI HALPERN

10 Cytoarchitectonic and Connectional Organization of the Lacertilian Telencephalon with Comments on Vertebrate Forebrain Evolution

ANN B. BUTLER

11 Parallels in the Organization of Auditory and Visual Systems in Crocodiles

MICHAEL B. PRITZ

12 Behavioral Studies of Telencephalic Function in Reptiles

ELLENGENE PETERSON

13 Functional Organization of the Avian Telencephalon

LARRY BENOWITZ

14 Morphological Correlates of Specialized Elaborations in Somatic Sensory Cerebral Neocortex

JOHN IRWIN JOHNSON, Jr.

15 Thalamocortical Relationships in Echidna (*Tachyglossus aculeatus*)

WALLY WELKER and RIÇHARD A. LENDE

16 A Comparative Survey of Visual Cortex Organization in Mammals

JON H. KAAS

1

On The Organization of the Telencephalon in Elasmobranchs

SVEN O. E. EBBESSON

I. Introduction

The interest in brain organization of elasmobranchs relates to the evolutionary history of the group. The best paleontological information suggests an origin in the early Devonian period, some 400 million years ago, or 250 million years before the African and American continents separated. The sharks evolved rapidly in Devonian times and continued their expansion through the Carboniferous and Permian periods. The available data suggest that the group was successful early and that relatively few selective pressures for structural modification have taken place since those early days.

Contrary to common belief only 10 years ago, recent studies have shown that brain organization in sharks is much more "advanced" in terms of connections than hitherto believed, that the brain size–body weight ratio in some sharks exceeds those of other anamniotes, and that some sharks are capable of learning complex visual discriminations rapidly (see Chapter 2 in this volume). These and other findings have revealed our ignorance about brain organizations of elasmobranchs and have provided new insights into brain evolution. Perhaps the most important recent revision of thought relates to the organization and functional role of the forebrain. Whereas the telencephalon has traditionally been considered an "olfactory lobe," recent experiments indicate an organization comparable to that of other vertebrates, including mammals.

This is a brief overview of telencephalic organization as we see it 12 years after the new neuroanatomical methods of Nauta (1957) were first applied to shark

SVEN O. E. EBBESSON • Department of Anatomy, Catholic University of Puerto Rico, Ponce, Puerto Rico 00731.

brains (Ebbesson, 1967; for an excellent review of brain organization as it was understood in 1963, see Aronson, 1963). These techniques allowed the first accurate tracing of neuronal pathways and involve the selective silver impregnation of degenerating axons and their terminals (Ebbesson, 1970).

II. Organization of Elasmobranchs

The cartilagenous fishes (class Chondrichthyes) are composed of two major groups, the Holocephali and the Elasmobranchii. The latter group is by far the larger and comprises the sharks, rays, and skates. Table I indicates the organization of the class and shows which groups have been studied in terms of their brain structure (from Northcutt, 1977).

III. Brain Weight–Body Weight Ratio

Brains of elasmobranchs are, on the whole, relatively large compared to brains of other nonmammalian forms. Brain weight–body weight ratios are in some cases comparable to those of birds and mammals (Ebbesson and Northcutt, 1976; Northcutt, 1977). The relatively large telencephalon in elasmobranchs is also noteworthy. The mammalian and the osteichthyan data presented in Fig. 1 have been taken from Jerison (1973), and the stippled polygon encloses the elasmobranch brain–body data reported by Ebbesson and Northcutt (1976) and Northcutt (1977), as

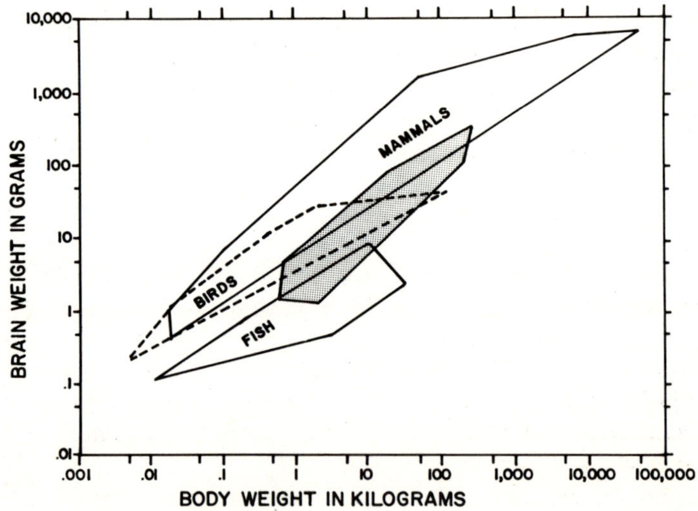

Figure 1. Brain and body weights for four vertebrate classes expressed as minimum convex polygons after Jerison (1973). Stippled polygon encloses elasmobranch brain–body ratios and overlaps polygons for bony fishes, birds, and mammals. From Ebbesson and Northcutt (1976), Northcutt (1977), and data recently collected by the author.

Table I. Elasmobranch CNS in Literature

- Class Chondrichthyes
  - Subclass Holocephali
    - *Callorhynchus antarcticus* (Kuhlenbeck and Niimi, 1969)
    - *Chimaera monstrosa* (Holmgren, 1922; Faucette, 1969)
    - *Hydrolagus colliei*[a] (Kuhlenbeck and Niimi, 1969)
  - Subclass Elasmobranchii
    - Superorder Squalomorphii
      - Order Hexanchiformes
        - *Chlamydoselachus anguineus* (Masai, 1961)
        - *Hexanchus* (Ariëns Kappers *et al.*, 1936)
        - *Notorynchus maculatus*[a]
        - *Heptranchias* (Johnston, 1911; Bäckström, 1924)
      - Order Squaliformes
        - *Etmopterus lucifer* (Okada *et al.*, 1969; Masai *et al.*, 1973)
        - *Etmopterus hillianus*[a]
        - *Squalus acanthias*[a] (Johnston, 1911; Holmgren, 1922; Bäckström, 1924; Leghissa, 1962; Smeets and Nieuwenhuys, 1976)
        - *Deania rostrata* (Okada *et al.*, 1969)
        - *Centroscyllium ritteri* (Okada *et al.*, 1969)
      - Order Pristiophoriformes
        - *Pristiophorus japonicus* (Okada *et al.*, 1969)
    - Superorder Batoidea
      - Order Rajiformes
        - *Rhinobatos productus*[a]
        - *Platyrhinoidis triseriata*[a]
        - *Raja clavata* (Johnston, 1911; Bäckström, 1924; Leghissa, 1962; Veselkin, 1965)
        - *Raja eglanteria*[a]
      - Order Pristiformes
        - No known literature
      - Order Torpediniformes
        - *Torpedo ocellata* (Bäckström, 1924; Hugosson, 1955; Leghissa, 1962; Bruckmoser, 1973; Bruckmoser and Dieringer, 1973; Platt *et al.*, 1974)
      - Order Myliobatiformes
        - *Potamotrygon motoro*[a]
        - *Myliobatis aquila* (Johnston, 1911; Ariëns Kappers *et al.*, 1936)
    - Superorder Squatinomorphii
      - No known literature
    - Superorder Galeomorphii
      - Order Heterodontiformes
        - *Heterodontus francisci*[a]
        - *Heterodontus japonicus* (Masai, 1962; Kusunoki *et al.*, 1973)

- Class Chondrichthyes (*continued*)
  - Subclass Elasmobranchii (*continued*)
    - Superorder Galeomorphii (*continued*)
      - Order Orectolobiformes
        - *Ginglymostoma cirratum*[a] (Ebbesson and Ramsey, 1968; Ebbesson and Heimer, 1970; Ebbesson and Schroeder, 1971; Ebbesson, 1972*a,b*; Cohen *et al.*, 1973; Ebbesson and Campbell, 1973; Schroeder and Ebbesson, 1974; Schroeder and Ebbesson, 1975)
      - Order Lamniformes
        - *Odontaspis* (Okada *et al.*, 1969)
        - *Mitsukurina owstoni* (Masai *et al.*, 1973)
        - *Alopias* (Okada *et al.*, 1969)
        - *Carcharodon carcharias* (Gilbert, 1963)
        - *Isurus oxyrinchus* (Gilbert, 1963; Okada *et al.*, 1969)
        - *Lamna* (Ariëns Kappers *et al.*, 1936)
      - Order Carcharhiniformes
        - *Scyliorhinus caniculus* (Haller, 1898; Edinger, 1901; Johnston, 1911; Dart, 1920; Bäckström, 1924; Beccari, 1930; Bruckmoser and Dieringer, 1973; Platt *et al.*, 1974; Smeets and Nieuwenhuys, 1976)
        - *Scyliorhinus retifer*[a]
        - *Scyliorhinus stellaris* (Johnston, 1911; Bäckström, 1924; Leghissa, 1962)
        - *Mustelus canis*[a] (Shaper, 1898; Houser, 1901; Bäckström, 1924; Gerlach, 1947; McCready and Boord, 1976)
        - *Mustelus laevis* (Bäckström, 1924; Leghissa, 1962; Platt *et al.*, 1974)
        - *Triakis scyllia*[a]
        - *Galeocerdo cuvieri*[a] (Ebbesson and Ramsey, 1968)
        - *Scoliodon* (Johnston, 1911; Masai, 1962)
        - *Carcharhinus floridanus*[a]
        - *Carcharhinus leucas*[a]
        - *Carcharhinus milberti*[a]
        - *Aprionodon isodon*[a]
        - *Negaprion brevirostris*[a] (Tester, 1963; Graeber and Ebbesson, 1972*a*)
        - *Prionace glauca*[a] (Aronson, 1963; Okada *et al.*, 1969)
        - *Sphyrna lewini*[a]
        - *Sphyrna tiburo*[a]
        - *Sphyrna zygaena* (Okada *et al.*, 1969)

[a] Studied by Northcutt (1977).

well as new data I have collected. In addition to the brain–body ratios comparable to those of birds and mammals, it is clear that elasmobranchs have approximately the same range of variation in brain size as do other major vertebrate classes. It is particularly clear from Northcutt's (1977) analysis that squalomorph sharks in general have lower brain–body ratios than galeomorph sharks. The batoids range throughout the polygon, but the rajiforms are characterized by low brain–body ratios and the more advanced myliobatiforms by the highest brain–body ratios presently known for elasmobranchs (Northcutt, 1977).

The significance of these facts alone is now known, but the data, evaluated together with our observations of the relatively dense packing of neurons and the massive and complex neuronal systems, suggest to me that sharks likely live a more complex life and are "cerebrally more capable" than has previously been thought.

IV. Telencephalic Organization in General

The brains of elasmobranchs share gross features of organization with other vertebrate groups, although the adult telencephalon of most sharks and rays shows

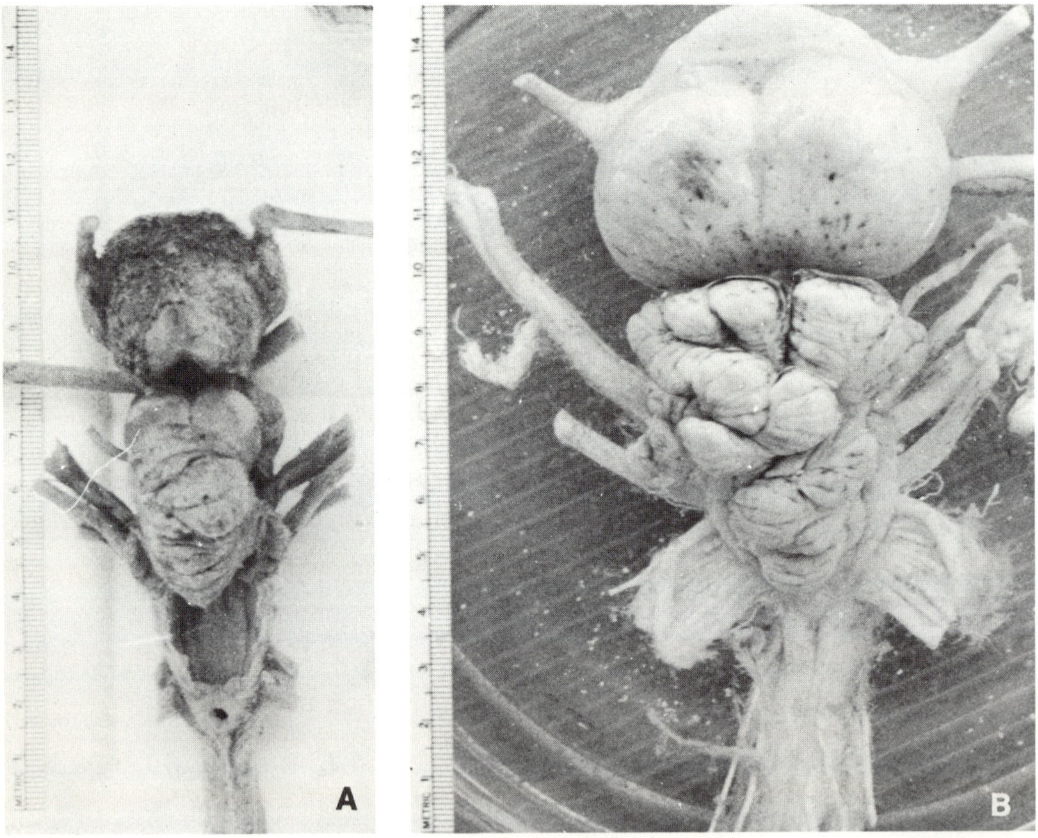

Figure 2. Photographs of the dorsal surface of a tiger shark brain (A) and a manta ray brain (B). The tiger shark weighed 568 kg and its brain 47.2 g. The manta weighed 248 kg and its brain 270 g.

a confounding organization in that the hemispheres are fused across the midline and that the major part of the lateral ventricles is obliterated by a massive development of large nuclear groups (Figs. 2–4). This appearance in cross sections is a unique feature of elasmobranchs and appears to have confused comparative neurologists from the very beginning.

The telencephalon in nurse sharks appears to have most features in common with that of other elasmobranchs. The hemispheres are fused in the midline, the lateral ventricles are compressed, and all cell aggregates, with the exception of the area superficialis basalis of Johnston (1911), appear as unlaminated cell groups, although they all must evolve from the embryonic lamination of the embryonic telencephalic vesicles (see Fig. 3). Since the significance and interrelationships at the various telencephalic masses are still poorly understood, only well-studied aggregates are labeled in Fig. 7. The literature predating the connectional studies in

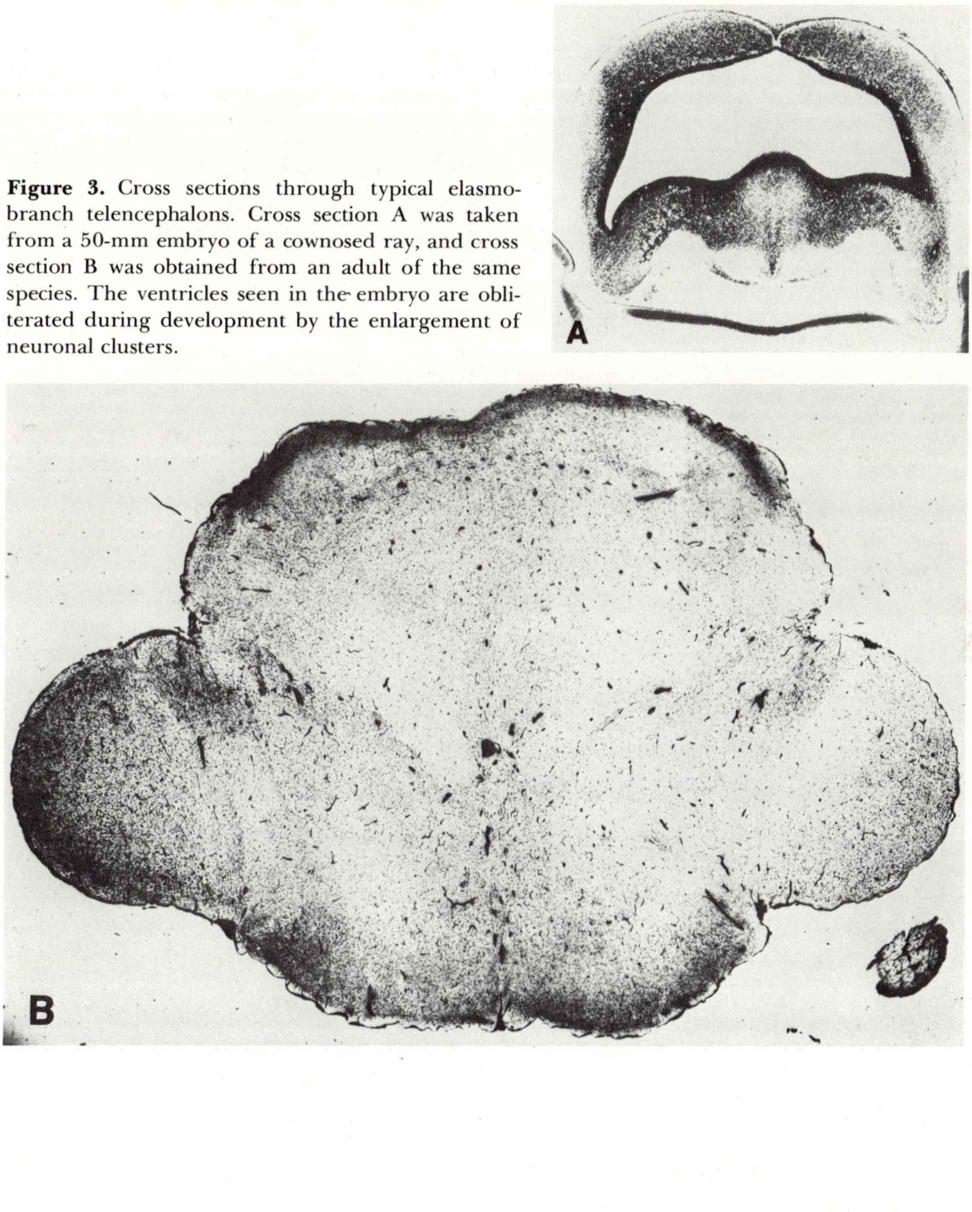

Figure 3. Cross sections through typical elasmobranch telencephalons. Cross section A was taken from a 50-mm embryo of a cownosed ray, and cross section B was obtained from an adult of the same species. The ventricles seen in the embryo are obliterated during development by the enlargement of neuronal clusters.

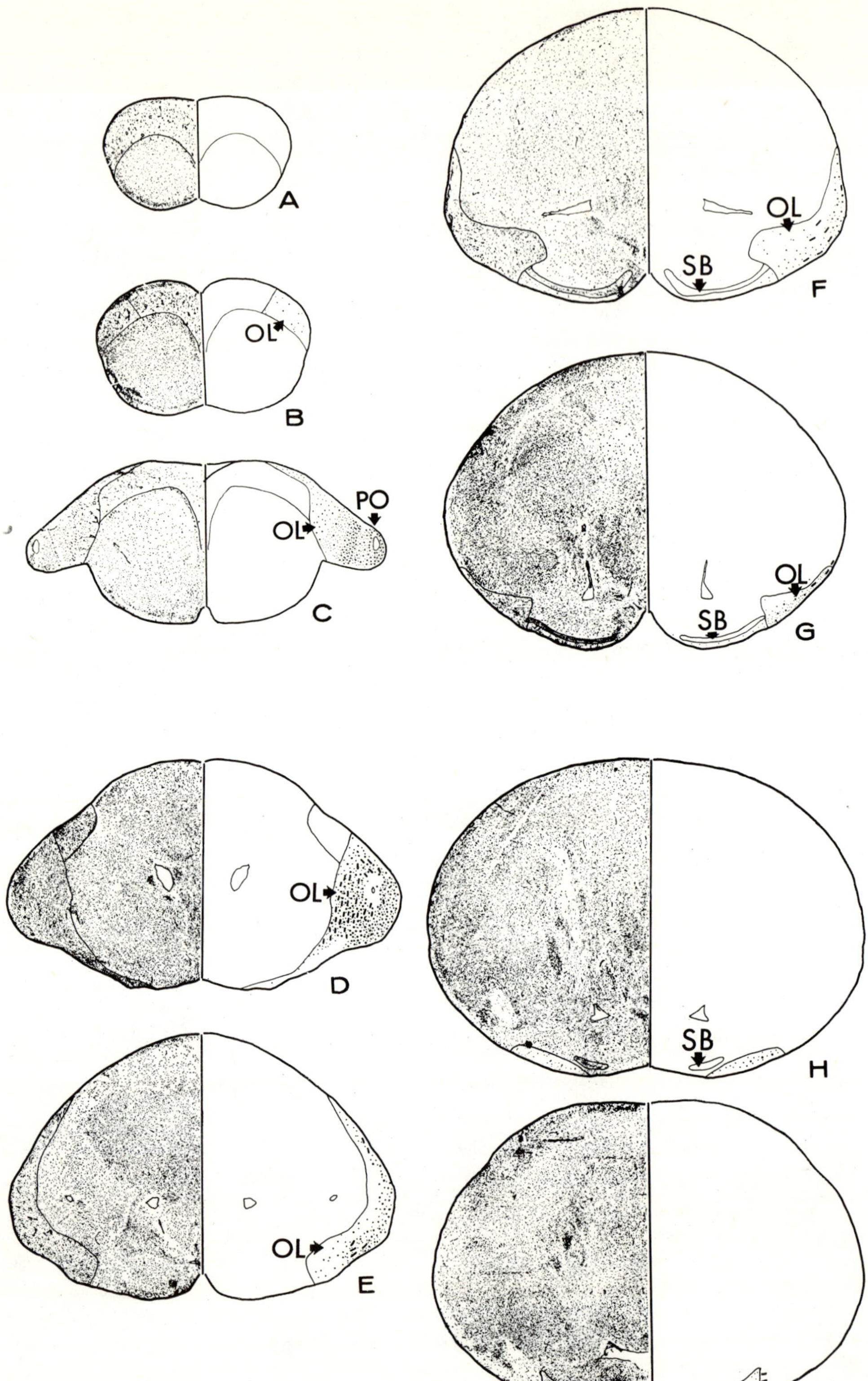
A
OL
B
PO
OL
C
OL
SB
F
OL
SB
G
OL
D
OL
E
SB
H
I

my laboratory has been reviewed elsewhere (Schroeder and Ebbesson, 1974) and will not be repeated here because of its questionable significance. Suffice it to say that almost every investigator has applied his or her own nomenclature to a given cell group depending on his or her interpretation of homologies.

Shark brains vary considerably among species, reflecting ancestry, mode of life, and sensory capabilities. At one extreme, heterodonts have small, poorly developed brains, whereas carcharinids, at the other extreme, have relatively large and well-differentiated brains associated with better development of the sensory systems. The most striking feature about shark brains is the comparatively large telencephalon, which until recently was thought to be concerned primarily with the olfactory system.

The sharks and rays show a unity of structure that suggests their common ancestry (Compagno, 1973). The skates and rays are, in effect, specialized sharks, having evolved from the primitive sharks. In these fishes the pectoral fins have become greatly enlarged and are used somewhat like wings. Gross brain morphology of sharks and rays is strikingly similar, especially if specimens of embryos are compared. Not only are embryonic brains of sharks and rays similar, but embryonic brains are also strikingly similar to the adult brains of the so-called primitive sharks (e.g., *Heterodontus*). In *Ginglymostoma* and other advanced sharks and rays, the basic vertebrate picture of a telencephalic vesicle with lateral ventricles is obliterated by a massive enlargement of the pallial mantle. The result is the creation of enormous, poorly differentiated nuclei, whose organization is poorly understood. The central telencephalic nucleus is such an aggregate; its role as a likely neopallial homologue did not become apparent until connectional studies revealed its similarity to neocortex.

Systematic surveys of neuronal connections in a broad sample of elasmobranch species have not been undertaken, and our present understanding of brain organization comes principally from an intensive examination of the brain of the nurse shark (*Ginglymostoma cirratum*) over the last 12 years. These studies have revealed that visual, olfactory, somatosensory, cerebellar, and tectal pathways are strikingly similar to those reported in other vertebrates (Ebbesson, 1967, 1972*b*; Ebbesson and Campbell, 1973; Ebbesson and Heimer, 1970). How typical the results of these

Figure 4. A: Frontal section through the nurse shark telencephalon about 0.5 mm from the rostral pole. A photomicrograph of the Nissl picture is shown on the left-hand half of A–I for the purpose of giving the orientation of the nuclear groups. Evidence of degenerating olfactory tract fibers was absent at this level. B: Frontal section about 1.0 mm caudal to A showing diffuse terminal degeneration in the lateral olfactory area (OL). In the drawing on the right-hand side, in this and C–I, the large dots and interrupted lines indicate degenerating fibers of passage and small dots show loci of terminal degeneration. C: Frontal section about 2.0 mm caudal to B, through the level of the olfactory peduncle (PO) and the lateral olfactory area (OL). D: Frontal section about 3.0 mm caudal to C illustrating the diffuse terminal degeneration seen in the lateral olfactory area (OL), here covering most of the lateral surface of the telencephalon. E: Frontal section about 3.0 mm caudal to D beginning to show the ventral shift of the lateral olfactory area (OL). F: Frontal section about 2.0 mm caudal to E and through the area superficialis basalis (SB). Note the shift of olfactory tract fibers to a more ventral position. G: Frontal section about 3.0 mm caudal to F showing a relatively small lateral olfactory area (OL) and evidence of a small amount of terminal degeneration ventral to area superficialis basalis (SB). H: Frontal section about 2.0 mm caudal to G showing the caudal tip of area superficialis basalis (SB) and an area of diffuse terminal degeneration just lateral to it. I: Section about 2.0 mm caudal to H showing the most caudally traced olfactory tract fibers.

observations are of other elasmobranchs is not known, although the general impression is that they are probably representative of the class because of the relative similarity of their gross morphological features.

Nauta's method for tracing neuronal connections was one of the major technical breakthroughs in neuroanatomical methodology. It was first applied to mammals but was later modified for other vertebrates (Ebbesson, 1970), including fishes (Ebbesson, 1967). The techniques involve lesioning an individual brain tract under general anesthesia, closing the wound, and letting the animal survive the operation for about 30 days. At this time, the animal is transcardially perfused with a fixative and the brain removed. The fixed brain is then frozen and sectioned serially. The sections are treated according to one or more variants of the original Nauta technique (Ebbesson, 1970). The resulting microscopic preparations reveal the course and destination of degenerated nerve fibers lesioned months earlier. By such techniques it has been possible to trace the course and termination of a considerable number of pathways. The whole picture is far from complete, however, because most brain structures have not been studied and numerous aspects of brain organization still remain unknown.

V. Olfactory Input

That olfaction is an important modality in most sharks is brought out by the large size of the olfactory epithelia and the related brain parts. The rhinencephalon of sharks is composed of the olfactory penduncle, the lateral olfactory area, and the area superficialis basalis of Johnston (see Fig. 4). These olfactory regions compose approximately the same percentage of forebrain bulk as in the rat. Histologically these regions are poorly differentiated compared to the olfactory cortex of land-dwelling vertebrates in which it is usually conspicuously laminated with several layers of cells possessing well differentiated dendrites oriented toward the brain surface. In most sharks, on the other hand, olfactory neurons appear relatively simple, their dendrites lacking any obvious preferred orientation, and they are not arranged in laminae except in the area superficialis basalis of Johnston (1911).

The olfactory tract distributes fibers diffusely to the well-restricted olfactory regions in the ipsilateral ventrolateral part of the brain (Ebbesson and Heimer, 1970) (Fig. 4). Only when large lesions of the lateral olfactory area (OL) were made was it possible to observe a contralateral connection (Ebbesson, 1972*b*). In this series of experiments, the lateral olfactory area was found to project heavily to the lateral portion of area superficialis basalis ipsilaterally, with a few fibers extending caudally to cross at the level of the optic chiasm and terminate in the contralateral area superficialis basalis and the lateral olfactory area. A few degenerating axons could also be traced into the contralateral olfactory tract.

These findings were in direct conflict with the view that the entire telencephalon in sharks had a bilateral input from the olfactory bulbs (e.g., Bäckström, 1924), making it essentially an olfactory structure. Later anatomical studies (Ebbesson, 1972*b*) and electrophysiological investigations (Cohen, Leonard, Duff, and Ebbesson, unpublished observations) have confirmed the limits of this system.

It would perhaps not be fair to say that these findings indicate a smaller role of olfaction in sharks than hitherto suggested. When one takes the available behavioral, physiological, and connectional data together, however, the impression is rather that sharks indeed have a great olfactory sensitivity but that the discrimination of a great variety of odors might not be possible if there is a correlation between brain differentiation and descriminative ability.

VI. Visual Input

Vision plays an important role in many shark species, and, although this modality is generally considered primarily useful at short range (Gilbert, 1963), it is clear both from the size of the eyes and related brain structures and from behavioral studies that vision is heavily relied on (Fig. 5 and Chapter 2). Gilbert (1963) has in many elegant contributions described the anatomy of the eye and the role of vision in sharks, and his publications are referred to for those aspects. The brain organization subserving vision has recently received considerable attention in our laboratory and will be reviewed here. Although most of our studies have involved the nurse shark, we have found the lemon shark (Graeber and Ebbesson, 1972*a*) and the tiger shark (Ebbesson, 1967) surprisingly similar in basic organization. The main difference appears to be a greater packing density of neurons in the nurse shark, with a concomitant greater differentiation of neuronal pools, a finding not understood at this time.

The brain structures subserving vision are (1) those that receive a retinal input and (2) those that receive secondary or tertiary inputs via the primary visual nuclei.

The optic tract projects almost entirely contralaterally to (1) the hypothalamus, (2) the dorsolateral optic complex (DLOC) of the thalamus, (3) the ventrolateral

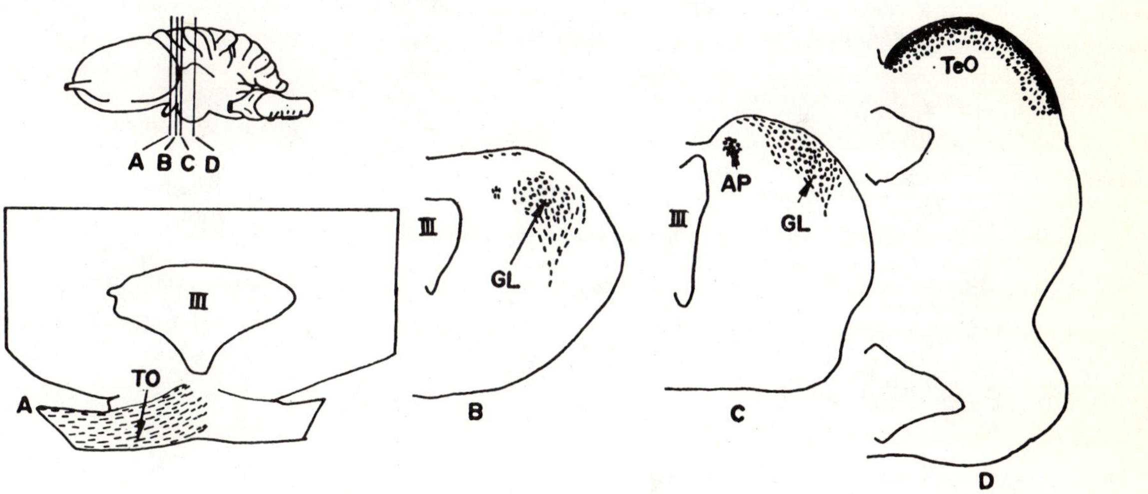

Figure 5. The degenerating fibers following unilateral eye enucleation can be traced with the Nauta technique to the contralateral hypothalamus (not shown), lateral geniculate nucleus (GL) (sometimes referred to as the dorsolateral optic nuclear complex, DLOC), the pretectal area (AP), and the optic tectum (TeO). TO, Optic tract; III, third ventricle.

optic nucleus (VLO), (4) the optic tectum, (5) the pretectal nuclei, and (6) in some species a projection to a ventromedial optic nucleus (VMO) (Ebbesson, 1972*a*; Ebbesson and Ramsey, 1968; Northcutt, 1976). Little is known about some of these connections, and only the retinal projections to the hypothalamus, the DLOC, and the optic tectum will be described below.

The optic nerve has been traced to the various targets in the brain with the Nauta (1957) and Fink–Heimer (1967) techniques in several species of sharks (Ebbesson, 1967; Ebbesson and Ramsey, 1968; Graeber and Ebbesson, 1972*a*). The optic nerve fibers undergo complete decussation, with the exception of a very small number of fibers that leave the tract ventral to the third ventricle and terminate in the ipsilateral hypothalamus. The contralateral projection to the hypothalamus is considerably larger and terminates in a cell group originally called "nucleus chiasmaticus" (Ebbesson, 1972*a*). This projection is thought to exist in all vertebrates (Ebbesson, 1972*a*), although striking evidence is lacking in many. In mammals this pathway plays an important role in circadian rhythms of the animal (Moore *et al.*, 1971), a finding not tested in other forms.

A very large portion of the optic nerve fibers terminate in the superficial layers of a well-developed optic tectum. Compared to the teleosts, sharks have poorly differentiated tectal cells and concomitant poor parcellation of cellular layers (Ebbesson *et al.,* 1975). There is also considerable overlap between retinal and telencephalic inputs. The significance of these findings is not understood, but, together with available behavioral data from nurse sharks in which complete tectal ablations did not effect pattern recognition (Graeber and Ebbesson, 1972*b*), it is suggested that the tectum in sharks is probably involved more in oculomotor functions and less in perceptual functions.

Retinal fibers sweep over the lateral surface of diencephalon and terminate in at least two readily identifiable thalamic cell clusters. The more ventral is smaller and very reminiscent of the ventral geniculate nucleus of other vertebrates (Ebbesson, 1972*a*) and has therefore tentatively been called the ventrolateral optic nucleus (VLO). It has inputs from the optic tectum and the telencephalon, as does its counterpart in other vertebrates.

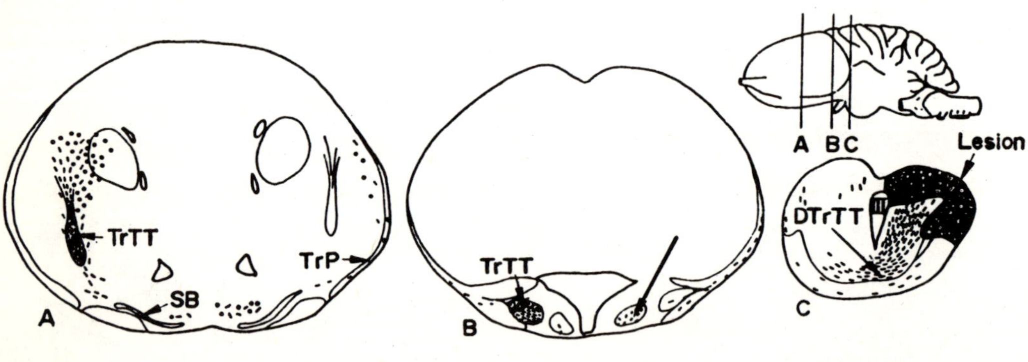

Figure 6. Degenerating axons are traced from a lesion in the thalamus (shown in frontal section in C) to the contralateral telencephalon via the thalamo-telencephalic tract (TrTT), which crosses in the decussation of the thalamo-telencephalic tract (DTrTT) ventral to the third ventricle (III). A bilateral ventromedial tract (see large arrow), terminating in the medial portion of the area superficialis basalis (SB), also degenerates following such a lesion, but this tract has a more caudal origin than the thalamus (see text). A few ipsilateral thalamo-telencephalic fibers are also shown in the tractus pallii (TrP).

Immediately dorsal to the VLO is the dorsolateral optic complex (DLOC), which receives not only a massive retinal input but a tectal one as well (Ebbesson, 1972*a*).

DLOC projects to the contralateral central telencephalic nucleus (CT) (Ebbesson and Schroeder, 1971; Cohen *et al.,* 1973). The DLOC in sharks is interesting because it has the combined connections of the two main, usually separate, visual systems. This finding has led to the speculation that the dorsal nucleus of the lateral geniculate body and the inferior part of the nucleus lateralis posterior of mammals may have evolved from a single nucleus (Ebbesson, 1972*a*). The DLOC-CT system is reminiscent of the geniculo-cortical connections of mammals and appears to play an important role in the vision since lesions of this system have severe effects on visual discrimination (see Chapter 2). The evidence for the DLOC-CT connection comes from anatomical and neurophysiological experiments.

After we had determined that the retina in the shark has major connections with the dorsal thalamus, we decided to explore whether the thalamus projects to nonolfactory telencephalic structures, a pattern characteristic of mammals. To this end, unilateral lesions were made in the diencephalon in a large sample of nurse sharks (Ebbesson and Shroeder, 1971; Schroeder and Ebbesson, 1974). In all cases of sharks with lesions in the dorsal thalamus, degenerating fibers could be traced to two well-defined cell aggregates in the contralateral half of the telencephalon and to a ventral telencephalic structure bilaterally (Fig. 6). The latter projection was found degenerating also in cases of lesions candal to the diencephalon. The origin of this pathway is still unknown.

Perhaps the most unexpected finding was the evidence for a major, principally crossed thalamo-telencephalic pathway. So far, the only other vertebrate form in which any contralateral thalamo-telencephalic connections have been observed is the owl (H. J. Karten and W. J. H. Nauta, personal communication). However, in that avian species, no more than approximately 25% of the thalamic efferents decussate, while in the nurse shark all thalamo-telencephalic fibers appear to cross with the exception of sporadic fibers in the ipsilateral tractus pallii. The contralateral thalamo-telencephalic projection is to a cell group we have identified as the central telencephalic nucleus (CT) and to a less well-defined region ventrolateral to it (Fig. 6).

The neurophysiological experiments confirming the visual input to the telencephalon were also carried out on nurse sharks (Cohen *et al.*, 1973). Optic nerve stimulation in the shark evokes short-latency telencephalic field potentials localized to the ipsilateral, posterior central telencephalic nucleus (Fig. 7).

VII. Representation of Other Sensory Systems in the Telencephalon

Although sharks can distinguish electrical fields, and at least some species depend on this modality to a yet undetermined extent, little is known about which brain parts are involved in this modality. Bullock and co-workers have evidence for both mesencephalic and telencephalic involvement (Platt *et al.*, 1974), but precise localization is not known.

In our stimulation of the supraophthalmic and maxillary branches of the trigeminal nerve in the nurse shark, evoked potentials were restricted to the ros-

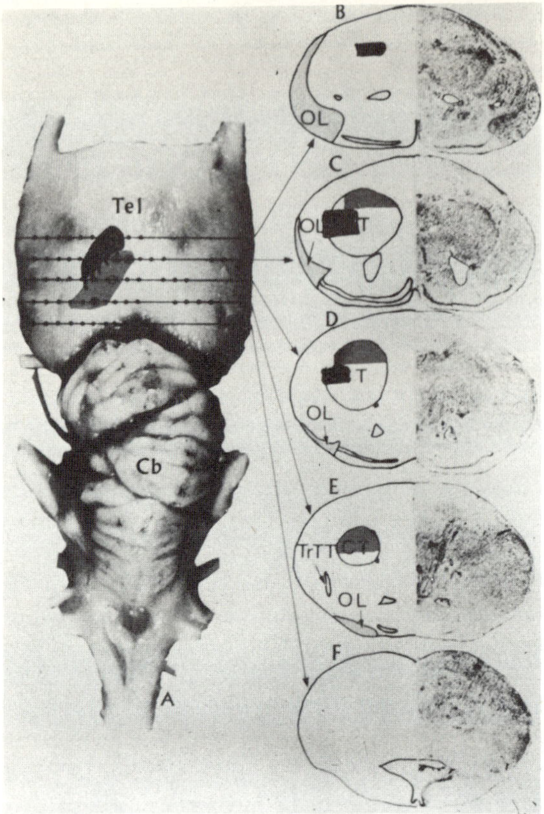

Figure 7. The visual (gray) and trigeminal (black) fields in the telencephalon of the nurse shark as revealed by electrophysiological studies.

troventral region of the central telencephalic nucleus (Cohen, Leonard, Ebbesson, and Jane, unpublished observation). This may represent evidence for localization of the electroreceptive modality since these nerves in the nurse shark may contain fibers from electroreceptors; however, only experiments involving natural stimulation can verify this point.

The lateral line systems are well developed in sharks but have as yet not been studied in sufficient detail to be described here. Suffice it to say that the lateral line nerves project principally onto the lateral line lobes. The projections of the latter structures have not been studied and therefore cannot be commented on.

The spinal sensory systems appear anatomically similar to those described in other vertebrates (Ebbesson, 1972*b*), but until electrophysiological studies have characterized the modalities in the telencephalon it is not possible to suggest any unusual features in the shark.

VIII. Telencephalic Efferent Pathways

Connections of the telencephalon with caudal centers have also been misunderstood and thought to be primarily related to the epithalamus and the hypothalamus (Aronson, 1963). Contradiction and confusion about these pathways are evident everywhere in the literature because the data available could not provide definitive answers, and bias of one sort or another has swayed interpretations. The tractus pallii of Edinger, for example, has been believed to be principally an ascending pathway by some (Catois, 1901), while others (Ariëns Kappers, 1906; Wallenberg, 1907) held the opposite point of view.

Our findings about telencephalic projections in the nurse shark differ in almost every respect from previous descriptions (Ariëns Kappers *et al.*, 1936). In an experiment involving some 50 sharks and telencephalic lesions of various sizes and locations (Ebbesson and Schroeder, 1971), connections with both epithalamic and hypothalamic centers, as shown by earlier workers, were found, but in addition massive connections with thalamus, optic tectum, and select neuronal aggregates at every level of the brainstem were discovered (Fig. 8). Since telencephalic projections to such levels in mammals originate predominantly in the cerebral cortex, we have reached the tentative conclusion that some of the telencephalic efferents in elasmobranchs represent pathways homologous to mammalian cortico-thalamic and cortico-bulbar pathways.

IX. Conclusion

Brains of sharks have, over the years, played important roles in the minds of comparative neurologists because of their numerous presumed primitive features.

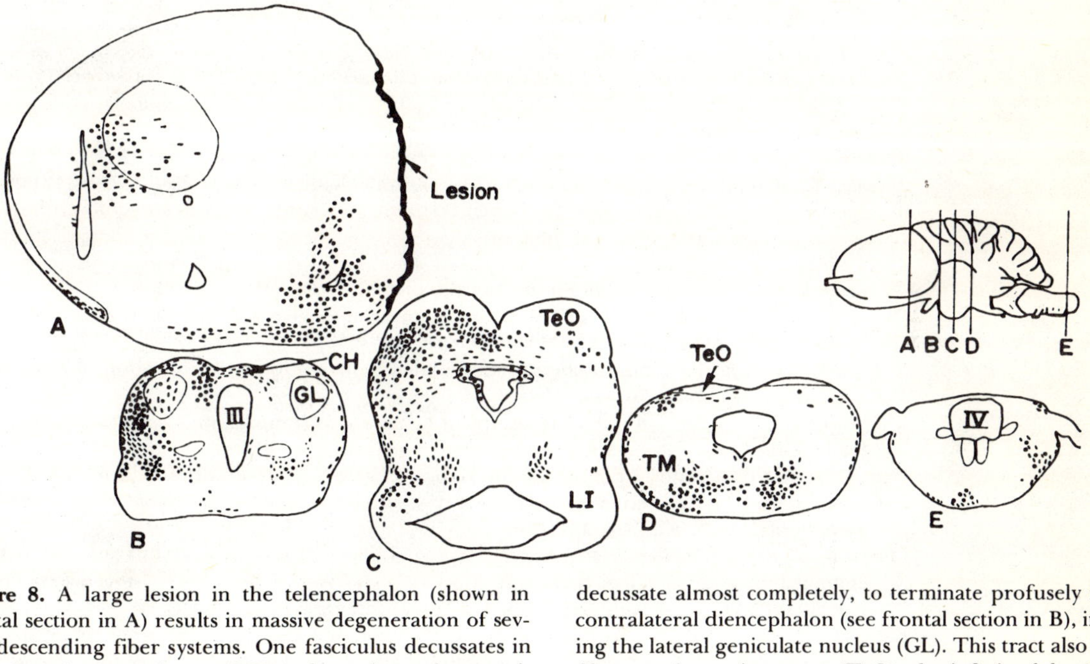

Figure 8. A large lesion in the telencephalon (shown in frontal section in A) results in massive degeneration of several descending fiber systems. One fasciculus decussates in the habenular commissure (CH) and terminates in an epithalamus; another bundle is bilateral and reaches the mesencephalic tegmentum (TM), and the fibers of a third tract decussate almost completely, to terminate profusely in the contralateral diencephalon (see frontal section in B), including the lateral geniculate nucleus (GL). This tract also issues fibers to the optic tectum (TeO), the inferior lobe (LI) of the hypothalamus, and more caudal brain stem nuclei (see frontal sections in D and E).

The presence of structures homologous to the neocortex of mammals was not known until a few years ago, because it had been supposed that the olfactory system dominated telencephalic functions. Other sensory information was thought to be processed principally in the brain stem. The assumed absence of neocortical equivalents in sharks and other anamniotes indicated that "higher" sensory functions did not exist or were handled by such structures as the optic lobes, which are unusually well developed in most anamniotes. The ascent of man and "higher" vertebrates was often correlated with a supposed invasion of nonolfactory modalities into the forebrain. During the last few years we have learned that sharks and other anamniotes have much more extensive sensory representation in the forebrain than hitherto believed and that sensory (and perhaps motor) neocortex probably exists in most vertebrate forms in one form or another but varies tremendously in cytoarchitecture from group to group, ranging in appearance from nonlaminar aggregates in some sharks and birds to the highly laminated cortex of mammals. The encephalization theory is, therefore, incorrect if one suggests a gradual evolutionary shift from tectum to cortex for processing sensory information. The basic systems were apparently present from the beginning, and various selective pressures resulted in the broad range of morphological features confronting the comparative neurologist today.

X. References

Ariëns Kappers, C. U., 1906, The structure of the teleostean and selachian brain, *F. Comp. Neurol.* **16:**1.

Ariëns Kappers, C. U., Huber, G. C., and Crosby E. C., 1936, *The Comparative Anatomy of the Nervous System of Vertebrates, Including Man,* Macmillan, New York.

Aronson, L. R., 1963, The central nervous system of sharks and bony fishes with special reference to sensory and integrative mechanisms, in: *Sharks and Survival* (P. W. Gilbert, ed.), pp. 165–241, Heath, Boston.

Bäckström, K., 1924, Contributions to the forebrain morphology in selachians, *Acta Zool.* **5:**123.

Beccari, N., 1930, I centri tegmentali dell' asse cerebrale dei Selaci, *Arch. Zool. Ital.* **14:**411.

Bruckmoser, P., 1973, Beziehungen zwischen Struktur and Funktion in der Evolution des Telencephalon, *Verh. Dtsch. Zool. Ges.* **66:**219.

Bruckmoser, P., and Dieringer, N., 1973, Evoked potentials in the primary and secondary olfactory projection areas of the forebrain in elasmobranchia, *J. Comp. Physiol.* **87:**65.

Catois, E. M., 1901, Recherches sur l'histologie et l'anatomie microscopique de l'encéphale chez les poissons, *Bull. Sci. Fr. Belg.* **36:**1.

Cohen, D. H., Duff, T. A., and Ebbesson, S. O., Electrophysiological identification of a visual area in shark telencephalon, *Science* **182:**492.

Compagno, L. J. V., 1973, Interrelationships of living elasmobranchs, in: *Interrelationships of Fishes* (P. H. Greenwood, R. S. Miles, and C. Patterson, eds.), pp. 15–61, Academic Press, London.

Dart, R. A., 1920, A contribution to the morphology of the corpus striatum, *J. Anat.* **55:**1.

Ebbesson, S. O. E, 1967, Retinal projections in two species of sharks (*Galeocerdo cuvieri and Ginglymostoma cirratum*), *Anat. Rec.* **157:**238.

Ebbesson, S.O.E., 1970, The selective silver impregnation of degenerating axons and their synaptic endings in non-mammalian species, in: *Contemporary Research Methods in Neuroanatomy* (W.J.H. Nauta and S.O.E. Ebbesson, eds.),pp. 132–161, Springer-Verlag, New York

Ebbesson, S. O. E., 1972*a*, A proposal for a common nomenclature for some optic nuclei in vertebrates and the evidence for a common origin of two such cell groups, *Brain Behav. Evol.* **6:**75.

Ebbesson, S.O.E., 1972*b*, New insights into the organization of the shark brain, *Comp. Biochem. Physiol.* **42A:**121.

Ebbesson, S. O. E., and Campbell, C.B.G., 1973, On the organization of cerebellar efferent pathways in the nurse shark (*Ginglymostoma cirratum*), *J. Comp. Neurol.* **152:**233.

Ebbesson, S.O.E., and Heimer L., 1970, Projections of the olfactory tract fibers in the nurse shark (*Ginglymostoma cirratum*), *Brain Res.* **17:**47.

Ebbesson, S.O.E., and Northcutt, R. G., 1976, Neurology of anamniotic vertebrates, in: *Evolution of Brain and Behavior in Vertebrates* (R. B. Masterton, M. E. Bitterman, C. B. G. Campbell, and N. Hotton, eds.), pp. 115–146, Lawrence Erlbaum Associates, Hillsdale, N.J.

Ebbesson, S.O.E., and Ramsey, J.S., 1968, The optic tracts in two species of sharks (*Galeocerdo cuvieri* and *Ginglymostoma cirratum*), *Brain Res.* **8:**36.

Ebbesson, S.O.E., and Schroeder, D.M., 1971, Connections of the nurse shark's telencephalon, *Science* **173:**254.

Ebbesson, S.O.E., Jane, J. A., and Schroeder, D.M., 1972, A general overview of major interspecific variations in thalamic organization, *Brain Behav. Evol.* **6:**92.

Ebesson, S. O. E., Schroeder, D. M., and Butler, A.B., 1975, The Golgi method and the revival of comparative neurology, in: *Golgi Centennial Symposium, Proceedings* (M. Santini, ed.), pp. 153–160, Raven Press, New York.

Edinger, L., 1901, Das Cerebellum von *Scyllium canicula*, *Arch. Mikrosk. Anat.* **58:**661.

Faucette, J.R., 1969, The olfactory bulb and medial hemisphere wall of the rat-fish, *Chimaera*, *J. Comp. Neurol.* **137:**377.

Fink, R.P., and Heimer, L., 1967, Two methods for selective silver impregnation of degenerating axons and their synaptic endings in the central nervous system, *Brain Res.* **4:**369.

Gerlach, J., 1947, Beiträge zur vergleichenden Morphologie des Selachierhirnes, *Anat. Anz.* **96:**79

Gilbert, P., 1963, The visual apparatus of sharks, in: *Sharks and Survival* (P.W. Gilbert, ed.), pp. 283–326, Heath, Boston.

Graeber, R.C., and Ebbesson, S. O. E., 1972*a*, Retinal projections in the lemon shark (*Negaprion brevirostris*), *Brain Behav. Evol.* **5:**461.

Graeber, R. C., and Ebbesson, S.O.E., 1972*b*, Visual discrimination learning in normal and tectal-ablated nurse sharks (*Ginglymostoma cirratum*), *Comp. Biochem. Physiol.* **42A:**131.

Haller, B., 1898, Vom Bau des Wirbelthiergehirns. I. *Salmo* und *Scyllium*, *Morphol. Jb.* **26:**345.

Holmgren, N., 1922, Points of view concerning forebrain morphology in lower vertebrates, *J. Comp. Neurol.* **34:**391.

Houser, G. L., 1901, The neurones and supporting elements of the brain of a selachian, *J. Comp. Neurol.* **11:**65.

Hugosson, R., 1955, Studien über die Entwicklung der longitudinalen Zellsäulen und der Anlagen der Gehirnnervenkerne in der Medulla oblongata bei verschiedenen Vertebrate, *Z. Anat. Entwicklungsgesch.* **118:**543.

Jerison, H. J., 1973, *Evolution of the Brain and Intelligence*, Academic Press, New York.

Johnston, J. B., 1911, The telencephalon of selachians, *J. Comp. Neurol.* **21:**1.

Kuhlenbeck, H., and Niimi, K., 1969, Further observations on the morphology of the brain in the holocephalian elasmobranchs *Chimaera* and *Callorhynchus*, *J. Hirnforsch.* **11:**267.

Kusunoki, T., Tsuda, Y., and Takashima, F., 1973, The chemoarchitectonics of the shark brain, *J. Hirnforsch.* **14:**13.

Leghissa, S., 1962, La struttura della corteccia mesencefalica dei ciclostomi selaci ed urodeli, *Acca. Sci. Ist. Bologna Classe Sci. Fisiche* **9:**123.

Masai, H., 1961, On the brain pattern of *Chlamydoselachus anguineus*, *Yokohama Med. Bull.* **12:**231.

Masai, H., 1962, On the external form of the brain of *Heterodontus japonicus*, *Yokohama Med. Bull.* **13:**249.

Masai, H., Sato, Y., and Aoki, M., 1973, The brain of *Mitsukurina owstoni*, *J. Hirnforsch.* **14:**493

McCready, P. J., and Boord, R. L., 1976, The topography of the superficial roots and ganglia of the anterior lateral line nerve of the smooth dogfish, *Mustelus canis*, *J. Morphol.* **150:**527.

Moore, R. Y., Karapas, F., and Lenn, N. J., 1971, A retinohypothalamic projection in the rat, *Anat. Rec.* **169:**382.

Nauta, W. J. H., 1957, Silver impregnation of degenerating axons, in: *New Research Techniques of Neuroanatomy* (W. F. Windle, ed.), pp. 17–26, Thomas, Springfield, Ill.

Northcutt, R. G., 1976, Retinofugal pathways in fetal dogfish pups, *Squalus acanthias:* An autoradiographic study, *Anat. Rec.* **184:**489.

Northcutt, R.G., 1977, Elasmobranch central nervous system organization and its possible evolutionary significance, *Am. Zool.* **17:**411.

Okada, Y., Aoki, M., Sato, Y., and Masai, H., 1969, The brain patterns of sharks in relation to habit, *J. Hirnforsch.* **11:**347.

Platt, C.J., Bullock, T.H., Czéh, G., Kovacevié, N., Konjevié, D., and Gojković, M., 1974, Comparison of electroreceptor, mechanoreceptor, and optic evoked potentials in the brain of some rays and sharks, *J. Comp. Physiol.* **95:**323.

Schroeder, D. M., and Ebbesson, S. O. E., 1974, Nonolfactory telencephalic afferents in the nurse shark (*Ginglymostoma cirratum*), *Brain Behav. Evol.* **9:**121.

Schroeder, D. M., and Ebbesson, S.O.E., 1975, Cytoarchitecture of the optic tectum in the nurse shark, *J. Comp. Neurol.* **160:**443.

Shaper, A., 1898, The finer structure of the selachian cerebellum (*Mustelus vulgaris*), *J. Comp. Neurol.* **8:**1.

Smeets, W. J. A. J., and Nieuwenhuys, R., 1976, Topological analysis of the brain stem of the sharks *Squalus acanthias* and *Scyliorhinus canicula, J. Comp. Neurol.* **165:**33.

Tester, A. L., 1963, Olfaction, gustation, and the common chemical sense in sharks, in: *Sharks and Survival* (P. W. Gilbert, ed.), pp. 255–282, Heath, Boston.

Veselkin, N. P., 1965, Electrical responses in skate brain to photic stimulation, *Fed. Proc. Tr. Suppl.* **24:**368.

Wallenberg A., 1907, Beiträge zur Kenntniss des Gehirns der Telostier und Selachier, *Anat. Anz.* **31:**369.

2

Telencephalic Function in Elasmobranchs

A Behavioral Perspective

RAYMOND CURTIS GRAEBER

I. Use of Sharks in Comparative Neuropsychology

A. Phylogenetic Advantages

Both comparative neurologists and psychologists have often been intrigued with the possibility of inferring past evolutionary trends in the relationship between the vertebrate brain and behavior. In general, two investigative approaches have been taken toward realizing this goal. Some workers have attempted to correlate the behavior patterns of different existing animal species with known structural differences in their central nervous systems. Others have chosen to compare the behavioral effects of similar types of selective brain damage among various related animal groups. In either case, the choice of subjects is critical.

Paleontological evidence indicates that most extant animal species are far removed in morphological development from their early ancestors. As Hodos and Campbell (1969) have emphasized, it is especially difficult to infer evolutionary trends without first considering the phylogenetic background of the species being compared. Even when the chosen species possess a common evolutionary lineage, the ability to draw inferences about historical phylogenetic events is still limited by

---

RAYMOND CURTIS GRAEBER • Department of Military Medical Psychophysiology, Division of Neuropsychiatry, Walter Reed Army Institute of Research, Washington, D.C. 20012. The opinions and assertions contained herein are the private views of the author and are not to be construed as official or as reflecting the views of the Department of the Army or the Department of Defense.

the many diversifications and adaptations which may have occured since the disappearance of their early ancestors. The experimenter is thus faced with the requirement of sorting out ancestral features from those derived within the lineage being examined (Campbell, 1976).

The task of obtaining appropriate experimental animals can be extremely difficult, especially if one wishes to study the transition from water-dwelling to land-dwelling vertebrates. Most paleontologists agree that the crossopterygians, or lobe-finned fishes, are the best candidates for tetrapod ancestry (Hotton, 1976). These fish flourished in the Devonian period, but rapidly diminished and, after the Paleozoic era, continued only in the form of an aberrant side branch of which a single form, the coelacanth *Latimeria,* survives in the Indian Ocean (Romer, 1967). Many investigators have attempted to fill this evolutionary gap by gathering data on modern teleosts such as the goldfish, *Carrasius auratus,* which is rapidly becoming the "standard species" for behavioral fish research. Although "no teleost fish ever was an ancestor of any amphibian, reptile, bird, or mammal" (Hodos and Campbell, 1969, p. 341), one might argue that since teleosts are descendents of the actinopterygians, or ray-finned fishes, they are at least cousins of the practically extinct crossopterygians. However, this strategy fails to consider the distance of the cousin relationship. Fossil records clearly indicate that modern teleosts did not appear until about 100 million years ago after evolving from two prior orders, the chondrosteans and the later holosteans (Romer, 1956).

Not only are teleosts very distant cousins of the crossopterygians, but they are also highly diverse, and, with over 20,000 different species, form the largest group of extant vertebrates (Romer, 1956; Marshall, 1971). Such diversity and variation in habitat have naturally been accompanied by a great deal of neural variation (Segaar, 1965) and specialization to include hypertrophy of certain primary sensory areas, the presence of large paired Mauthner's cells in the reticular formation, and pronounced structural differences among brains even within a single genus of fish (Herrick, 1962; Aronson, 1963). In addition, the organization of the teleostean forebrain is basically different from that of most other vertebrates, making topographical comparisons useless and homologizing difficult (Segaar, 1965; Bernstein, 1970). This difference results from the eversion of the dorsolateral walls of the neural tube in the embryological formation of the teleost forebrain as opposed to the evagination and inversion of these walls in the embryological development of all other vertebrates (Aronson, 1963; Bernstein, 1970).

In view of these phylogenetic and anatomical considerations, teleosts can be considered less than ideal subjects for studying early trends in the evolution of forebrain function in vertebrates. This is not to say that comparing data from various teleosts, as well as other poikilotherms, should not enhance our understanding of vertebrate brain evolution and adaptation, but rather, that it may prove more worthwhile to place greater emphasis on studying the brain–behavior relationship in cartilaginous fish, or elasmobranchs.

Although comparative anatomists have recognized the conceptual advantages of studying sharks ever since the end of the nineteenth century (Ariëns Kappers *et al.,* 1936), there has been no such recognition by comparative neuropsychologists. Realizing this in his 1963 review, Aronson regretfully pointed out the almost total lack of any behavioral research on shark brain function. Despite his expressed concern at that time, there have been very few additional papers published on the topic since then. The recent findings will be reviewed later, but first, in hopes of exceeding Aronson's colleague conversion rate, it may prove worthwhile to review the reasons why sharks should be considered more useful subjects for studying early phylogenetic trends in the brain–behavior relationship.

The earliest representatives of the elasmobranchs first appeared in the late Devonian period, about 280 million years ago, much earlier than the teleosts and slightly after the first crossopterygians (Romer, 1956). Despite their ancient lineage, modern sharks closely resemble their early ancestors, unlike bony fishes, and are therefore a rather unique group of animals (Romer, 1956; Herrick, 1962; Schaeffer, 1967). In this regard, Romer (1956) has stated that "modern sharks are typical representatives of . . . the Chrondrichthyes" and "except for skeletal degeneration, the sharks appear to be in general 'proper' fishes of a fairly primitive type" (pp. 40–41).

Examination of the fossil record indicates that shark history can be divided into three successive stages: (1) the cladoselachian stage characteristic of the late Devonian and Carboniferous periods (about 280–210 million years ago), (2) the hybodont stage extending from the Carboniferous to the Triassic period (250–150 million years ago), and (3) the modern stage beginning in the Jurassic period with the appearance of today's sharks (Romer, 1968*a,b*). The most significant aspect of this genealogy is that it forms a linear progression without any diverging side-branches, so that elasmobranchs constitute a concise and well-defined group of fish which has retained many of its ancestral anatomical and physiological features (Moy-Thomas, 1939). This lack of divergence most likely results from sharks being highly successful, well-adapted organisms ever since their first appearance on earth almost 300 million years ago (Budker, 1971). The remarkable success of sharks has therefore worked to the advantage of comparative researchers by reducing the need for more recent evolutionary structural changes.

It must be cautioned, however, that fossil records can supply direct information concerning only skeletal structures. Even if these are shown to have undergone only minor evolutionary modification, the same is not necessarily true for corresponding soft tissues (Hodos, 1970). Nevertheless, studies of the internal anatomy of fossilized brain cases can reveal much about the nature of their former contents. Until recently, it had been assumed that the Paleozoic (cladoselachian) shark braincase resembled that of modern forms in having an extremely short posterior (i.e., otic) region, but new fossil evidence indicates that this region was greatly elongated in ancient sharks (Romer, 1968*a*). Because the size and shape of sharks' brains often do not correspond to the inner dimensions of their chondocranial cavities (Masai, 1962; Stensiö, 1963), one is again faced with the dilemma of ascertaining to what extent neurological change accompanied the skeletal modification. Except for this reduction of the postorbital process, the major features of the modern shark braincase were already present during the hybodont stage of shark evolution (Schaeffer, 1967).

B. Neuroanatomical Features

Although the paleontological approach provides certain obvious advantages for those studying the evolution of gross structural alterations in external brain form, a more detailed understanding of evolutionary change in central neural organization can be gained by examining the morphology of modern shark brains. Such analyses reveal that the shark brain lacks the specializations seen in the brains of teleosts (Herrick, 1962; Aronson, 1963). Moreover, the brain of the adult shark differs far less from the simple neural tube of its embryo than do the brains of other vertebrates (Herrick, 1962), yet the shark is phylogenetically the first living vertebrate to possess central myelinated fibers (Ariëns Kappers *et al.*, 1936).

Despite this general simplicity, the shark brain has recently been shown to have much more in common with brains of other vertebrates than was previously believed (Ebbesson, 1972*a*). For instance, although the shark forebrain has always been considered primarily olfactory in function and composition (Ariëns Kappers *et al.*, 1936; Aronson, 1963; Nieuwenhuys, 1967), experimental studies employing modifications of the Nauta and Fink–Heimer silver impregnation techniques have demonstrated a very limited olfactory area (Ebbesson and Heimer, 1970; Ebbesson, 1972*a*). In addition, descending projections have been found extending from the telencephalon to many lower regions such as the thalamus, epithalamus, hypothalamus, optic tectum, and brain stem (Ebbesson and Schroeder, 1971; Graeber, unpublished observations), while ascending pathways have been demonstrated from diencephalic regions into the telencephalon (Ebbesson and Schroeder, 1971; Schroeder and Ebbesson, 1974). These connections indicate that the shark telencephalon is much more comparable to those of birds and tetrapods than was previously thought and that it may perform substantial nonolfactory functions. Related studies have also shown that the major connections of both the thalamus and tectum are essentially similar to those of other vertebrates (Ebbesson, 1971, 1972*a*). The previous inability to detect these pathways in "normal shark material" can be traced to their characteristic poorly myelinated, fine-caliber fibers (Polyak, 1957, p. 301; Bakay and Lee, 1966).

Examination of the cytoarchitecture of the shark brain reveals that nuclear groups are poorly differentiated, with vague boundaries lying between them (Nieuwenhuys, 1967; Schroeder and Ebbesson, 1974). For instance, the optic tectum, the dorsolateral optic complex of the thalamus, and the telencephalic olfactory region all lack the stratification into cellular layers characteristic of their counterparts in other living vertebrates. Nissl-stained sections also demonstrate that the boundaries between various regions of the telencephalon and thalamus are vague and poorly defined (Holmgren, 1922; Ebbesson and Heimer, 1970; Schroeder and Ebbesson, 1974). Additional evidence for the more generalized organization of the shark brain is the manner in which both olfactory and retinal afferents terminate embedded among fibers of passage rather than in select nuclear regions (Ebbesson and Ramsey, 1968; Ebbesson and Heimer, 1970). Electron microscopic studies have further revealed that the shark neuropil possesses only astrocytic glia; however, these glia contribute to the formation of both myelin sheaths and the blood–brain barrier and consequently perform the dual roles assigned to different glial cells in mammals (Bakay and Lee, 1966). Thus, while the basic organization of the shark brain resembles that of other vertebrates, including mammals, its many primitive features and relative lack of specialization suggest that sharks have maintained an unusually consistent pattern of neuroanatomical organization throughout their evolutionary history.

These features of shark brain morphology contrast vividly with the recent discovery that elasmobranchs are characterized by brain–body weight ratios equal to those of some mammals and birds, in some cases 400% higher than those of all other anamniotes (Ebbesson and Northcutt, 1976; Northcutt, 1977). Although an adequate explanation of these higher ratios is still lacking, the data show that they are primarily due to higher forebrain and cerebellar weights, particularly among galeomorphs, and are not a result of the shark's lack of a dermal skeleton. In summary, Ebbesson and Northcutt state that "Our data do not support the traditional concept of encephalization. Instead they suggest that several levels of brain–body ratios exist and that these levels have been reached independently by a number of vertebrate taxa at different times" (1976, p. 123).

The traditional interpretation is that higher brain–body weight ratios indicate an increased complexity of information processing and motor control. If this is true of sharks, then it is possible that the ancestral forms of elasmobranchs were capable of more complex central neural processing than previously believed. The pervasiveness of high ratios among the extant species of elasmobranchs so far examined suggests that the characteristic is not peculiar to a few divergent side-branches but rather is common to all. It is tempting to speculate that the brains of many living anamniotic vertebrates, except for elasmobranchs, represent an evolutionary trend away from a generalized ancestral brain capable of processing fairly complex information from a variety of sensory systems toward a more specialized brain designed for unusually sophisticated informational analysis particular to a few highly developed sensory systems. The increasing evidence for multimodal telencephalic functioning in sharks supports this possibility (Cohen *et al.,* 1973; Veselkin and Kovacevic, 1973; Platt *et al.,* 1974). The present lack of an adequate phylogenetic explanation should not inhibit behavioral scientists from exploring the variations in behavior which accompany these higher brain–body weight ratios in sharks. The advantages conferred by the lack of elaboration in the shark brain may accelerate our understanding of basic brain–behavior relationships.

C. Behavioral Repertoire

One reason for the relative lack of behavioral research on sharks is the widespread unfamiliarity of comparative neuropsychologists with the rapidly growing literature on shark sensory systems, instinctive response patterns, and learning capabilities. Many individuals still labor under the outdated belief that sharks are simplistic fish with a very circumscribed behavioral repertoire characterized by stereotyped response patterns and poor coordination. A brief overview of some recent behavioral investigations may help to correct this false impression and underscore the feasibility of studying shark behavior.

A large proportion of the functional research on sharks has concentrated on their sensory systems and can be divided into two major types of experiments: those examining natural responses to variations in sensory stimulation and those using learned responses to analyze different sensory capacities.

1. Orientation

Representative of the more naturalistic studies are those which have demonstrated the attractiveness of low-frequency, pulsed sounds to many shark species

(Nelson and Gruber, 1963; Banner, 1968, 1972; Myrberg *et al.*, 1969; Nelson *et al.*, 1969; Myrberg, 1972; Nelson and Johnson, 1972). These investigations have utilized field situations to demonstrate that intermittently pulsed sounds are more effective than regularly pulsed sounds in attracting sharks and that the optimal effect is obtained as mean pulse rate is increased up to 20 pulses per second. The sharks' behavior is characterized by orientation toward the transducer while still swimming in the acoustically far field, beyond the limit of visibility, and then swimming directly toward the sound source. Thus Nelson and Gruber (1963) claim that sharks, unlike teleosts (see van Berjeijk, 1964), possess true directional hearing and are not dependent on sound-gradient searching to localize its source.

In a series of elegant studies combining laboratory observation of unlearned responses with electrophysiological recordings, Kalmijn (1966, 1971) has demonstrated the presence of directional electroreception in sharks. With a threshold of 0.01 $\mu V/cm^2$, the shark's ampullae of Lorenzini posses the greatest known electrical sensitivity in the animal world. Using this system to detect the bioelectric potentials produced by prey, both *Raja clavata* and *Scyliorhinus cannicula* are able to locate flatfish buried under the sand from distances up to 15 cm away. Other evidence has suggested a possible role of electroreception in shark navigation and open-ocean orientation by the shark's response to variations in the earth's magnetic fields (Kalmijn, 1973, 1974).

Research on chemosensory orientation in sharks extends back to Parker and Sheldon's classic work on the importance of olfactory cues in predation by *Mustelus* (Sheldon, 1909, 1911; Parker, 1910, 1914; Parker and Sheldon, 1913). Tester (1963) has since clarified their original findings by demonstrating that sharks are attracted to a chemical source originating from prey living in an independent tank, thereby ruling out the possible contribution of sonic cues. He also has reported that the intensity and topography of the shark's response pattern depend on the level of excitement or distress exhibited by the prey fish. Hobson (1963) extended these findings to field situations using water siphoned from a tank containing a "distressed" grouper to attract gray sharks from as far as a quarter mile away.

As might be expected, the effectiveness of such stimuli depends on prevailing water currents (Kleerekoper *et al.*, 1975). Some species of sharks have apparently undergone an adaptation of their chemical localization mechanism which allows them to compensate for this factor. Although Parker (1914) originally described gradient searching (klinotaxis) as the basis of the dogfish's chemosensory directional response, it now appears that this may be the case only for benthic feeders and not for all sharks. Hodgson and Mathewson (1971) have experimentally shown that the nurse shark (*Ginglymostoma cirratum*), like the dogfish *Mustelus*, relies on true gradient searching to localize a chemical source; however, the carcharhinid *Negaprion breviostris* (lemon shark) reacts rheotactically to chemical stimuli by swimming up against the strongest prevailing current regardless of the location of the chemical source. Under most natural conditions, these two different reponse patterns would be highly adaptive to the species involved. Nurse sharks are benthic feeders (Tanaka, 1973) that encounter currents constantly disrupted by bottom topography, making rheotaxis inappropriate for their food localization. Lemon sharks, by comparison, are a more active littoral species preying mostly on fish (Springer, 1950) whose chemical traces would typically be carried to the shark from an upstream position. A dependence on klinotaxis would merely slow the carcharhinid's arrival at the prey's location.

Most research involving learning has been designed to investigate shark sensory capacities, especially vision or audition. Following Clark's (1959) initial demonstration that sharks could learn to bump a target for food reward, there have been a variety of studies using classical or instrumental conditioning techniques to investigate brightness, color, and form discrimination, in addition to dark adaptation, visual sensitivity, and critical-flicker-fusion frequency (Aronson *et al.,* 1967; Clark, 1961; Graeber, 1972; Graeber and Ebbesson, 1972*a*; Gruber, 1967, 1975; Tester and Kato, 1966). In general, these studies corroborate other findings from feeding (Gilbert, 1962) and from anatomical (Gruber *et al.,* 1963, 1975; Hamasaki and Gruber, 1965; Stell, 1972) and physiological studies (Hamasaki and Bridges, 1965; Kuchnow and Gilbert, 1967; Cohen *et al.,* 1977) indicating that sharks have a more sensitive, functional visual system than previously suspected and that at least some species possess both scotopic and photopic vision.

There is already considerable agreement that sharks can learn to discriminate black–white, brightness levels, horizontal–vertical stripes, and various shapes, including squares vs. circles and upright vs. inverted equilateral triangles. The electrophysiological and anatomical evidence suggest that they should also be able to discriminate hue, but so far no studies of color discrimination have adequately controlled for confounding differences in luminosity (Clark, 1961, 1963; Tester and Kato, 1966). While there are known species differences regarding the ease of conditioning (Clark, 1963; Tester and Kato, 1966), it appears that sharks can be instrumentally conditioned to perform both simultaneous and successive visual discriminations. There can also be dramatic individual differences in the aversiveness produced by equilvalent levels of electric shock administered to sharks (e.g., Tester and Kato, 1966), suggesting perhaps that food reward is the preferable means of motivating learning performance.

Instrumental conditioning employing food reward or shock avoidance has likewise been used to determine hearing thresholds and frequency discrimination abilities in several species of sharks (Kritzler and Wood, 1961; Nelson, 1967; Kelly and Nelson, 1975). One study has supplemented this method with respondent conditioning using caudal shock to condition a bradycardia response to pure tones (Kelly and Nelson, 1975). This latter procedure provides the experimenter with strict control over the distance between the subjects and the sound source. Similarly, Gruber (1967; Gruber and Schneiderman, 1975) has demonstrated rapid classical conditioning of the shock-induced nictitating membrane response in lemon sharks using a light flash conditioned stimulus. As in auditory research, being able to use a restrained shark can provide a methodological advantage in visual psychophysical experiments where precise control of the effective stimulus is desirable.

3. Ethology and Naturalistic Response Patterns

In their recent discussion of approaches to studying shark behavior, Gruber and Myrberg (1977) have provided a timely summary of current ethological research on sharks, including their social organization, daily movements, and courtship activities. While only a couple of species have been examined, there are now reliable quantitative descriptions of the swimming patterns and body postures which occur in response to dominance hierarchies and social stimuli (Allee and Dickinson,

1954; Myrberg and Gruber, 1974). In support of less precise field observations (Eibl-Eibesfeldt and Haas, 1959; Hobson, 1963), these group studies also reveal a surprising lack of intraspecific aggression in the presence of limited food supplies. If anything, sharks appear to increase their attempts to avoid each other when environmental conditions become more crowded or competitive. A tendency to avoid direct aggression is also seen in the agonistic threat display by the gray reef shark (*Carcharhinus menisorrah*) when rapidly approached by a human diver. Johnson and Nelson (1973) describe this behavior as primarily defensive and as characterized by distinct, stereotyped exaggerated movements and posturing which increase in intensity with increased escape-route restriction and more direct head-on approaches by the diver.

By effectively combining laboratory and field studies Nelson and his colleagues have also examined the circadian rhythms of shark activity. Using telemetry devices, they have successfully plotted the swimming patterns of blue sharks (*Prionace glauca*) living near Santa Catalina Island, California. As might be expected, the sharks' movements are highlighted by a distinct shoreward migration at dusk followed by a sudden increase in nonlinear swimming patterns and a return to deeper offshore water several hours later (Nelson, 1974). Likewise, systematic visual field observations of bottom-dwelling horn (*Heterodontus francisci*) and swell (*Cephaloscyllium ventriosum*) sharks in the same vicinity have revealed a marked pattern of nocturnal activity and diurnal resting (Nelson and Johnson, 1970). Laboratory studies have indicated an endogenous control of circadian rhythmicity in both species accompanied by differences in the distribution of nocturnal activity bouts and in the phase lability to shifts in the timing of the light–dark synchronizer (Nelson and Johnson, 1970; Finstad and Nelson, 1975). Endogenous factors may also be responsible for the infradian rhythms which have been documented in the feeding behavior of juvenile lemon sharks (Graeber, 1974).

The combination of ethological observations with current neurophysiological methods potentially offers a significant opportunity for the fruitful analysis of brain–behavior relationships. Demski (1977) has initiated an examination of the responses to electrical brain stimulation in chronically implanted, free-swimming nurse (*G. cirratum*) and sharpnose (*Rhizoprionodon terraenovae*) sharks. Depending on the site of stimulation, he has been able to elicit organized response patterns as well as more specific motor reflexes. The latter were reported as early as 1913 by Polimanti in *Scyllium*. Future experiments utilizing more naturalistic response opportunities may permit the specification of anatomical substrates underlying the more basic behavior patterns of sharks.

II. The Reign of Olfaction

A. Origins of the "Smell Brain"

During the first half of this century, comparative neurologists viewed the elasmobranch telencephalon as a diffusely organized structure with relatively few interconnecting pathways. Its traditional function has been to serve exclusively as an olfacto-gustatory correlation center (Houser, 1901; Ariëns Kappers, 1906; Johnston, 1911; Herrick, 1922; Bäckström, 1924). The early neuroanatomical findings, based on "normal" material, reflected the prevailing views of zoologists regarding shark sensory capacities, particularly those of Parker and Sheldon, who demonstrated the dogfish's (*Mustelus canis*) critical dependence on smell for locating prey (Parker, 1910; Sheldon, 1911; Parker and Sheldon, 1913). The functional roles of the other known senses, such as vision, appeared to be secondary and less demanding of higher level, i.e., telencephalic, integrating mechanisms, a view in agreement with the apparent restriction of visual input to the midbrain optic tectum and the lack of tectal differentiation in sharks compared to teleosts (Houser, 1901; Ariëns Kappers *et al.,* 1936).

This tradition has been continued by more recent authors (e.g., Aronson, 1963, 1970; Nieuwenhuys, 1967; Lineaweaver and Backus, 1973), who describe the shark forebrain as a comparatively rudimentary structure consisting of poorly interrelated areas devoted primarily to sensation, especially olfaction. Voronin *et al.* (1968) state that the elasmobranch telencephalon lacks distinct nuclear groups and is devoid of any neural basis for associative processes, a finding consistent with the view that sharks are primitive fish whose behavior is often "clumsy" and mainly composed of instinctive, stereotyped response patterns (Aronson, 1963).

The belief that the telencephalon plays no role in shark vision is fairly well supported by the findings of previous behavioral studies studies (Ten Cate, 1935; Healy, 1957). Steiner (1886, 1888) was the first to examine the swimming behavior of sharks (*Scyliorhinus cannicula*) following selective ablation of the telencephalon. He reported that no deficits appeared in the normally existing functions of the animal, including vision, but that spontaneous food-seeking ceased, presumably because of the loss of olfaction. Similar experiments were subsequently conducted by Bethe (1899) and Loeb (1891). They also observed that operated sharks continued to maintain normal balance and move spontaneously in the aquarium without bumping into the sides. Therefore, they concluded that telencephalic ablation produces no disturbances in motility, equilibrium, or vision.

Polimanti (1911, 1913) reached the same conclusion after studying the results of both unilateral and bilateral telencephalic ablations in the spotted dogfish, *S. cannicula* and the smooth dogfish, *Mustelus laevis.* He found that the former produced neither circling or turning movements and that complete removal did not prevent spontaneous feeding. However, Polimanti further noted that, if the ablation included the nucleus of the terminal nerve, the shark readily bumped its snout against the aquarium walls. He explained this behavior as resulting from the loss of pressure sensation caused by lateral line dysfunction. Rizzolo (1929) repeated these experiments on smooth dogfish (*Galeus canis*). He confirmed the general finding of no visual or motor deficits and demonstrated that telencephalic removal did not disturb the shark's ability to immediately right itself when placed on its back at the water's surface. Its posture remained upright both while swimming and while resting on the bottom.

Although these behavioral findings were based solely on nonsystematic descriptive observations, there is no reason to question their validity. In fact, some modern functional studies performed by Russian neuroscientists support the widespread belief that the elasmobranch telencephalon is not involved in vision. Baru (cited in Karamyan, 1956) found that telencephalically ablated sharks did not differ from unoperated controls in the ability to learn or retain classically conditioned reflexes to light onset. Similarly, both Veselkin (1964) and Karamyan *et al.* (1966) were unable to obtain evoked potentials in the elasmobranch telencephalon following photic stimulation or electrical stimulation of the optic nerve.

B. Multimodal Representation

The reign of olfaction over the elasmobranch telencephalon was initially questioned by the discovery that the bulk of the nurse shark's (*Ginglymostoma cirratum*) telencephalon does not receive any primary or higher-order olfactory fibers (Ebbesson and Heimer, 1970; Ebbesson, 1972*a*). Furthermore, the use of experimental neuroanatomical techniques revealed previously unknown retinal projections to the dorsolateral thalamus ("lateral geniculate nucleus" of Houser, 1901) of lemon, nurse, and tiger sharks (Ebbesson and Ramsey, 1968; Graeber and Ebbesson, 1972*b*). The large extent of this diencephalic visual input suggested the remote possibility of a second-order visual pathway from the thalamus to some area in the telencephalon devoid of olfactory input. This hypothesis was confirmed morphologically by Ebbesson and Schroeder (1971; Schroeder and Ebbesson, 1974), who demonstrated that experimental lesions in the dorsolateral thalamus of nurse sharks produce terminal degeneration in the central nucleus of the contralateral telencephalon. Additional anatomical work has shown that the traditional shark visual center, the optic tectum, also provides substantial ipsilateral input into the dorsolateral thalamus in such a manner as to overlap with many of the terminal areas receiving direction retinal projections (Ebbesson, 1971, 1972*b*; Ebbesson *et al.*, 1972).

In all fairness it should be mentioned that Johnston (1911) was the first to describe a thalamo-telencephalic tract ("tractus thalamo-corticalis") in sharks, running from the dorsal thalamic centers, include the lateral geniculate nucleus, to a caudal telencephalic cell group which he labeled the "somatic area." Herrick (1922) concurred with Johnston's observations, but Ariens Kappers *et al.* (1936) were less certain, especially regarding the ascending direction of this pathway.

Electrophysiological evidence in support of telencephalic visual function in elasmobranchs was forthcoming soon after completion of the neuroanatomical experiments. Two groups of investigators independently obtained telencephalic evoked potentials in response to electrical stimulation of the optic nerves in nurse sharks (Cohen *et al.*, 1973) and rays (Veselkin and Kovacevic, 1973). Cohen and his colleagues recorded short-latency (20–23 msec) field potentials localized within the posterior portion of the ipsilateral central telencephalic nucleus after stimulating the optic nerve with 0.1 msec monophasic square waves. The physiologically responsive area was found to overlap with that previously shown by Ebbesson and Schroeder to receive fibers from the thalamic visual region. The absence of any responsiveness in the contralateral telencephalon confirmed the morphological picture of an almost completely crossed ascending thalamo-telencephalic pathway.

In general, these findings were substantiated by Veselkin and Kovacevic (1973) in the telencephali of the rays *Dasyatis pastinaca, Raja clavata*, and *Torpedo ocellata.* They found ipsilateral responses to optic nerve stimulation in all three species of rays but not in the shark *Scyllium (Scyliorhinus cannicula)*. The responses in the former were localized in the posterior telencephalon, slightly more medially than those reported by Cohen and his colleagues in the nurse shark. These telencephalic responses were retained in rays after complete destruction of the optic tectum and sectioning of the stem between the mesencephalon and diencephalon. Therefore, it tentatively appears that the contralateral thalamotelencephalic tract is primarily relaying information derived from the retinal input to the dorsal thalamus rather than that derived from the overlapping tectal input.

Although there were no visual responses in *S. cannicula,* evoked potentials were recorded in the same telencephalic region following electrical stimulation of the contralateral dorsal thalamus. Thus Veselkin and Kovacevic conclude that the absence of visual responsivity is due to functional differences and not to morphological ones. This negative finding may be the most important aspect of their study in that it implies that this species of shark, and perhaps other dogfish as well, is unique among elasmobranchs and lacks the physiological basis for telencephalic visual involvement. If true, this would explain the lack of visual deficits described in the previously cited behavioral work of Steiner (1886, 1888), Loeb (1891), Bethe (1899), Polimanti (1911, 1913), and Rizzolo (1929). All these early studies were conducted on various species of dogfish, most often *Scyllium* (i.e., *Scyliorhinus cannicula*).

Subsequent experiments by Platt *et al.* (1974) clearly substantiate that the elasmobranch telencephalon receives multimodal sensory input. Through the combined use of electrical nerve stimulation and natural stimuli, they have confirmed the presence of electrosensory and mechanosensory responses in the telencephali of the ray *Torpedo* and the sharks *Scyliorhinus* and *Mustelus.* As the authors point out, they failed to discover any more than doubtful telencephalic evoked potentials to light-flash stimulation probably because they were recording exclusively on the side of the telencephalon contralateral to the stimulated eye. At the time, they did not realize the crossed nature of the thalamotelencephalic pathway. Bruckmoser and Dieringer's (1973) electrophysiological confirmation of a highly restricted secondary olfactory area in *Scyliorhinus* and *Torpedo* lends added credence to the emerging view of sensory systems converging within the elasmobranch telencephalon.

III. Telencephalic Involvement in Visual Discrimination

Except for olfaction, the central visual system is currently the most thoroughly studied sensory processing system in the elasmobranch forebrain. While the details of its anatomy and physiology are far from completely understood, there is sufficient available information to guide the design of behavioral experiments aimed at elucidating its functional character. By combining this newly gained information with modern techniques of behavioral analysis, we can begin to reexamine the findings of the turn-of-the-century comparative neurologists concerning telencephalic functioning in cartilaginous fish (Graeber, 1978).

So far, only one such set of experiments has been completed. Their impetus came from the discovery that free-swimming nurse sharks with complete tectal ablations could still learn to perform simple visual discriminations (Graeber *et al.*, 1973). The fact that these sharks learned the visual tasks almost as rapidly as unoperated controls reinforces the conclusion that the optic tectum is not, as traditionally believed, the sole central neural locus underlying visuomotor behavior in elasmobranchs. The central telencephalic nucleus, with its visual input from the thalamus, is the next most logical candidate for providing the neural substrate necessary to guide such behavior.

A. Experimental Evidence

The basic design for the telencephalic experiments has followed that used for studying the effects of tectal ablations. Juvenile nurse sharks were trained either before or after surgery to discriminate a series of visual target pairs in a fixed-trial instrumental conditioning situation. They were required to swim down the approach alley of a modified Y-maze and to choose a target by crossing a line drawn on the bottom of the pool perpendicular to a 6-inch baffle separating the target doors. If the correct target was chosen, the guillotine-style door opened and the shark received a piece of cut fish as a reward. If the incorrect target was chosen, the door remained closed and the shark had to correct itself before receiving a reward. Care was taken to control for any olfactory or sonic cues which might bias target choices. After completion of each trial, the subject swam back through a corridor to the start-pen. The discrimination was considered learned when the subject had made at least 17 correct choices within three consecutive training sessions of six trials each ($p < 0.01$; Bogartz, 1965). More detailed descriptions of the training pool and procedures, including that used for determining target position, are available elsewhere (Graeber, 1972; Graeber and Ebbesson, 1972*a*; Graeber *et al.*, 1978).

The first behavioral evidence for telencephalic visual function in elasmobranchs resulted from attempts to train naive operated sharks to discriminate black vs. white (BW) and horizontal vs. vertical (HV) black and white stripes (Graeber *et al.*, 1972, 1978). Nurse sharks suffering severe bilateral damage to the central telencephalic nuclei (CN) experienced great difficulty learning, or were unable to learn, these tasks. The performance of two of these subjects is shown in Fig. 1. Note that neither animal achieved criterion on the BW or HV task. However, the performance latencies, shown in the upper half of each data set, indicate that the sharks were not suffering from any motivational impairment such as that described by Steiner (1886, 1888) in his original studies of telencephalic ablation in *Scyllium*. Both animals exhibited a progressive decrease in median correct response latency which approached an asymptote halfway through BW training. The stable low latencies substantiate the sharks' ability to successfully learn the general response requirements of the training procedure, including the rapid correction of errors. Nevertheless, their choice performance, especially that of NS-186, continued to vary about the chance level throughout the more than 500 trials of BW training. Time restrictions limited to 22 sessions the amount of training which could be carried out on the more difficult HV discrimination task.

The visual nature of the postoperative learning deficit is revealed by the successful performance of NS-186 on a nonvisual position task (LR) in which the correct target of the HV pair was always located on the left, or nonpreferred, side. Here, the shark reached criterion after only 54 trials, performing perfectly during the last three sessions. When the positions of the horizontally and vertically striped targets were subsequently reversed, the shark continued to select the left-sided target, thereby confirming that it had not relied on target-associated visual cues to reach criterion.

In an attempt to reduce the initial learning requirement for telencephalically ablated sharks, a second set of nurse sharks was trained on the discriminations before surgery (Graeber *et al.*, 1978). This postoperative retention procedure produced no improvement in discrimination performance.

The results for the shark receiving the greatest amount of damage (about 95%

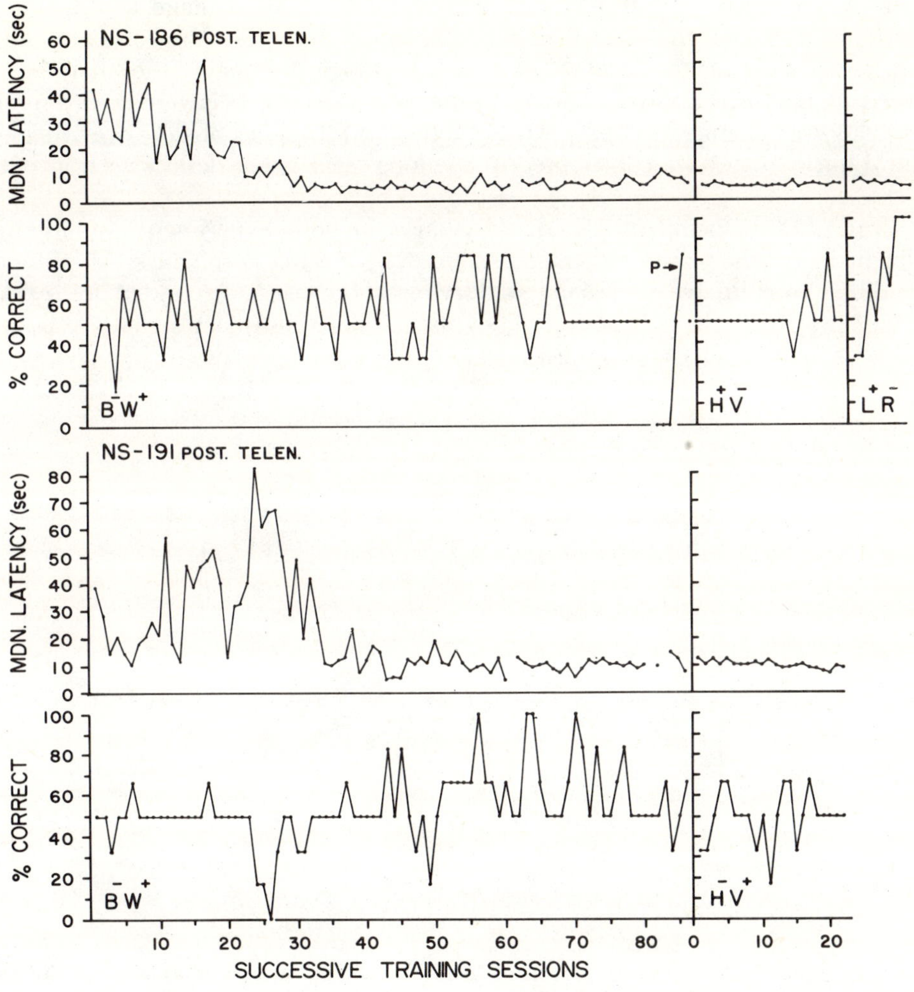

Figure 1. Visual discrimination performance for two sharks following extensive damage to telencephalic central nuclei. Upper function for each shark indicates median daily correct response latency from leaving the start-pen to choosing the correct target (marked with plus sign). P indicates placement of correct target on nonpreferred side for all daily trials to correct position habit.

of the CN destroyed bilaterally) are plotted in Fig. 2. Before surgery, this shark learned both the BW and HV tasks very quickly and retained the discriminations almost perfectly after 28 days of no additional training. Following surgery, its performance on BW remained consistently at the chance level for all 48 training sessions. During this time the shark continued to eat and swim well. Subsequently, an effort was made to teach the subject a light–dark (LD) discrimination at night. The results for this task are shown in the lower half of Fig. 2. It appears that the animal was at least able to detect the general location of the light, because responding usually exceeded chance but never dropped below it; however, no signs of improvement were noted after more than 6 weeks of training.

The other sharks in this experiment exhibited varying degrees of postoperative savings or loss in relearning the preoperatively acquired discriminations depending on the amount of damage to the telencephalic visual region. Those subjects with relatively superficial dorsal ablations, inflicting only 10% damage to the central telencephalic nuclei, manifested either near-perfect retention or very substantial savings. Considering the location of their neurological damage, they may be regarded as operated control subjects whose postoperative behavior rules out the possibility that damage to the portion of the dorsal telencephalon overlying the central nuclei may have contributed to the long-term visual deficits seen in other sharks.

Just prior to being sacrificed, the sharks in both experiments were tested individually for their responsiveness to sudden light onset in the dark. All of them, including those unable to learn the discrimination tasks, responded by quickly turning away from the light source. They also exhibited normal pupillary responses to changes in ambient light intensity.

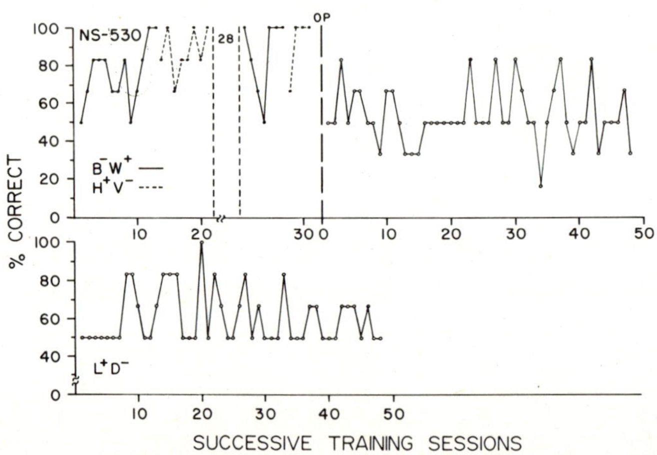

Figure 2. Visual discrimination performance before and after surgery (OP) resulting in 95% destruction of the central telencephalic nuclei. Twenty-eight days of no training is indicated by space between the pair of vertical dashed lines. Lower plot describes performance on light–dark (LD) discrimination task following BW postoperative training.

B. Nature of the Deficit

The successful performance of shark NS-186 on the position task, along with the stable low latencies exhibited on the visual tasks by CN-lesioned sharks, serves to eliminate two possible interpretations of the postoperative telencephalic deficit. Both are suggested by the teleost literature. The first is that telencephalic lesions interfere with a postulated nonspecific arousal function of the fish telencephalon (Aronson and Kaplan, 1968; Aronson, 1970). This view is supported by those behavioral studies reporting decreased spontaneous activity and increased response latency and variability in teleosts with telencephalic ablations (Aronson and Herberman, 1960; Kaplan and Aronson, 1967; Dewsbury and Bernstein, 1969; Overmier and Curnow, 1969). Although the sharks with central telencephalic lesions initially manifested such behavior, they eventually ceased doing so and instead consistently began to respond quickly in spite of continued choice errors. When given a task now requiring visual discrimination, NS-186 immediately demonstrated its ability to learn rapidly and perform correctly.

A second interpretation that might be offered stems from the work of Savage and Overmier. They have argued that telencephalic ablation in teleosts interferes with short-term memory and disrupts reinforcement mechanisms in instrumental learning situations (Savage, 1968*a,b,* 1969*a,b*; Savage and Swingland, 1969; Flood and Overmier, 1971; Overmier and Savage, 1974). Such deficits, if present in the operated nurse sharks, should have equally affected both position learning and visual discrimination learning. Furthermore, there was little basis for delay of reinforcement in the training situation. The maximal amount of delay was the time required for the shark to cross the choice line and swim forward the 30–40 cm to contact the fish reward, rarely more than a second. The delays used in the pertinent teleost experiments are usually 5 sec long and require the fish to turn around and swim back away from the choice area to obtain the reward (e.g., Savage and Swingland, 1969). One might further claim that, in the present study, escaping from the choice alley itself served as a major source of immediate reinforcement. This possibility is suggested by the occasional observation of sharks, both operated and unoperated, swimming quickly down the alley, responding correctly, and then swimming posthaste back to the start-pen after having ignored the fish reward.

At this point, it should be noted that the comparison of results derived from bony fish with those derived from elasmobranchs, although seductive, can be treacherous and fraught with misconceptions unless the systematic and neuroanatomical differences between these two groups of fishes are kept clearly in mind. Often reviewers of behavioral work have neglected this requirement and have characterized elasmobranch brain function on the basis of teleost experiments. Until we have accumulated a sufficient behavioral data base on sharks and rays, it would be best to avoid any further comparisons with teleostean brain function.

Based on Steiner's (1886, 1888) original findings on the spotted dogfish, there is reason to believe that lesions elsewhere in the nurse shark's telencephalon might lead to the sort of behavioral disorders described above for teleosts, particularly those indicative of decreased arousal. The results gathered from operated control sharks do not support this possibility. As shown in Fig. 3, control sharks, with anterior telencephalic lesions equivalent in size to the experimental lesions in the posterior telencephalon, experienced no difficulty learning the visual discriminations. Their range of performance was equivalent to that of unoperated sharks (see Graeber and Ebbesson, 1972*a*), one of which is described in Fig. 4. A third operated control animal reached criterion on both tasks within the range of trials of the other two subjects.

The control ablations severely damaged the rostral third of the telencephalon in all three sharks and included large portions of the lateral olfactory area. This resulted in an initial postoperative anorexia in all three sharks, which lasted for no more than 2 weeks. As Polimanti (1911, 1913) found in his forebrain-ablated spotted and smooth dogfish, these sharks subsequently manifested no deficits in spontaneous feeding or performance speed. Their median correct response latency consistently remained below 10 sec. The success of these control subjects in learning the visual discriminations also underscores the localized nature of the posterior telencephalic ablations which produced the visuomotor deficits in the experimental sharks.

The exact nature of the postoperative visuomotor deficit remains elusive at the present time. Although several nonvisual explanations have already been discussed and rejected, there persists the question of specificity of dysfunction. What neural component(s) underlying visually guided behavior was (were) disrupted by damage to the central telencephalic nuclei? It is clear that even those sharks unable to learn or relearn a simple BW discrimination could still detect light. The lack of

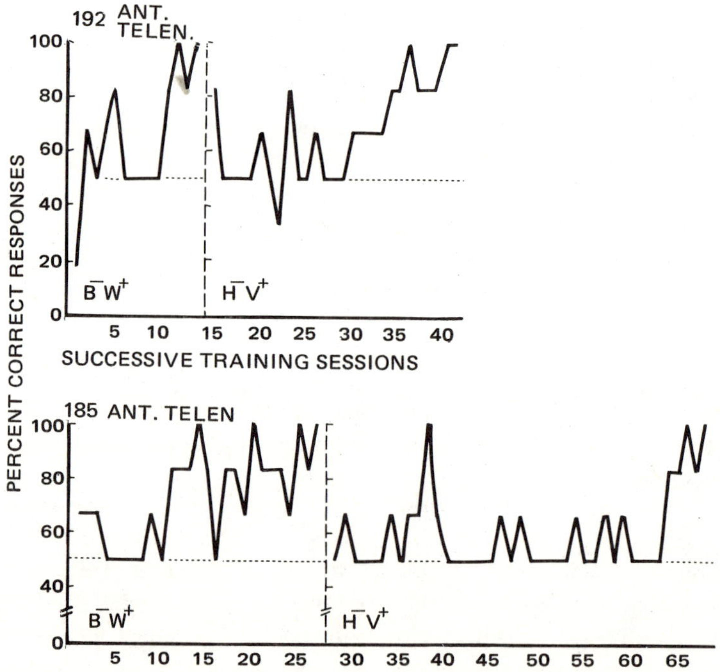

Figure 3. Visual discrimination performance for two control subjects following surgery which removed portions of anterior telencephalon.

a total sensory loss is also supported by Baru's (cited in Karamyan, 1956) finding that telencephalically ablated sharks do not differ from their unoperated counterparts in the ability to acquire classically conditioned reflexes to light onset.

There is still the more important question of whether the observed deficit involves primarily a disruption of visual identification mechanisms or an inability to localize a visual stimulus in space. While some argument can be made for a disruption of visual localization (see Graeber *et al.*, 1978), further research needs to be conducted in which the response requirements of the discrimination task are manipulated. The preliminary findings of Thomas and Jane (personal communication) suggest that any localization deficit, if present, is specific to vision and not common to other sense modalities. This conclusion is based on a nurse shark with almost total destruction of the CN that retained the ability to discriminate the location of a low-frequency continuously pulsed sound source while remaining unable to relearn the HV stripes discrimination.

The possibility of a less-than-total pure sensory deficit seems slim in light of the CN-lesioned sharks' inability to reach criterion on BW. Such an explanation, although not unprecedented, would require an extremely severe sensory loss that appears unlikely in view of the amount of central visual system remaining in the thalamus and midbrain. Future classical conditioning experiments using various levels of luminous flux as conditioned stimuli (see Gruber and Schneiderman, 1975) may be the best way to investigate this alternative.

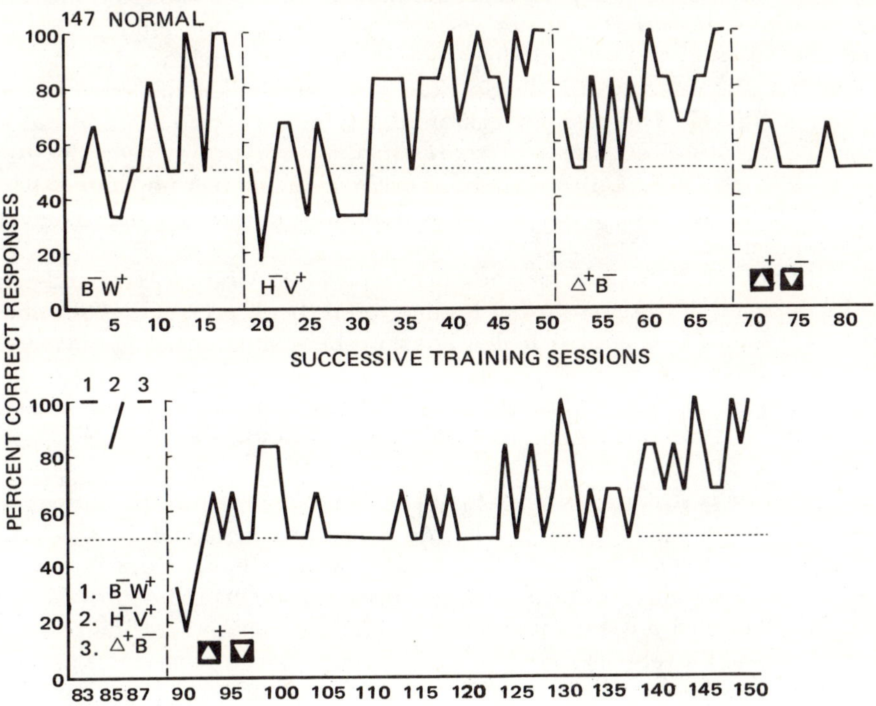

Figure 4. Visual discrimination performance of an unoperated nurse shark on a successive series of tasks. Retention tests are shown on far left side of lower panel.

C. Performance Characteristics of Normal Sharks

While descriptions of visual discrimination learning by unoperated sharks may not provide any direct evidence regarding telencephalic function, such observations may offer indirect clues to prompt further neurological experiments. A reexamination of Fig. 4 reveals some interesting facts about the ability of free-swimming nurse sharks to learn and retain these discriminations. First, as is typical of almost all unoperated and operated control sharks, NS-147 required more training sessions to learn the stripes discrimination than to learn BW. Second, after undergoing additional training on two equilateral triangle problems, the shark retained perfectly all three previously learned tasks, thus confirming the adequacy of the chosen criterion of learned discriminations. Finally, along with a few other sharks, it learned to discriminate an upright from an inverted solid white triangle on a black background. Although this task is a fairly difficult form discrimination for some vertebrate species, it would be premature to conclude whether or not the shark was really discriminating form *per se* or merely distinguishing one consistent target feature, e.g., flux density across the lower third of each target.

One of the more intriguing behaviors witnessed during training is the manner in which sharks approach the target. For example, during both triangle training periods subject NS-147 maintained a strong left-going position habit for a number of sessions, but as training progressed it learned to swerve suddenly to the right just in front of the baffle whenever the correct target was on the right side. Development of these position preferences, especially during training on the more difficult problems such as HV stripes and triangles, is common among both unoperated and operated sharks, including those with tectal or telencephalic lesions. Many, but not all, subsequently develop the disjointed mode of approach and choice seen in NS-147. The possible relation of this indirect approach and sudden swerving to the natural responses of sharks in field studies has been discussed elsewhere (Graeber, 1978). Unfortunately, its occurrence among unoperated sharks further complicates the interpretation of lesion-induced visuomotor deficits involving orientation errors.

Another potentially significant approach behavior is vicarious trial-and-error (VTE). Again, it usually occurs during training on difficult problems. The subject swims up the center of the approach alley but slows down upon nearing the targets, and then, sometimes halting, slowly moves its head from side to side before making a choice. This behavior typically occurs on several trials for no more than a day or two; however, it is almost always associated with a sudden increase in correct responding.

This behavior is strikingly similar to VTE reported in mammals undergoing simultaneous discrimination training. The comparison suggests that the shark may be searching for additional cues before responding or may be temporarily trapped in an approach–avoidance conflict. A more theoretical interpretation of VTE in mammals has been that it is a manifestation of ongoing cognitive cortical processes whereby an animal actively develops problem solving strategies instead of passively depending on simple associative learning. Whether a more parsimonious explanation is appropriate for VTE in sharks remains to be seen. Given the surprisingly high brain/body weight ratios in sharks and their multimodal telencephalon, it is likely that they will continue to respond in the laboratory in a manner traditionally thought to be characteristic of "higher" vertebrates. The challenge will be to experimentally define the extent of the similarities and to determine how they relate to forebrain organization in elasmobranchs.

IV. References

Allee, W. C., and Dickinson, J. C., 1954, Dominance and subordination in the smooth dogfish, *Mustelus canis* (Mitchill), *Physiol. Zool.* **27:**356.

Ariëns Kappers, C. U., 1906, The structure of the teleostean and selachian brain, *J. Comp. Neurol. Psychiat.* **16:**1.

Ariëns Kappers, C. U., Huber, G. C., and Crosby, E. C., 1936, *Comparative Anatomy of the Nervous System of Vertebrates, Including Man,* Macmillan, New York (reprinted 1967, Hafner, New York, 3 vols.).

Aronson, L. R., 1963, The central nervous system of sharks and bony fishes with special reference to sensory and integrative mechanisms, in: *Sharks and Survival* (P. W. Gilbert, ed.), pp. 165–241, Heath, Boston.

Aronson, L. R., 1970, Functional evolution of the forebrain in lower vertebrates, in: *Development and Evolution of Behavior: Essays in Memory of T. C. Schneirla* (L. R. Aronson, E. Tobach, D. S. Lehrman, and J. S. Rosenblatt, eds.), pp. 75–107, Freeman, San Francisco.

Aronson, L. R., and Herberman, R., 1960, Persistence of a conditioned response in the cichlid fish, *Tilapia macrocephalia,* after forebrain and cerebellar ablations, *Anat. Rec.* **138:**322.

Aronson, L. R., and Kaplan, H., 1968, Function of the teleostean forebrain, in: *The Central Nervous and Fish Behavior* (D. Ingle, ed.), pp. 107–125, University of Chicago Press, Chicago.

Aronson, L. R., Aronson, F. R., and Clark, E., 1967, Instrumental conditioning and light-dark discrimination in young sharks, *Bull. Mar. Sci.* **17:**249.

Bäckström, K., 1924, Contributions to the forebrain morphology in selachians, *Acta Zool.* **5:**123.

Bakay, L., and Lee, J. C., 1966, Ultrastructural changes in the edematous central nervous system, *Arch. Neurol.* **14:**644.

Banner, A., 1968, Attraction of young lemon sharks, *Negaprion brevirostris,* by sound, *Copeia* **1968:**871.

Banner, A., 1972, Use of sound in predation by young lemon sharks, *Negaprion brevirostris* (Poey), *Bull. Mar. Sci.* **22:**251.

Bernstein, J. J., 1970, Anatomy and physiology of the central nervous system, in: *Fish Physiology,* Vol. IV: *The Nervous System, Circulation, and Respiration* (W. S. Hoar and D. J. Randall, eds.), pp. 1-90, Academic Press, New York.

Bethe, A., 1899, Die Lokomotion des Haifisches (*Scyllium*) und ihre Beziehung zu den einselnen Gehirnteilen und zum Labyrinth, *Pfluegers Arch.* **76:**470.

Bogartz, R. S., 1965, The criterion method: Some analyses and remarks, *Psychol. Bull.* **64:**1.

Bruckmoser, P., and Dieringer, N., 1973, Evoked potentials in the primary and secondary olfactory projection areas of the forebrain in elasmobranchs, *J. Comp. Physiol.* **87:**65.

Budker, P., 1971, *The Life of Sharks,* Columbia University Press, New York.

Campbell, C. B. G., 1976, What animals should we compare? in: *Evolution, Brain, and Behavior: Persistent Problems* (R. B. Masterton, W. Hodos, and H. Jerison, eds.), pp. 107–113, Erlbaum Associates, Hillsdale, N.J.

Clark, E., 1959, Instrumental conditioning of lemon sharks, *Science* **136:**217.

Clark, E., 1961, Visual discrimination in lemon sharks, *Symp. Papers 10th Pacific Sci. Congr. Honolulu* **10:**175.

Clark, E., 1963, The maintenance of sharks in captivity, with a report on their instrumental conditioning, in: *Sharks and Survival* (P. W. Gilbert, ed.), pp. 115–149, Heath, Boston

Cohen, D. H., Duff, T. A., and Ebbesson, S. O. E., 1973, Electrophysiological identification of a visual area in shark telencephalon, *Science* **182:**492.

Cohen, J. L., Gruber, S. H., and Hamasaki, D. F. 1977, Spectral sensitivity and Purkinje shift in the retina of the lemon shark, *Negaprion brevirostris* (Poey), *Vision Res.* **17:**787.

Demski, L, 1977, Electrical stimulation of the shark brain, *Am. Zool.* **17:**487.

Dewsbury, D. A., and Bernstein, J. J., 1969, Role of the telencephalon in the performance of conditioned avoidance responses by goldfish, *Exp. Neurol.* **23:**445.

Ebbesson, S. O. E., 1971, Projections of the optic tectum in the nurse shark *(Ginglymostoma cirratum* Bonnaterre), *Proc. Soc. Neurosci. 1st Annu. Meet.* **1971:**109.

Ebbesson, S. O. E., 1972*a*, New insights into the organization of the shark brain, *Comp. Biochem. Physiol.* **42A:**121.

Ebbesson, S. O. E., 1972*b*, A proposal for a common nomenclature for some optic nuclei in vetebrates and the evidence for the common origin of two such cell groups, *Brain Behav. Evol.* **6:**75.

Ebbesson, S. O. E., and Heimer, L., 1970, Projections of the olfactory tract fibers in the nurse shark (*Ginglymostoma cirratum*), *Brain Res.* **17:**47.

Ebbesson, S. O. E., and Northcutt, R. G., 1976, Neurology of anamniotic vertebrates, in: *Evolution of Brain and Behavior in Vertebrates* (R. B. Masterton, M. E. Bitterman, C. B. G. Campbell, and N. Hotton, eds.), pp.115–146, Erlbaum Associates, Hillsdale, N.J.

Ebbesson, S. O. E., and Ramsey, J. S., 1968, The optic tracts of two species of sharks (*Galeocerdo cuvier* and *Ginglymostoma cirratum*), *Brain Res.* **8:**36.

Ebbesson, S. O. E., and Schroeder, D. M., 1971, Connections of the nurse shark's telencephalon, *Science* **173:**254.

Ebbesson, S. O. E., Jane, J. A., and Schroeder, D. M., 1972, A general overview of major interspecific variations in thalamic organization, *Brain Behav. Evol.* **6:**92.

Eibl-Eibesfeldt, I., and Haas, H., 1959, Erfahrungen mit haien, *Z. Tierpsychol.* **16:**733.

Finstad, W. O., and Nelson, D. R., 1975, Circadian activity rhythm in the horn shark, *Heterodontus francesci:* Effect of light intensity, *Bull. S. Calif. Acad. Sci.* **74:**20.

Flood, N. B. and Overmier, J. B., 1971, Effects of telencephalic and olfactory lesions on appetitive learning in goldfish, *Physiol. Behav.* **6:**35.

Gilbert, P. W., 1962, The behavior of sharks, *Sci. Am.* **207:**60.

Graeber, R. C., 1972, Visual discrimination learning in sharks (*Negaprion brevirostris* and *Ginglymostoma cirratum*): Effects of central nervous system lesions, 191 pp., Doctoral dissertation, University of Virginia.

Graeber, R. C., 1974, Food intake patterns in captive juvenile lemon sharks, *Negaprion brevirostris, Copeia* **1974:**554.

Graeber, R. C., 1978, Behavioral studies correlated with central nervous system integration of vision in sharks, in: *Sensory Biology of Elasmobranchs* (E. S. Hodgson and R. F. Mathewson, eds.), pp. 195–225, U.S. Government Printing Office, Washington, D.C.

Graeber, R. C., and Ebbesson, S. O. E., 1972*a*, Visual discrimination learning in normal and tectal-ablated nurse sharks (*Ginglymostoma cirratum*), *Comp. Biochem. Physiol.* **42A:**131.

Graeber, R. C., and Ebbesson, S. O. E., 1972*b*, Retinal projections in the lemon shark (*Negaprion brevirostris*), *Brain Behav. Evol.* **5:**461.

Graeber, R. C., Schroeder, D. M., Jane, J. A., and Ebbesson, S. O. E., 1972, The importance of telencephalic structures in visual discrimination learning in nurse sharks, *Proc. Soc. Neurosci. 2nd Annu. Meet.* **1972:**100.

Graeber, R. C., Ebbesson, S. O. E., and Jane, J. A., 1973, Visual discrimination in sharks without optic tectum, *Science* **180:**413.

Graeber, R. C., Schroeder, D. M., Jane, J. A., and Ebbesson, S. O. E., 1978, Visual discrimination following partial telencephalic ablations in nurse sharks (*Ginglymostoma cirratum*), *J. Comp. Neurol.* **180:**325.

Gruber, S. H., 1967, A behavioral measurement of dark adaptation in the lemon shark, *Negaprion brevirostris,* in: *Sharks, Skates, and Rays* (P. W. Gilbert, R. F. Mathewson, and D. P. Rall, eds.), pp. 479–490, Johns Hopkins University Press, Baltimore.

Gruber, S. H., 1975, Duplex vision in elasmobranchs: Histological, electrophysiological and psychophysical evidence, in: *New Approaches to the Study of Vision in Fishes* (M. A. Ali, ed.), pp. 525–540, Plenum Press, New York.

Gruber, S. H., and Myrberg, A. A., 1977, Approaches to the study of the behavior of sharks, *Am. Zool.* **17:**471.

Gruber, S. H., and Schneiderman, N., 1975, Classical conditioning of the nictitating membrane response of the lemon shark (*Negaprion Brevirostris*), *Behav. Res. Methods Instrum.* **7:**430.

Gruber, S. H., Hamasaki, D. H., and Bridges, C. D. B., 1963, Cones in the retina of the lemon shark (*Negaprion brevirostris), Vision Res.* **3:**397.

Gruber, S. H., Gulley, R. L., and Brandon, J., 1975, Duplex retina in seven elasmobranch species, *Bull. Mar. Sci.* **25:**353.

Hamasaki, D. H., and Bridges, C. D. B., 1965, Properties of the electroretinogram in three elasmobranch species, *Vision Res.* **5:**483.

Hamasaki, D. H., and Gruber, S. H., 1965, The photoreceptors of the nurse shark, *Ginglymostoma cirratum,* and the sting ray, *Dasyatis sayi, Bull. Mar. Sci.* **15:**1051.

Healey, E. G., 1957, The nervous system, in: *The Physiology of Fishes* (M. E. Brown, ed.), pp. 1–119, Academic Press, New York.

Herrick, C. J., 1922, Functional factors in the morphology of the forebrain of fishes, in: *Libro en Honor de D. Santiago Ramón y Cajal*, Vol. I, pp. 143–204, Jiménez y Molina, Madrid.

Herrick, C. J., 1962, *Neurological Foundations of Animal Behavior,* Hafner, New York.

Hobson, E. S., 1963, Feeding behavior in three species of sharks, *Pac. Sci.* **17:**171.

Hodgson, E. S., and Mathewson, R. F., 1971, Chemosensory orientation in sharks, *Ann. N.Y. Acad. Sci.* **188:**175.

Hodos, W., 1970, Evolutionary interpretations of neural and behavioral studies of living vertebrates, in: *The Neurosciences: A Second Study Program* (F. O. Schmitt, ed.), pp. 26–39, Rockefeller University Press, New York.

Hodos, W., and Campbell, C. B. G., 1969, Scala naturae: Why there is no theory in comparative psychology, *Psychol. Rev.* **76:**337.

Holmgren, N., 1922, Points of view concerning forebrain morphology in lower vertebrates, *J. Comp. Neurol.* **34:**391.

Hotton, N., 1976, Origin and radiation of the classes of poikilothermous vertebrates, in: *Evolution of Brain and Behavior in Vertebrates* (R. B. Masterton, M. E. Bitterman, C. B. G. Campbell, and N. Hotton, eds.), pp.1–24, Erlbaum Associates, Hillsdale, N.J.

Houser, G. L., 1901, The neurons and supporting elements of the brain of a selachian, *J. Comp. Neurol.* **11:**65.

Johnson, R. H., and D. R. Nelson, 1973, Agonistic display in the gray reef shark, *Carcharhinus menisorrah,* and its relationship to man, *Copeia* **1973:**76.

Johnston, J. B., 1911, The telencephalon of selachians, *J. Comp. Neurol.* **21:**1.

Kalmijn, A. J., 1966, Electro-perception in sharks and rays, *Nature (London)* **212:**1232.

Kalmijn, A. J., 1971, The electric sense of sharks and rays, *J. Exp. Biol.* **55:**371.

Kalmijn, A. J., 1973, Electro-orientation in sharks and rays: Theory and experimental evidence, *Scripps Inst. Oceanogr. Contrib.* **73-39:**1.

Kalmijn, A. J., 1974, The detection of electric fields from inanimate and animate sources other than electric organs, in: *Handbook of Sensory Physiology,* Vol. III/3 (A. Fessard, ed.), pp. 147–200, Springer-Verlag, New York.

Kaplan, H., and Aronson, L. R., 1967, Effect of forebrain ablation on the performance of a conditioned avoidance response in the teleost fish, *Tilapia h. macrocephalia, Anim. Behav.* **15:** 438.

Karamyan, A. I., 1956, *Evolution of the Function of the Cerebellum and Cerebral Hemispheres,* Medgiz, Leningrad (transl. by Israel Program for Scientific Translations, Jerusalem, 1962).

Karamyan, A. I., Vesselkin, N. P., Belekhova, M. G., and Zagorul'ko, T. M., 1966, Electrophysiological characteristics of tectal and thalamocortical divisions of the visual system in lower vertebrates, *J. Comp. Neurol.* **127:**559.

Kelly, J. C., and Nelson, D. R., 1975, Hearing thresholds of the horn shark, *Heterodontus francisci, J. Acoust. Soc. Am.* **58:**905.

Kleerekoper, H., Gruber, D., and Matis, J., 1975, Accuracy of localization of a chemical stimulus in flowing and stagnant water by the nurse shark, *Ginglymostoma cirratum, J. Comp. Physiol.* **98:** 257.

Kritzler, H., and Wood, L., 1961, Provisional audiogram for the shark, *Carcharhinus leucas, Science* **133:**1480.

Kuchnow, K. P., and Gilbert, P. W., 1967, Preliminary in vivo studies on pupillary and tapetal pigment responses in the lemon shark, *Negaprion brevirostris,* in: *Sharks, Skates, and Rays* (P. W. Gilbert, R. F. Mathewson, and D. P. Rall, eds.), pp. 465–477, Johns Hopkins University Press, Baltimore.

Lineaweaver, T. H., and Backus, R. H., 1973, *The Natural History of Sharks,* Doubleday, Garden City, N.Y.

Loeb, J., 1891, Ueber den Anteil des Hörnerven an den nach Gehirnverletzung auftretenden

Zwangslagen und assozienten Stellungsanderungen der Bulbi und Extremitäten, *Pflüegers Arch.* **50:**66.

Marshall, N. B., 1971, *Explorations in the Life of Fishes,* Harvard University Press, Cambridge, Mass.

Masai, H., 1962, On the external form of the brain of *Heterodontus japonicus, Yokohama Med. Bull.* **13:**249.

Moy-Thomas, J. A., 1939, The early evolution and relationships of the elasmobranchs, *Biol. Rev.* **14:**1.

Myrberg, A. A., 1972, Using sound to influence the behavior of free-ranging marine animals, in: *Behavior of Marine Animals—Current Perspectives in Research,* Vol. 2 (H. E. Winn and B. L. Olla, eds.), pp. 435–468, Plenum Press, New York.

Myrberg, A. A., and Gruber, S. H., 1974, The behavior of the bonnethead shark, *Sphyrna tiburo, Copeia* **1974:**358.

Myrberg, A. A., Banner, A., and Richard, J. D., 1969, Shark attraction using a video-acoustic system, *Mar. Biol.* **2:**264.

Nelson, D. R., 1967, Hearing thresholds, frequency discrimination, and acoustic orientation in the lemon shark, *Negaprion brevirostris* (Poey), *Bull. Mar. Sci.* **17:**741.

Nelson, D. R., 1974, Ultrasonic telemetry of shark behavior, *Naval Res. Rev.* **27:**1.

Nelson, D. R., and Gruber, S. H., 1963, Sharks: Attraction by low-frequency sounds, *Science* **142:**975.

Nelson, D. R., and Johnson, R. H., 1970, Diel activity rhythms in the nocturnal, bottom-dwelling sharks, *Heterodontus francisci* and *Cephaloscyllium ventriosum, Copeia* **1970:**732.

Nelson, D. R., and Johnson, R. H., 1972, Acoustic attraction of Pacific reef sharks; effect of pulse intermittency and variability, *Comp. Biochem, Physiol.* **42A:**85.

Nelson, D. R., Johnson, R. H., and Waldrop, L. G., 1969, Responses in Bahamian sharks and grouper to low-frequency pulsed sounds, *Bull. S. Calif. Acad. Sci.* **68:**131.

Nieuwenhuys, R., 1967, Comparative anatomy of olfactory centres and tracts, in: *Progress in Brain Research,* Vol. 23 (Y. Zotterman, ed.), pp. 1–64, Elsevier, Amsterdam.

Northcutt, R. G., 1977, Elasmobranch central nervous system organization and its possible evolutionary significance, *Am. Zool.* **17:**411.

Overmier, B. J., and Curnow, P. F., 1969, Classical conditioning, pseudoconditioning and sensitization in "normal" and forebrainless goldfish, *J. Comp. Physiol. Psychol.* **68:**193.

Overmier, B. J., and Savage, G. E., 1974, Effects of telencephalic ablation on trace conditioning of heart rate in goldfish, *Exp. Neurol.* **42:**339.

Parker, G. H., 1910, Olfactory reactions in fishes, *J. Exp. Zool.* **8:**535.

Parker, G. H., 1914, The directive influence of the sense of smell in the dogfish, *Bull. U.S. Bur. Fisheries* **33:**61.

Parker, G. H., and Sheldon, R. E., 1913, The sense of smell in fishes, *Bull. U.S. Bur. Fisheries* **32:**33.

Platt, C. J., Bullock, T. H., Czéh, G., Kovačević, D., and Gojković, M., 1974, Comparison of the electroreceptor, mechanoreceptor, and optic evoked potentials in the brains of some rays and sharks, *J. Comp. Physiol.* **95:**323.

Polimanti, O., 1911, Contributi alla fisiligia del sistema nervoso centrale e del movimento dei pesci, I. Selacoidei, *Zool. Jahrb.* **30:**473.

Polimanti, O., 1913, Contributions a la physiolgie du systeme nerveaux central et du mouvement des poissons, *Arch. Ital. Biol.* **59:**383.

Polyak, S., 1957, *The Vertebrate Visual System,* University of Chicago Press, Chicago.

Rizzolo, A., 1929, A study of equilibrium in the smooth dogfish (*Galeus canis Mitchill)* after removal of different parts of the brain, *Biol. Bull.* **57:**245.

Romer, A. S., 1956, *The Vertebrate Body,* Saunders, Philadelphia.

Romer, A. S., 1967, Major steps in vertebrate evolution, *Science* **158:**1629.

Romer, A. S., 1968*a, Notes and Comments on Vertebrate Paleontology,* University of Chicago Press, Chicago.

Romer, A. S., 1968*b, The Procession of Life,* World Press, Cleveland.

Savage, G. E., 1968*a*, Function of the forebrain in the memory system of the fish, in: *The Central Nervous System and Fish Behavior* (D. Ingle, ed.), pp. 127–138, Chicago University Press, Chicago.

Savage, G. E., 1968*b*, Temporal factors in avoidance learning in normal and forebrainless goldfish, *Nature (London)* **218:**1168.

Savage, G. E., 1969*a*, Some preliminary observations on the role of the telencephalon in food-reinforced behavior in the goldfish, *Carassius auratus, Anim. Behav.* **17:**760.

Savage, G. E., 1969*b*, Telencephalic lesions and avoidance behavior in the goldfish (*Carassius auratus*), *Anim. Behav.* **17:**362.

Savage, G. E., and Swingland, I. R., 1969, Positively reinforced behavior and the forebrain in goldfish, *Nature (London)* **221:**878.

Schaeffer, B., 1967, Comments on elasmobranch evolution, in: *Sharks, Skates and Rays* (P. W. Gilbert, R. F. Mathewson, and D. P. Rall, eds.), pp. 3–35, John Hopkins University Press, Baltimore.

Schroeder, D. M., and Ebbesson, S. O. E., 1974, Nonolfactory telencephalic afferents in the nurse shark (*Ginglymostoma cirratum*), *Brain Behav. Evol.* **9:**121.

Segaar, J., 1965, Behavioral aspects of degeneration and regeneration in fish brain: A comparison with higher vertebrates, in: *Progress in Brain Research,* Vol. 14 (Y. Zotterman, ed.), pp. 143–231, Elsevier, Amsterdam.

Sheldon, R. E., 1909, The reactions of dogfish to chemical stimuli, *J. Comp. Neurol.* **19:**273.

Sheldon, R. E., 1911, The sense of smell in selachians, *J. Exp. Zool.* **10:**51.

Springer, S., 1950, Natural history notes on the lemon shark, *Tex. J. Sci.* **2:**349.

Steiner, I., 1886, Ueber das Centralnervensystem des Haifisches und des *Amphioxus lanceolatus* und über die halbcirkelförmigen Canäle des Haifisches, *Sitzungsber. Akad. Wiss, Berlin* **1886:**495.

Steiner, I., 1888, *Die Functionem des Zentralnervensystems und ihre Phylogneese. 2. Abt. Die Fische,* Vieweg, Braunschweig.

Stell, W. K., 1972, The structure and morphologic relations of rods and cones in the retina of the spiny dogfish, *Squalus, Comp. Biochem, Physiol.* **42A:**141.

Stensiö, E., 1963, The brain and the cranial nerves in fossil, lower craniate vertebrates, *Skrift. Norske Videnskaps-Akad. Mat.-Naturv. Klasse Ny Ser.* **13:**1.

Tanaka, S. K., 1973, Suction feeding by the nurse shark, *Copeia* **1973:**606.

Ten Cate, J., 1935, Physiologie des Zentralnervensystem der Fische, *Ergeb. Biol.* **11:**335.

Tester, A. L., 1963, Olfaction, gustation, and the common chemical sense in sharks, in: *Sharks and Survival* (P. W. Gilbert, ed.), pp. 255–282, Heath, Boston.

Tester, A. L., and Kato, S., 1966, Visual target discrimination in blacktip sharks (*Carcharhinus melanopterus)* and grey sharks (*C. menisorrah), Pacific Sci.* **20:**461.

van Bergeijk, W. A., 1964, Directional and nondirectional hearing in fish, in: *Marine Bio-Acoustics* (W. N. Tavolga, ed.), pp. 281–299, Pergamon Press, New York.

Veselkin, N. P., 1964, Electrical responses in skate brain to photic stimulation, *Fiziol. Zh. SSSR im. I. M. Sechenova* **50:**268 [Translated in *Fed. Proc. Fed. Am. Soc. Exp. Biol.* **24:**368 (1965)].

Veselkin, N. P., and Kovacevic, N., 1973, Nonolfactory afferent projections of the telencephalon of elasmobranchii, *Z. Evol. Biokim. Fiziol.* **9:**585.

Voronin, L. G., Gusselnikova, K. G., Gusselnikov, V. I., and Supin, A. J., 1968, On the problem of the evolution of the vertebrate afferent systems, in: *Progress in Brain Research,* Vol. 22 (Y. Zotterman, ed.), pp. 541–565, Elsevier, Amsterdam.

3

New Observations on the Organization and Evolution of the Telencephalon of Actinopterygian Fishes

R. GLENN NORTHCUTT and MARK R. BRAFORD, Jr.

I. Introduction

A. The Fishes

The Osteichthyes comprise at least three groups of bony fishes which are generally believed to share a common ancestor: the Crossopterygii, the Dipnoi, and the Actinopterygii. The intergroup relationships have long been disputed by paleontologists, and there is no consensus at the present time. It is usually argued either that the Crossopterygii and the Dipnoi are more closely related to one another than either is to the Actinopterygii (Romer, 1966; Gardiner, 1973) or that the three have been distinct groups since their earliest appearance (Schaeffer, 1969; Miles in Moy-Thomas, 1971). Jarvik (1968), however, has favored a closer affinity between the Crossopterygii and the Actinopterygii than between either of these groups and the Dipnoi.

The Crossopterygii are represented by a single living member, *Latimeria,* but a separate, now-extinct line gave rise to the land vertebrates. The Dipnoi or lungfish are likewise represented by relict populations assigned to three genera. The Actinopterygii or ray-finned fish, however, form a major vertebrate radiation consisting of 20,000 or more living species. Among the actinopterygians three levels of

R. GLENN NORTHCUTT and MARK R. BRAFORD, Jr. • Division of Biological Sciences, University of Michigan, Ann Arbor, Michigan 48109.

organization or grades are traditionally recognized: Chondrostei, Holostei, and Teleostei. The chondrosteans include the sturgeons and paddlefish. The living holosteans consist of two genera, *Amia* and *Lepisosteus.* The vast remainder of the actinopterygians are teleosts. They have been grouped into three divisions by Greenwood *et al.* (1966).* Division I includes the eels, eel-like fish, and perhaps the herringlike fish. In Division II there are two very specialized groups, the osteoglossiforms and the mormyriforms, both of which display unusually highly differentiated forebrains. The bulk of the teleosts belong to Division III.

The relationships of the polypteriforms, *Polypterus* and *Erpetoichthys* (formerly *Calamoichthys*), are uncertain (Schaeffer, 1973). At present, there are two opinions regarding their affinities: (1) that they are a specialized group of chondrosteans (Romer, 1966; Gardiner, 1967; Miles in Moy-Thomas, 1971) and (2) that they represent a distinct and independent group of osteichthyans—the Brachiopterygii (Holmgren and Stensiö, 1936; Jarvik, 1947, 1968; Lehman, 1966). We will try to show in this chapter that the telencephalon of the polypteriforms shares many derived characters with that of the other actinopterygians and that the organization of the dorsal part of their telencephalon is unique. We thus consider it likely that the polypteriforms constitute a separate group *within* the Actinopterygii.

B. The Telencephalon

The organization of the telencephalon of the actinopterygians is strikingly different from that of land vertebrates and even from that of the other osteichthyans. In land vertebrates and the Dipnoi, the dorsal and ventral portions of the lateral walls of the embryonic telencephalon undergo an inward bending or inversion. This is followed by various evagination processes resulting in a pair of hemispheres enclosing lateral ventricles. In contrast, the telencephalon of adult actinopterygians generally consists of two solid masses flanking a median ventricular space. The situation in *Latimeria* is intermediate (Nieuwenhuys, 1965).† Representatives of the various telencephalic configurations seen in ectothermic vertebrates are shown in Fig. 1.

Several early workers (Rabl-Rückhard, 1884; Edinger, 1896; Goldstein, 1905) considered the paired masses of the actinopterygians to be homologous to the basal telencephalon or subpallium of land vertebrates. They regarded the overlying membranous ependyma as the pallial homologue. Gage (1893) and later Studnicka (1896) concluded that the paired masses contain both pallial and subpallial homologues and that the overlying ependyma is a greatly expanded tela chorioidea. They further suggested that the unusual configuration of the actinopterygian telencephalon results from an outward bending or eversion of the dorsal portion—the pallial anlage—of the lateral wall. A major consequence of such a simple eversion process would be a mediolateral reversal of the pallium relative to its

* Also see Greenwood (1973) for a slightly modified interpretation of the interrelationships of the major groups of teleosts.

† For more detailed considerations of the various processes which occur during the development of the telencephalon of amniotes, see Holmgren (1922), Holmgren and van der Horst (1925), Källén (1951), and especially Nieuwenhuys (1964, 1965).

orientation in the inverted condition (Fig. 2). Subsequently, a number of embryological and comparative morphological studies have confirmed the presence of a pallium and a subpallium in these fishes (e.g., Johnston, 1911; Holmgren, 1922; Kuhlenbeck, 1929; Källén, 1951; Nieuwenhuys, 1962*a*); however, the position of the boundary between them is disputed. The eversion hypothesis has been generally, but not universally, accepted by later workers. As a consequence of these various disagreements, the cell groups in the telencephalon have received several divergent interpretations.

One group of workers, which might be called the "directly comparable school"

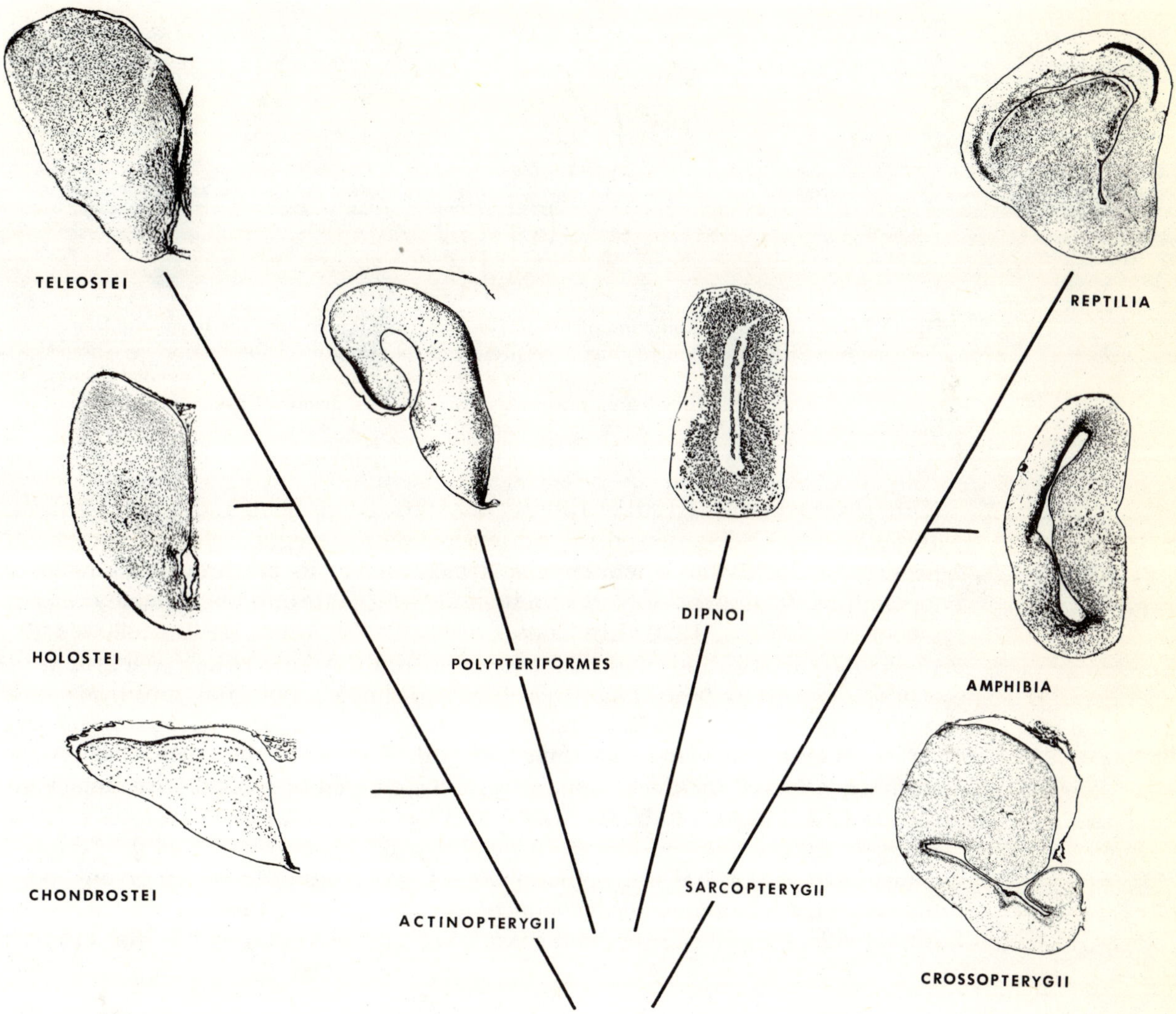

Figure 1. Cladogram of telencephalic variation in bony fishes and their derivatives. No general agreement exists on the number of distinct radiations; two to four may exist depending on the affinities of Polypteriformes and Dipnoi. Each taxon is represented by a transverse section through one-half of the telencephalon stained to reveal the number and distribution of neuronal cell bodies.

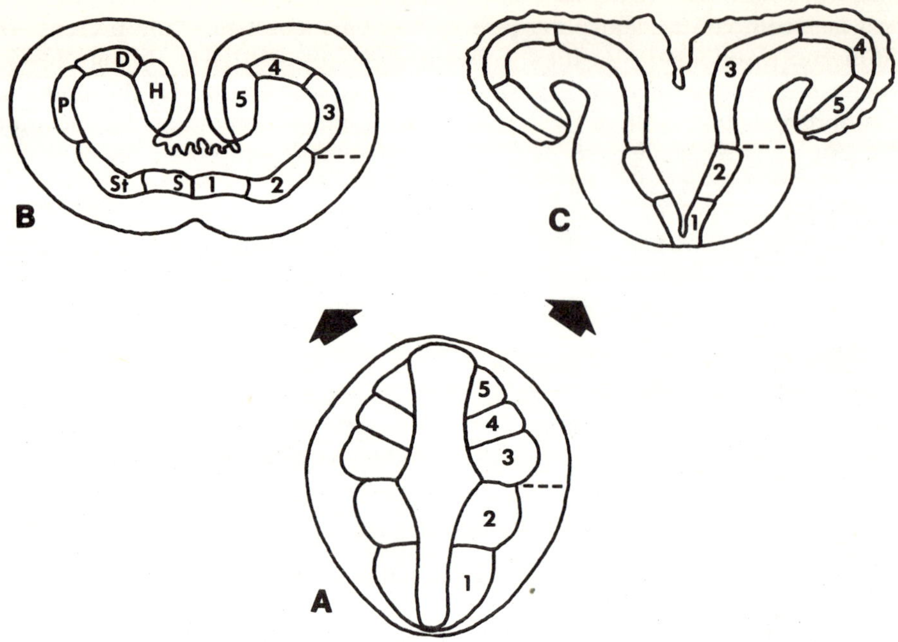

Figure 2. Schematic representation of the way in which the topology of the major subdivisions of the embryonic telencephalon (A) might be preserved following inversion in land vertebrates (B) and eversion in *Polypterus* (C). D, Dorsal pallium; H, hippocampal complex or medial pallium; P, piriform or lateral pallium; S, septal nuclei; St, striatum; 1–5, major telencephalic subdivisions or columns.

(Droogleever-Fortuyn, 1961; Crosby *et al.*, 1967; Schnitzlein, 1964, 1968; Wright, 1967; Morgan, 1975), denied the existence and/or the significance of an eversion process and held the actinopterygian telencephalon to be directly comparable, topographically, to that of land vertebrates. A second group, the "simple eversion school" (Holmgren, 1922; Kuhlenbeck, 1929, 1973; Miller, 1940), followed the suggestion of Gage and Studnicka and compared the telencephalic cell groups of actinopterygians to those of land vertebrates by simple topological transformations. A third group, the "eversion–rearrangement school" (Sheldon, 1912; Herrick, 1921), while not denying that some outward bending of the telencephalic walls occurs, considered the thickening of the walls followed by a plastic rearrangement of various cell groups to be the most important morphogenetic processes.* Their interpretation of the cell masses turns out to be similar to that of the "directly comparable school" but with some mixing of cells from different embryonic populations. Finally, students of the "noncomparable school" (Källén, 1951; Nieuwenhuys, 1962*b*, 1963, 1967*a*) accept the eversion hypothesis but contend—for different

* Herrick, however, accepted a simple eversion process for *Polypterus* which shows no thickening but rather a lengthening of the lateral walls during development (see Holmgren, 1922; Nieuwenhuys *et al.*, 1969). Braford and Northcutt (1974) have flirted with some of the notions of the "eversion–rearrangement school" in an attempt to relate the pallial organization of *Polypterus* to that of the teleosts.

reasons—that the actinopterygian pallium cannot be directly compared to those of land vertebrates. They do, nevertheless, homologize the subpallial masses to those of land vertebrates. Specifically, Källén states that in most vertebrates the cells of the pallium divide at an early embryonic stage into a periventricular and a migrated layer, the latter subsequently differentiating into three pallial areas. On the other hand, in the nonevaginated portion of the pallium of chondrosteans and holosteans and in the whole of the teleost pallium there is a continuous cell proliferation from the matrix zone, forming a uniform pallial anlage which only at a late embryonic stage divides into three parts. Thus he believes the two sets of pallial areas are not comparable. Nieuwenhuys has argued that the pallial areas of these fish are the result of a differentiation which has taken place entirely within the actinopterygian line. This argument is based, at least in part, on the progressive increase in the number of pallial cytoarchitectonic areas he was able to recognize in the series: polypteriforms (one uniform area), chondrosteans (three areas), holosteans (three areas), and teleosts (three to seven areas, depending on the species). We will return to this argument later in this chapter. It should be noted that from the interpretations of both the "eversion–rearrangement" and the "noncomparable" schools it follows that the actinopterygian pallial areas cannot be compared to those of land vertebrates as strict homologues. The various interpretations of the telencephalon of teleosts are summarized schematically in Fig. 3.

The interpretations of these four "schools" are of more than historical importance: At least some elements of each have been espoused within the last decade. An understanding of the organization of the telencephalon of the actinopterygians is hampered by a lack of reliable information concerning the character and connectivity patterns of the constituent cell populations. In this chapter we will present some new data which bear on the problem. In particular, we will analyze the normal morphology of the telencephalon in five actinopterygian species, the projections of the olfactory bulb in three of these species, and histochemical data in three of them.

II. Species Studied

The species used in this study are listed in Table I. Although there are a total of nine species in the list, no differences were evident between members of the same genus, and the brain of *Erpetoichthys* is essentially indistinguishable from that of its close relative *Polypterus* (Fig. 4). Thus our five representatives are *Polypterus,* a polypteriform; *Scaphirhynchus*, a chondrostean; *Lepisosteus* (Fig. 5), a holostean which displays a much lesser degree of pallial eversion than the other holostean *Amia; Salmo,* a teleost showing a slight eversion relative to that seen in most teleosts; and *Lepomis* (Fig. 6), a more typical teleost. *Salmo* and *Lepomis* are both members of the largest branch of teleosts, Division III of Greenwood *et al.* (1966). The salmonids are sufficiently generalized to be considered as the basal stock from which Division III teleosts arose, whereas *Lepomis* (family Centrarchidae) is an advanced teleost

In addition to the above species which were studied in detail, the brains of numerous other actinopterygians were frequently examined and compared. These

Table I. Species Studied

Actinopterygii	
Polypteriformes	
Polypterus palmas	Bichir
Polypterus ornatipinnis	Bichir
Erpetoichthys calabaricus	Reed fish
Chondrostei	
Scaphirhynchus platorynchus	Shovelnose sturgeon
Holostei	
Lepisosteus osseus	Longnose gar
Lepisosteus productus	Spotted gar
Teleostei	
Salmo gairdneri	Rainbow trout
Lepomis cyanellus	Green sunfish
Lepomis cyanellus × *Lepomis macrochirus*	Green sunfish–bluegill hybrid

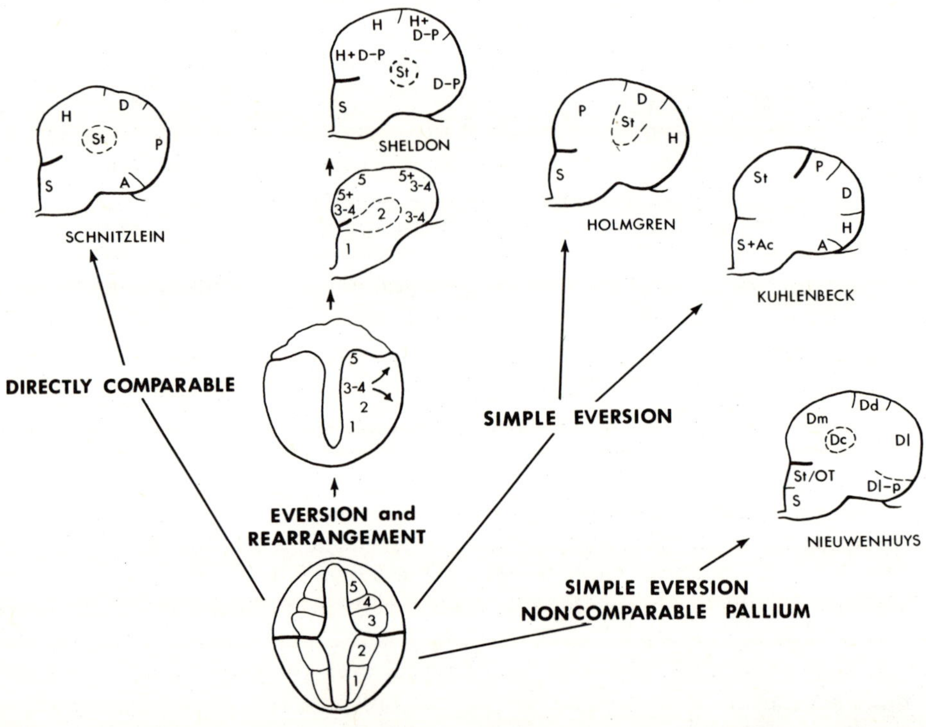

Figure 3. Schematic representations of teleost telencephalic homologies based on the interpretations of different schools of thought regarding the major developmental processes involved (Schnitzlein, 1968; Sheldon, 1912; Holmgren, 1920; Kuhlenbeck, 1973; Nieuwenhuys, 1963). A, Amygdala; Ac, nucleus accumbens; D, dorsal pallium; Dc, central zone of area dorsalis telencephali; Dd, dorsal zone of area dorsalis telencephali; Dl, lateral zone of area dorsalis telencephali; Dl-p, posterior part of lateral zone; Dm, medial zone of area dorsalis telencephali; H, hippocampal complex; OT, olfactory tubercle; P, piriform pallium; S, septal nuclei; St, striatum; 1–5, major telencephalic subdivisions or columns.

include representatives of the following genera: *Aequidens, Amia, Carassius, Gnathonemus, Hemichromis, Ictalurus, Osteoglossum, Polyodon,* and *Toxoides.*

III. Quantitative Considerations

The brains of the five actinopterygian representatives and that of *Amia calva* (the other holostean) were fixed in AFA and dissected while immersed in fixative. Each brain part was blotted immediately prior to weighing on a Mettler analytical balance (model H 10). Ten repeated measurements of small brains (0.03 g) varied by ±0.3%, whereas those on small brain parts (0.003 g) varied by ±1.6%. AFA fixation results in about a 9% reduction in brain weight, and the weights reported are corrected for this loss. Body weights are of fresh material.

In Table II we have reported body weight, total brain weight, weight of the telencephalon proper (excluding the olfactory bulbs), and weight of the olfactory bulbs. In the species studied, the percentages of the total brain weight accounted

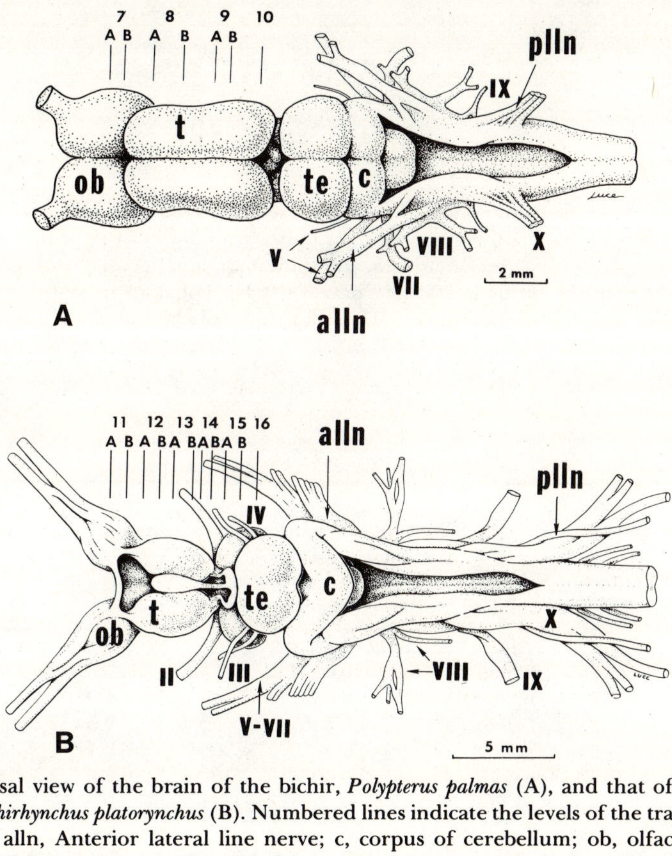

Figure 4. Dorsal view of the brain of the bichir, *Polypterus palmas* (A), and that of the shovelnose sturgeon, *Scaphirhynchus platorynchus* (B). Numbered lines indicate the levels of the transverse sections in Figs. 7–16. alln, Anterior lateral line nerve; c, corpus of cerebellum; ob, olfactory bulb; plln, posterior lateral line nerve; t, telencephalon; te, optic tectum; II, optic nerve; III, oculomotor nerve; IV, trochlear nerve; V, profundus and trigeminal nerves; VII, facial nerve; VIII, acousticovestibular nerve; IX, glossopharyngeal nerve; X, vagal nerve.

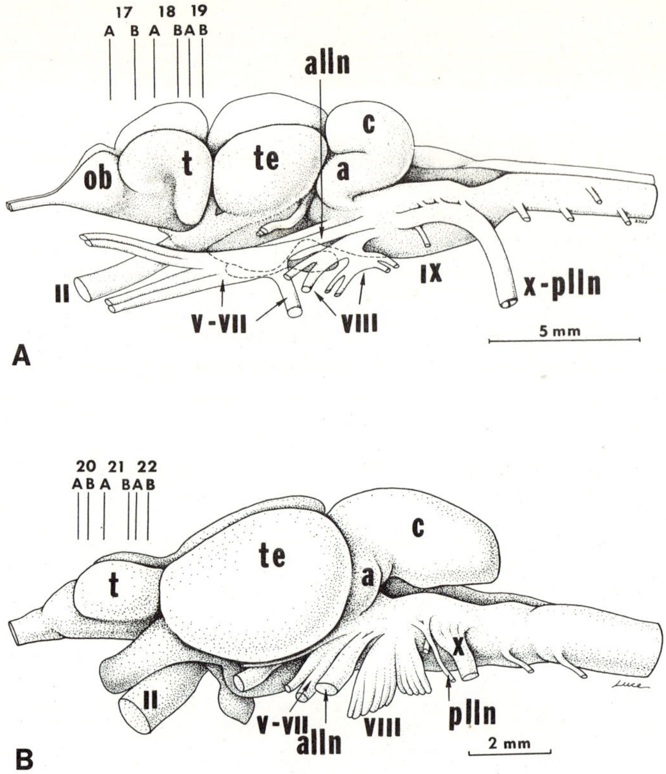

Figure 5. Dorsolateral view of the brain of the longnose gar, *Lepisosteus osseus* (A), and that of the rainbow trout, *Salmo gairdneri* (B). Numbered lines indicate the levels of the transverse sections in Figs. 17–22. A, Auricle of the cerebellum; alln, anterior lateral line nerve; c, corpus of cerebellum; ob, olfactory bulb; plln, posterior lateral line nerve; t, telencephalon; te, optic tectum; II, optic nerve; V–VII, trigemino-facial complex; VIII, acoustico-vestibular nerve; IX, glossopharyngeal nerve; X, vagal nerve.

Table II. Quantitative Data

	A	*B*	*C*	*D*	*E*	*F*	*G*	*H*
	Body weight (g)	Brain weight (g)	Weight of telen-cephalon proper (g)	Weight of olfactory bulbs (g)	$\frac{B}{A^{2/3}} \times 10^4$	$\frac{C}{A^{2/3}} \times 10^4$	$\frac{D}{A^{2/3}} \times 10^4$	*D* : *C*
Polypterus	75[a]	0.0963	0.0365	0.0114	54	21.0	6.0	1:3.5
Scaphirhynchus	510	0.2567	0.0316	0.0341	40	4.9	5.3	1:0.93
Amia	727	0.4026	0.0777	0.0363	50	9.5	4.5	1:2.1
Lepisosteus	1065	0.6550	0.1360	0.0393	63	13.1	3.8	1:3.5
Salmo	280	0.4279	0.0257	0.0086	100	6.0	2.0	1:3.0
Lepomis	82	0.1337	0.0180	0.0011	71	9.5	0.6	1:15.8

[a] This body weight is certainly not maximal for *Polypterus palmas*, but we have found several female specimens of this size to be gravid. As a check, we measured the body and brain weights of a large museum specimen of *Polypterus congicus*. This animal was preserved in 70% ethanol, and no corrections were made for fixation. Its body weight was 630 g and its brain weight 0.3230 g. Thus its brain–body ratio (column E) is 44—a figure between that of the chondrosteans and that of the holosteans.

for by the olfactory bulbs are as follows: *Polypterus,* 12%; *Scaphirhynchus,* 13%; *Amia,* 9%; *Lepisosteus,* 6%; *Salmo,* 2%; and *Lepomis,* 0.8%. Such data fail to take into account the possible independent hypertrophy or atrophy of other brain parts and thus do not give the most accurate assessment of the relative development of individual brain parts in various species. More meaningful statistics can be obtained by calculating brain–body or brain part–body ratios. Using a "quick" method (Jerison, 1973) to correct for body weight with a coefficient of allometry of 2/3 (see Ridet *et al.,* 1975; Bauchot *et al.,* 1977), we have calculated the relative weights of the whole brain, the telencephalon proper, and the olfactory bulbs. The figures obtained have been multiplied by 10^4 (simply to avoid decimals) and entered in Table II, columns E, F, and G. These numbers can be translated into the "encephalization indices" of Ridet *et al.* and Bauchot *et al.* by multiplying the former by approximately 0.8. In column H we have shown the ratios of the weights of the olfactory bulbs to the weights of the telencephalon proper.

When corrected for body size, the size of the brain shows a progressive increase from chondrosteans to holosteans to teleosts. The brain–body ratio of *Polypterus,* however, reaches that of the holostean grade. If the telencephala are compared, the following order is seen: *Scaphirhynchus* < *Salmo* < *Amia* < *Lepomis* < *Lepisosteus* < *Polypterus.* No clear trend is apparent. For the olfactory bulbs the order is: *Lepomis* < *Salmo* < *Lepisosteus* < *Amia* < *Scaphirhynchus* < *Polypterus,* which is a progressive decrease from *Polypterus* to the advanced teleost.

The ratios in column H might be taken as rough estimators of the relative amounts of the telencephalon which are concerned with nonolfactory functions. Here, it is noteworthy that in *Scaphirhynchus* the olfactory bulbs are actually slightly larger than the telencephalon and that in *Lepomis* there is a great reduction in the size of the bulbs relative to that of the telencephalon.

Although it is not possible to draw many conclusions from these limited data, one finding is surprising: The telencephalon of *Polypterus* is by far the largest of any of the species studied. Even though other data which we have show that some other teleosts possess a larger telencephalon than does *Polypterus,* the fact that the telencephalon of this species is larger than that of the chondrosteans, holosteans, and numerous teleosts suggests that *Polypterus* represents a separate radiation of actinopterygian fishes with respect to brain–body evolution.

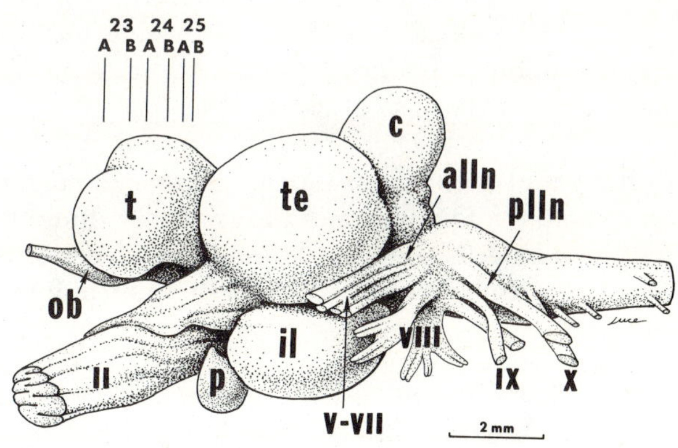

Figure 6. Lateral view of the brain of the green sunfish, *Lepomis cyanellus.* Numbered lines indicate the levels of the transverse sections in Figs. 23–25. alln, Anterior lateral line nerve; c, corpus of cerebellum; il, inferior lobe of the hypothalamus; ob, olfactory bulb; p, pituitary gland; plln, posterior lateral line nerve; t, telencephalon; te, optic tectum; II, optic nerve; V–VII, trigemino-facial complex; VIII, acoustico-vestibular nerve; IX, glossopharyngeal nerve; X, vagal nerve.

IV. Normal Morphology

In the following sections we will describe the normal morphology of the olfactory bulb, the subpallium, and the pallium of our five actinopterygian representatives. In these descriptions we will consider the boundary between the subpallium and the pallium to be that generally recognized (e.g., Källén, 1951; Nieuwenhuys, 1963), but alternative interpretations will be taken up in the general discussion.

A. Olfactory Bulb

1. General Description

As numerous workers (e.g., Källén, 1951; Nieuwenhuys, 1964) have pointed out, in the chondrosteans, the holosteans, and several of the teleosts a rostral evagination occurs, producing the bulbar ventricles. This evagination is to be compared to the bulbar evagination in land vertebrates and the Dipnoi and *not* to the evagination which produces the hemispheres—a process separable from and temporally independent of the bulbar evagination. In most teleosts, however, the olfactory bulbs are formed by solid thickenings of the rostroventral telencephalic walls. In these forms the bulbar ventricles consist of only shallow pits on the caudomedial surface of the bulbs. Several teleosts (e.g., members of Division II, the cyprinids, and silurids) display pedunculated bulbs attached to the telencephalon proper by long, slender stalks. These olfactory peduncles are hollow and enclose extensions of the telencephalic ventricles which end at the caudal poles of the bulbs.

The nomenclature used in the following description of the olfactory bulbs is that of Nieuwenhuys (1967*b*). The olfactory bulbs of all five species studied are attached directly to the telencephalon proper and enclose ventricles, although those of *Salmo* (Fig. 20A) and *Lepomis* are relatively small and extend only into the caudalmost part of the bulbs. The bulbs display the general pattern of concentric laminae in the following centripetal order: (1) layer of primary olfactory fibers comprising the olfactory nerve (ON), (2) glomerular layer (GL), (3) external cellular layer (ECL), (4) layer of secondary olfactory fibers (SOF), (5) internal cellular layer (ICL), and, where a ventricle is present, (6) the ependyma. See Figs. 7A,B, 8A, 11A,B, 17A, 20A,B, and 23A, and Table III. These laminae do not always have sharply defined boundaries—the constituents of the ECL, in particular, being intermixed with those of adjacent layers.

The ON is thicker along the ventral and lateral aspects of the bulb than it is dorsally and medially. Caudally, as more and more of its axons terminate in the glomeruli, the ON becomes progressively thinner on all sides, generally disappearing first along the dorsal and medial surfaces of the bulbs. Likewise, the GL drops out first dorsally and medially as the bulbar formation is replaced caudally by the subpallium.

The ECL contains both large mitral cells and smaller elements. The mitral cells do not generally form a continuous lamina but show a marked tendency to appear in small groups or clumps, as we have specifically indicated in *Lepisosteus*

(Fig. 17A). They are intermingled with the smaller elements of the ECL, the outer portion of the SOF, and the glomeruli. In *Polypterus* the mitral cells appear to be more evenly dispersed, and only in this species do the smaller elements of the ECL form a well-defined lamina deep to the glomeruli (Figs. 7A,B). In the others there are only scattered small cells in this lamina.

The SOF becomes larger at caudal levels as the axons of bulbar cells accumulate to form the medial and lateral olfactory tracts. The source of these axons is probably predominantly the large mitral cells. However, in Golgi preparations of the sturgeon *Acipenser,* Johnston (1898, 1901) also traced axons of small mitral cells and various other types of small cells of the ECL and the ICL into the olfactory tracts. For more detailed considerations of the various cell types and synaptologies found in the olfactory bulbs of actinopterygians, see Catois (1902), Sheldon (1912), Holmgren (1920), the review of Nieuwenhuys (1967*b*), and Ichikawa (1976).

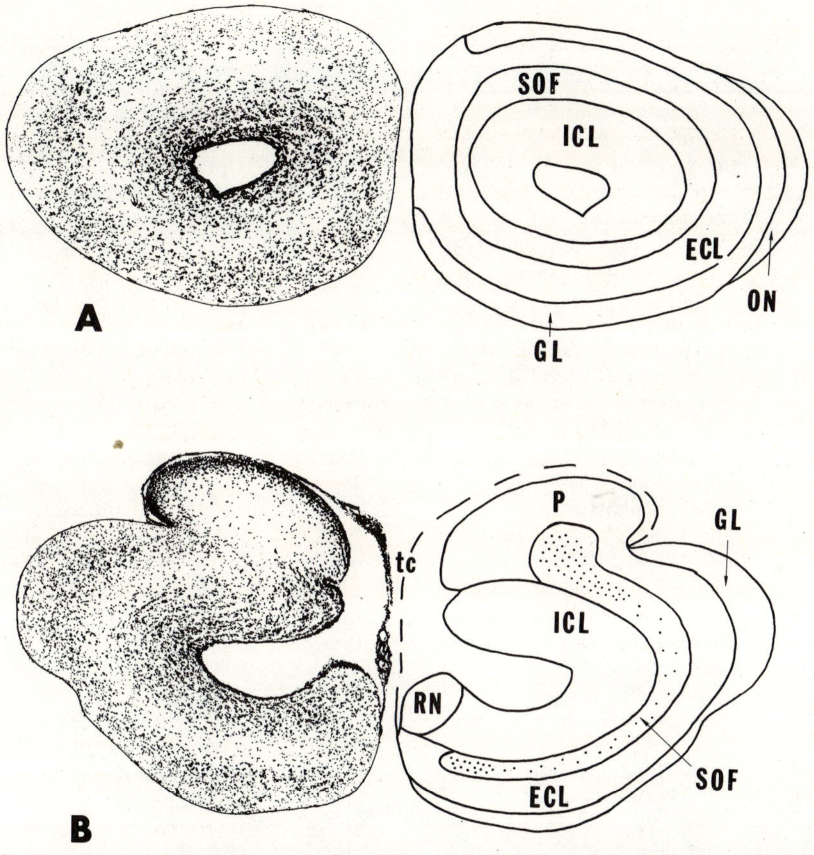

Figure 7. Transverse sections through the olfactory bulb (A) and rostral telencephalon (B) of *Polypterus.* In this and the following 18 figures (Figs. 8–25) the left side is a high-contrast photograph of a transverse section stained with cresyl violet. On the right, the major cell groups are indicated and the distribution of degenerating particles following olfactory bulb removal (if performed for that species) is shown with stippling for terminal fields and dashes for degenerating fibers. Where only stippling is shown (Figs. 7–10), we were not able to clearly distinguish between axons of passage and terminal fields. Abbreviations for Figs. 7–25 are listed in Table III.

The ICL is composed of granule cells and other small cells. At the junction of the olfactory bulb with the telencephalon proper, this layer continues caudally, lying lateral to the periventricular cells of the subpallium.

2. Special Features

There are several special features of the caudal portion of the olfactory bulbs which are present in some but not all of the five species studied.

In *Polypterus* and *Scaphirhynchus* the caudomedial portion of the bulbar evagination is devoid of glomeruli and thus is considered a part of the telencephalon proper (Nieuwenhuys, 1963). In *Polypterus* we have previously (Braford and Northcutt, 1974) termed a conspicuous cell mass in this region the retrobulbar nucleus (RN, Fig. 7B), and here we apply the same name to a somewhat smaller group of cells in the same position in *Scaphirhynchus* (Fig. 11B).

In *Lepisosteus* three "special" cell groups are present in the caudal olfactory

Table III. Abbreviations for Figs. 7–25

AC	Anterior commissure	NOT	Nucleus of the olfactory tract
D	Area dorsalis telencephali	NT	Nucleus taenia
Dc	Central zone of D	OC	Optic chiasm
Dc-1,2,3,4	Parts of Dc	OHT	Olfacto-hypothalamic tract
Dd	Dorsal zone of D	ON	Olfactory nerve
Dd+Dl	Dorsal zone plus lateral zone of D	OT	Optic tract
Dd+Dl-d	Dorsal zone plus dorsal part of lateral zone of D	P	Pallium
		PP	Periventricular preoptic nucleus
Dl	Lateral zone of D	PPm	Magnocellular part of PP
Dl-d	Dorsal part of lateral zone of D	PPp	Parvocellular part of PP
Dl-p	Posterior part of lateral zone of D	PT	Pretectum
Dl-v	Ventral part of lateral zone of D	P1-d	Dorsal part of first pallial zone
Dm	Medial zone of D	P1-v	Ventral part of first pallial zone
Dm-1,2,3,4	Parts of Dm	P2	Second pallial zone
Dp	Posterior zone of D	P3	Third pallial zone
E	Entopeduncular nucleus	RN	Retrobulbar nucleus
Ec	Caudal entopeduncular nucleus	SCO	Subcommissural organ
Ed	Dorsal entopeduncular nucleus	SOF	Secondary olfactory fiber layer of the olfactory bulb
Er	Rostral entopeduncular nucleus		
Ev	Ventral entopeduncular nucleus	SM	Stria medullaris
ECL	External cellular layer of olfactory bulb	T	Tectum
		tc	Tela chorioidea
FR	Fasciculus retroflexus	TH	Thalamus
GL	Glomerular layer of olfactory bulb	TN	Terminal nerve
		V	Area ventralis telencephali
H	Habenula	Vc	Commissural nucleus of V
ICL	Internal cellular layer of olfactory bulb	Vd	Dorsal nucleus of V
		Vi	Intermediate nucleus of V
IL	Inferior lobe	Vl	Lateral nucleus of V
MC	Mitral cells	Vn	'Nother nucleus of V
MTP	Median nucleus of the posterior tuber	Vp	Postcommissural nucleus of V
		Vs	Supracommissural nucleus of V
NI	Interstitial nucleus of the medial longitudinal fasciculus	Vv	Ventral nucleus of V
		VT	Ventral thalamus

bulb. The first appears in the dorsocaudal part of the ECL and consists of cells morphologically similar to but considerably larger than the mitral cells of the rest of the bulb. It is unclear at present whether this group might constitute an accessory olfactory bulb. Schnitzlein (1964) so labeled the dorsomedial aspect of the caudal bulb in *Amia*, as did Story (1964) in the chondrostean *Polyodon*, the latter noting that the mitral cells there were smaller than those in the main bulb. The existence of an accessory olfactory bulb in actinopterygians remains an unresolved issue. We note that Broman (1920) and Parsons (1970) have suggested that the olfactory epithelium of these fishes resembles the vomeronasal rather than the olfactory epithelium of land vertebrates. If this is so, it would follow that the entire olfactory bulb of actinopterygians is homologous to the accessory olfactory bulb of tetrapods. We are inclined to reject this notion on the basis of the data on efferent connections of the bulb, which we will present below. The second group in *Lepisosteus* appears on the superficial edge of the ECL laterally and consists of cells slightly smaller and somewhat less darkly stained with cresyl violet than the mitral cells. It continues caudally immediately deep to the olfactory tract fibers, from which it receives an input. We have termed this group the nucleus of the olfactory tract (NOT, Fig. 17B). The same group is present in the other holostean, *Amia,* but has no clear homologue in the other species studied. The third group appears laterally, superficial to a caudal contingent of mitral cells. This group, consisting of small, deeply staining cells in clusters, is a part of the telencephalon proper which has been carried rostrally by the bulbar evagination. We have termed it the lateral subpallial nucleus (Vl, Fig. 17B) after Nieuwenhuys's (1963) designation of an identically situated mass in *Amia* (see below).

In *Lepomis* a collection of very large cells are scattered along a fiber bundle which runs on the ventromedial surface of the olfactory bulb (TN, Fig. 23A). This is the "kaudale Zellgruppe des Bulbus" of Holmgren (1920) and "*x*" of Ariëns Kappers *et al.* (1936, p. 1270). The cells and the associated fiber bundle appear to be separate from the olfactory bulb and may constitute a nervus terminalis system.

Following Herrick's (1910, 1924) analyses of other vertebrates, many workers have designated at least the caudal portion of the ICL of the bulb as the anterior olfactory nucleus in actinopterygians (Sheldon, 1912; Droogleever-Fortuyn, 1961; Schnitzlein, 1964; Wright, 1967; Chanconie and Clairambault, 1975; Morgan, 1975). Although the subependymal portion of the ICL appears more lightly stained than the remainder of the layer, we can find no convincing cytoarchitectural grounds for such a designation in the five species studied. We prefer to consider the entire mass as the ICL, at least for the present (cf. Nieuwenhuys, 1967*b*, pp. 57–58).

B. Area Ventralis Telencephali (V) or Subpallium

Our observations on the subpallium and the nomenclature we have used are in close agreement with those of Nieuwenhuys (1963). Although the subpallia of the five species studied show considerably less morphological variation than that displayed by their pallia, they are sufficiently diverse to warrant a separate description for each species.

1. *Polypterus* (Figs. 4A, 7–10)

We have previously described the subpallium of *Polypterus* (Bradford and Northcutt, 1974), but to facilitate comparisons we will outline the main features here.

In the rostral subpallium three major cell groups are recognized: the ventral and dorsal subpallial nuclei (Vv and Vd) in a periventricular position and the lateral subpallial nucleus (Vl) in a migrated position (Figs. 8A,B and 9A). Vv extends from the retrobulbar nucleus rostrally to the commissural ridge caudally. Its ventral portion consists of a mass of cells densely packed near the ependymal surface, whereas its dorsal portion displays a laminated pattern, especially at caudal levels.

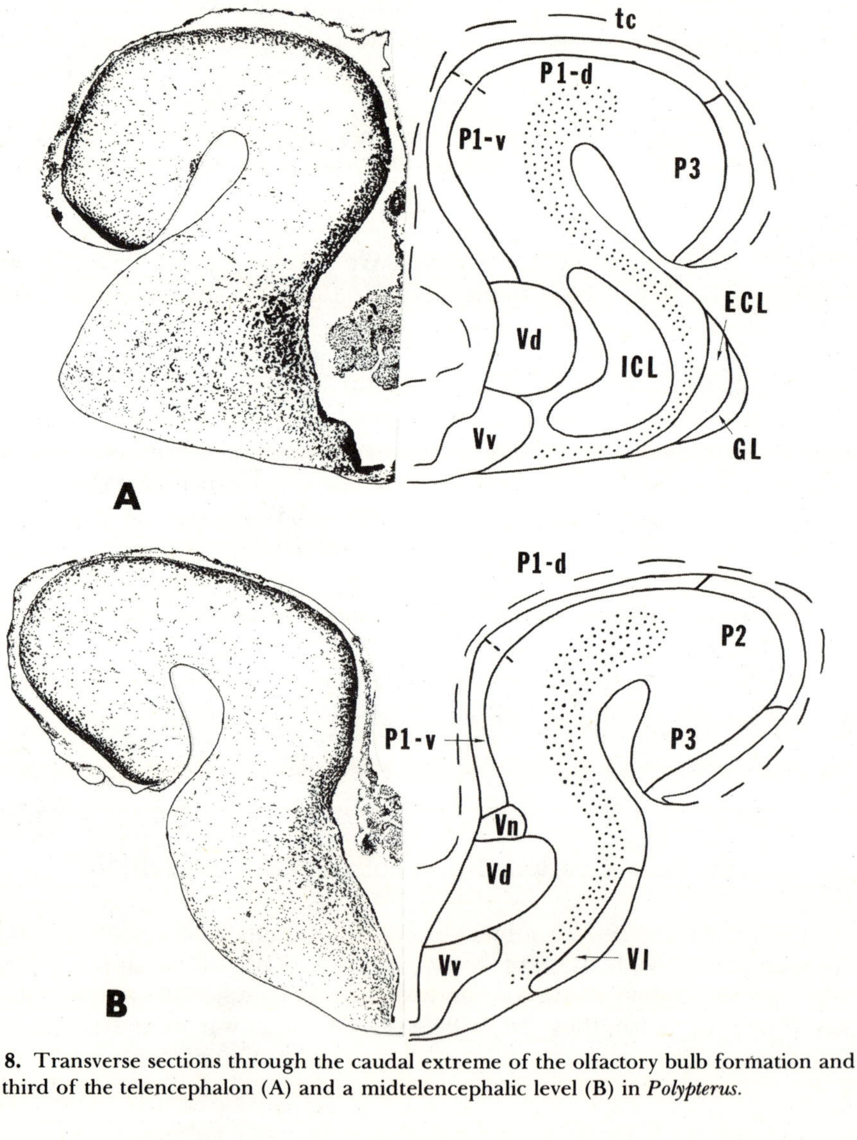

Figure 8. Transverse sections through the caudal extreme of the olfactory bulb formation and the rostral third of the telencephalon (A) and a midtelencephalic level (B) in *Polypterus*.

Intercalated between Vv and the pallium is a crescent-shaped group of deeply staining cell clusters, Vd. Caudally, the dorsal part of Vd is characterized by the presence of a diffuse bundle of transversely oriented fibers. A number of larger cells are also present here (Fig. 8B), constituting a small mass termed Vn (= V 'nother?) by Nieuwenhuys (1963). We will reconsider Vn later in this chapter. Vl appears on the lateral surface of the subpallium slightly behind the caudalmost part of the olfactory bulb formation and extends to about the level of the commissural ridge.

In the caudal subpallium three periventricular groups and three migrated groups are present. Just rostral to the commissural ridge Vd is displaced slightly laterally by the supracommissural nucleus (Vs, Fig. 9A), which rapidly replaces it

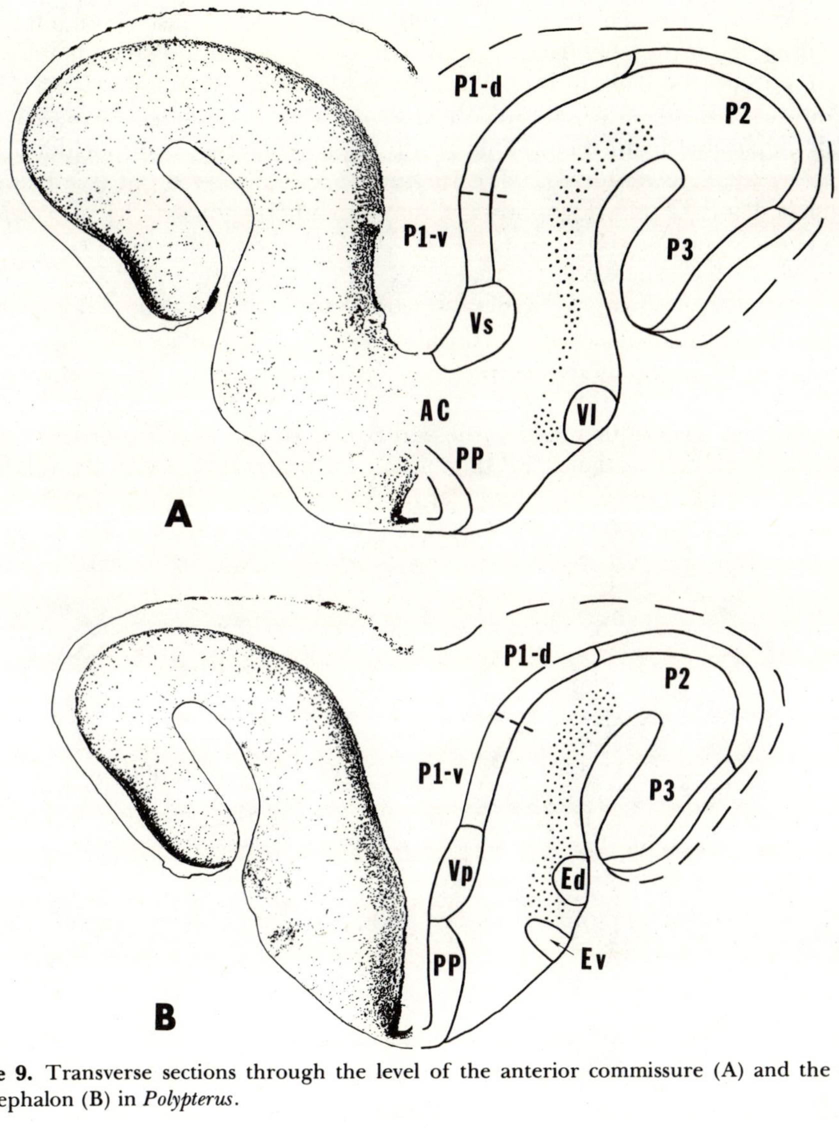

Figure 9. Transverse sections through the level of the anterior commissure (A) and the caudal telencephalon (B) in *Polypterus*.

at more caudal levels. Vs is caudally continuous with the postcommissural nucleus (Vp, Fig. 9B). At postcommissural levels the preoptic recess of the third ventricle appears ventrally in the midline surrounded by the small-celled portion of nucleus preopticus periventricularis (PP, Fig. 9A), which lies subjacent to Vp. The so-called entopeduncular complex lies in a migrated position in the caudal subpallium (Figs. 9B and 10). The ventral and dorsal entopeduncular nuclei (Ev and Ed) are cytologically similar and consist of small cells. The caudal entopeduncular nucleus (Ec) contains slightly larger cells and extends caudally into the thalamus.

2. ***Scaphirhynchus*** (Figs. 4B, 11–16)

In the rostral subpallium three nuclei are present in a periventricular position, from ventral to dorsal: Vv, a group of small cells packed against the ependyma (Fig. 11B); Vd, a circular group of slightly larger cells in clusters migrated very slightly away from the ependyma; and Vn, a loosely organized circular mass lying between Vd and the pallium (Fig. 12A). An additional substantial cell mass lies in contiguity with the lateral edge of Vn and the dorsolateral aspect of Vd but is generally separable from them. This group appears to have been included in Vd in *Acipenser* by Nieuwenhuys (1963). In view of its olfactory input (see below) we have termed it Vl and suggest that it may be homologous to Vl of *Polypterus,* although it has not migrated as far from the ependyma in *Scaphirhynchus.* In a position which does correspond to that of Vl in *Polypterus*, we find in *Scaphirhynchus* only a very scattered group of small cells, which at some levels extend dorsolaterally along the meningeal surface for a considerable distance (unlabeled, Figs. 12A,B).

In the caudal subpallium, as in *Polypterus,* Vd is replaced by Vs at about the level of the commissural ridge (Fig. 13A). In *Scaphirhynchus* Vs consists of rows of cells oriented at an oblique angle to the ventricular surface. Vs is replaced caudally by Vp, which ventrally adjoins PP (Fig. 13B). In a migrated position caudally, we can identify only a single entopeduncular nucleus (E, Figs. 13B and 14A). It consists

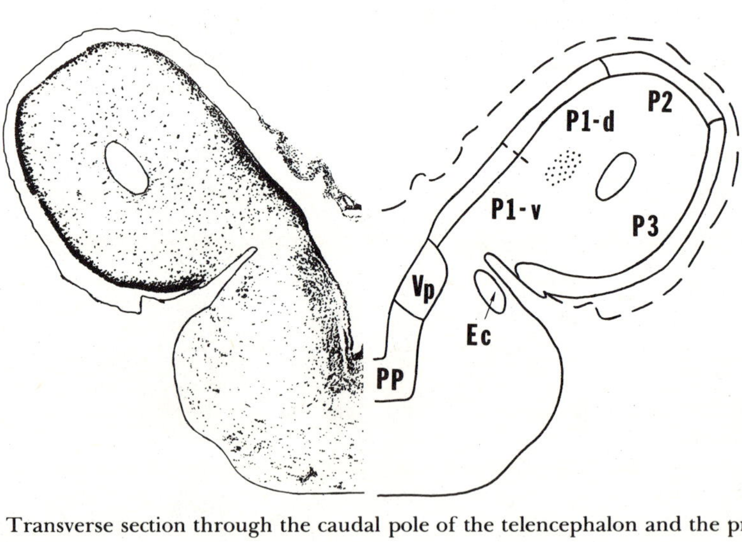

Figure 10. Transverse section through the caudal pole of the telencephalon and the preoptic area in *Polypterus*.

of small cells and continues into the thalamus, where its caudal pole lies interstitial to the most medial fibers of the optic tract.

3. *Lepisosteus* (Figs. 5A, 17–19)

In addition to the nucleus of the olfactory tract described above, Vv, Vd, Vn, and Vl are present in the rostral subpallium of *Lepisosteus* (Fig. 17B). Vv and Vd are similar to those of *Polypterus* and *Scaphirhynchus.* Clusters of small, darkly staining cells lie dorsal to Vd in *Lepisosteus.* These cells and the more rostrolateral mass which extends into the bulbar evagination (see above) become continuous, forming a large, uniform, C-shaped cell mass. We have termed the periventricular portion of this group Vn and the more lateral portion Vl. They are homologous to the dorsal portion of Vd (n.s.d-l) and Vl, respectively, of Nieuwenhuys (1969) in *Amia.* These groups largely disappear at the level of the commissural ridge, but scattered dorsolateral elements persist for some distance caudally (Fig. 18A).

Slightly rostral to the commissural ridge, Vd lies a short distance away from the ependymal surface and soon becomes indistinct. Out of this "disorganized" area, a prominent Vs arises caudally, dorsal to the commissure (Fig. 18A). Vs. is replaced at more caudal levels by a smaller Vp, which is again continuous ventrally with PP (Fig. 18B). In *Lepisosteus* Vp is laterally continuous with a mass of small

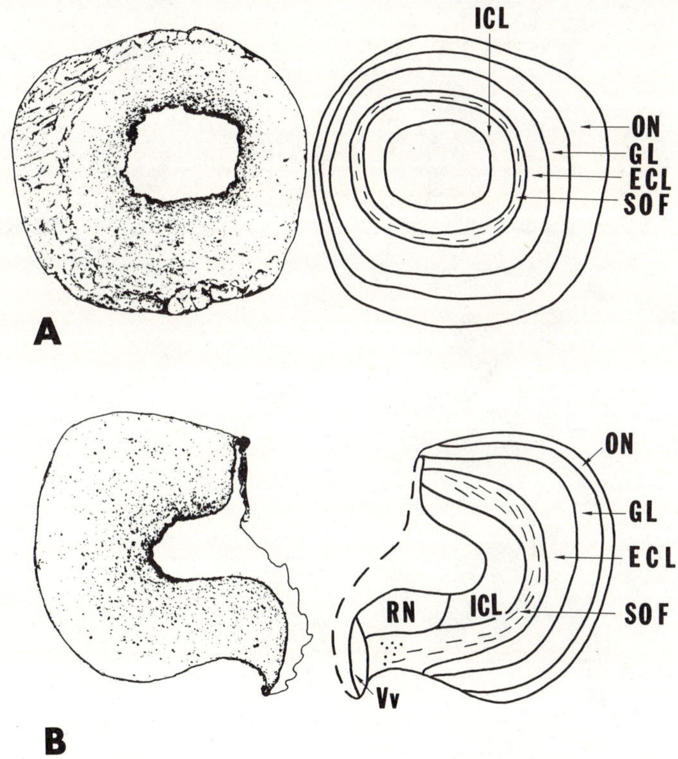

Figure 11. Transverse sections through middle (A) and caudal (B) levels of the olfactory bulb in *Scaphirhynchus.*

cells which has been termed the intermediate subpallial nucleus (Vi) in *Amia* and some teleosts by Nieuwenhuys (Fig. 19A). Two entopeduncular nuclei are present (Figs. 18B and 19A): a large rostral group (Er) composed of small cells and comparable to Ev plus Ed of *Polypterus,* and a caudal one (Ec) consisting of slightly smaller cells and extending into the thalamus in the same manner as that described for Ec in *Polypterus* and E in *Scaphirhynchus.*

4. *Salmo* (Figs. 5B, 20–22)

In the rostral subpallium Vv and Vd lie in a periventricular position with no cells intervening between Vd and the pallium (Figs. 20B and 21A). Vl (Fig. 21A) consists of an elongated group of scattered cells which extends along the meningeal surface in much the same manner as the unlabeled cell group in *Scaphirhynchus* (Fig. 12A,B). At commissural levels Vd lies slightly away from the ependymal surface (Fig. 21B) and is gradually replaced at more caudal levels by the much more scattered cells of Vs (Figs. 21B and 22A). At about the same level a number of scattered cells are present in the center of the subpallium, at the lateral edge of the commissural fibers. At some levels these cells form enough of a condensation

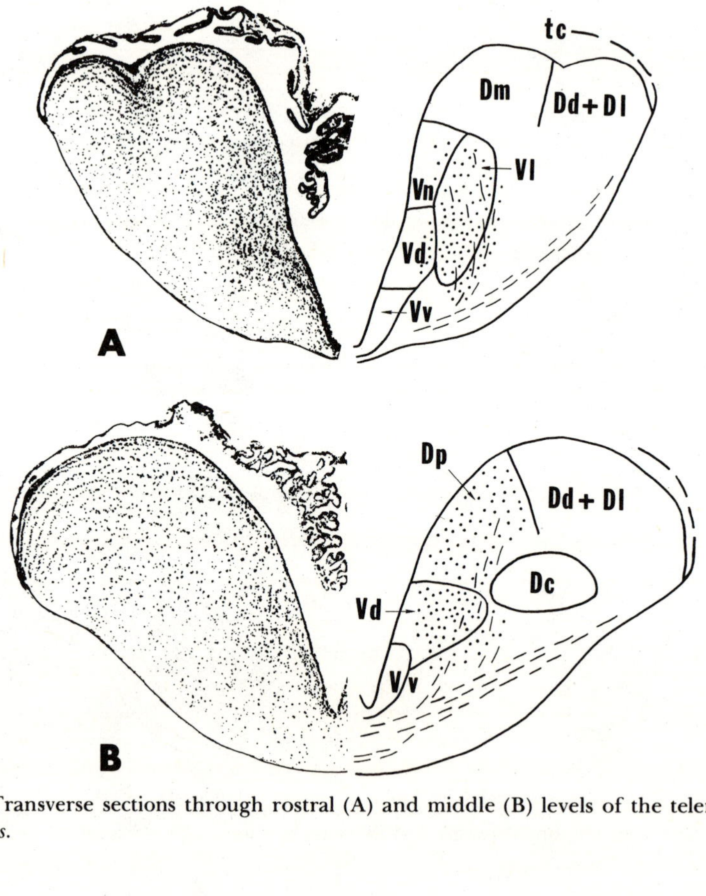

Figure 12. Transverse sections through rostral (A) and middle (B) levels of the telencephalon of *Scaphirhynchus.*

to be considered a nuclear group which we have termed the commissural subpallial nucleus (Vc, Figs. 21B, 22A). Just caudal to the commissure, PP lies ventrally in a periventricular position (Fig. 22A). More caudally, it expands in a dorsal direction to become ventrally adjacent to Vp, which in *Salmo* is a very indistinct and cell-poor group (Fig. 22B). The single entopeduncular nucleus (E) contains small, very tightly packed cells and does not extend caudally into the thalamus (Fig. 22B).

5. *Lepomis* (Figs. 6, 23–25)

At rostral levels two cell groups are present in a periventricular position (Fig. 23B): Vv and Vd. In a migrated position rostrally, a relatively few cells constitute a small Vl in *Lepomis* (Figs. 23B and 24A). Just rostral to the commissural ridge, a group of larger, more darkly staining cells appears dorsolateral to Vl (Fig. 24A). This group, Vc, occupies a central position at commissural levels (Fig. 24B). At about this level, as in the other species studied, Vd is replaced from its medial side by Vs (Fig. 24A). PPp surrounds the preoptic recess. A large Vp is present ventrally adjacent to Vs but with no significant continuity with PPp (Figs. 24B and 25A,B). There is a single entopeduncular nucleus (E) comparable to that seen in *Salmo* (Fig.

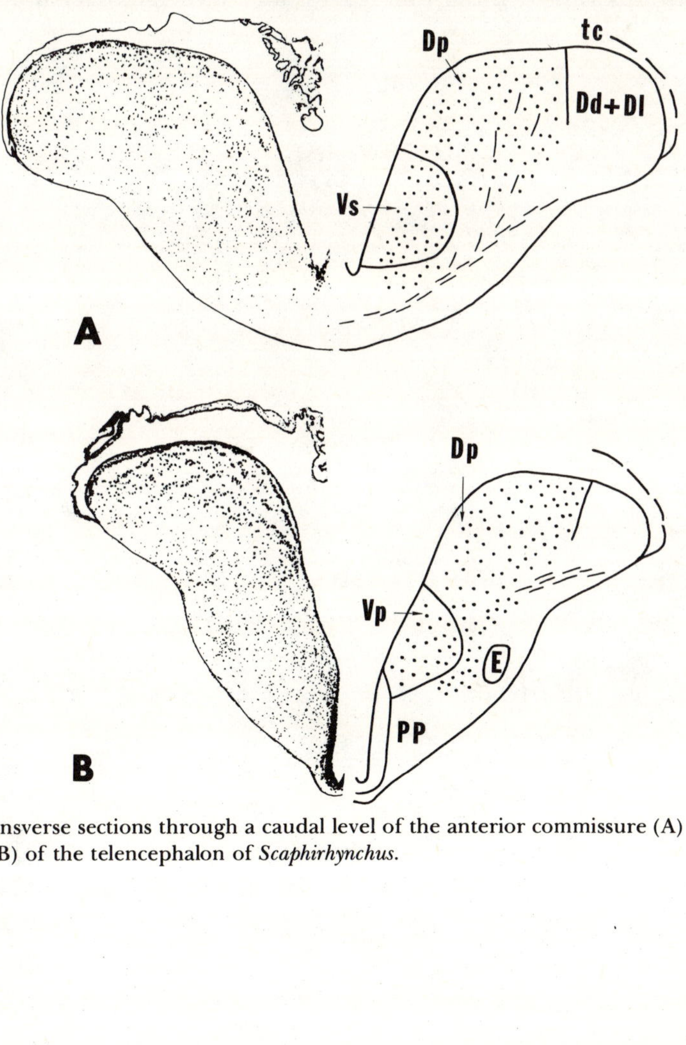

Figure 13. Transverse sections through a caudal level of the anterior commissure (A) and a rostral preoptic level (B) of the telencephalon of *Scaphirhynchus*.

25A,B). Ventrolateral to Vp and dorsal to E lies another small cell mass which is laterally continuous with Dp of the pallium. We have termed it Vi (cf. *Lepisosteus*, Fig. 19A).

C. Area Dorsalis Telencephali (D) or Pallium

As Nieuwenhuys (1962*b*, 1963) has emphasized, the pallium of actinopterygians displays remarkable morphological variation. Although comparisons of the subpallia of our five representatives are not without some difficulties, on the basis of presently available information it is simply impossible to compare their pallial areas with even that degree of certainty. We will describe the pallium of each species and indicate by our terminology those areas which appear to be homologous.

The nomenclature of the following account, with the notable exception of that for *Polypterus*, is patterned after Nieuwenhuys (1963). Except in *Polypterus*, where he considered the pallium to be a uniform structure throughout, Nieuwenhuys divided the actinopterygian area dorsalis (D) into three longitudinal zones along the ependymal surface, from medial to lateral: Dm, Dd, and Dl. In a central position he identified an additional zone, Dc. We have generally recognized, and in some cases subdivided, these four zones and have given separate status to a

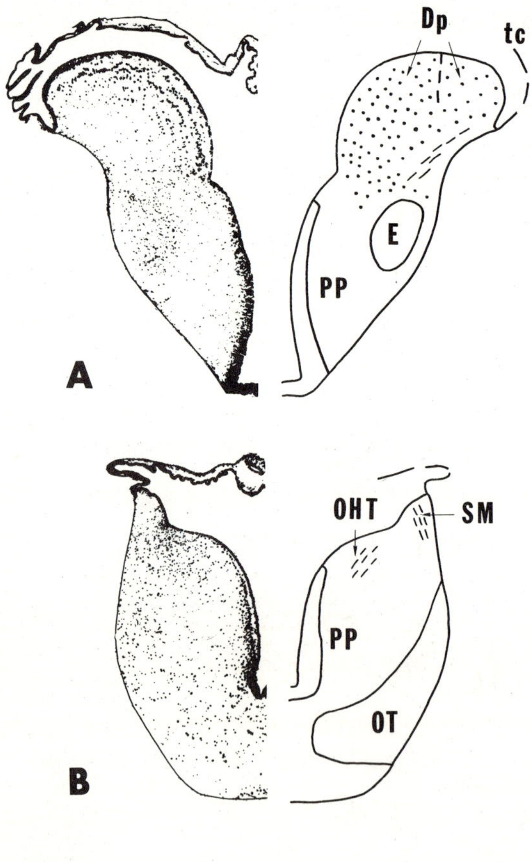

Figure 14. Transverse sections through the caudal pole of the telencephalon (A) and rostral diencephalon (B) of *Scaphirhynchus*.

posterior zone, Dp, which corresponds at least in part to Dlp (the posterior part of Dl) of Nieuwenhuys.

1. *Polypterus*

The organization of the pallium of *Polypterus* is so different from that of any other actinopterygian that we have used a new nomenclature for it (Braford and Northcutt, 1974). The eversion of the pallium of *Polypterus* is a simple one and proceeds without the thickening of the walls and the migration of cell masses seen in the other actinopterygians. The vast majority of cell bodies form a thin sheet against the ependyma. Certain regional differences in the staining properties and thickness of this pallial sheet allow us to make a division into three major longitu-

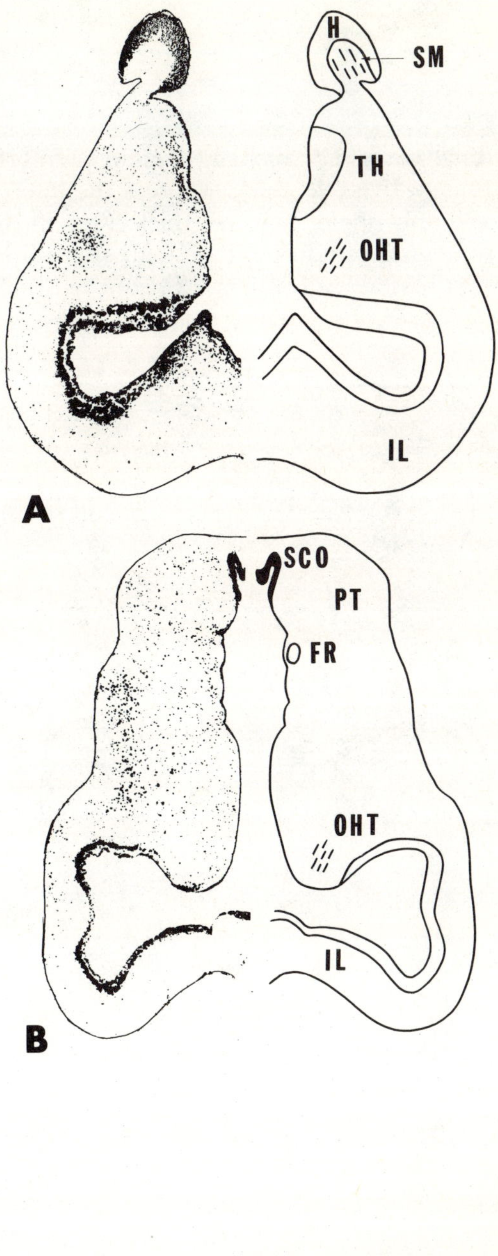

Figure 15. Transverse sections through midthalamic (A) and pretectal (B) levels in *Scaphirhynchus* illustrating the course of the olfacto-hypothalamic tract.

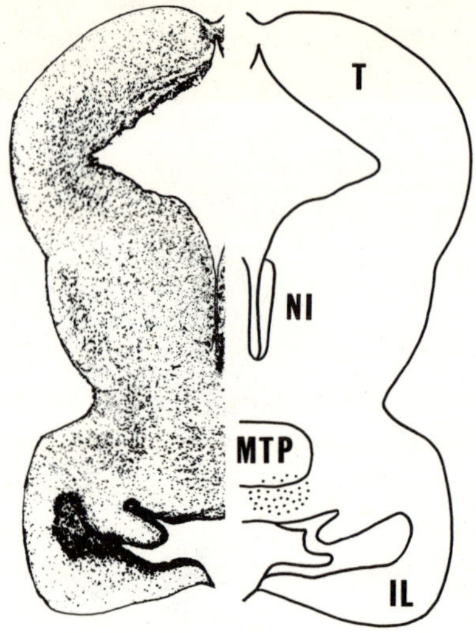

Figure 16. Transverse section through a caudal hypothalamic level in *Scaphirhynchus* illustrating the termination of the olfacto-hypothalamic tract near a midline hypothalamic nucleus (MTP).

dinal zones. The medial (P1) and lateral (P3) zones are more intensely stained and four to five cells thick, whereas the intercalated dorsal zone (P2) is lightly stained and only one or two cells thick (Figs. 8–10). The transitions between the zones are sometimes gradual rather than sharp and are especially difficult to recognize at very rostral levels where P2 seems to be absent (Fig. 7B). There are a few migrated

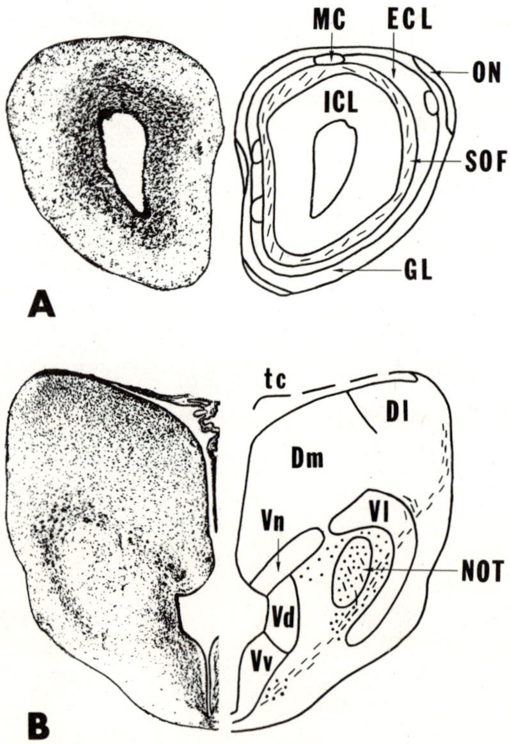

Figure 17. Transverse sections through the caudal olfactory bulb (A) and rostral telencephalon (B) in *Lepisosteus*.

cells, predominantly in P3, but no central zone (Dc) is present. We have subdivided P1 into dorsal (P1-d) and ventral (P1-v) subzones on the basis of a greater cell density in P1-v. One might suggest from a superficial inspection that the three major longitudinal zones in *Polypterus*—P1, P2, and P3—correspond to the three longitudinal zones in the other actinopterygians—Dm, Dd, and D1, respectively. For reasons which will become apparent later in this chapter, this is not the case.

2. *Scaphirhynchus*

Rostrally in a medial position just dorsal to the subpallium lies a zone of cells which is less regularly laminated than the remainder of the pallium (Fig. 12A). This mass is Dm, but, unlike the situation in *Lepisosteus* and the teleosts described below, Dm does not extend the full length of the pallium in *Scaphirhynchus*. Rather, it is gradually replaced from its medial aspect by Dp at successively more caudal levels (Fig. 12B). Dm and, more caudally, Dp are bordered laterally by a rather uniformly laminated zone which we have termed Dd + Dl (Figs. 12 and 13). This

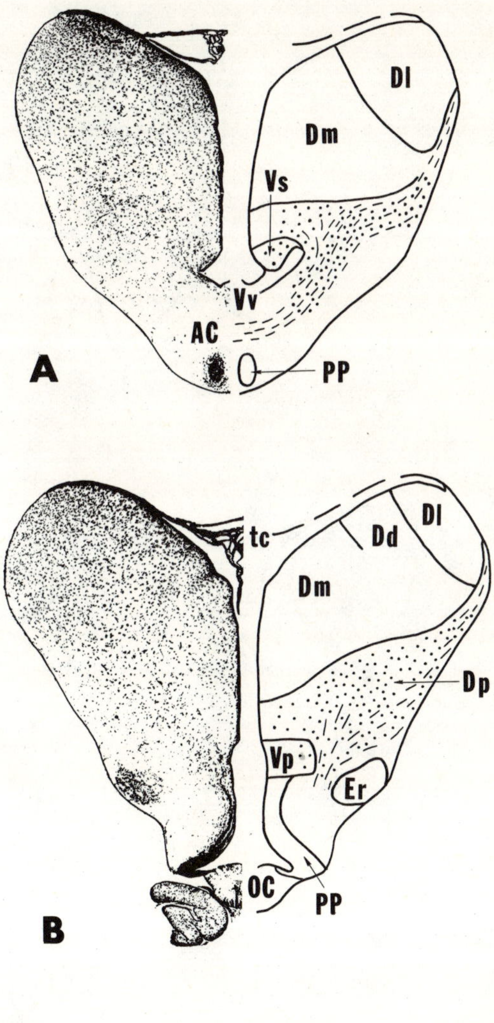

Figure 18. Transverse sections through the level of the anterior commissure (A) and rostral preoptic area (B) in *Lepisosteus*.

zone gradually diminishes caudally and is eventually replaced by Dp in the caudal pole (Fig. 14A). At this level Dp consists of two zones which show slight morphological differences, the lateral one containing more migrated cells. At midtelencephalic levels a group of large, scattered cells in a migrated position constitutes the central zone, Dc (Fig. 12B).

3. *Lepisosteus* and the Teleosts

The pallium of *Lepisosteus* is a cytoarchitectonic nightmare, and the pallium of *Salmo* differs sufficiently from that of other teleosts that comparisons are difficult. Therefore, we will first describe the pallium of *Lepomis* in which the cell groups are relatively distinct and then make comparisons with the other two species.

a. *Lepomis*. The pallium of *Lepomis* is organized into two major longitudinal

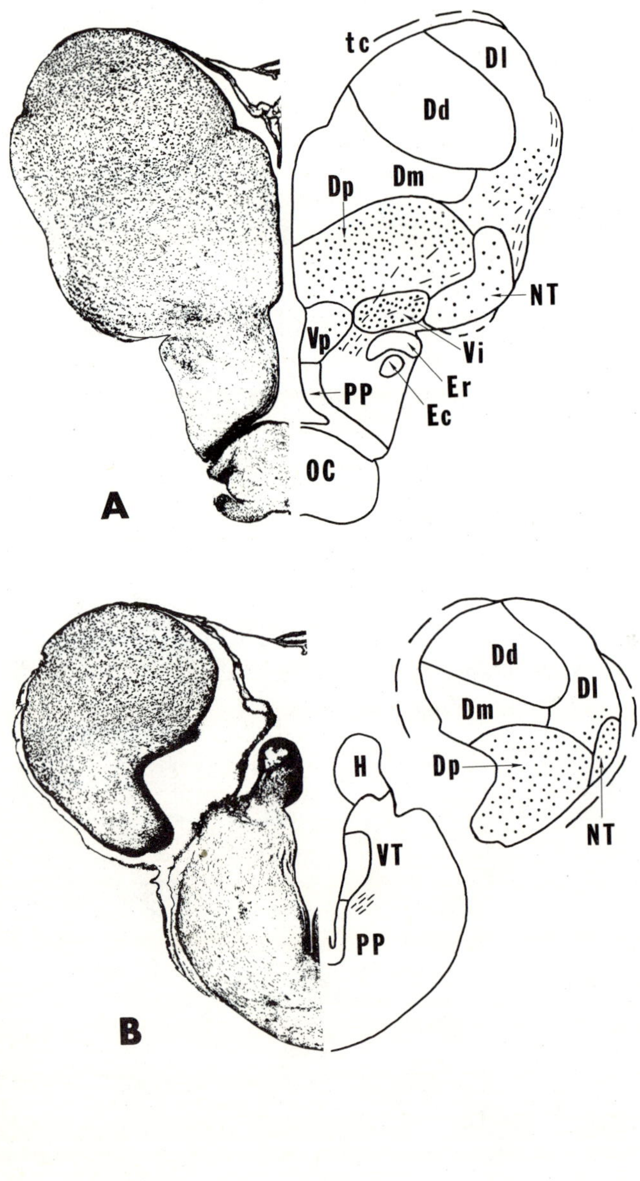

Figure 19. Transverse sections through the caudal third (A) and caudal pole (B) of the telencephalon in *Lepisosteus* illustrating olfactory terminal fields.

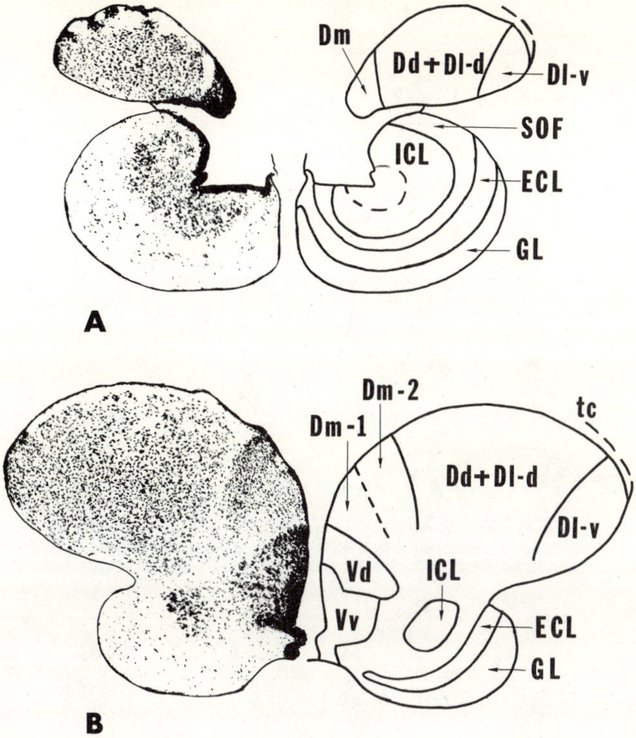

Figure 20. Transverse sections through the caudal olfactory bulb (A) and rostral telencephalon (B) in *Salmo*.

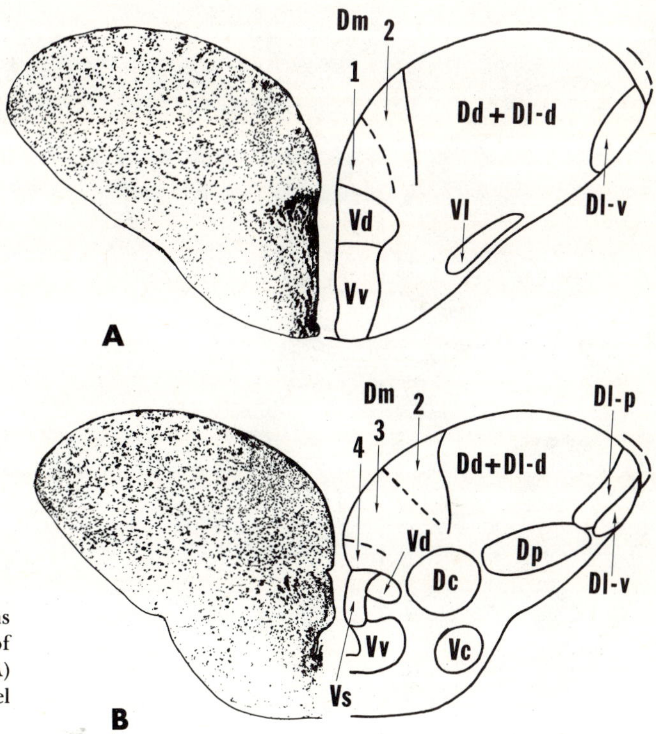

Figure 21. Transverse sections through the maximal extent of the rostral subpallial areas (A) and anterior commissure level (B) in *Salmo*.

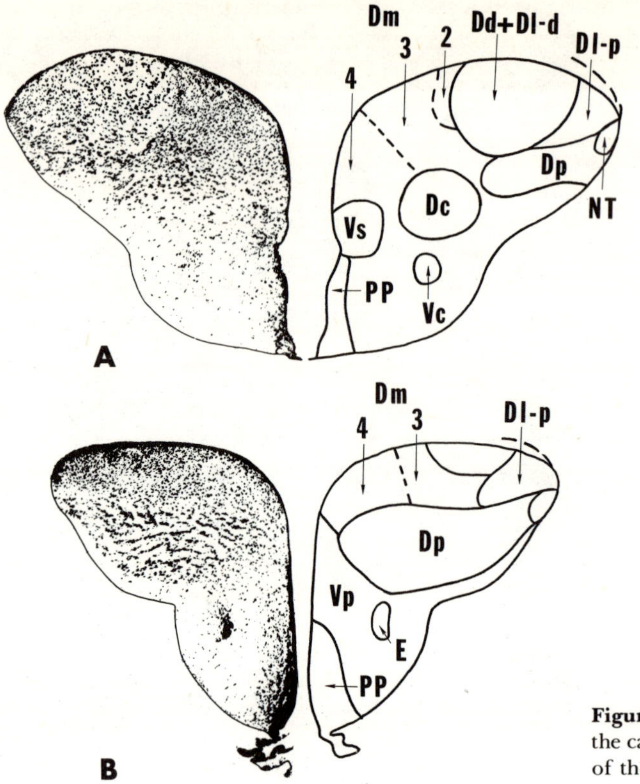

Figure 22. Transverse sections through the caudal third (A) and caudal pole (B) of the telencephalon in *Salmo*.

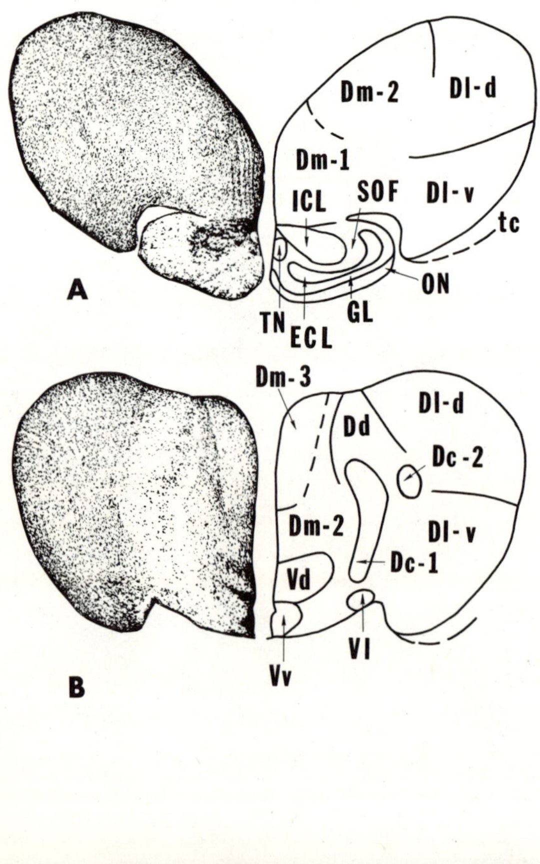

Figure 23. Transverse sections through the caudal olfactory bulb and rostral telencephalon (A) and rostral ventral telencephalon (B) in *Lepomis*.

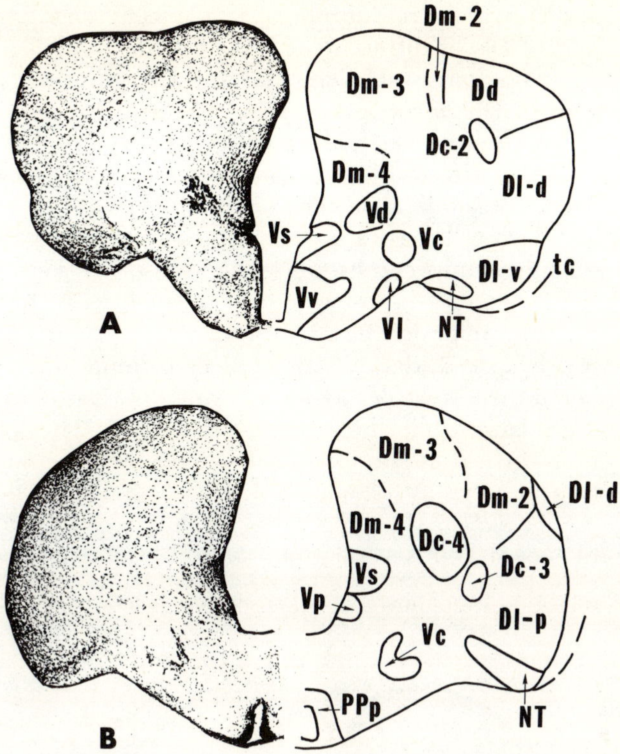

Figure 24. Transverse sections through a level just rostral to the lamina terminalis (A) and through the level of the anterior commissure (B) in *Lepomis*.

zones along the ependymal surface: a dorsomedial Dm and a lateral Dl. Dm and Dl are separated at midrostral levels by a small third zone, Dd. The caudoventral pole is occupied by a fourth zone, Dp, and the central core of the pallium by migrated groups of large neurons, Dc.

At the rostral pole of the telencephalon proper, the pallium lies immediately dorsal to the olfactory bulb (Fig. 23A). Two subzones of Dm are present: a ventral, distinctly laminated group of small cells, Dm-1; and a more dorsal, subependymal group of larger cells, Dm-2 (Fig. 23A). Between the levels of Fig. 23A and Fig. 23B, a group of large cells lies deep to Dm-1. These cells are smaller and less darkly stained than those of Dc and are considered to be a part of Dm. More caudally, Dm-1 is replaced by Dm-2, and the rostral pole of Dm-3 lies in a dorsomedial position separating the periventricular portions of Dm-2 (Fig. 23B). Slightly more caudally, Dm-4 appears ventral to Dm-3, replacing the ventral part of Dm-2 (Fig. 24A). Dm-3 consists of scattered cells and Dm-4 of clusters of cells which form discontinuous laminae. Dm-4, Dm-3, and the dorsal remnant of Dm-2 extend to the caudal pole of the telencephalon in a dorsomedial position (Figs. 24A,B and 25A,B).*

Dl is a large zone which can be divided into at least three parts, two of which are present rostrally: Dl-d, a dorsal subzone consisting of medium-sized cells which have a tendency to be oriented in columns perpendicular to the ependymal surface,

* Bannister (1973) has recognized two divisions of Dm in the European minnow, *Phoxinus phoxinus*. His D.m. 1 appears to be equivalent to our Dm-1 plus Dm-2, whereas his D.m. 2 corresponds to our Dm-3 plus Dm-4.

and Dl-v, a ventral subzone of smaller cells (Figs. 23A,B and 24A). The most ventral part of Dl-v is differentiated from the rest of it by the presence of cell clusters. At about commissural levels, Dl-d and Dl-v drop out and are replaced by a posterior zone of Dl, Dl-p (Figs. 24B and 25A,B). Our Dl-p does not correspond to Dlp of Nieuwenhuys (1963), but our Dp does.

At midrostral levels, Dm and Dl are separated by a small zone of small cells which constitute a Dd (Figs. 23B and 24A).

Two cell masses occupy the caudoventral pallium: a narrow band of darkly staining clumped cells, nucleus taenia (NT) (Figs. 24A,B and 25A,B); and dorsal to it an extensive posterior zone of small cells, Dp (Fig. 25A,B).

In a migrated position in the core of the pallium are several groups of large, widely spaced, darkly staining cells forming the central zone, Dc. We have numbered them, rostrocaudally, 1 through 4 (Figs. 23B–25). The cells of Dc-1 and Dc-4 are larger than those of Dc-2 and Dc-3. The four central groups appear to be more or less in continuity with, and possibly related to, certain adjacent periventricular zones as follows: Dc-1, Dd; Dc-2, Dl-d; Dc-3, D1-p; Dc-4, Dm-3.

b. *Salmo*. The general organization of the pallium of *Salmo* is similar to that of *Lepomis,* but several important differences exist:

1. The pallium of *Salmo* is much less everted than that of *Lepomis,* and thus

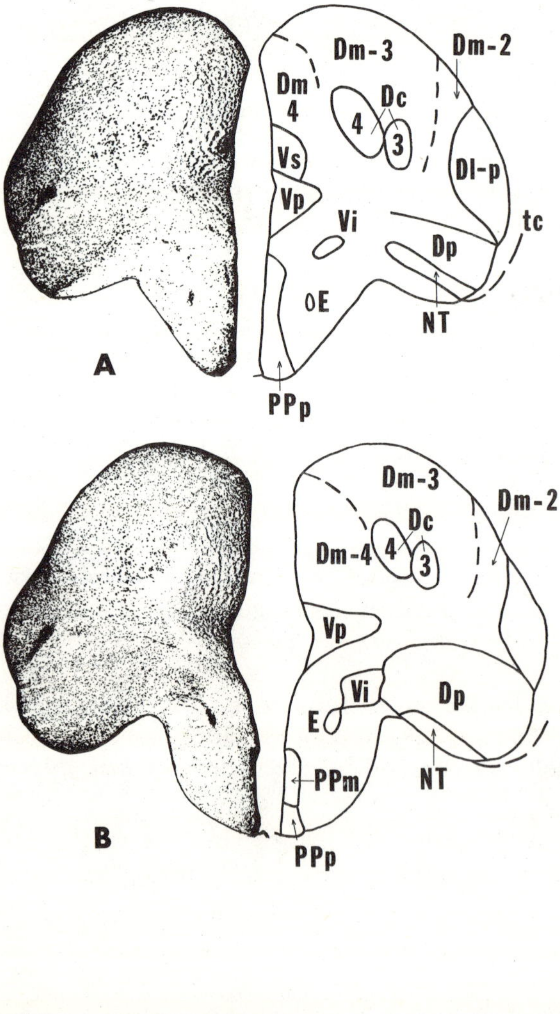

Figure 25. Transverse sections through the level of the pallial amygdala (A) and caudal pole of the telencephalon (B) in *Lepomis.*

in *Salmo* the point of attachment of the tela chorioidea is dorsolateral rather than ventrolateral as it is in *Lepomis* and most teleosts (compare Figs. 20B and 23A).

2. No separate Dd can be recognized in *Salmo* on the basis of cytoarchitectonic differences. We have followed the suggestion of Nieuwenhuys (1963) and considered the large, dorsally situated mass (Figs. 20A–22A) to represent both Dd and Dl-d. The columnar arrangement characteristic of Dl-d in *Lepomis* is particularly evident in the lateral part of this area in Fig. 21A. Histochemical differences (see below) further suggest that our Dd + Dl-d is divisible into more than one group.
3. In *Salmo* only one major collection of large, migrated cells constitutes a Dc (Figs. 21B and 22A). A few slightly smaller cells lie lateral to Dc and may represent a second Dc group.
4. The arrangement of the cells of Dp in *Salmo* differs markedly from that in *Lepomis.* In *Lepomis* the cells are small, lightly stained, and evenly spaced; in *Salmo* they are larger, darkly stained, and in clumps forming transversely oriented laminae (Figs. 21B and 22A,B). It should also be noted that in *Salmo* Dp extends medially, nearly reaching the ependymal surface (Fig. 22B; cf. *Scaphirhynchus,* Figs. 12B–14A, and *Lepisosteus,* Figs. 18B and 19A,B).

c. *Lepisosteus.* The pallium of *Lepisosteus* is less well differentiated than that of either of the two teleosts. Although it is clear that there are some differences in the arrangement of cells within our major zones (e.g., the dorsal and ventral parts of Dm in Fig. 17B) and that histochemical data support further division (see below), we have not been able to consistently subdivide Dm and Dl in *Lepisosteus*. Several further differences are apparent:

1. As in *Salmo,* the pallium of *Lepisosteus* is relatively slightly everted as the tela is attached dorsolaterally (e.g., Fig. 17B).
2. Zone Dd (Figs. 18B and 19A,B), as we have reckoned it, lies caudally and is relatively large in *Lepisosteus*—much larger than the Dd we have recognized in *Lepomis.* Further study may indicate that a part of this Dd is comparable to Dl-d in other species or that some other revision of its boundaries is appropriate.
3. No concentration of large, migrated cells representing a Dc in *Lepisosteus* could be identified. However, the more centrally located cells in the core of the pallium are larger than their periventricular neighbors. They are probably homologous to Dc in the other species.
4. Dp is very extensive in *Lepisosteus* and reaches the ependymal surface medially (Figs. 18A,B and 19A,B). Its cells are very similar to those in Dp of *Lepomis.*

D. Summary and Discussion

1. Olfactory Bulb

The structure of the olfactory bulbs is less variable than that of the remainder of the telencephalon in the five species studied. All display the same general pattern of laminar organization which is generally typical for the bulbs of all vertebrates.

In addition to the special features discussed above, two other differences are noteworthy. In *Polypterus, Scaphirhynchus,* and *Lepisosteus* the bulbar ventricles are large, extending far forward into the bulbs, whereas in the teleosts they are much smaller and reach only the caudalmost parts of the bulb. The small cells of the external cellular layer (ECL) form a well-defined, robust lamina only in *Polypterus.*

2. Area Ventralis Telencephali

The subpallial cell groups which we have recognized in the five species are summarized in Table IV. Vv, Vd, and Vs are present and readily identifiable in all five species. The same is true for Vp, with the qualification that it is poorly developed in *Salmo*. Vc is present only in the teleosts, Vi only in *Lepisosteus* and *Lepomis,* and NOT only in *Lepisosteus* (and *Amia*). With regard to Vn and Vl, the situation is somewhat more complicated. It is clear that the two groups form a continuous, uniform mass in *Lepisosteus,* as well as in *Amia.* In the teleosts no periventricular portion is present, and the migrated group, designated Vl, is relatively small. In *Polypterus* the migrated group (Vl) is well developed, and only a small periventricular Vn can be identified. The histochemical results presented below provide some basis for a reinterpretation of Vn in *Polypterus.* In *Scaphirhynchus* three groups are involved: periventricular Vn, a partially migrated Vl, and a submeningeal group, unnamed. This last group is morphologically most similar to Vl in the teleosts. Additional information is needed to understand the relationships of the Vn's and Vl's in these fishes. In all five species an entopeduncular nucleus (Ec or E) is present caudally. More rostrally located groups have been labeled entopeduncular in *Polypterus* (Ed and Ev) and *Lepisosteus* (Er), but they have no correlates in the other three species studied.

3. Area Dorsalis Telencephali

The area dorsalis shows more diversity in the species studied than does the area ventralis. Perhaps most notable is that the pallium of *Polypterus* is organized differently from that of all the other actinopterygian species. Its general shape—a thin elongated sheet—contrasts to the thickened, shorter mass of the other species. Furthermore, unlike the situation in the other actinopterygians, the pallium of *Polypterus* contains very few migrated cells. If we consider the major pallial zones identified in the other actinopterygians—Dm, Dd, Dl, Dp, and Dc—we are at a loss

Table IV. Summary of Cell Masses in the Subpallium

	RN	Vv	Vd	Vn	Vl	Vc	Vs	Vp	Vi	E	
Polypterus	+	+	+	+[a]	+		+	+		Ed, Ev	Ec
Scaphirhynchus	+	+	+	+	+[b]		+	+			E
Lepisosteus[c]		+	+	+	+		+	+	+	Er	Ec
Salmo		+	+		+[b]	+	+	+[d]			E
Lepomis		+	+		+[b]	+	+	+	+		E

[a] Vn in *Polypterus* may be comparable to Dm in the other actinopterygians rather than to Vn in *Scaphirhynchus* and *Lepisosteus*, and Dm may be part of the subpallium. See text.
[b] In addition to the cell group labeled Vl in *Scaphirhynchus*, a second smaller group is present more superficially. This latter group is comparable to Vl in *Salmo* and *Lepomis*. See text.
[c] NOT is present only in *Amia* and *Lepisosteus*.
[d] Vp is poorly developed in *Salmo*.

to recognize them in *Polypterus,* and this is reflected in our different terminology for the pallium of *Polypterus*. On cytoarchitectonic grounds, it is clear that no Dc is present in *Polypterus,* and it is unclear to what P1, P2, and P3 of *Polypterus* correspond in the other species studied, although the data on olfactory projections presented below shed some light on the situation.

With regard to the other species studied, some general trends in the relative development of the various pallial zones are apparent in the series *Scaphirhynchus–Lepisosteus–Salmo–Lepomis:*

1. *Dm hypertrophies and becomes more differentiated.* In *Scaphirhynchus* it is confined to rostral levels. In the holostean and the teleosts it extends the full length of the telencephalon, occupying a large extent of the dorsomedial and dorsal ependymal surface. One uniform cytoarchitectonic zone is present in *Scaphirhynchus.* In *Lepisosteus*, although we were not able to consistently subdivide Dm, it is clear that several subzones are present. In the teleosts four separate cytoarchitectonic divisions can be recognized.
2. *Dd becomes differentiable as a separate zone but is relatively small.* No separate Dd can be recognized in *Scaphirhynchus,* or *Salmo,* on cytoarchitectonic grounds. In *Lepisosteus* a relatively large Dd has been recognized, and in *Lepomis* it is of moderate size but clearly differentiable from surrounding zones.
3. *Dl hypertrophies and becomes more differentiated.* In *Scaphirhynchus* and *Lepisosteus* only a single zone can be recognized for Dl, and in the former it is not separable from Dd. In *Salmo* three zones can be recognized, but one (Dl-d) is not separable from Dd. In *Lepomis* three clearly separate zones are seen, and Dl-v in particular, and Dl-p to some extent, are hypertrophied relative to the situation in *Salmo*.
4. *Dp is reduced.* Dp is very extensive in *Scaphirhynchus* and extends completely across the ventrocaudal pallium in *Lepisosteus*. In *Salmo* it nearly reaches the ependymal surface medially, whereas in *Lepomis* and other advanced teleosts examined it is restricted to the ventrolateral portion of the caudal pallium.
5. *Dc becomes more differentiated and more complex.* In *Scaphirhynchus* a somewhat indistinct collection of large cells represents a single Dc. In *Lepisosteus* some larger cells are present centrally, but no clearly recognizable condensation of such cells is seen. In *Salmo* one and possibly two Dc groups are present. In *Lepomis* Dc is remarkably large and distinct and consists of four separate cellular condensations.

4. Discussion

In spite of the various differences in the subpallium noted above, the general pattern of its organization in all five species is very similar. This actinopterygian pattern is partly the result of the lack of an inversion (Fig. 2) of the ventral telencephalon in these fishes. Similarly, the general pattern of pallial morphology in all species studied is characterized by an extensive ependymal surface overlain by a greatly expanded tela chorioidea which encloses the telencephalic ventricle. The lateral or outward bending of the pallium constitutes an eversion as defined by Nieuwenhuys (1962*a*) and is unique to the actinopterygian fishes. The actinopterygian pattern of subpallial organization and pallial eversion is not shared with the other bony fishes, *Latimeria* and the Dipnoi, although parts of the telencephalon of *Latimeria* are everted (Nieuwenhuys, 1965, 1969; Nieuwenhuys and Hickey, 1965; Schnitzlein and Crosby, 1967). Furthermore, since this pattern is not found in either the agnathans (Johnston, 1902; Heier, 1948) or the cartilaginous fishes (Johnston, 1911; Holmgren, 1922; Faucette, 1969*a,b;* Kuhlenbeck and Niimi, 1969; Nieuwenhuys, 1969; Northcutt, 1977), it must be a derived rather than a primitive condition. The polypteriforms display this same pattern of subpallial organization and pallial eversion, and thus, on the basis of telencephalic characters, they are considered to be actinopterygians. The peculiar organization of the pallium of the polypteriforms, however, separates them from all other actinopterygians.

V. Olfactory Bulb Projections

A. Methods

The efferent projections of the olfactory bulb were studied with degeneration techniques in three species. Following unilateral aspiration lesions of the olfactory bulb, animals were allowed to survive from 5 to 29 days as follows: *Polypterus,* 5, 10, 16, 16, 23, 29; *Scaphirhynchus* 5, 6, 7, 7, 10, 16; and *Lepisosteus*, 6, 7, 8, 12, 16. The animals were perfused with 10% formalin, and the brains were removed and stored in formalin for at least 1 week. Following gelatin embedding, frozen sections were cut at 25 μm in transverse or horizontal planes. The sections were processed according to Fink–Heimer procedure II (Fink and Heimer, 1967) to demonstrate degenerating axons and terminals. In all three species the olfactory bulbs are sessile, that is, they are attached directly to the telencephalon proper. Consequently, in order to avoid damage to the telencephalon proper, our aspiration lesions frequently spared the caudalmost part of the bulb. In addition, a completely separate analysis of the medial and lateral olfactory tracts (see Finger, 1975, in *Ictalurus,* which has pedunculated bulbs) was not feasible in these species. To simplify the descriptions in the following account, we have referred to medial and lateral olfactory tracts, but at some levels a clear separation cannot be made.

B. Results

1. *Polypterus*

Although previously described (Braford and Northcutt, 1974), the projections of the olfactory bulb in *Polypterus* will be briefly summarized here.

In the caudal bulb degenerating fibers collect at the ventromedial and dorsal edges of the SOF to form the medial and lateral olfactory tracts, respectively (Fig. 7B). The medial olfactory tract runs in a superficial position in the ventrolateral subpallium. Rostrally, it extends toward but does not reach the cell bodies of Vv, although it may engage their dendrites (Fig. 8A). At more caudal levels it lies medially adjacent to Vl (Fig. 8B). Dense accumulations of degenerating debris are seen on the medial and, more caudally, the ventromedial aspects of Vl (Fig. 9A).

The lateral olfactory tract projects to a region between Ev and Ed in the caudal subpallium (Fig. 9B) and massively to both the dorsal and ventral portions of area P1 of the pallium (Figs. 8A,B and 9A,B). Rostrally, the degeneration occupies the superficial third of this "medial" pallial area, sparing a thin submeningeal strip occupied by tractus pallii. Caudally, the band of degeneration narrows slightly and diminishes both in density and dorsoventral extent as the caudal pole of the pallium is approached (Fig. 10).

The degeneration patterns described above are all ipsilateral to the lesion in the olfactory bulb. A sparse but consistently present patch of argyrophilic material was found between Ev and Ed on the contralateral side. However, no degenerating fibers were seen crossing the midline in either the anterior or the habenular commissure, nor were degenerating fibers observed to the contralateral olfactory bulb.

In summary, the major targets of the olfactory tracts in *Polypterus* are Vl, Ev and Ed, and P1, and probably Vv. Golgi preparations indicate that the dendrites of the periventricular subpallial cell groups extend into the path of the degenerating olfactory bulb efferents and may receive inputs.

2. *Scaphirhynchus*

Degenerating fibers leave the SOF of the bulb dorsally and ventromedially and distribute widely to the telencephalon. The medial olfactory tract gives rise to a small terminal field lateral to Vv (Fig. 11B), but most of its fibers continue caudally, cross in the anterior commissure (Figs. 12B and 13A), and distribute to the contralateral telencephalon. Dorsally directed fibers enter Vd, Vn, and Vl. Scattered terminals are seen in the lateral parts of Vd and Vn rostrally (Fig. 12A), and considerably denser ones are seen in Vl (Fig. 12A) and the lateral part of Vd more caudally (Fig. 12B). In the caudal subpallium both Vs (Fig. 13A) and Vp (Fig. 13B) are in receipt of olfactory input, the projection to Vs being the heavier of the two. The terminal field in Vp extends lateral to the boundary of the nucleus—between it and E.

At very rostral levels (Fig. 12A) the pallium is free of degeneration, but at commissural levels (Fig. 12B) Dm is replaced by Dp, which receives a large olfactory input. At successively caudal levels (Figs. 13A,B and 14A), Dp, which is coincident with the olfactory terminal field in the pallium, extends more and more laterally and finally occupies the entire caudal pole of the pallium.

Two bundles of degenerating fibers can be traced into the thalamus. One enters the stria medullaris (Fig. 14B), decussates in the habenular commissure, and distributes to the contralateral telencephalon. The other continues in a caudoventral direction through the medial thalamus as the olfacto-hypothalamic tract (OHT, Figs. 14B and 15A,B) and terminates in the caudalmost hypothalamus near the midline just ventral to the median nucleus of the posterior tuber (MTP, Fig. 16). This projection is bilateral. The olfactory projections to the contralateral telencephalon are symmetrical to the ipsilateral ones, but sparser. A large number of degenerating fibers enter the SOF of the contralateral bulb and terminate on mitral cells and more sparsely on the most superficial cells of the ICL.

In summary, the major olfactory targets in *Scaphirhynchus* include at least parts of all of the subpallial cell groups (except the retrobulbar nucleus), an extensive Dp, the caudal hypothalamus, and the contralateral bulb.

3. *Lepisosteus*

At rostral levels the medial olfactory tract courses ventromedially toward Vv and runs along its lateral edge. A small terminal field is seen just lateral to Vv (Fig. 17B), but the majority of these fibers continue ventromedially, cross more caudally in the anterior commissure (Fig. 18A), and distribute contralaterally. Some fibers of the medial tract appear to contribute to more caudal terminal fields on the ipsilateral side, but they cannot be clearly separated from lateral olfactory tract fibers.

As it enters the subpallium, the lateral olfactory tract courses lateral to and among the cells of NOT and medial to Vl. Some terminals are seen in NOT, and a prominent band of them lies along the concave border of Vl and extends medially, ventral to Vn, where it is somewhat less dense (Fig. 17B). The more lateral part of this terminal field widens and continues caudally to about the level of the anterior commissure. Dense terminals occupy an unnamed region in the central subpallium and extend medially into Vs (Fig. 18A).

At more rostral levels a large fascicle penetrates Vl dorsolaterally (Fig. 17B) and continues in that direction into the pallium where it takes up a superficial position. This fascicle continues caudally for some distance before terminating in the ventral part of the caudal pallium (Figs. 18B and 19A,B). While this large terminal field extends completely across the ventral pallium, the greatest density of terminals is seen in the central part of Dp, as well as ventral to it throughout Vi. Slightly less dense terminations are found in the remainder of Dp and in D1 dorsolateral to Dp. Relatively sparse terminals are present in the lateral portion of Vp and in NT.

A prominent fascicle continues caudally, running medial to the entopeduncular complex (Fig. 19A). It courses through the thalamus (Fig. 19B) and terminates, as in *Scaphirhynchus,* near the midline in the caudalmost hypothalamus.

The contralateral connections are, in general, symmetrical to, but considerably more sparse than, the ipsilateral ones. A sparse projection is seen to the contralateral olfactory bulb terminating predominantly in the superficial part of the ICL. At least most of the crossed fibers reach their destinations via the anterior commissure, for the evidence of degeneration in the habenular commissure consists of a total of one or two fibers in all of our material.

To summarize, in *Lepisosteus* very dense terminal fields are seen in Vi and the core of Dp. Moderately dense terminations are seen adjacent to Vv, Vl, and Vn and within NOT, Vs, the remainder of Dp, a small part of Dl, and the caudal hypothalamus. Sparser terminations are seen in the lateral part of Vp and in NT, as well as in symmetrical regions of the contralateral telencephalon and in the contralateral olfactory bulb.

1. Teleosts

We have not studied the projections of the olfactory bulbs in *Salmo* or *Lepomis*. There are, however, two reports in the literature on olfactory bulb projections in other teleosts: Scalia and Ebbesson (1971), moray eel, *Gymnothorax funebris*, family Muraenidae, Division I; and Finger (1975), bullhead catfish, *Ictalurus nebulosus*, family Ictaluridae, Division III. The results of these two studies are in general agreement. Three major terminal fields were seen bilaterally in the telencephalon proper: (1) a medial terminal field in the subpallium (Vv, Scalia and Ebbesson; apparently more dorsally in V, Finger); (2) a lateral terminal field in the pallium (Dp, Scalia and Ebbesson; nucleus taenia, Dp, and perhaps a part of Dl, Finger); and (3) a posterior or central–posterior terminal field (perhaps part of Dc, both studies). In addition, Finger reported a bilateral projection to the caudal hypothalamus and a projection to the contralateral olfactory bulb.

2. Comparisons

In the series chondrosteans–holosteans–teleosts the trend is clearly a reduction in olfactory input to the telencephalon. In *Scaphirhynchus* there are relatively few telencephalic territories which do not receive some olfactory afference. The situation in *Lepisosteus* is intermediate between that in *Scaphirhynchus* and that in the teleosts, but it is closer to the teleosts.

With respect to the pallium, the major target in all of these fishes is Dp. The size of Dp is progressively reduced in the series *Scaphirhynchus*–*Lepisosteus*–*Salmo*–*Lepomis*. Dp is most likely homologous to the lateral or piriform pallium of land vertebrates. Thus certain previous interpretations of the actinopterygian pallium are no longer tenable. In particular, the interpretations of the simple eversion school—Holmgren and Kuhlenbeck—which place the piriform pallium in a dorsomedial or dorsal position, respectively, are incompatible with the data on olfactory input.

In *Polypterus* the pallial olfactory target is located dorsomedially. In the topographically corresponding position in the other actinopterygians we find Dm—at least at rostral levels. If we examine the position of Dp in the other actinopterygians more closely, it seems likely that *Scaphirhynchus*, *Lepisosteus*, and *Salmo* display transitional stages between *Polypterus* and the advanced teleosts with respect to the position of Dp. Dp lies exactly where it would be expected to in *Polypterus* on the basis of an eversion of the pallium—that is, just dorsal to the subpallium (see Fig. 2). In *Scaphirhynchus*, at rostral levels Dm lies in this position, but at midtelencephalic levels Dp lies immediately dorsal to the subpallium. In *Lepisosteus*, although Dm extends the whole length of the telencephalon, when Dp makes its appearance caudally it lies adjacent to the subpallium along the medial ependymal surface. In *Salmo* Dp lies in a similar position but has apparently migrated slightly away from the medial ependyma. In the advanced teleosts Dp lies more laterally and is smaller. The hypothesis, then, is that the major pallial olfactory target—Dp or P1—has decreased in size, moved caudally, and migrated away from the medial ependyma.

It must be borne in mind that the surface of the caudal pole of the telencephalon is also ependymal. So the most probable correct statement of the situation is that the ependymal zone which gives rise embryonically to Dp has moved caudally and laterally in the series.

The above data clearly show that the telencephalon of all actinopterygians contains significant territories which are not in receipt of secondary olfactory afference. To gain some insight into the nature of these other areas, we have undertaken a series of histochemical studies in three of our five representative species and a study of ascending input to the telencephalon in *Polypterus*. We will describe the results of these studies in the following section.

VI. Histochemistry

A. Introduction

The regional distribution in brain tissue of neural transmitters, enzymes involved in their metabolism, and other enzymes and compounds can provide additional information for characterizing neuronal populations. The regional distributions of enzymes involved in the metabolism of transmitter substances are sometimes correlated with the distribution of the transmitter. Monoamine and GABA distributions both parallel those of their synthesizing enzymes (tyrosine hydroxylase, L-aromatic amino acid decarboxylase, tryptophan hydroxylase, and glutamate decarboxylase), but there is no such correlation with the distribution of their degradative enzymes [catechol-*O*-transferase, monoamine oxidase (MAO), GABA-transaminase, and succinic semialdehyde dehydrogenase]. In contrast, in the acetylcholine system such a general correlation exists for both the synthesizing (choline acetyltransferase) and the degradative [acetylcholinesterase (AChE)] enzymes (Jacobowitz and Palkovits, 1974; Fahn, 1976). This does not mean, however, that the presence of AChE necessarily implies the presence of a cholinergic system. Even when the distributions of enzymes do not correlate with those of their transmitters, these distributions can still be useful as markers of neuronal populations. For example, the regional distributions of MAO are similar in the telencephalons of vertebrates belonging to several different classes (mammals: Bogdanski *et al.*, 1957; Shimizu *et al.*, 1959; Hashimoto *et al.*, 1962; birds: Kusunoki, 1969; reptiles: Kusunoki, 1971; amphibians: Northcutt, 1974). The distributions of other enzymes which are assumed to be ubiquitous in cells—such as the mitochondrial enzyme succinate dehydrogenase (SDH)—are nonuniform in the brain. High concentrations of SDH are correlated with regions of sensory input in the telencephalon of mammals and reptiles (Friede, 1960; Pritz and Northcutt, 1977).

The telencephalic distributions of three enzymes—monoamine oxidase (MAO) (Figs. 26–28), acetylcholinesterase (AChE) (Figs. 29–31), and succinate dehydrogenase (SDH) (Figs. 32–34)—were studied in three species: *Polypterus* (or *Erpetoichthys), Lepisosteus,* and *Salmo.*

B. Methods

Specimens of *Polypterus palmas* ($n = 4$), *Erpetoichthys calabaricus* ($n = 2$), *Lepisosteus osseus* ($n = 4$), and *Salmo gairdneri* ($n = 4$) were killed by decapitation. In some cases the animals were anesthetized in a solution of ethyl-*m*-aminobenzoate (MS-222) prior to decapitation. MS-222 does not appear to affect the intensity of the enzymatic reactions which we examined. Following decapitation, the brains were placed in plastic embedding molds containing a commercially prepared, water-soluble resin (Tissue-Tek II, Lab-Tek Products). Quick-freeze was achieved by immersing the embedded brains in 2-methyl butane cooled to −70°C in a dry ice and ethanol bath. Transverse sections were cut at 25 μm on a Harris cryostat at −20°C and collected on chrome-alum-treated slides.

The methods used to demonstrate various enzymatic activities were as follows: the method of Glenner *et al.* (1957) for MAO, the method of Koelle (Gomori, 1952) for AChE, and the method of Pearse (1960) for SDH. Incubation times ranged from 30 min to 3 hr at 25–40°C. The following times were finally selected as optimal: MAO, 40 min; AChE, 3 hr; SDH, 40 min. As a control for the specificity of cholinesterases demonstrated, additional sections were incubated in the reaction mixture with butyrylthiocholine rather than acetylthiocholine. No cholinesterases were demonstrated by this method. As a control for the specificity of MAO, sections were incubated in the reaction mixture, from which tryptamine hydrochloride had been omitted. In these cases no reaction was seen. No specific inhibitors of AChE or MAO were employed as further controls.

The regional distributions of enzymatic reactions were analyzed by projecting individual sections and tracing the outlines of the sections and the boundaries of the reactive zones. In previous studies of the distributions and relative activities of these enzymes in the telencephalon of amphibians and reptiles (Northcutt, 1974, 1978), the relative activities have been reported in terms of optical density or absorbance. However, the actinopterygians which we examined demonstrate such low telencephalic concentrations—particularly of AChE—that optical densities could not be satisfactorily measured. Two lines of evidence lead us to believe that these low telencephalic concentrations of AChE are real rather than due to failure of the Koelle method to demonstrate more intense reactions. First, other brain regions, such as the optic tectum and the medulla, exhibit high AChE concentrations with the same or shorter incubation times. Second, bioassay of AChE activity (Northcutt and Shephard, unpublished observations) reveals that AChE activity in the forebrain of actinopterygians is four- to fivefold less than that in the midbrain. Our designation of high, moderate, and low activities of the enzymes thus refers to the relative intensities of staining *within* the telencephalon without reference to other brain regions, which in many cases show considerably higher concentrations than any area in the telencephalon. These relative intensities and their distributions are plotted in Figs. 26–34. In these figures the levels of the transverse sections correspond to those of the figures in which cytoarchitectonic boundaries are shown (i.e., *Polypterus*, Figs. 7–10; *Lepisosteus*, Figs. 17–19; and *Salmo*, Figs. 20–22). To further facilitate comparisons among the species, we have summarized the distributions of the three enzymes within the various telencephalic cell groups in Table V.

Table V. Summary of Enzyme Distribution in the Telencephalon

	MAO			AChE			SDH		
	High	Moderate	Low	High	Moderate	Low	High	Moderate	Low
Polypterus	GL	ECL				ECL	GL	ECL	SOF
	SOF	Vd				Mitral cells	P1	Vv	
	RN	Vl				(c)[a]	P2	Vd	
	Vv	Vs				SOF	P3	Vn	
	Vd	P1				ICL		Vl	
	Vn	P2				Vv		Vs	
	PP	P3				Vn		Vp	
	P3					Vs		PP	
						Vp		Ec	
						PP		P1	
						Ec		P3	
Lepisosteus	NOT	GL	ECL	ECL (c)	Vv	ICL	GL	Vp	Vv
	Vl	Vv	ICL	NOT (c)	Vp	Vn	ECL	Vi	Vd
	Vp	Vn	Vd	Dp (c)	PP	Vs	NOT	PP	Vn
	Vi	Vs	Dm		Dm	Vp	Dl	Dm	Vl
	PP	Dm	Dl		Dl	Vi		Dd	Vs
		Dl	Dp			Dm		Dl	PP
		Dp				Dl		Dp	Er
		NT				Dp		NT	Dm
						NT			Dd
									Dp
									NT
Salmo	GL	SOF	Vd	Vc	ICL	Vd	ECL	ICL	Dm-1
	ECL	ICL	PP	PP	Vv	Dd + Dl-d	ICL	Dm-3	Dm-2
	PP	Vl	Dd + Dl-d	Dm-3	Vl	Dp	Vc	Dd + Dl-d	Dm-4
	Dm-3	PP		Dp (c)	Vs		Dd + Dl-d	Dl-p	Dd + Dl-d
	Dd + Dl-d	Dm-1		Dc (c)	Dm-4		Dp	Dp	
	Dl-v	Dm-2			Dd + Dl-d			Dc	
	Dl-p	Dm-3							
		Dd + Dl-d							
		Dl-v							
		Dl-p							

[a] (c) indicates high AChE activity in cell bodies but not in the surrounding neuropil. With the Koelle method, AChE activity in neuropil areas tends to obscure the possible presence of AChE in cell bodies within those areas.

Several generalizations can be made about the histochemical results. In many cases the distributions of the enzymes studied coincide with, and thus confirm, our cytoarchitectonic boundaries. In several cases the histochemical data suggest further subdivisions of large zones which we were not able to consistently subdivide on solely cytoarchitectonic grounds (e.g., Dm in *Lepisosteus* and Dd + Dl−d in *Salmo*). Detailed cross-species comparisons of the histochemical findings are difficult to make, although some similarities are apparent. Finally, as Table V indicates, the telencephalic distributions of the three enzymes are very complicated, and a complete discussion of these results is beyond the scope of this chapter. We will consider the results for each of the three enzymes separately, calling attention to those we consider to be of particular interest and making some comparisons with similar studies in other vertebrates.

1. MAO

As we mentioned above, the distributions of MAO have been found to be generally similar in vertebrates of several different classes. In the telencephalon of all vertebrates studied, high or moderate concentrations of MAO have been reported in the following regions (see references above): preoptic area, septal area, part of the amygdala (or archistriatum), and dorsal striatum* (paleostriatum augmentatum, caudoputamen). Additionally, in amniotes moderate to high MAO concentrations are seen in the hippocampal complex.

If we first consider the high-MAO regions in *Polypterus* (Fig. 26), we find a distribution which is generally comparable to that seen in other vertebrates—provided that certain interpretations of the cell masses are made based on their topological position. The high-MAO regions are as follows (excluding olfactory bulb structures): preoptic area, retrobulbar nucleus, Vv, Vd, Vn, and P3. On the basis of topological position, the retrobulbar nucleus, Vv, and Vd (or parts thereof) can reasonably be homologized to the septal region; Vn is tentatively compared to the striatum (see below); and P3 is comparable to the medial pallium of amphibians and possibly the hippocampal complex of amniotes.

Although the preoptic area also shows high MAO concentrations in both *Lepisosteus* and *Salmo* (Figs. 27C,D,E and 28E,F), the remainder of the high-MAO areas in these two species are less readily comparable to other vertebrates, and we cannot make any reasonable interpretation of them at the present time. We note that in *Salmo* there is a remarkably large area of high MAO activity rostrally in Dd + Dl−d (Fig. 28A,B), but we do not know whether this is typical for teleosts.

2. AChE

In the telencephalon of all vertebrates studied, the concentration of AChE in the subpallium is much higher than it is in the pallium. The highest concentrations of AChE are localized in the dorsal striatum (paleostriatum augmentatum, caudo-

* The use of the term "dorsal striatum" in amphibians and reptiles follows that of Northcutt (1974, 1978). In reptiles it does *not* refer to the dorsal ventricular ridge.

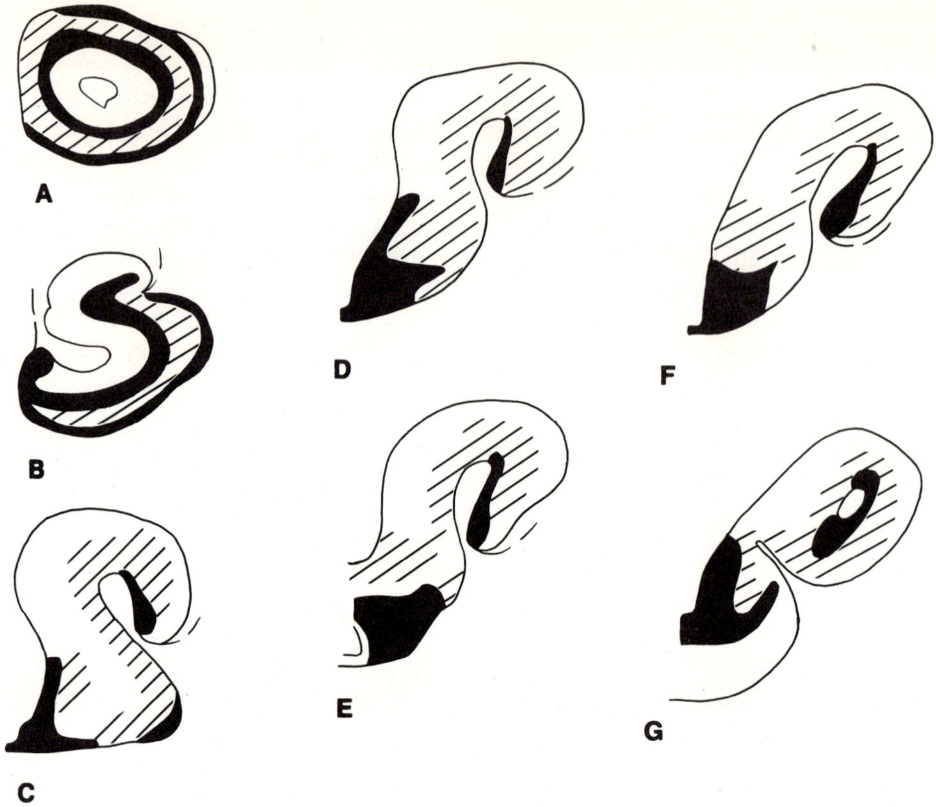

Figure 26. MAO, *Polypterus*. Plot of regional distribution and relative intensities of monoamine oxidase activity in the telencephalon of *Polypterus*. Solid black areas indicate high intensities, whereas hatched areas indicate moderate intensities. Various levels of the telencephalon charted here are identical to those illustrated in Figs. 7–10. Tabular summary of active telencephalic areas is presented in Table V.

putamen), nucleus accumbens, olfactory tubercle, and nucleus of the diagonal band of Broca (Koelle, 1954; Shen *et al.,* 1955; Ishii, 1957; Kusunoki, 1969, 1971; Parent and Olivier, 1970; Jacobowitz and Palkovits, 1974; Northcutt, 1974; McGeer and McGeer in Fahn, 1976).

The single most surprising finding that we report in this chapter* is the presence of a large area of high AChE concentration in the pallium of *Salmo,* specifically in Dm-3 (Fig. 31D,E). Dm-4 displays moderate AChE concentrations (Fig. 31D,E,F). Similarly, in *Lepisosteus,* moderate AChE concentrations are present in the caudal part of Dm (Fig. 30E,F). Although we have not included a description of our AChE results in *Lepomis* in this chapter, high concentrations are also present caudally in Dm in this species.

One interpretation of this finding is that the caudal part of Dm is not pallial, but rather subpallial, and specifically homologous to the dorsal striatum (paleostriatum augmentatum, caudoputamen) of tetrapods. The following considerations support this hypothesis:

* See also Northcutt and Braford (1977).

1. Caudal Dm displays high AChE concentrations.
2. In *Lepomis* the caudal part of Dm is heavily innervated by catecholaminergic fibers as revealed by the Falck–Hillarp method (Parent *et al.*, 1977).
3. High levels of AChE combined with dopaminergic innervation are diagnostic for the dorsal striatum in reptiles, birds, and mammals (Parent and Olivier, 1970). Thus the histochemical evidence that caudal Dm is homologous to dorsal striatum will be strengthened if further study reveals its catecholaminergic innervation to be dopaminergic.
4. If the boundary between the subpallium and the pallium were actually dorsal to Dm rather than ventral to it—as has been suggested by Kuhlenbeck (1929, 1973; see Fig. 3)—the topological position of Dm would be appropriate for the dorsal striatum, i.e., the dorsalmost subpallial cell mass.

Although most of the available evidence supports this hypothesis, there are two problems. First, only the caudal parts of Dm display high AChE activity. Dm-

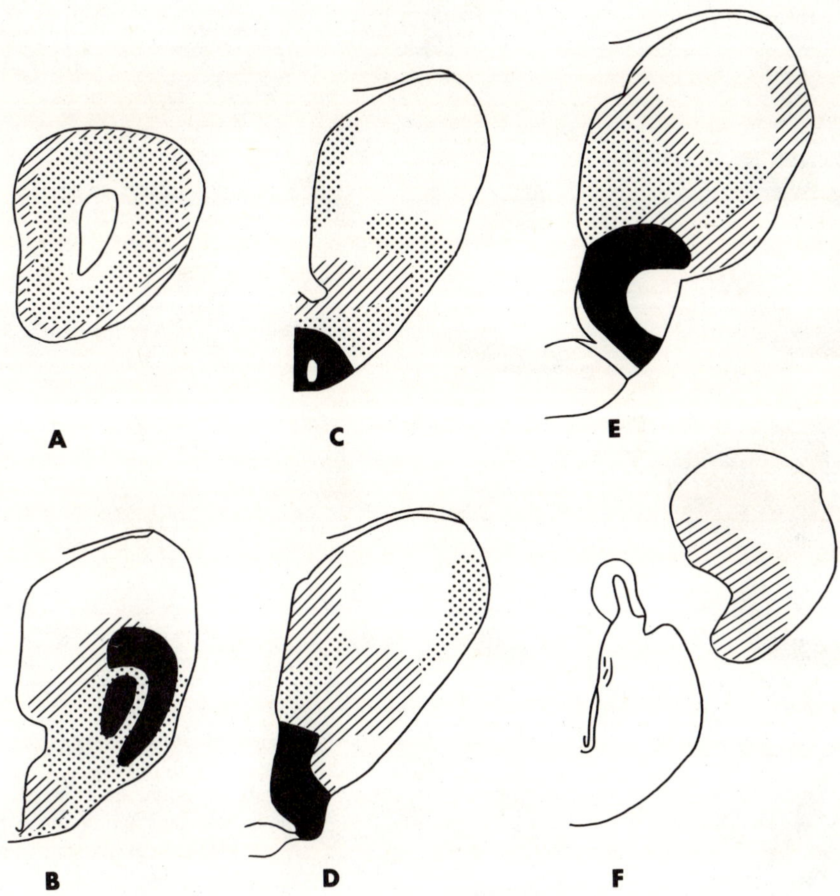

Figure 27. MAO, *Lepisosteus.* Plot of regional distribution and relative intensities of monoamine oxidase activity in the telencephalon of *Lepisosteus.* Solid black areas indicate high intensities, hatched areas moderate intensities, and stippled areas low intensities. The charted telencephalic levels are identical to those in Figs. 17–19. Tabular summary of active areas is presented in Table V.

1 and Dm-2 are free of such activity and receive no substantial catecholaminergic innervation. This suggests at least two possibilities: (1) The rostral part of Dm is *not* homologous to the dorsal striatum, or (2) populations of different cell types, which are intermingled and together constitute the dorsal striatum of land vertebrates, are segregated into different subdivisions of Dm in teleosts. The second problem is that no Dm is present in *Polypterus.* All the AChE-positive areas in the telencephalon of *Polypterus* display low concentrations (Table V and Fig. 29). Of these areas, Vn is topologically comparable to Dm. It is possible that the entire Vn-Vl complex in *Polypterus* has migrated away from the ependymal surface, forming the relatively large Vl (see above). Thus Vn in *Polypterus* would not be comparable to the other Vn's but rather would be the best candidate for a Dm and dorsal striatal homologue. This interpretation seems preferable to arguing that no such formation is present in *Polypterus*.

It is possible to entertain other interpretations of the homologies of Dm. One can argue that Dm is homologous to the hippocampal complex of tetrapods (see the "directly comparable" school, Fig. 3). However , although the hippocampus of land vertebrates does display moderate AChE activity, it is never as high as that of

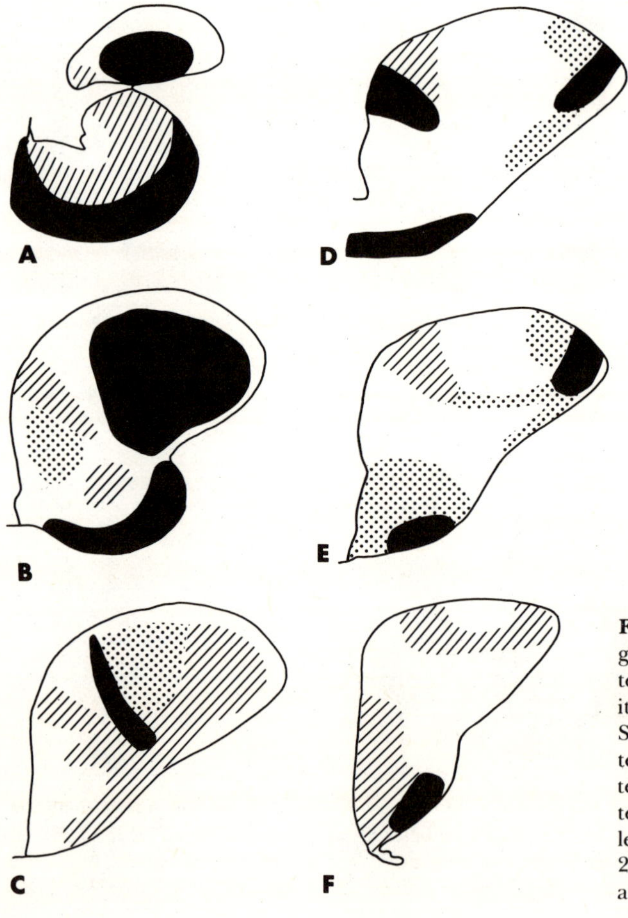

Figure 28. MAO, *Salmo.* Plot of regional distribution and relative intensity of monoamine oxidase activity in the telencephalon of *Salmo.* Solid black areas indicate high intensities, hatched areas moderate intensities, and stippled areas low intensities. The charted telencephalic levels are identical to those in Figs. 20–22. Tabular summary of active areas is presented in Table V.

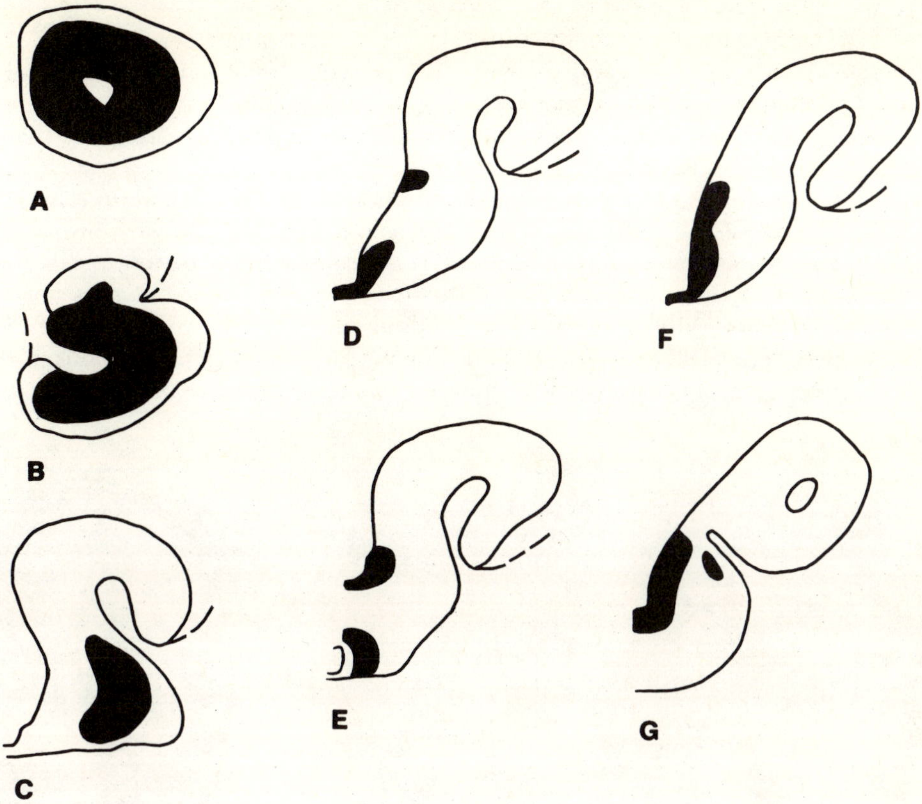

Figure 29. AChE, *Polypterus.* Plot of regional distribution of acetylcholinesterase activity in the telencephalon of *Polypterus.* Solid black areas indicate regions of activity. Telencephalic levels are identical to those of Figs. 7–10. Tabular summary of active areas is presented in Table V.

the caudoputamen. Furthermore, the topological position of Dm cannot be reconciled with that of the hippocampal complex (Fig. 2). Another possibility that should be considered is that Dm is not homologous to either the caudoputamen or the hippocampal formation. This could be the case if histochemical changes have occurred within homologous cell populations in the course of evolution. A definitive answer will be possible only when the connections of Dm and other telencephalic cell groups are analyzed.*

3. SDH

The distribution of the mitochondrial enzyme SDH is nonuniform in brain tissue (see Friede, 1966). In the telencephalon high SDH concentrations are cor-

* We note here that there is only one experimental study of the efferent connections of the telencephalon in actinopterygians—Vanegas and Ebbesson (1976). They reported on the projections of the entire telencephalon of two teleosts (a beryciform, *Holocentrus,* and a perciform, *Eugerres*), describing major ipsilateral pathways to the thalamus, hypothalamus, inferior lobe, and optic tectum. They found no long descending connections to the rhombencephalon or spinal cord.

related with sensory areas. In the cerebral cortex of guinea pigs the highest levels of SDH activity are found in the upper layers of the primary sensory areas, that is, somatosensory, auditory, and visual cortices (Friede, 1960); and in the dorsal ventricular ridge of crocodiles regions showing high SDH concentrations are correlated with terminal fields of ascending auditory and visual pathways from the thalamus (Pritz and Northcutt, 1977).

An examination of the regional distribution of SDH in *Polypterus* (Fig. 32 and Table V) reveals an extremely good correlation with the known sensory inputs (Braford and Northcutt, 1977). High SDH concentrations are seen in the glomerular layer of the olfactory bulb and in P1—major targets of the olfactory nerve and secondary olfactory fibers, respectively. Additionally, the neuropil areas of P2 and P3 display high SDH concentrations. Following large diencephalic lesions in *Polypterus,* ascending fibers were traced into the telencephalon and found to terminate

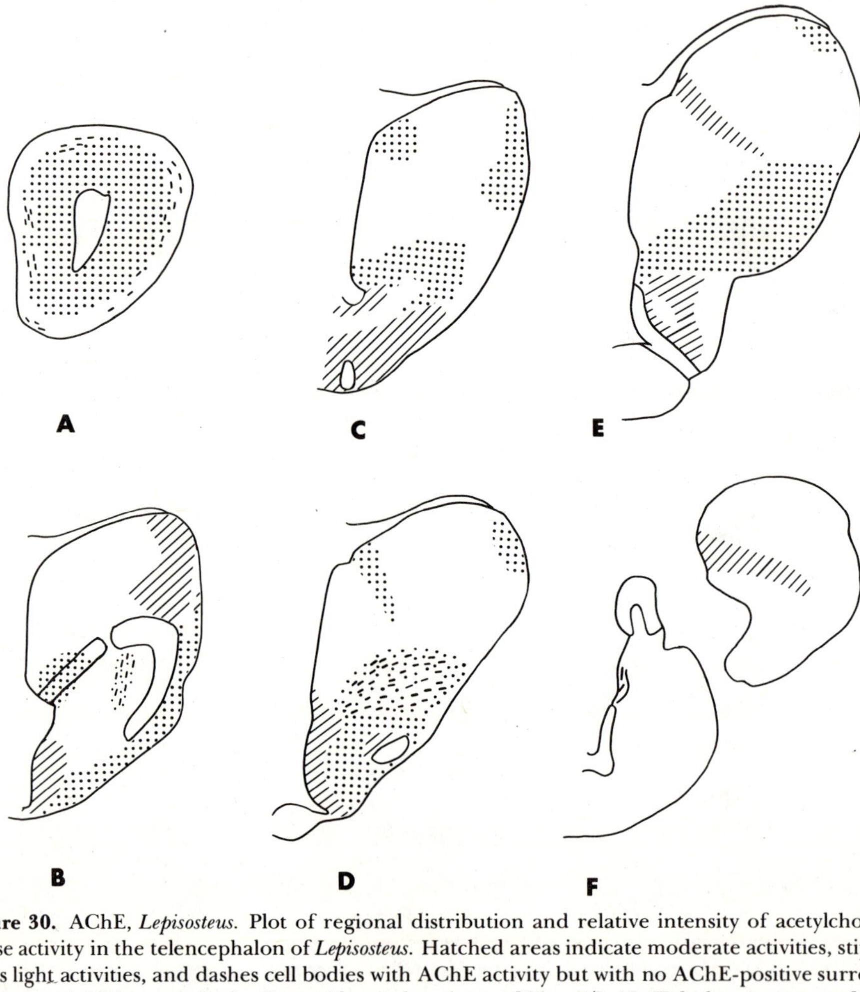

Figure 30. AChE, *Lepisosteus.* Plot of regional distribution and relative intensity of acetylcholinesterase activity in the telencephalon of *Lepisosteus.* Hatched areas indicate moderate activities, stippled areas light activities, and dashes cell bodies with AChE activity but with no AChE-positive surrounding neuropil. Telencephalic levels are identical to those of Figs. 17–19. Tabular summary of active areas is presented in Table V.

heavily in P2 and P3 (Fig. 35). The combined pallial distribution of the olfactory bulb and ascending projections coincides in precise detail with the high-SDH areas (compare Fig. 32 with Figs. 7–10 and 35). The areas of moderate SDH activity in the subpallium also correspond closely to the areas which receive olfactory or ascending inputs.

In *Lepisosteus* (Fig. 33 and Table V) high and moderate SDH concentrations generally correlate with areas of known sensory input: glomerular layer and external cellular layer of the olfactory bulb (primary olfactory targets); NOT, Vi, Vp, NT, and Dp (secondary olfactory targets). On the basis of these correlations, one can predict that the other high SDH areas probably receive sensory input. These areas include the rostral part of Dl (*Lepisosteus*, Fig. 33B) and Vc and parts of Dd + Dl-d and Dp (*Salmo,* Fig. 34B–F).

VII. General Discussion

At the end of each of the three previous sections in this chapter, we have summarized and discussed the findings of that section. Rather than repeat those

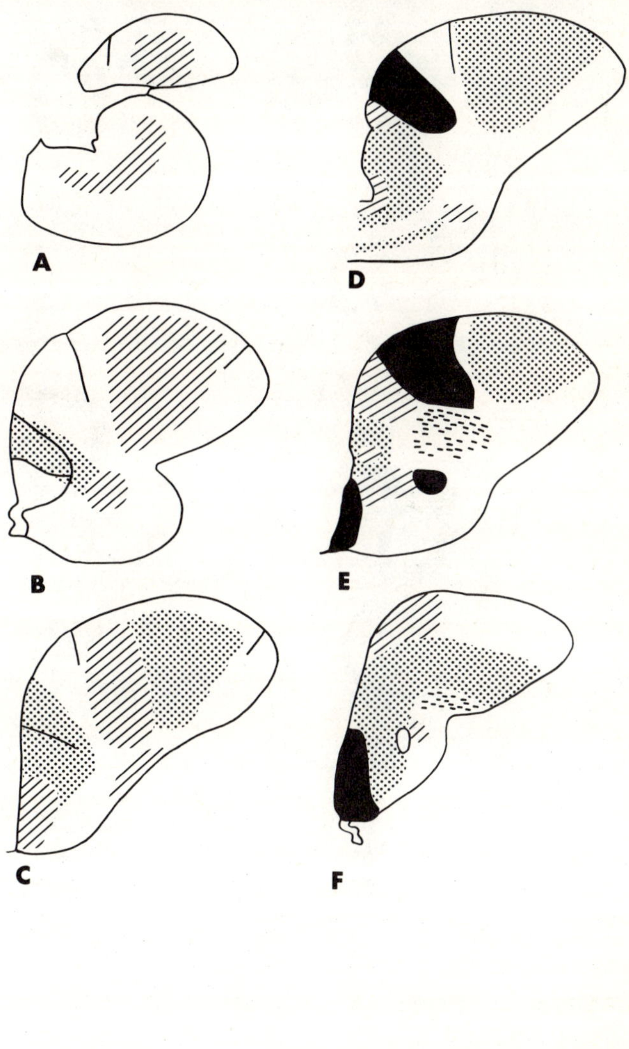

Figure 31. AChE, *Salmo.* Plot of regional distribution and relative intensity of acetylcholinesterase activity in the telencephalon of *Salmo.* Solid black areas indicate high intensities, hatched areas moderate intensities, and stippled areas light activities. Dashes indicate cell bodies with AChE activity. Telencephalic levels are identical to those of Figs. 20–22. Tabular summary of active areas is presented in Table V.

discussions here, we will briefly reconsider the various earlier interpretations of the telencephalon of actinopterygians in the light of our findings, offer an interpretation of our own, and conclude with some remarks on the evolution of the actinopterygian telencephalon.

A. Previous Interpretations of the Telencephalon

1. *Polypterus*

For reasons presented above, we believe the polypteriforms constitute a separate group within the actinopterygians. Because their telencephalon is relatively simply organized and more readily comparable to the telencephalon of land vertebrates than that of the other actinopterygians, we will consider them separately.

Three interpretations of the pallium of *Polypterus* have been advocated in the literature: (1) that it is topographically directly comparable to the pallium of land vertebrates (P1 = hippocampal complex, P2 = dorsal pallium, P3 = piriform

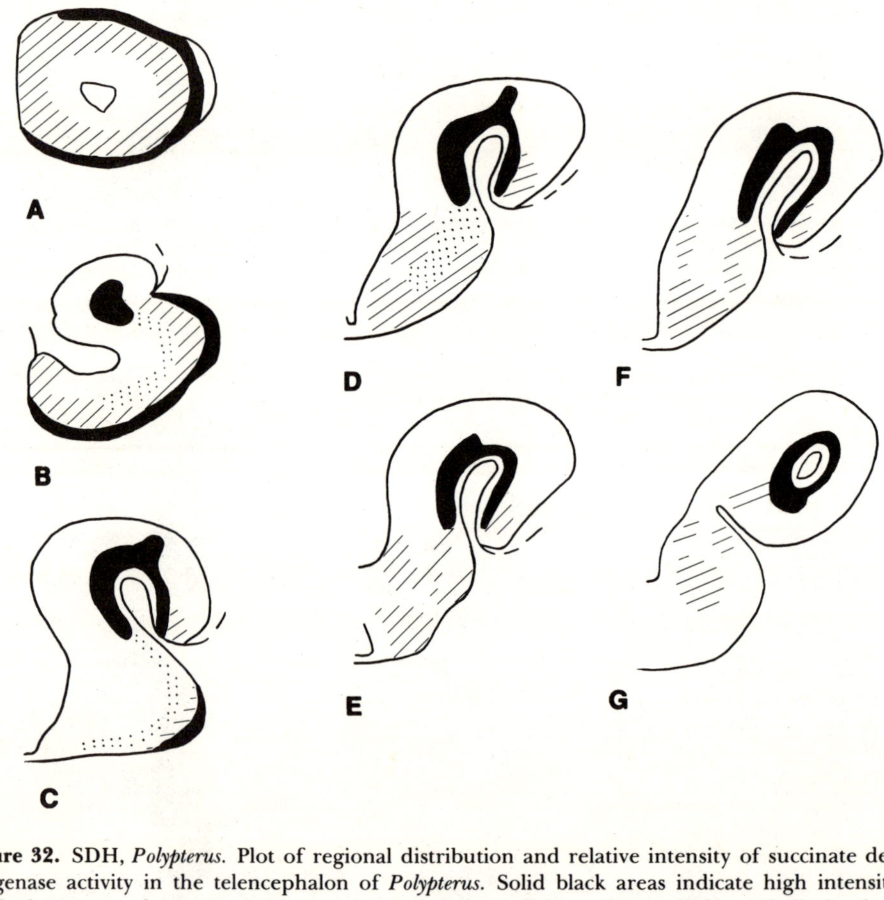

Figure 32. SDH, *Polypterus.* Plot of regional distribution and relative intensity of succinate dehydrogenase activity in the telencephalon of *Polypterus.* Solid black areas indicate high intensities, hatched areas moderate intensities, and stippled areas light activities. Telencephalic levels are identical to those of Figs. 7–10. Tabular summary of active areas is presented in Table V.

pallium + amygdala; Wright, 1967); (2) that it has undergone a simple eversion with a resultant mediolateral reversal of the pallial areas relative to their positions in land vertebrates (P1 = piriform pallium, P2 = dorsal pallium, P3 = hippocampal complex; Holmgren, 1922); and (3) that it has undergone a simple eversion but that the entire pallium consists of one uniform area (Nieuwenhuys, 1963, 1967*b*). The evidence, as we read it, unequivocally supports the interpretation of Holmgren and can be summarized as follows:

1. The adult form of the pallium of *Polypterus* is achieved embryologically by a simple eversion (Holmgren, 1922; Nieuwenhuys *et al.*, 1969). The pallium elongates, and very few cells migrate away from the ependymal zone.
2. The olfactory bulb projects massively to area P1 of the pallium and to no other pallial area. This is incompatible with Wright's interpretation of P1 as hippocampal and P3 as piriform and with Nieuwenhuys's concept of a single uniform pallial area.

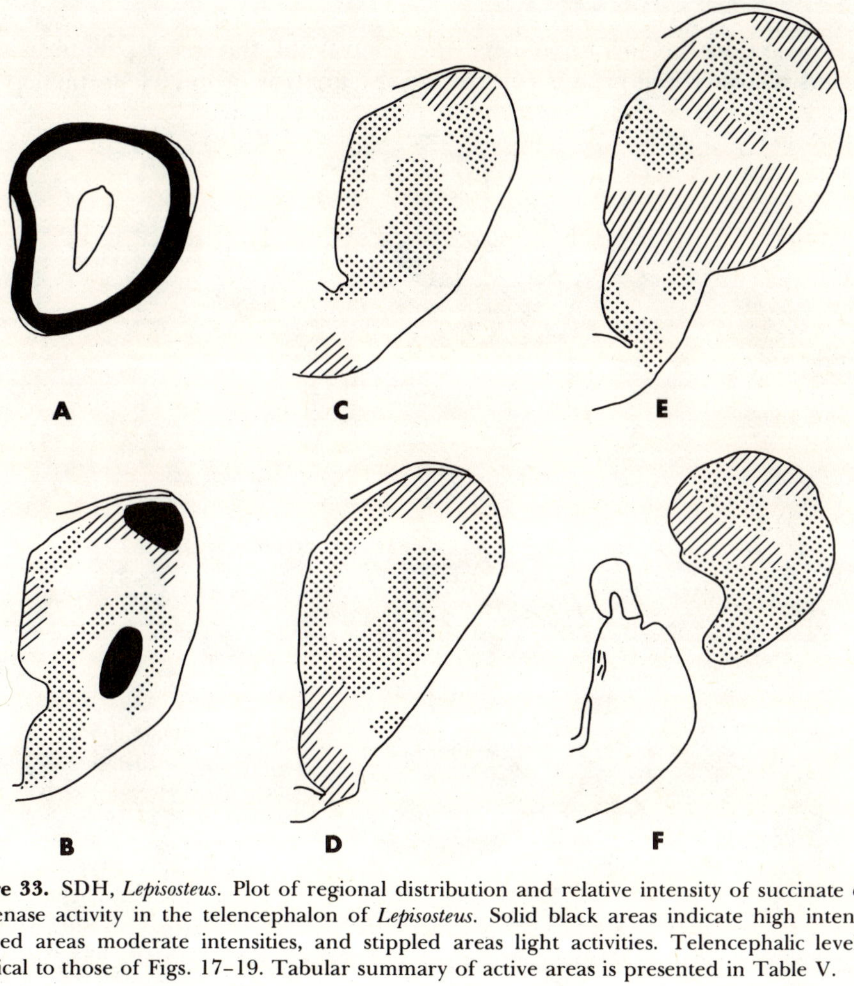

Figure 33. SDH, *Lepisosteus.* Plot of regional distribution and relative intensity of succinate dehydrogenase activity in the telencephalon of *Lepisosteus.* Solid black areas indicate high intensities, hatched areas moderate intensities, and stippled areas light activities. Telencephalic levels are identical to those of Figs. 17–19. Tabular summary of active areas is presented in Table V.

3. The remainder of the pallium (P2 and P3) receives a large ascending input(s) which projects extremely sparsely, if at all, to P1. Although the nature and the source of this input remain to be determined, its presence is compatible with Holmgren's interpretation of P2 as dorsal pallium and P3 as medial pallium or hippocampal complex (cf. amphibians: Kicliter and Northcutt, 1975; Scalia and Colman, 1975). The presence of high MAO concentrations in P3 further supports its correspondence to the medial pallium of tetrapods.

With regard to the subpallium of *Polypterus,* the directly comparable school (Wright) and the simple eversion schools (Holmgren and Nieuwenhuys) have equally divergent interpretations. The former interprets the cell masses as though an inversion similar to that seen in land vertebrates had occurred, whereas the latter assume that the subpallium retains its original, embryonic position in the neural tube (see Fig. 2). These interpretations of the subpallium of *Polypterus* and one of our own are summarized in Table VI.

2. The Other Actinopterygians

In the chondrosteans, holosteans, and teleosts the thickened pallium with its numerous migrated cell groups complicates the analysis of the telencephalon. We

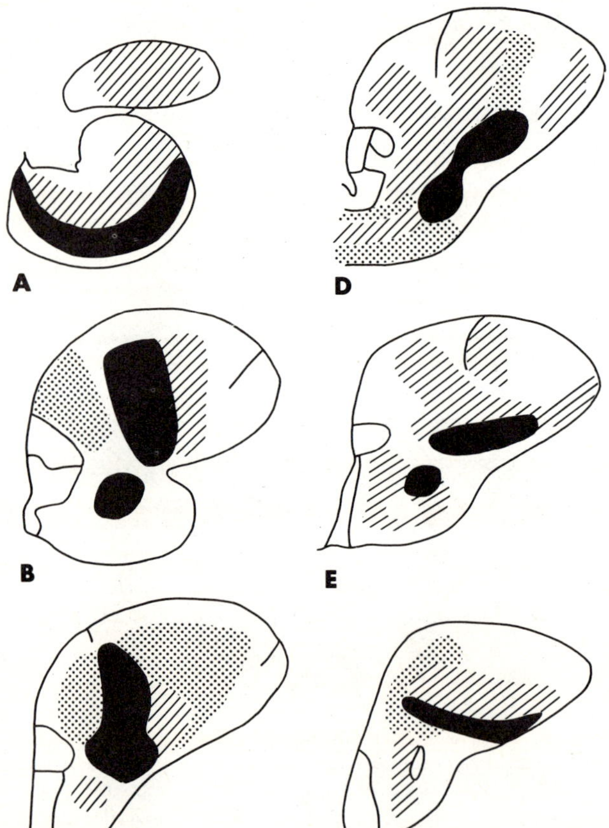

Figure 34. Plot of regional distribution and relative intensity of succinate dehydrogenase activity in the telencephalon of *Salmo.* Solid black areas indicate high intensities, hatched areas moderate intensities, and stippled areas light activities. Telencephalic levels are identical to those of Figs. 20–22. Tabular summary of active areas is presented in Table V.

Table VI. Various Proposals for Subpallial Homologies between *Polypterus* and Land Vertebrates

Nomenclature of this chapter	This chapter	Nieuwenhuys (1967*a*)	Wright (1967)
Vv	Medial septal nucleus	Lateral septal nucleus	Medial septal nucleus (ventral part) + lateral septal nucleus
Vd	Lateral septal nucleus	Olfactory tubercle + striatum	Medial septal nucleus (dorsal part)
Vn	Striatum		Medial septal nucleus (dorsal part)
Vl	Olfactory tubercle	Medial septal nucleus	Olfactory tubercle
Vs and Vp	Amygdala	Amygdala	Medial septal nucleus + bed nucleus of hippocampal commissure
Migrated cells of P1	(Pallium)	(Pallium)	Striatum
Part of P3	(Pallium)	(Pallium)	Amygdala

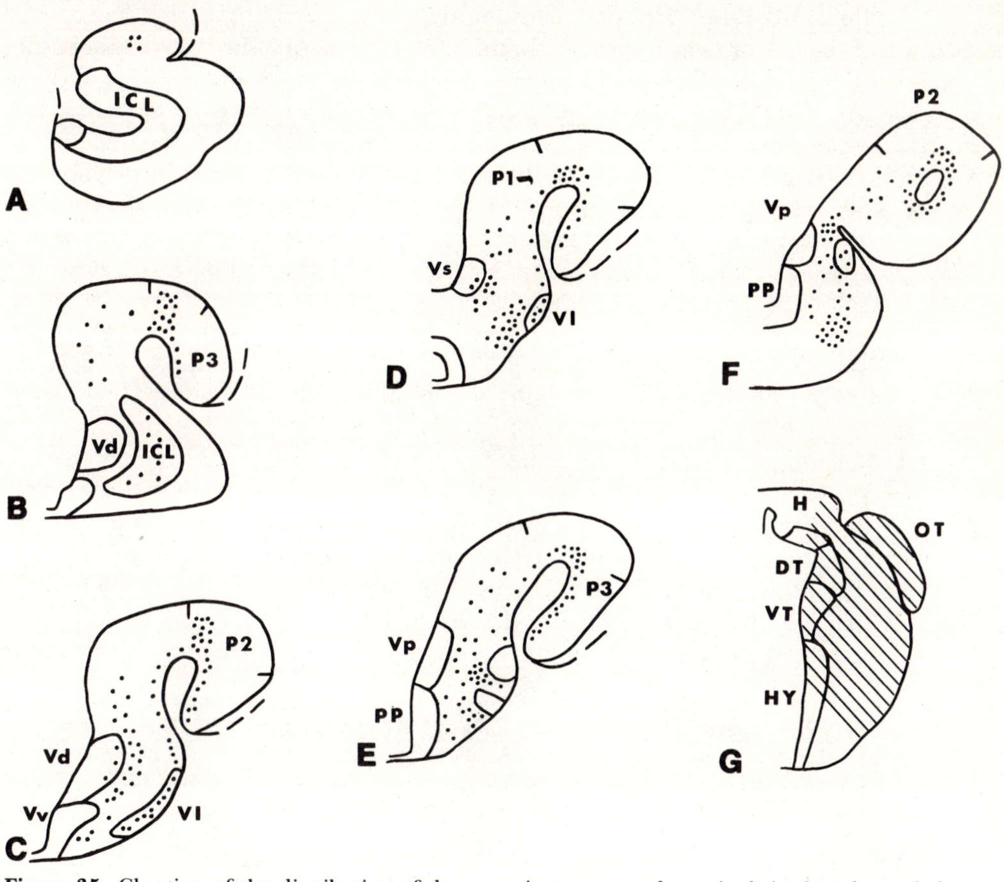

Figure 35. Charting of the distribution of degenerating axons and terminals in the telencephalon of *Polypterus* following unilateral ablation of the diencephalon. Hatched area indicates the maximal extent of the diencephalic ablation. Survival time 12 days. Telencephalic levels are identical to those of Figs. 7B–10.

will briefly reconsider the interpretations of the four schools as they apply to teleosts. (See Fig. 3.)

a. Simple Eversion School. As we noted in the section on the discussion of the olfactory bulb projections, the interpretations of the simple eversion school (Holmgren, 1922; Kuhlenbeck, 1929, 1973) are not compatible with the position of the olfactory targets in the pallium of teleosts—they are not located dorsomedially or dorsally.

b. Directly Comparable School. The position of the olfactory input to the pallium in teleosts does apparently correspond to the area designated as piriform by the directly comparable school, although this is only partially true for *Scaphirhynchus* and *Lepisosteus*, in which the pallial olfactory target extends medially to the ependymal surface (Figs. 12B–14A, 18, and 19). Even in teleosts, we cannot accept the full interpretation of the telencephalon offered by the directly comparable school because we cannot see how such an arrangement could have developed. How, for example, can the hippocampal complex lie dorsally adjacent to the medial septum along the *ependymal* surface when, in land vertebrates, the two structures come into contiguity only by virtue of an inversion—a process for which there is no evidence in actinopterygians?*

c. Noncomparable School. Nieuwenhuys's argument for a simple eversion but with a pallial organization not comparable to that of other vertebrates is an interesting one. It is based on his interpretation of the number of pallial areas in various actinopterygians: one in *Polypterus,* three in the chondrosteans and holosteans, and three to seven in the teleosts. He reasoned that if the pallium of *Polypterus* was uniform throughout, then the progressive increase in pallial areas in the other actinopterygian grades had to be the result of a line of differentiation which had taken place wholly within the actinopterygians. Therefore, any resemblance between the pallium of actinopterygians and that of land vertebrates must be the result of independent evolution. We now know that the pallium of *Polypterus* is not uniform and contains at least three separate populations. Thus, as we will argue below, since this pattern of multiple pallial divisions is common to actinopterygians, other osteichthyans, and land vertebrates, their pallia are most probably comparable.

d. Eversion–Rearrangement School. It seems probable to us that an eversion and some sort of rearrangement occur in the development of the teleost telencephalon. This rearrangement may not involve an actual mixing of cells from separate embryonic populations, as Sheldon (1912) advocated, but merely some shifting of cell groups without loss of their integrity. The latter notion is the simpler of the two. It predicts that experimentally determined fiber connections of individual telencephalic cell groups in actinopterygians should closely resemble those of in-

* Morgan (1974*a,b*), in a study of the embryology of the telencephalon of the marine catfish *Galeichthys felis,* supports the directly comparable school. Although he notes that some of their homologies "may be questioned on the basis of topographical relationships," he believes these conditions are explicable by recognizing the telencephalon of actinopterygians as "nonevaginated, rather than everted." His description of the embryological development conforms well to those of similar studies in other actinopterygians (e.g., Nieuwenhuys, 1962*a*), but he emphasizes the dorsally directed growth of the pallium and not the "extreme eversion" as the reason for the ventrolateral attachment of the tela chorioidea. It seems to us that Morgan's observations are consistent with an eversion as defined by Nieuwenhuys (1962*a*) and that the disagreement over what to call the process is at least partly one of semantics.

dividual telencephalic cell groups in land vertebrates. On the other hand, if mixtures of cell populations are present in the actinopterygian telencephalon, then the connections of one cellular "group" would be expected to resemble those of several different groups in land vertebrates.

In summary, whereas some elements of the interpretations of all of the four schools seem to fit some of the data, none of the interpretations is wholely satisfactory. Thus we propose a new hypothesis concerning the organization of the actinopterygian telencephalon.

B. A New Hypothesis

Members of the other schools might term us the "eclectic school" in that several aspects of our interpretation have been advanced by various other schools. We would admit only, however, to being *de facto* eclectic—that is, our interpretation has not been arrived at by taking this notion from one school and that notion from another, but rather is based on a series of assumptions, enunciated below, the data in the literature, and the new data we have presented in this chapter.

Our interpretation of the actinopterygian telencephalon is based on the following assumptions:

1. Since the actinopterygians are believed to share a common ancestor with the other osteichthyans (some of which gave rise to land vertebrates), the telencephalon of actinopterygians can be compared to that of other vertebrates.
2. Topological relationships among various neuronal populations do not change in a disorderly or inexplicable manner.
3. Variation does exist in many telencephalic characters, and trends from ancestral to derived conditions can be recognized. Increasing complexity of the telencephalon as measured by an increase in the number of recognizable cell groups characterizes the series polypteriforms–chondrosteans–holosteans–basal teleosts–advanced teleosts. This is *not* to say that the condition in the polypteriforms evolved into the condition in the chondrosteans, etc. In the words of Holmgren (1922): "The living species of the groups of vertebrates represent the upper tips of the widely branched vertebrate phylum, and thus they are not to be derived from each other. In the same way it is impossible to derive brain structures of one of these groups from those of another. This is a rule against which comparative neurology has sinned very much."
4. The general patterns of neuronal connectivity are conservative among vertebrates. For example, the olfactory bulb cannot project solely to the piriform pallium in one group of vertebrates and solely to the hippocampal formation in another.
5. The histochemical properties of homologous neuronal populations are similar among vertebrates.
6. The fundamental process involved in the development of the telencephalon of actinopterygians is an eversion as defined by Nieuwenhuys (1962*a*).

It is possible to argue with any and all of the above assumptions. However, we believe that they are the simplest possible ones to make on the basis of presently available information, and thus are the ones that should be made until one or more of them is shown to be incorrect.

Our hypothesis of proposed telencephalic homologies between ray-finned fishes and land vertebrates is summarized in Table VII. The rostral ventral telencephalon, exclusive of the olfactory bulb formations, consists of three major nuclei: Vv, Vd, and Vn + Vl. We believe Vv and Vd are homologous to the medial and lateral septal nuclei of land vertebrates based on their topological positions and the fact that Vv receives an olfactory input from the medial olfactory tract, as does the medial septal nucleus in amphibians (Northcutt and Royce, 1975). However, there is a more extensive olfactory projection to the olfactory tubercle via the lateral olfactory tract in land vertebrates.* A comparable situation also exists in actinopterygians. Vn + Vl receives the largest olfactory input of all the rostral ventral telencephalic areas, and that input is via a lateral olfactory tract. Finally, if Vn + Vl originate embryonically from the ependymal surface in a position between Vd and Dm (see *Lepisosteus,* Fig. 17B), then Vn + Vl occupy an identical position to that of the olfactory tubercle of land vertebrates. The caudal ventral telencephalon of ray-finned fishes contains five nuclei: Vs, Vc, Vp, Vi, and NT. Two of these nuclei (Vs and Vc) occupy the lamina terminalis in the vicinity of the anterior commissure, replace Vd caudally, and do not receive olfactory input. Based on this topology and the absence of olfactory input, they are possibly homologous to the subpallial (pars medialis) amygdala of amphibians (Northcutt, 1974). Similarly, Vp, Vi, and NT form a transitional series from Dp (the main pallial olfactory target) to the preoptic area (Fig. 19A) and all receive olfactory input. A part of the amygdala in amphibians is characterized by similar relationships. In amphibians the ventral continuation of the lateral pallium is termed the pallial (pars lateralis) amygdala and grades over into the preoptic area (Northcutt, 1974; Kokoros and Northcutt, 1977). It receives a specialized olfactory input via the accessory olfactory tract (Scalia, 1972; Northcutt and Royce, 1975).

Earlier in this chapter we have argued that parts of Dm (Dm-3 and perhaps Dm-4) may be homologous to the dorsal striatum (caudoputamen) based on high AChE concentrations and the presence of catecholamines. This proposed homology also satisfies topological criteria. In amphibians the striatum is bordered by the lateral septal nucleus (Vd) and the lateral pallium (Dp). In *Polypterus* and *Scaphirhynchus* the main pallial olfactory target (P1 or Dp) also lies dorsal to the striatum (Vn or Dm). This pallial olfactory area migrates laterally in the actinopterygian series until it occupies a lateral and caudal position in advanced teleosts.

It follows from this interpretation of Dm that parts of Dc could be homologized, on topological grounds, to the ventral striatum (globus pallidus) of land vertebrates. The presence of AChE in the cell bodies of Dc neurons, but not in the surrounding neuropil, also supports such an interpretation.

We believe that Dp is homologous to the lateral pallium of land vertebrates based on its initial topological position in *Polypterus* and *Scaphirhynchus* and its

* In amphibians the olfactory-recipient portion of the ventromedial telencephalon (presumably homologous to the olfactory tubercle in amniotes) has been included in the medial septal nucleus by Northcutt and Royce (1975) and in the nucleus of the diagonal band of Broca by Kicliter and Ebbesson (1976).

strong olfactory input. A logical extension of this interpretation is that Dd and Dl-d topologically correspond to the dorsal pallium and that Dl-v and Dl-p correspond to the medial pallium of land vertebrates. We have grouped Dd with Dl-d in our comparisons because in teleosts such as *Salmo* no distinct cytoarchitectonic boundary can be distinguished and because both of these areas possess high SDH concentrations and hypertrophy together in advanced teleosts.

At the present stage of analysis, several interpretations exist within our hypothesis for at least two of the cell groups—Dm and Dc. Our analysis of Dm is far from satisfactory, particularly regarding Dm-1 and -2. Dm-1 and -2 could be homologized to part of the striatum or subpallial amygdala on the basis of topology. The absence of AChE and the low catecholamine activity do not support a striatal interpretation; however, they do not exclude a subpallial amygdalar interpretation. Dc is also a problematic group. No distinct Dc is recognizable in *Polypterus* or *Lepisosteus.* A single Dc is seen in *Scaphirhynchus,* one and possibly two are seen in *Salmo,* and four separate groups are seen in *Lepomis.* Several interpretations are possible. First, in *Polypterus,* where no Dc is present, it is possible that the cells of Dc and Dm are present in Vn as a field homology. This interpretation would suggest that Dc arose by migration from Dm phylogenetically and became subdivided at the advanced teleost grade of organization. Second, in *Lepisosteus*, although we have not recognized a separate Dc, there is an increase in the size of neurons in Dm, Dd, and Dl as they are traced from the ependymal surface toward the center of the telencephalic wall. In addition, in *Lepomis* the various subdivisions of Dc seem to be associated with different periventricular groups (see above). This suggests that Dc does not consist of a single neuronal population in all actinopterygians but is formed, at least in some of them, by migrations from several different periventricular zones. Finally, a combination of these two may have occurred, and thus Dc may represent both a migration from Dm, giving rise to a distinct striatal division, and migrations from Dd and/or Dl.

Our speculative interpretation of the teleost telencephalon, like those of the previous schools, clearly goes beyond the data. We have proposed it as an hypothesis which can be tested and hope that it will be useful as a framework for future analyses.

Table VII. Proposed Telencephalic Homologies between Ray-Finned Fishes and Land Vertebrates

Actinopterygian fishes	Land vertebrates
Vv	Medial septal nucleus
Vd	Lateral septal nucleus
Vn + Vl	Olfactory tubercle
Vs + Vc	Basal amygdala
Vp + Vi + NT	Pallial amygdala
Dm (in part)	Dorsal striatum (caudoputamen)
Dc (in part)	Ventral striatum (globus pallidus)
E	Nucleus entopeduncularis
Dp	Lateral pallium
Dd + Dl-d	Dorsal pallium
Dl-v + Dl-p	Medial pallium

C. Evolutionary Considerations

The actinopterygian fishes constitute a large and separate vertebrate radiation. The morphological variation of the telencephalon of these fishes is extreme. In this chapter we have not examined the most complex and highly differentiated teleost telencephalons. These are found in several unrelated groups, including the coral reef beryciforms (e.g., family Holocentridae), the swamp eels (family Synbranchidae), and especially three families of Division II—the Notopteridae, Mormyridae, and Osteoglossidae (van der Horst, 1917; Weston, 1937; Meader, 1939; Nieuwenhuys, 1962*b*, 1963). In discussing this great diversity, Nieuwenhuys (1963) concluded that the range of variation in the telencephalon among actinopterygian fishes is greater than that seen within the Chondrichthyes, Dipnoi, Amphibia, or Reptilia and that the pallium of the Osteoglossidae seems to be further differentiated than that of any reptile. He noted that C. L. Herrick (1891) had gone even further in stating "that the axial lobe [of the telencephalon] of a fish is more complex than that of other animals, not even excepting the bird." Whether or not these conclusions are correct, it is clear that there is no basis for considering ray-finned fishes primitive in relation to other vertebrate groups, as is often done in such so-called "evolutionary" sequences as fish–amphibian–reptile–bird–mammal. Rather, certain trends characterize the evolution within the actinopterygians. These trends include increase in brain size, reduction in olfaction, expansion of the dorsal striatum, and expansion and differentiation of the nonolfactory pallium. Similar, independently evolved trends are seen within other vertebrate radiations. In the Chondrichthyes, increase in brain size and expansion of the nonolfactory pallium have been documented (Northcutt, 1977). Increase in brain size and expansion of the dorsal striatum and the nonolfactory pallium occur within reptiles (Northcutt, 1978) and birds (Stingelin, 1958). In mammals, increase in brain size, decrease in olfaction, and expansion of the dorsal striatum and nonolfactory pallium characterize several lines (Stephan and Andy, 1964; Stephan and Pirlot, 1970; Jerison, 1973; Welker, 1976). These trends, or some of them, occur one or more times in various lines within these classes of vertebrates but do not necessarily characterize an entire class.

Our summary of the trends within the actinopterygians is undoubtedly too simple minded, for little of the variation among the 20,000 or more species has been sampled, and almost no quantitative data on brain parts are available at the present. Moreover, we lack the detailed information on cellular changes and changes in connectivity patterns which is needed to characterize accurately the various trends in the evolution of the telencephalon and assess their functional significance. In a general way, increase in the size of brains or brain parts and increase in the number of units must be related to increases in the information-processing capacity of nervous tissue (Jerison, 1973; Welker, 1976). This, in turn, will undoubtedly be reflected in increasing complexity of behaviors.

Given that there are inherent constraints on the ways that neuronal populations can change, it seems probable that certain ways of solving certain problems have been "discovered" independently by different groups of vertebrates in the course of evolution. We need much more information on the organization and function of central nervous systems and on the natural history and behavioral capabilities of all vertebrates before we can understand either these solutions or the problems that they solve.

ACKNOWLEDGMENTS. We gratefully acknowledge Mr. Ronald G. Nicholes for his excellent histochemical preparations, and we thank the Museum of Zoology, Division of Biological Sciences, The University of Michigan, for the brain of a specimen of *Polypterus congicus*. Research supported by NSF (GB-40134) and NIH (NS 11006) grants to R. G. N. and NINDS (NS 02560) postdoctoral fellowship to M. R. B.

VIII. References

Ariëns Kappers, C. U., Huber, G. C., and Crosby, E. C., 1936, *The Comparative Anatomy of the Nervous System of Vertebrates, Including Man,* reprinted 1960, Hafner, New York.

Bannister, L. H., 1973, Forebrain structure in *Phoxinus phoxinus,* a teleost of the cyprinid family, *J. Hirnforsch.* **14:**413.

Bauchot, R., Bauchot, M. L., Platel, R., and Ridet, J. M., 1977, Brains of Hawaiian tropical fishes; brain size and evolution, *Copeia* **1977:**42.

Bogdanski, D. F., Weissbach, H., and Udenfriend, S., 1957, The distribution of serotonin, 5-hydroxytryptophan decarboxylase, and monoamine oxidase in brain, *J. Neurochem.* **1:**272.

Braford, M. R., Jr., and Northcutt, R. G., 1974, Olfactory bulb projections in the bichir, *Polypterus, J. Comp. Neurol.* **156:**165.

Braford, M. R., Jr., and Northcutt, R. G., 1977, Telencephalic afferents and SDH distribution in *Polypterus, Neurosci. Abstr.* **3:**89.

Broman, I., 1920, Das Organon vomero-nasale Jacobsoni—ein Wassergeruchsorgan! *Anat. Hefte Abt. I* **58:**137 (cited after Parsons, 1970).

Catois, E. H., 1902, Recherches sur l'histologie et l'anatomie microscopique de l'encéphale chez poissons, *Bull. Sci. Fr. Belg.* **36:**1.

Chanconie, M., and Clairambault, P., 1975, Développement du télencéphale de *Salmo irideus* Gib, *J. Hirnforsch.* **16:**75.

Crosby, E. C., DeJonge, B. R., and Schneider, R. C., 1967, Evidence for some of the trends in the phylogenetic development of the vertebrate telencephalon, in: *Evolution of the Forebrain* (R. Hassler and H. Stephan, eds.), pp. 117–135, Plenum Press, New York.

Droogleever-Fortuyn, J., 1961, Topographical relations in the telencephalon of the sunfish, *Eupomotis gibbosus, J. Comp. Neurol.* **116:**249.

Edinger, L., 1896, *Vorlesungen über den Bau der nervösen Zentralorgane*, Vogel, Leipzig.

Fahn, S., 1976, Regional distribution studies of GABA and other putative neurotransmitters and their enzymes, in: *GABA in Nervous Function* (E. Roberts, T. N. Chase, and D. B. Tower, eds.), pp. 169–186, Raven Press, New York.

Faucette, J. R., 1969*a*, The olfactory bulb and medial hemisphere wall of the rat-fish, *Chimaera, J. Comp. Neurol.* **137:**377.

Faucette, J. R., 1969*b*, The accessory olfactory bulbs and the lateral telencephalic wall of the rat-fish, *Chimaera, J. Comp. Neurol.* **137:**407.

Finger, T. E., 1975, The distribution of the olfactory tracts in the bullhead catfish, *Ictalurus nebulosus, J. Comp. Neurol.* **161:**125.

Fink, R. P., and Heimer, L., 1967, Two methods for selective silver impregnation of degenerating axons and their synaptic endings in the central nervous system, *Brain Res.* **4:**369.

Friede, R. L., 1960, Histochemical investigations on succinic dehydrogenase in the central nervous system. IV. A histochemical mapping of the cerebral cortex of the guinea pig, *J. Neurochem.* **5:**156.

Friede, R. L., 1966, *Topographic Brain Chemistry,* Academic Press, New York.

Gage, S. P., 1893, *The Brain of Diemyctilus viridescens from Larval to Adult Life and Comparison with the Brain of Amia and Petromyzon,* pp. 259–314, Wilder Quarter Century Book, Ithaca, N.Y.

Gardiner, B. G., 1967, Further notes on palaeoniscoid fishes with a classification of the Chondrostei, *Bull. Br. Mus. Nat. Hist. (Geol.)* **14:**143-206.

Gardiner, B. G., 1973, Interrelationships of teleostomes in: *Interrelationships of Fishes* (P. H. Greenwood, R. S. Miles, and C. Patterson, eds.), Suppl. No. 1, *Zoological Journal of the Linnaean Society,* Vol. 53, pp. 105–135, Academic Press, New York.

Glenner, G. G., Burtner, H. J., and Brown, G. W., 1957, The histochemical demonstration of monoamine oxidase activity by tetrazolium salts, *J. Histochem. Cytochem.* **5:**591.

Goldstein, K., 1905, Untersuchungen über das Vorderhirn und Zwischenhirn einiger Knochenfische (nebst einigen Beiträgen über Mittelhirn und Kleinhirn derselben), *Arch. Mikrosk. Anat.* **66:**135.

Gomori, G., 1952, *Microscopic Histochemistry: Principles and Practice,* University of Chicago Press, Chicago.

Greenwood, P. H., 1973, Interrelationships of osteoglossomorphs, in: *Interrelationships of Fishes* (P. H. Greenwood, R. S. Miles, and C. Patterson, eds.), Suppl. No. 1, *Zoological Journal of the Linnaean Society,* Vol. 53, pp. 105–135, Academic Press, New York.

Greenwood, P. H., Rosen, D. E., Weitzman, S. H., and Myers, G. S., 1966, Phyletic studies of teleostean fishes, with a provisional classification of living forms, *Bull. Am. Mus. Nat. Hist.* **131:**341.

Hashimoto, P. H., Maeda, T., Torii, K., and Shimizu, N., 1962, Histochemical demonstration of autonomic regions in the central nervous system of the rabbit by means of a monoamine oxidase staining, *Med. J. Osaka Univ.* **12:**425.

Heier, P., 1948, Fundamental principles in the structure of the brain; a study of the brain of *Petromyzon fluviatilis, Acta Anat. Suppl.* **8:**1.

Herrick, C. J., 1910, The morphology of the forebrain in amphibia and reptilia, *J. Comp. Neurol.* **20:**413.

Herrick, C. J., 1921, A sketch of the origin of the cerebral hemispheres, *J. Comp. Neurol.* **32:**429.

Herrick, C. J., 1924, The nucleus olfactorius anterior of the opossum, *J. Comp. Neurol.* **37:**317.

Herrick, C. L., 1891, Contributions to the morphology of the brains of bony fishes. II. Studies on the brains of some American freshwater fishes (cont.), *J. Comp. Neurol.* **1:**333.

Holmgren, N., 1920, Zur Anatomie und Histologie des Vorder- und Zwischenhirns der Knochenfische, *Acta Zool.* **1:**137.

Holmgren, N., 1922, Points of view concerning forebrain morphology in lower vertebrates, *J. Comp. Neurol.* **34:**391.

Holmgren, N., and Stensiö, E. A., 1936, Kranium und Visceralskelett der Akranier, Cyclostomen und Fische, in: *Handbuch der vergleichenden Anatomie der Wirbeltiere* Vol. 4 (L. Bolk, E. Göppert, E. Kallius, and W. Lubosch, eds.), pp. 233–500, Urban and Schwarzenberg, Berlin.

Holmgren, N., and van der Horst, C. J., 1925, Contribution to the morphology of the brain of *Ceratodus, Acta Zool.* **6:**59.

Ichikawa, M., 1976, Fine structure of the olfactory bulb in the goldfish, *Carassius auratus, Brain Res.* **115:**53.

Ishii, Y., 1957, The histochemical studies of cholinesterase in the central nervous system. I. Normal distribution in rodents, *Arch. Histol. Jpn.* **12:**587.

Jacobowitz, D. M., and Palkovits, M., 1974, Topographic atlas of catecholamine and acetylcholinesterase-containing neurons in the rat brain. I. Forebrain (telencephalon, diencephalon), *J. Comp. Neurol.* **157:**13.

Jarvik, E., 1947, Notes on the pit-lines and dermal bones of the head in *Polypterus, Zool. Bidr. Uppsala* **25:**60.

Jarvik, E., 1968, Aspects of vertebrate phylogeny, *Nobel Symp.* **4:**497.

Jerison, H. J., 1973, *Evolution of the Brain and Intelligence,* Academic Press, New York.

Johnston, J. B., 1898, The olfactory lobes, forebrain, and habenular tracts of *Acipenser, Zool. Bull.* **1:**221.

Johnston, J. B., 1901, The brain of *Acipenser, Zool. Jahrb. Abt. Anat. Ontog. Tiere* **15:**59.

Johnston, J. B., 1902, The brain of *Petromyzon, J. Comp. Neurol.* **12:**1.

Johnston, J. B., 1911, The telencephalon of ganoids and teleosts, *J. Comp. Neurol.* **21:**489.

Källén, B., 1951, Embryological studies on the nuclei and their homologization in the vertebrate forebrain, *K. Fysiogr. Saellsk. Handl.* **62:**1.

Kicliter, E., and Ebbesson, S. O. E., 1976, Organization of the "nonolfactory" telencephalon, in:

Frog Neurobiology (R. Llinás and W. Precht, eds.), pp. 946–972, Springer-Verlag, New York.

Kicliter, E., and Northcutt, R. G., 1975, Ascending afferents to the telencephalon of ranid frogs: An anterograde degeneration study, *J. Comp. Neurol.* **161:**239.

Koelle, G. B., 1954, The histochemical localization of cholinesterases in the central nervous system of the rat, *J. Comp. Neurol.* **100:**211.

Kokoros, J. J., and Northcutt, R. G., 1977, Telencephalic efferents of the tiger salamander *Ambystoma tigrinum tigrinum* (Green), *J. Comp. Neurol.* **173:**613.

Kuhlenbeck, H., 1929, Die Grundbestandteile des Endhirns im Lichte der Bauplanlehre, *Anat. Anz.* **67:**1.

Kuhlenbeck, H., 1973, *The Central Nervous System of Vertebrates*, Vol. 3, Part II: *Overall Morphologic Pattern,* Karger, New York.

Kuhlenbeck, H., and Niimi, K., 1969, Further observations on the morphology of the brain in the holocephalian elasmobranchs *Chimaera* and *Callorhynchus, J. Hirnforsch.* **11:**265.

Kusunoki, T., 1969, The chemoarchitectonics of the avian brain, *J. Hirnforsch.* **11:**477.

Kusunoki, T., 1971, The chemoarchitectonics of the turtle brain, *Yokohama Med. Bull.* **22:**1.

Lehman, J.-P., 1966, Actinopterygii, in: *Traité de Paléontologie,* Tome 4, Vol. 3 (J. Pivateau, ed.), pp. 1–242, Masson et Cie., Paris.

Meader, R. G., 1939, The forebrain of bony fishes, *K. Ned. Akad. Wet. Proc. Sect. Sci.* **42:**657.

Miller, R. N., 1940, The telencephalic zonal system of the teleost *Corydora paliatus, J. Comp. Neurol.* **72:**149.

Morgan, G. C., Jr., 1974*a*, The early development of the telencephalon of the marine catfish, *Galeichthys felis, J. Hirnforsch.* **15:**427.

Morgan, G. C., Jr., 1974*b*, The late embryology and maturation of the telencephalon of the marine catfish, *Galeichthys felis, J. Hirnforsch.* **15:**449.

Morgan, G. C., Jr., 1975, The telencephalon of the sea catfish *Galeichthys felis, J. Hirnforsch.* **16:**131.

Moy-Thomas, J. A., 1971, *Palaeozoic Fishes,* 2nd ed., revised by R. S. Miles, Saunders, Philadelphia.

Nieuwenhuys, R., 1962*a*, The morphogenesis and the general structure of the actinopterygian forebrain, *Acta Morphol. Neerl. Scand.* **5:**65.

Nieuwenhuys, R., 1962*b*, Trends in the evolution of the actinopterygian forebrain, *J. Morphol.* **111:**69.

Nieuwenhuys, R., 1963, The comparative anatomy of the actinopterygian forebrain, *J. Hirnforsch.* **6:**171.

Nieuwenhuys, R., 1964, Further studies on the general structure of the actinopterygian forebrain, *Acta Morphol. Neerl. Scand.* **6:**65.

Nieuwenhuys, R., 1965, The forebrain of the crossopterygian *Latimeria chalumnae* Smith, *J. Morphol.* **117:**1.

Nieuwenhuys, R., 1967*a*, The interpretation of cell masses in the teleostean forebrain, in: *Evolution of the Forebrain* (R. Hassler and H. Stephan, eds.), pp. 32–39, Plenum Press, New York.

Nieuwenhuys, R., 1967*b*, Comparative anatomy of olfactory centres and tracts, *Progr. Brain Res.* **23:**1.

Nieuwenhuys, R., 1969, A survey of the structure of the forebrain in higher bony fishes (Osteichthyes), *Ann. N.Y. Acad. Sci.* **167:**31.

Nieuwenhuys, R., and Hickey, M., 1965, A survey of the forebrain of the Australian lungfish *Neoceratodus forsteri, J. Hirnforsch.* **7:**433.

Nieuwenhuys, R., Bauchot, R., and Arnoult, J., 1969, Le développement du télencéphale d'un poisson osseux primitif, *Polypterus senegalus* Cuvier, *Acta Zool.* **50:**101.

Northcutt, R. G., 1974, Some histochemical observations on the telencephalon of the bullfrog, *Rana catesbeiana* Shaw, *J. Comp. Neurol.* **157:**379.

Northcutt, R. G., 1977, Elasmobranch central nervous system organization and its possible evolutionary significance, *Am. Zool.* **17:**411.

Northcutt, R. G., 1978, Forebrain and midbrain organization in lizards and its phylogenetic significance, in: *Behavior and Neurology of Lizards* (N. Greenberg and P. D. MacLean, eds.), pp. 11–64, Department of Health, Education, and Welfare, NIMH, Rockville, Md.

Northcutt, R. G., and Braford, M. R., Jr., 1977, Acetylcholinesterase distribution in the telencephalon of the rainbow trout, *Anat. Rec.* **187:**669.

Northcutt, R. G., and Royce, G. J., 1975, Olfactory bulb projections in the bullfrog *Rana catesbeiana, J. Morphol.* **145:** 251.

Parent, A., and Olivier, A., 1970, Comparative histochemical study of the corpus striatum, *J. Hirnforsch.* **12:**73.

Parent, A., Dubé, L., Braford, M. R., Jr., and Northcutt, R. G., 1977, Histofluorescence study of the monoamine-containing neurons in the brain of the sunfish, *Lepomis gibbosus, Neurosci. Abstr.* **3:**93.

Parsons, T. S., 1970, The origin of Jacobson's organ, *Forma Functio* **3:**105.

Pearse, A. G. E., 1960, *Histochemistry, Theoretical and Applied,* 2nd ed., Little, Brown, Boston.

Pritz, M. B., and Northcutt, R. G., 1977, Succinate dehydrogenase activity in the telencephalon of crocodiles correlates with the projection areas of sensory thalamic nuclei, *Brain Res.* **124:**357.

Rabl-Rückhard, H., 1884, Das Gehirn der Knochenfische, *Biol. Centralbl.* **4:**499, 528.

Ridet, J. M., Gueze, P., Platel, R., and Bauchot, R., 1975, L'allométrie pondérale encéphalo-somatique chez les Poissons Téléostéens des côtes réunionnaises, *C. R. Acad. Sci. Ser. D* **280:**109.

Romer, A. S., 1966, *Vertebrate Paleontology,* 3rd ed., University of Chicago Press, Chicago.

Scalia, F., 1972, The projection of the accessory olfactory bulb in the frog, *Brain Res.* **36:**409.

Scalia, F., and Colman, D. R., 1975, Identification of telencephalic-afferent thalamic nuclei associated with the visual system of the frog, *Neurosci. Abstr.* **1:**46.

Scalia, F., and Ebbesson, S. O. E., 1971, The central projections of the olfactory bulb in a teleost *(Gymnothorax funebris), Brain Behav. Evol.* **4:**376.

Schaeffer, B., 1969, Adaptive radiation of the fishes and the fish–amphibian transition, *Ann. N.Y. Acad. Sci.* **167:**5.

Schaeffer, B., 1973, Interrelationships of chondrosteans, in: *Interrelationships of Fishes* (P. H. Greenwood, R. S. Miles, and C. Patterson, eds.), Suppl. No. 1, *Zoological Journal of the Linnaean Society,* Vol. 53, pp. 207–226, Academic Press, New York.

Schnitzlein, H. N., 1964, Correlation of the habit and structure in the fish brain, *Am. Zool.* **4:**21.

Schnitzlein, H. N., 1968, Introductory remarks on the telencephalon of fish, in: *The Central Nervous System and Fish Behavior* (D. Ingle, ed.), pp. 97–100, University of Chicago Press, Chicago.

Schnitzlein, H. N., and Crosby, E. C., 1967, The telencephalon of the lungfish, *Protopterus, J. Hirnforsch.* **9:**105.

Sheldon, R. E., 1912, The olfactory tracts and centers in teleosts, *J. Comp. Neurol.* **22:**177.

Shen, S. C., Greenfield, P., and Boell, E. J., 1955, The distribution of cholinesterase in the frog brain, *J. Comp. Neurol.* **102:**717.

Shimizu, N., Morikawa, N., and Okada, M., 1959, Histochemical studies of monoamine oxidase of the brain of rodents, *Z. Zellforsch.* **49:**389.

Stephan, H., and Andy, O. J., 1964, Quantitative comparisons of brain structures from Insectivores to Primates, *Am. Zool.* **4:**59.

Stephan, H., and Pirlot, P., 1970, Volumetric comparisons of brain structures in bats, *Z. Zool. Syst. Evolutionsforsch.* **8:**200.

Stingelin, W., 1958, *Vergleichend morphologische Untersuchungen am Vorderhirn der Vögel auf cytologischer und cytoarchitektonischer Grundlage,* Helbing und Lichtenhahn, Basel.

Story, R. H., 1964, The olfactory bulbar formation and related nuclei of the paddlefish *(Polyodon spathula), J. Comp. Neurol.* **123:**285.

Studnicka, F. K., 1896, Beiträge zur Anatomie und Entwicklungsgeschichte des Vorderhirns der Cranioten, *S.-B. Akad. Boehm. Wiss. Math.-Nat. Kl.,* Pt. 2.

van der Horst, C. J., 1917, The forebrain of Synbranchidae, *K. Ned. Acad. Wet. Proc. Sect. Sci.* **20:**216.

Vanegas, H., and Ebbesson, S. O. E., 1976, Telencephalic projections in two teleost species, *J. Comp. Neurol.* **165:**181.

Welker, W., 1976, Brain evolution in mammals: A review of concepts, problems, and methods, in: *Evolution of Brain and Behavior in Vertebrates* (R. B. Masterton, M. E. Bitterman, C. B. G. Campbell, and N. Hotton, eds.), pp. 251–344, Lawrence Erlbaum Associates, Hillsdale, N.J.

Weston, J. K., 1937, Notes on the telencephalon of *Mormyrus* and *Gnathonemus, K. Ned. Acad. Wet. Proc. Sect. Sci.* **40:**894.

Wright, J. D., 1967, The telencephalon of the bichir, *Polypterus, Ala. J. Med. Sci.* **4:**252.

4

The Telencephalon of Teleosts

DOLORES M. SCHROEDER

I. Introduction

The structure of the teleost forebrain (and that of other actinopterygians) is unusual in that there are no lateral ventricles and the two hemispheres are solid lobes separated by a slitlike ventricle. The lobes are covered with an ependymal membrane which is attached to the dorsolateral margins of the hemispheres. One suggestion has been that this forebrain structure is the result of a process of eversion during development (Gage, 1893; Holmgren, 1922; Miller, 1940; Källén, 1947, 1951), whereas the forebrains of most other vertebrates develop by inversion followed by an evagination (Fig. 1B). The proposed eversion growth process would rearrange the functional organization of the dorsal telencephalon, and thus the hippocampal pallium would be in a lateral position, the general cortex dorsal, and the pyriform pallium dorsomedial (Fig. 1C), departing markedly from the arrangement found in inverted–evaginated brains, where the hippocampal pallium is dorsomedial and the pyriform pallium lateral (Fig. 1B).

Another interpretation has been that the topography of the teleost pallium is similar to that of other vertebrates, i.e., the hippocampus is medial and the pyriform is lateral (Fig. 1D) (Sheldon, 1912; Droogleever-Fortuyn, 1961; Crosby *et al.,* 1966; Schnitzlein, 1964, 1977; Singh, 1969; Morgan, 1975). Support for this view comes from a recent embryological study on the telencephalon of *Galeichthys felis* (see Table I for list of common names) wherein Morgan (1974*a,b*) concluded that the growth of the hemispheres is directed primarily dorsally into the ventricle, rather than laterally as would be expected if there was extreme eversion. Although he found a slight folding out of the hemispheres, this did not affect the vertical

---

DOLORES M. SCHROEDER • Medical Sciences Program, Indiana University School of Medicine, Bloomington, Indiana 47401.

arrangement of the proliferative zones of nuclei. Morgan concluded that the hemispheres of Actinopterygii are nonevaginated rather than everted structures and are therefore homologous to those of other vertebrates.

Although Nieuwenhuys (1963, 1967) believes that the actinoptergyian brain everted, he refuses to homologize the pallium as hippocampal, general, or pyriform and states that these areas differentiated entirely within the actinopterygian line and therefore cannot be homologized to areas in any other vertebrate.

II. Terminology

The conflict over the type of development of the teleostean telencephalon is reflected in the variety of terminology for various telencephalic areas. The outline taken from the work of Finger (1975) gives a comparison of nomenclature of several investigators (Table II). The recent trend has been to use the nomenclature of Nieuwenhuys (1963), which avoids the labels of "pyriform" or "hippocampus" and substitutes topological and descriptive terms (Segaar, 1965; Fiedler, 1967; Demski and Knigge, 1971; Bannister, 1973; Chanconie and Clairambault, 1975; Finger, 1975; Peter and Gill, 1975; Peter *et al.,* 1975). This postpones the question of homologies until more experimental data become available on the connections and cytoarchitecture of the telencephalon of teleosts. The stereotaxic atlas on the forebrain of *Carassius auratus* (Peter and Gill, 1975) and *Fundulus heteroclitus* (Peter *et al.,* 1975) will encourage studies by electrophysiologists as well as anatonomists using either silver stains for degenerating fibers, autoradiography, or horseradish peroxidase for tracing pathways.

III. Gross Anatomy and Cytoarchitecture

There is considerable anatomical variation within the basic structure of the telencephalon of teleosts. The hemispheres may consist of small lobes without

Table I. Species and Common Names of Fish Discussed in This Chapter

Ameiurus nebulosus	Brown bullhead	*Gymnothorax funebris*	Green moray eel
Betta splendens	Siamese fighting fish	*Hemichromis*	Jewel fish
		Holocentrus	Squirrelfish
Carassius auratus	Goldfish	*Ictalurus nebulosus*	Bullhead catfish
Corydora paliatus	Peppered corydora	*Ictalurus punctatus*	Channel catfish
Crenilabrus	Wrasses	*Lebistes reticulatus*	Guppy
Cyprinus carpio	Carp	*Lepomis cyanellus*	Green sunfish
Diplodus	Sea breams	*Macropodus opercularis*	Paradise fish
Eugerres	Mojarra	*Micropterus salmoides*	Largemouth bass
Esox lucius	Great Northern pike	*Phoxinus phoxinus*	Minnow
Fundulus heteroclitus	Killifish	*Plecostomus*	Plecostomus catfish
Galeichythys felis	Marine catfish	*Polypterus palmas*	Bichir
Gasterosteus aculeatus	Three-spined stickleback	*Tilapia mossambica*	East African mouthbreeder

fissures, or they may have deep fissures and several large lobes. Several brains with a relatively large telencephalon are illustrated in Fig. 2, and a small telencephalon, in Fig. 3. The olfactory bulbs are closely applied to the hemispheres in most teleosts, but in Ostariophysi (carp families), Anacanthini (cod families), and Mormyrids (elephant fish), the olfactory bulb remains by the nasal sacs and the olfactory tracts elongate (Aronson and Kaplan, 1968).

The gross anatomy and cytoarchitecture of the telencephalon of species representing the order *Ostariophysi* have been studied extensively. These include *Ameiurus* (Johnston, 1911), *Cyprinus* (Sheldon, 1912), *Corydora* (Miller, 1940), *Carassius* (Schnitzlein, 1964; Peter and Gill, 1975); *Hypostomus* (Schnitzlein *et al.*, 1973), *Phoxinus* (Bannister, 1973), *Galeichthys* (Morgan, 1974*a,b,* 1975), and *Ictalurus* (Finger, 1975).

Ictalurus punctatus is used here as an example to illustrate some of the basic features of the teleost forebrain. The side and top views of the brain (Fig. 4) indicate the relative size of the telencephalon in respect to other major brain structures. (The olfactory bulbs are a considerable distance from the brain, and only the olfactory tracts are included in this figure.)

In the transverse Nissl-stained sections of the catfish telencephalon, only the major areas are labeled (Fig. 5). To compare these labels with the ones used by other authors, consult Table II, Nieuwenhuys (1963), and Peter and Gill (1975). The telencephalon may be divided into dorsal and ventral areas. The dorsal area is highly variable among teleosts (Figs. 2, 3, 7, and 8), whereas the ventral area is quite consistent in its internal organization.

The dorsal area consists of medial, dorsal, and lateral cellular fields surrounding a central field. The area dorsalis pars medialis (Dm) extends throughout the length of the telencephalon, occupying the dorsomedial section. The rostral Dm consists of small neurons arranged in diffuse laminae (Fig. 5A). One type of neuron extends its dendrites primarily toward the center (Fig. 6B) while another type extends its dendrites laterally (parallel to the ventricular surface) and medially

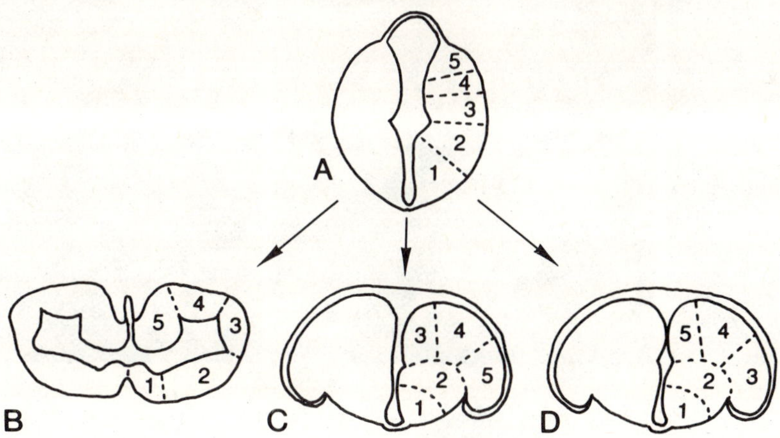

Figure 1. Representation of the way in which the topology of the fundamental subdivisions of an embryonic telencephalon (A) might be preserved after evagination (B), eversion (C), or nonevagination (D). 1, Septal region; 2, striatum; 3, pyriform pallium; 4, general pallium; 5, hippocampal pallium.

(Bannister, 1973; Ito, 1973). Bannister (1973) describes these axons as entering the anterior commissure and fasciculus lateralis telencephali (flt). In the caudal regions of Dm the cell bodies are larger and their axons extend to the lateral lobes of the hypothalamus, to the nucleus preopticus, and to the corresponding contralateral regions via the anterior commissure (Bannister, 1973).

Area dorsalis pars dorsalis (Dd) is a small region between the sulcus ypsiliforms and Dm. The multipolar cells are similar to those of Dm (Ito, 1973).

Area dorsalis pars lateralis (Dl) consists of a large lateral area of rostral telencephalon and decreases in size caudally. Although nuclear groups are evident, no

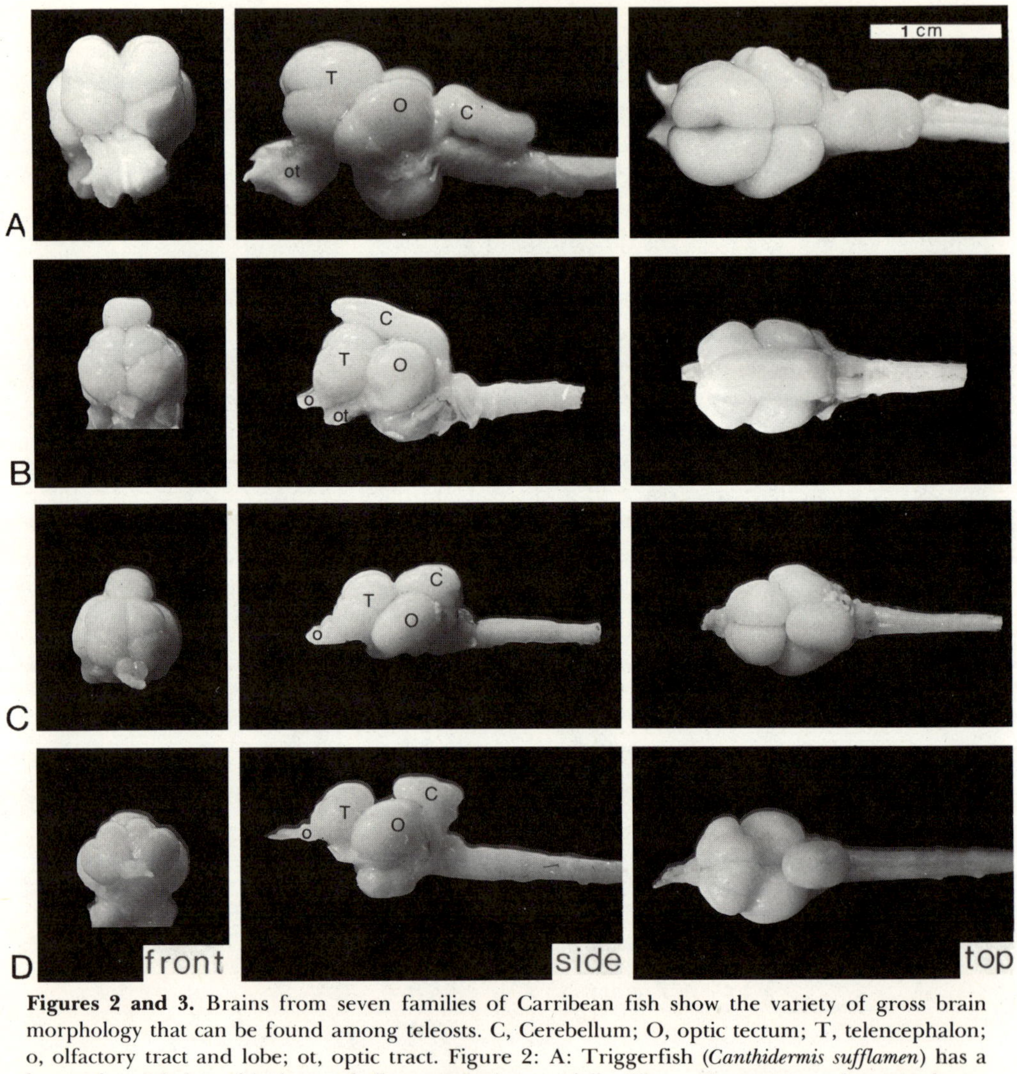

Figures 2 and 3. Brains from seven families of Carribean fish show the variety of gross brain morphology that can be found among teleosts. C, Cerebellum; O, optic tectum; T, telencephalon; o, olfactory tract and lobe; ot, optic tract. Figure 2: A: Triggerfish (*Canthidermis sufflamen*) has a large telencephalon with the cerebellum projecting caudally. The optic tracts are also quite large. B: Surgeon fish (*Acanthurus bahianus*) has a large telencephalon with several lobes, and the cerebellum overlies the telencephalon and optic tectum. C: Yellow tail snapper (*Ocyurus chysurus*) demonstrates the olfactory bulbs at the base of the large telencephalon. (The optic tracts were removed.)

attempt can be made to label them without additional experimental material. There are several neuronal cell types in Dl. The neurons located at the periphery have their dendrites parallel to the surface and extending medially (Fig. 6A) or occasionally branching from a thick process (Fig. 6C, right). Medially located cells have dendrites radiating from the soma in all directions (Fig. 6C, middle). Ito (1973) remarked that the cells in Dl have wider dendritic fields and more spines than those in Dm and Dd. Connections are with ipsilateral dorsal and ventral areas of the telencephalon, with the contralateral Dl via the anterior commissure, and with the hypothalamus (Bannister, 1973). Experimental material indicates that the ol-

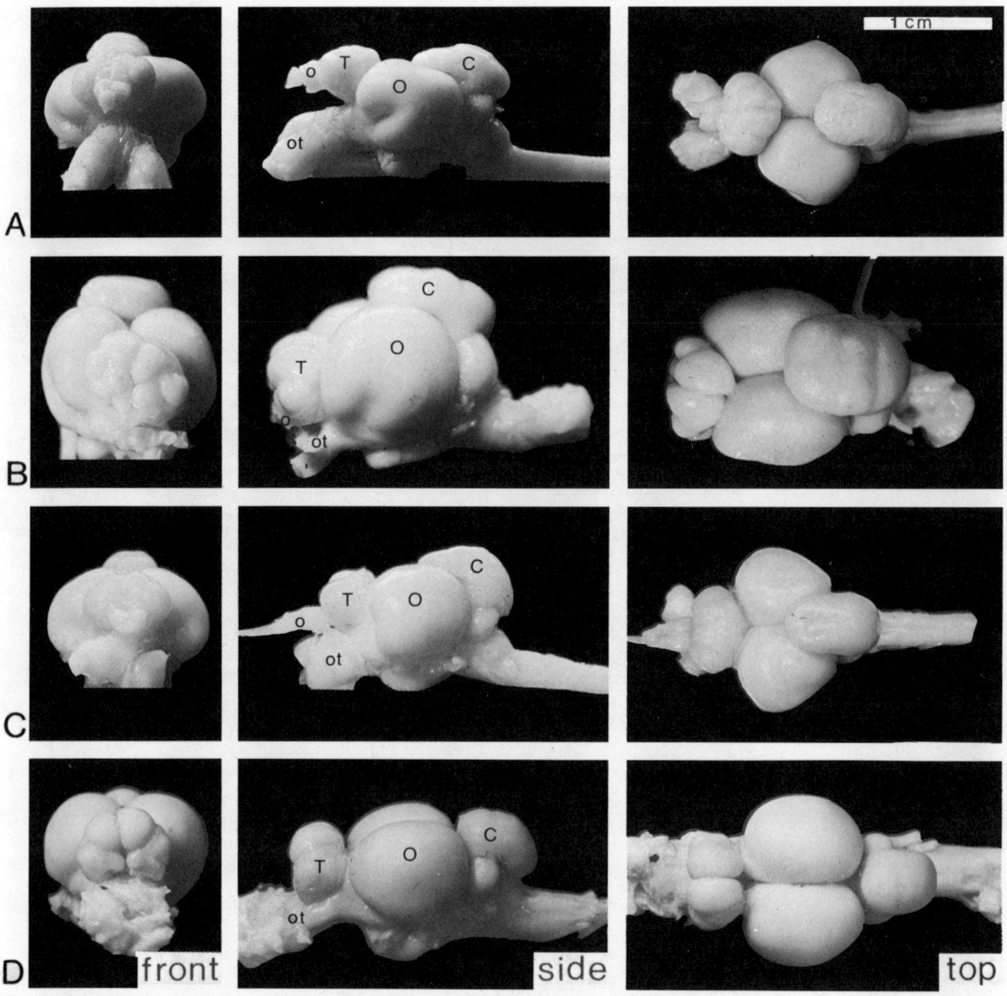

D: Red hind (*Epinephalus guttatus*) belongs to the grouper family, and the olfactory lobes are at the base of the telencephalon with large ventral lobes. Figure 3: A: Big-eyed scad (*Selar crumenophthalmus*) has a small telencephalon but very large optic tracts and optic tectum. B: Wahoo (*Acanthocybium solanderi*) belongs in the family with tunas and mackerels, and the large optic tectum overshadows the telencephalon. C: Blue runner (*Caranx fusus*) has a brain quite similar to that of the big-eyed scad, to which it is related. D: Great barracuda (*Sphyraena barracuda*), like the previous large predators, has a large optic tectum and small telencephalon (the olfactory lobes were torn away).

Table II. Comparison of Teleost Nomenclatures[a]

Nieuwenhuys (1963)	Goldstein (1905)	Ariëns-Kappers (1906)	Johnston (1911)
I. Area dorsalis (D)		Pars pallialis	Primord. hippocampi
1. Pars lateralis (Dl)	With region IV1 = lob. olf. post. p. lateralis	N. teniae (plus portions of a. olf. lat. and paleopallium)	
2. Pars dorsalis (Dd)		Portion of area olf. lat.	
3. Pars medialis (Dm)	With region II = striatum	Striatum	
II. Area dorsalis centralis (Dc)	With regions I2 and I3 = striatum	Striatum	Striatum
III. Area dorsalis pars lateralis posterior (Dlp) (also n. teniae)	N. teniae	N. teniae	Area superficialis basalis
IV.	Area olf. lateralis		
1. Area ventralis dorsalis (Vd)	With region I1 = lob. olf. post p. lat.	Lat. connect. lat. olf. area and epistriatum	Unnamed
2. Area ventralis intermedius (Vi)	Lob. olf. post. p. med.	Epistriatum	N. olf. medialis
3. With region V = area ventralis lateralis (V1)	Unnamed	N. olf. ant. p. precomm.	N. olf. lateralis
V. With region IV3 = area ventralis lateralis (V1)	Unnamed	N. circumstrialis	Area somatic
VI. Area ventralis ventralis (Vv)	Unnamed	N. precomm. p. inf.	Corpus precommissuralis
Sheldon (1912)	**Herrick (1922)**	**Holmgren (1922)**	**Droogleever-Fortuyn (1961)[b]**
I.	Area of dorsalis	Primord. pallii	Lobar
1. N. olfact. lateralis (lob. pyrif. plus n. taeniae)	Pars lateralis	Pars lateralis (primord. hippocampi)	Basolateral amygdala
2. N. olfact. lateralis	Pars dorsolateralis	Pars dorsolateralis (general pallium)	Gen. primord. cortex
3. N. olfact. dorsalis (primord. hippocampi)	Pars dorsomedialis	Pars medialis (lobus pyriformis)	Main part of primord. hippocampi
II. Paleostriatum	Area olfact.-somatica	Primord. pallii pars dorsolat. (= p. striatalis)	Striate body
III. N. teniae	N. occipitobasalis	N. teniae	Unnamed
IV.	Area olf. lateralis		
1. Corp. precomm. p. intermed. lateral division	Pars lateralis	N. olf. lat. p. lat.	Corticomedial amygdala
2. Corp. precomm. p. intermed. medial division	Pars medialis	N. precomm. pars. super.	Medial septal
3. N. comm. lateralis	Pars ventralis	N. olf. lat. p. vent.	Prepiriform area
V. N. entopeduncularis	Area somatica	Unnamed	N. entopeduncularis
VI. Corp. precommissuralis pars comm. plus p. medianus	Area olf. medialis	N. precommissuralis pars inferior	N. of the diagonal band

[a] Modified from Finger (1975).
[b] This terminology is also used by Schnitzlein (1964), Crosby *et al.* (1966), Singh (1969), and Morgan (1975).

factory tract projects to the ventral part of Dl in *Gymnothorax* (Fig. 7) (Scalia and Ebbesson, 1971), *Cyprinus* (Ito, 1973), and *Ictalurus* (Fig. 8) (Finger, 1975).

Area dorsalis pars lateralis posterior (Dlp) is the ventrolateral extension of Dl and is most prominent in caudal regions (Fig. 5B,C). Within this area, nucleus teniae can be distinguished caudal to the anterior commissure and immediately lateral to the external sulcus. Dlp has neurons that are bipolar (Fig. 6F, bottom) or with dendrites either emerging from the soma only at one side (Fig. 6E), or radiating in all directions (Fig. 6F, top). Ito (1973) indicated that in Dlp the cells are small and have short spine-poor dendrites emerging in all directions. Finger (1975) described dendrites of Dlp neurons as orienting toward the incoming olfactory tract fibers and the spiny dendrites of some nucleus teniae neurons either extending around somas within the nucleus or spreading dorsally and ventrally. Dpl receives extensive input from the olfactory tract (Figs. 7 and 8), with nucleus teniae receiving a dense terminal projection in *Ictalurus* (in areas caudal to Fig. 8). Connections of Dlp are to corresponding contralateral regions via the anterior commissure, nucleus preopticus parvocellularis, and other ventral telencephalic areas.

Area dorsalis pars centralis (Dc) is the central region of the telencephalon, consists of scattered large cells, and extends throughout the length of the telencephalon. These large somas have thick dendrites with many spines (Fig. 6D) (Sheldon, 1912; Bannister, 1973; Ito, 1973). Olfactory projections have been traced to its caudoventral areas (Scalia and Ebbesson, 1971; Ito, 1973; Finger, 1975). Axons of Dc neurons spread collaterals within Dc and extend across the commissure to the contralateral Dc (Bannister, 1973).

Turowski and Danner (1977) describe some neurons in the dorsal telencephalon of *Salmo irideus* which are generally very similar to the ones described for

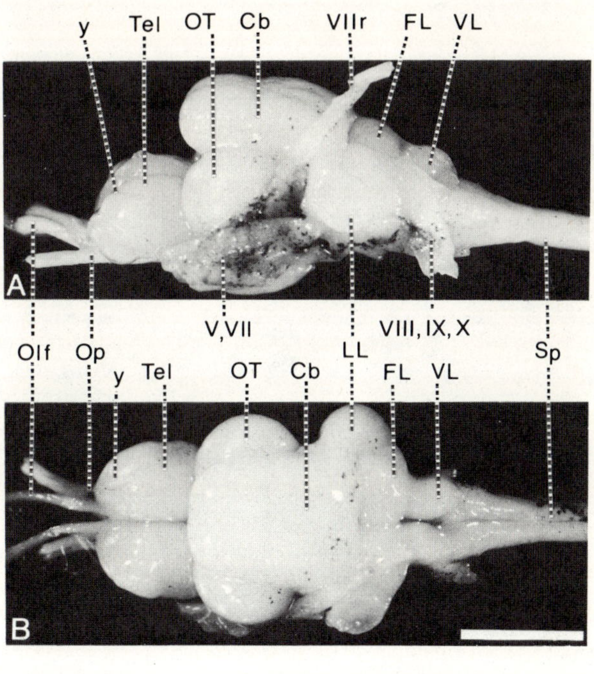

Figure 4. Side view (A) and top view (B) of the *Ictalurus punctatus* brain. Calibration bar is 5 mm. Cb, Cerebellum; Fl, facial lobe; LL, lateral line lobe; Olf, olfactory tract; Op, optic tract; OT, optic tectum; Sp, spinal cord; Tel, telencephalon; VL, vagus lobe; y, sulcus ypsiliformis; V–VII, trigeminal and facial cranial nerves (includes anterior lateral line nerve); VIII, IX, X, cranial nerves (including posterior lateral line nerve), VIIr, recurrens branch of facial nerve.

Ostariophysi, to resemble the pyramidal neurons. They conclude that these cytological data indicate that the dorsal telencephalon is homologous to limbic areas of other vertebrates.

Area ventralis is subdivided into two major zones: area ventralis pars dorsalis (Vd) and area ventralis pars ventralis (Vv). Vd, the larger one, is ventral to Dm and dorsal to Vv. It can be divided into several subdivisions. Just dorsal to the anterior commissure is the supracommissural area (Vs) (Fig. 5C). Caudal to the anterior commissure is the postcommissural zone (Vp), which in some species has a lateralward extension, pars intermedia (Vi). Pars lateralis (Vl, Fig. 5) is the lateral portion of Vd.

Area ventralis pars ventralis (Vv) is along the ventralmost portion of the ventricle (Fig. 5A,B,C). At the level of the anterior commissure and caudal to it, nucleus preopticus appears (Fig. 5B,C).

The neurons in area ventralis are quite small. In the dorsal division they are arranged in lamellae, and in the ventral area they are quite dense near the ventricles

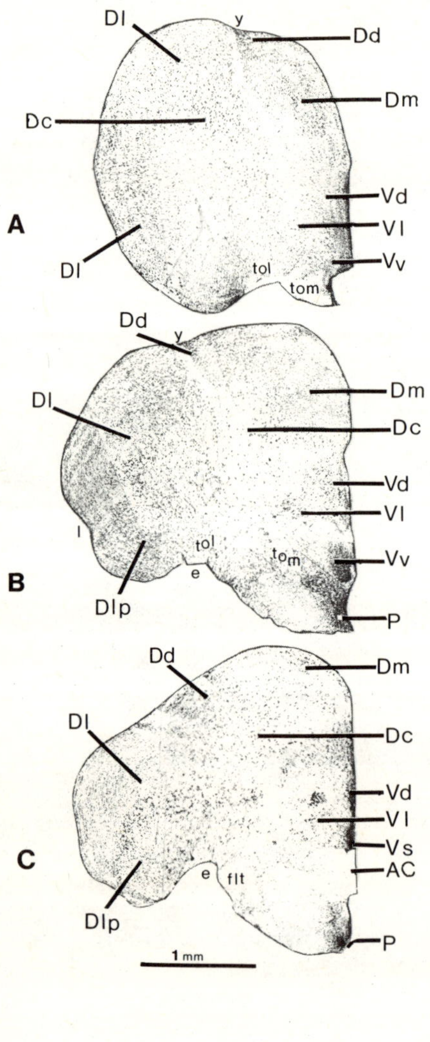

Figure 5. Transverse sections through the telencephalon of *Ictalurus punctatus*. Cresylecht violet stain. (A) Rostral, (B) middle, and (C) caudal regions. AC, Anterior commissure; Dc, area dorsalis pars centralis; Dd, area dorsalis pars dorsalis; Dl, area dorsalis pars lateralis; Dlp, area dorsalis pars lateralis posterior; Dm, area dorsalis pars medialis; e, sulcus externus; flt, fasciculus lateralis telencephali; l, sulcus lateralis; P, area preoptica; tom, tractus olfactorius medialis; tol, tractus olfactorius lateralis; Vd, area ventralis pars dorsalis; Vl, area ventralis pars lateralis; Vs, area ventralis pars supracommissuralis; Vv, area ventralis pars ventralis; y, sulcus ypsiliformis.

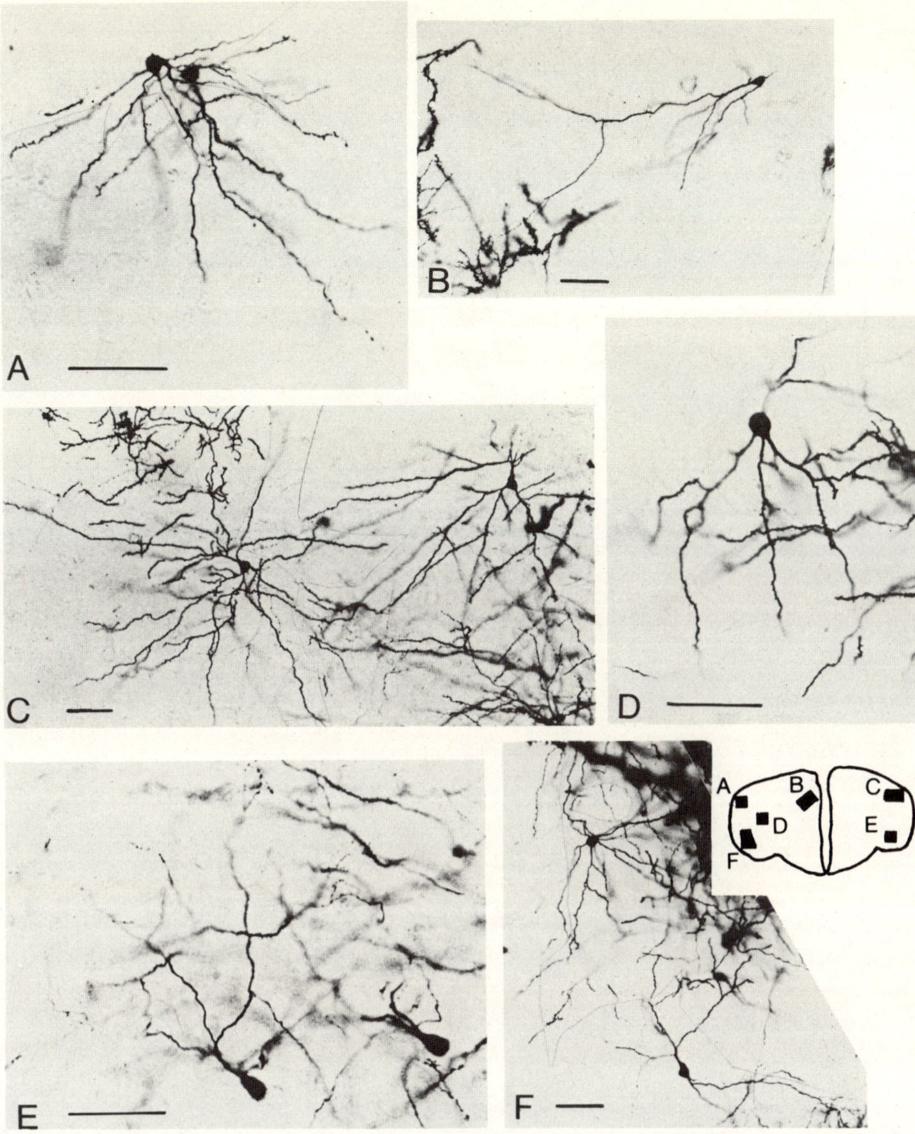

Figure 6. Golgi-impregnated neurons of the dorsal telencephalon of *Ictalurus punctatus*. Golgi–Kopsch procedure. Calibration bar is 0.05 mm. Inset shows the location of the neurons. A: Two neurons at the edge of the telencephalon in area dorsalis pars lateralis show the pattern that many peripherally located neurons have. The dendrites extend laterally and parallel to the ventricle and medially. B: A small cell in the medial edge of area dorsalis pars medialis has dendrites extending primarily toward the center of the telencephalon. The initial segment of the axons can be seen projecting toward the medial surface. C: Two dendritic patterns of neurons located in area dorsalis pars lateralis show the dendrites emerging either from the soma from all sides (right) or in part from a thick dendritic trunk (left). D: The neurons in area dorsalis pars centralis have large somas, and the thick dendrites are covered with spines. E: Some neurons in area dorsalis pars lateralis posterior have flask-shaped somas. F: Some neurons in area dorsalis pars lateralis posterior have dendrites radiating either in all directions from the soma (top) or branching from dendritic trunks (lower).

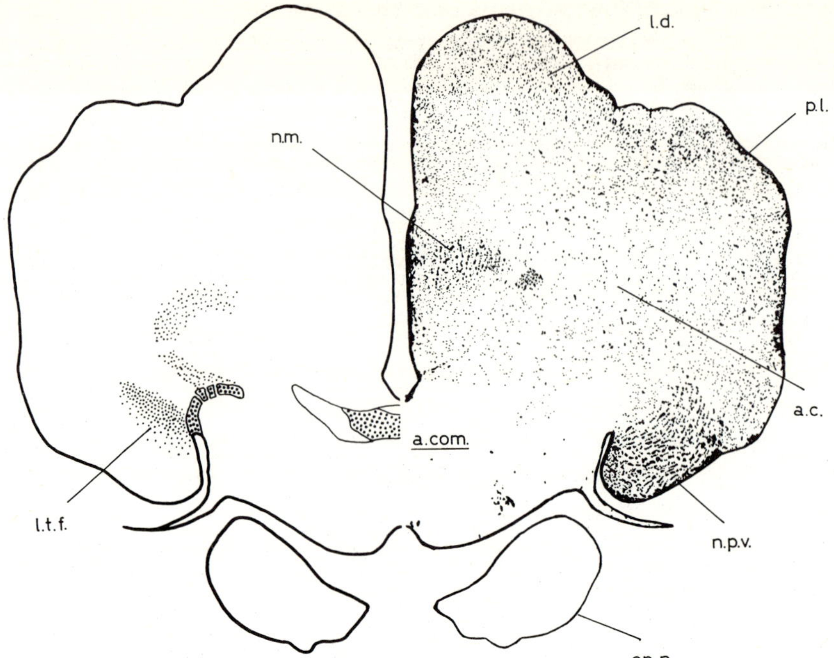

Figure 7. Olfactory tract projection in *Gymnothorax funebris*. The transverse section is at the level of the anterior commissure. a.c., Area centralis; a. com., anterior commissure; l.d., dorsal lobe; l.t.f., lateral terminal field; n.m., nucleus medianus; n.p.v., nucleus posteroventralis; op.n., optic nerve; p.l., posterolateral cortex. From Scalia and Ebbesson (1971).

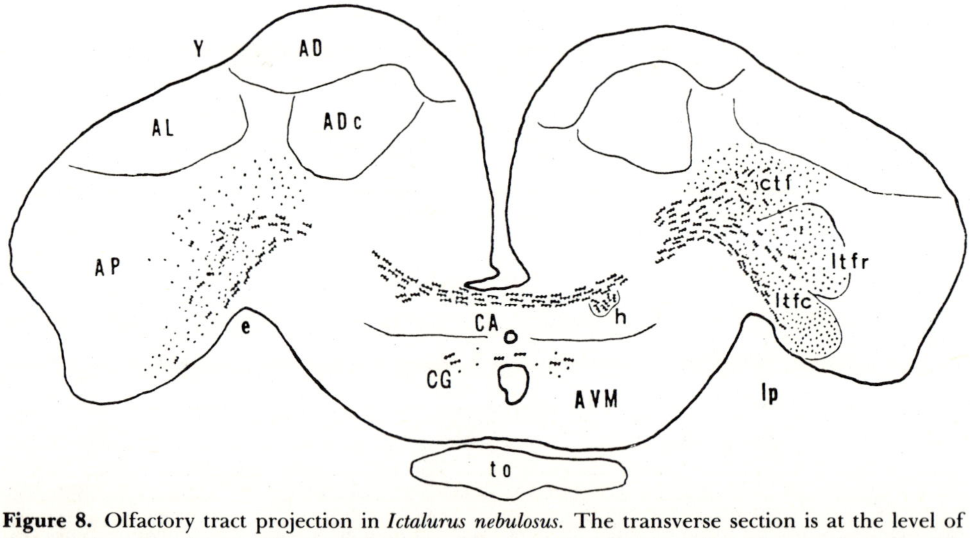

Figure 8. Olfactory tract projection in *Ictalurus nebulosus*. The transverse section is at the level of the anterior commissure. AD, Area dorsalis; ADc, area dorsalis centralis; AL, area lateralis; AP, area posterior; AVM, area ventralis medialis; CA, commissura anterior; CG, commissura olfactoria interbulbaris of Goldstein; ctf, commissural terminal field; e, sulcus endorhinalis; h, hypothalamic branch of medial olfactory tract; Ip, side ipsilateral to the lesion; ltfc, lateral terminal field pars caudalis; ltfr, lateral terminal field pars rostralis; to, tractus opticus; Y, sulcus ypsiliformis. From Finger (1975).

and dispersed laterally. Bannister (1973) noted that the dendritic pattern differs between Vd and Vv neurons. The former possess two or three main dendrites which branch irregularly in tangential plane or are oriented obliquely in a dorsolateral direction, whereas the ventrally located cells either are in the periventricular zone and are flask shaped with dendrites projecting laterally or are laterally located with their dendrites oriented parallel to fibers around them. The dendrites of area ventralis neurons have few if any spines (Ito, 1973).

Connections of area ventralis consist of olfactory tract projections which are very limited (Fig. 8). The efferents are to the medial hypothalamus via medial forebrain bundle.

The major afferent and efferent fiber tracts of the teleostean telencephalon are the olfactory tracts and basal forebrain bundles. The projections of the medial and lateral olfactory tract have been demonstrated with experimental methods and will be discussed later in this chapter. The descriptions of the basal forebrain bundles are according to Sheldon (1912), Schnitzlein (1962; Schnitzlein *et al.,* 1973), Nieuwenhuys (1963), and Bannister (1973).

The lateral forebrain bundle (fasciculus lateralis telencephali, flt) is the major fiber system of the telencephalon in teleosts. The fibers originate from all parts of area dorsalis (except Dlp and nucleus teniae), collect at the medial wall of sulcus externus, and proceed caudally to the diencephalon. Two distinct components are present in flt: the dorsal portion, consisting predominantly of myelinated fibers, and the ventral portion of fine unmyelinated fibers. The dorsal portion terminates in nucleus dorsolateralis of dorsal thalamus, area pretectalis, and nucleus rotundus, and the ventral portion terminates in nucleus preglomerulosus and nucleus glomerulosus but primarily in the lateral lobes of the hypothalamus. Johnston (1911) believed that flt had only ascending fibers from the hypothalamus to area dorsalis. Although Nieuwenhuys (1963) suggests that a portion of flt decussates in the

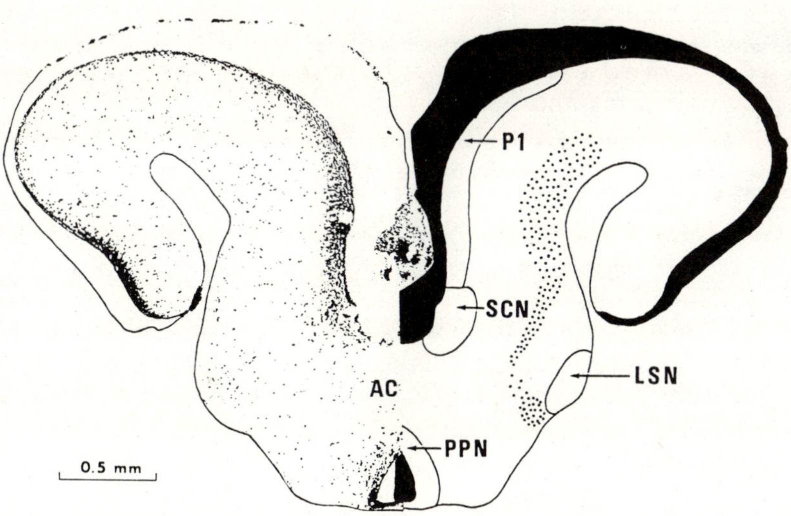

Figure 9. Olfactory tract projection in *Polypterus*. The transverse section is at the level of the anterior commissure. LSN, Lateral subpallial nucleus; Pl, "medial" pallial area; PPN, periventricular preoptic nucleus; SCN, supracommissural nucleus. From Braford and Northcutt (1974).

anterior commissure, this was not observed by Schnitzlein (1962) or Bannister (1973).

The medial forebrain bundle (fasciculus medialis telencephali, fmt) consists of short and long axons interconnecting the area ventralis with the medial hypothalamus, particularly nucleus preopticus and the cell masses immediately ventral to nucleus glomerulosus. Most of the fibers in fmt appear to be descending.

IV. Olfactory Tract Projections

Since the olfactory tract projects to the pyriform rather than the hippocampal pallium in all vertebrates where it has been examined with experimental methods, a closer examination of this tract in Actinopterygii with experimental methods should help to clarify the functional organization of their telencephalon. Experimental material on the olfactory tract projection of a chondrostean, *Polypterus* (Braford and Northcutt, 1974), and three teleosts, *Gymnothorax* (Scalia and Ebbesson, 1971), *Cyprinus* (Ito, 1973), and *Ictalurus* (Finger, 1975), is available. In *Polypterus* (Fig. 9) the olfactory tract projects primarily to the medial pallium (P1), which makes it homologous to that of the lateral or pyriform pallium of inverted forebrains. The olfactory tract projections of teleosts differ from *Polypterus* and also from each other. In *Gymnothorax* (Fig. 7) the lateral olfactory tract terminates in the lateral terminal field of the ventrolateral pallium (Dlp) and, together with the medial olfactory tract, in the posterior terminal field in the posterior lobe (Dc). Part of the medial tract terminates in the medial terminal field in the ventromedial area (Vv) and part crosses to terminate in the same area on the contralateral side as well as in the contralateral olfactory bulb. A similar pattern was described in *Ictalurus* (Fig. 8) and *Cyprinus*; however, projections to the contralateral side were more extensive than in *Gymnothorax,* with the lateral olfactory tract crossing partly in the anterior and habenular commissures and the medial tract in the anterior commissure. Scalia and Ebbesson (1971) suggest that the lateral, posterior, and medial terminal fields correspond to prepyriform cortex, amygdala, and olfactory tubercle of other vertebrates. Thus the pyriform lobe would be located in the *lateral* portion of the pallium rather than the medial portion.

Thus in *Polypterus* the major olfactory tract projection is to the dorsomedial pallium, whereas in teleosts the projection is to the ventrolateral part of the pallium. Braford and Northcutt (1974) concluded that "(1) the eversion of the pallium in teleosts is not a simple one and is accompanied by more complicated morphogenetic movement; (2) the migrations of cell populations within the developing teleost pallium obscure their sites of origin from the germinal matrix; and (3) during later stages of development differential proliferations of certain cell populations result in changes in their relative topographical positions. The three processes are not mutually exclusive and may all contribute to the formation of the pallium in teleosts" (p. 177).

V. Nonolfactory Efferent and Afferent Projections

Only recently have experimental techniques been applied to trace the efferents and afferents of the teleosts' telencephalon. Vanegas and Ebbesson (1976) made large unilateral lesions in the telencephalic lobe of *Eugerres* and *Holocentrus* and traced the degenerating fibers with the silver methods. Terminations were found in the contralateral telencephalic lobe and in the ipsilateral deep layers of the optic tectum, caudal hypothalamus, dorsomedial optic nucleus, medial region of the prethalamic nucleus of *Holocentrus* (thought to be homologous to nucleus rotundus), and bilaterally in nucleus rotundus of *Eugerres*. Injections of tritiated proline into the telencephalon of *Micropterus salmoides* showed a similar projection pattern to tectum and diencephalon as described by Vanegas and Ebbesson (Friedlander, 1978).

Telencephalic efferents to the tectum were examined by Ito and Kishida (1977) by injecting horseradish peroxidase into the superficial or deep layers of the optic tectum of *Cyprinus carpio*. Labeled cells in the telencephalon were seen only in the animals with deep tectal injections and were located in area dorsalis pars centralis (Dc) of the ipsilateral telencephalon. Their axons descend in the medial part of the lateral forebrain bundle and enter the tectum via the dorsomedial margin. The projections of the telencephalon to the deep layers of the tectum are consistent with the findings of Vanegas and Ebbesson and those reported for a variety of other vertebrates.

To investigate a possible source of afferents to the telencephalon, Ito and Kishida (1978) injected horseradish peroxidase into the telencephalon of *Cyprinus carpio*. They found labeled cells only in the nucleus preglomerulosus pars lateralis of the diencephalon.

The interconnections of the telencephalon with visual regions in the diencephalon, pretectum, and tectum were examined by Friedlander (1978) with electrophysiological techniques. Working with *Micropterus salmoides,* he described the response properties of the visually activated neurons and then examined their response to the stimulating electrodes placed on the telencephalon. Orthodromic responses of visually driven units in diencephalic–pretectal–tectal units were found in all regions tested except the dorsomedial thalamus. Both excitatory and inhibitory effects were seen, and some were capable of causing long-lasting effects on these cells as well as modifying their response to visual stimulation. Antidromic activation was found only in the dorsomedial thalamus.

In summary, experimental techniques indicate that the telencephalon of teleosts projects to various diencephalic and mesencephalic regions. Fewer data are available on ascending systems, and they imply that only a few diencephalic regions may be involved.

VI. Behavior following Ablations

The functions of the teleostean telencephalon have been examined with behavioral studies. These have been reviewed by Ten Cate (1935), Healey (1957), Aronson (1963), Segaar (1965), and Aronson and Kaplan (1968). Among the effects of the removal of the forebrain in fish are an increased threshold for elicitation of aggression in the sunfish, stickleback, and jewel fish (Noble, 1937; Hale, 1956; Segaar, 1961); reduction of fighting intensity in wrasses (Fiedler, 1967); disruption of some aspects of reproductive behavior in the East African mouthbreeder, stickleback, and jewel fish (Noble, 1937; Aronson, 1948; Segaar, 1960) and paradise fish (Davis *et al.*, 1976; Kassel *et al.*, 1976; Schwagmeyer *et al.*, 1977); impairment of avoidance learning in the goldfish and mouthbreeder (Kaplan and Aronson, 1967; Savage, 1969; Overmier and Gross, 1974); reduction of gill cover response, efficiency of food retrieval, and activity level in Siamese fighting fish (Shapiro *et al.*, 1974); depression of all reproductive cycle behavior of East African mouthbreeders regardless of their closeness to spawning (Overmier and Gross, 1974); and influence on schooling in goldfish (Kumakura, 1928), minnows (Hosch, 1936; Berwein, 1941), and jewel fish (Noble, 1936).

Forebrain ablation, however, does not influence classical conditioning (Overmier and Starkman, 1974), abolish color vision in the goldfish (Bernstein, 1962), or influence the degree of aggressive and feeding behavior in sea breams (Fiedler, 1967).

Some of the behavioral results after forebrain lesion strengthen the notion that functional analogies exist between the teleost forebrain and the mammalian limbic system and striatum (Segaar, 1965; Overmier and Gross, 1974), as has been suggested by anatomical studies (Droogleever-Fortuyn, 1961; Schnitzlein, 1964). Forebrain-ablated goldfish had a deficit in long-term memory (Peeke *et al.*, 1972), but short-term memory was apparently unaffected (Peeke *et al.*, 1972; Overmier and Savage, 1974). The disruption of the limbic system and striatal function in mammals has also been shown to interfere with formation of memory (Brunner *et al.*, 1970; Herz and Peeke, 1971; Kesner and Doty, 1968; McIntyre, 1970).

Aronson and Kaplan (1968) interpret a major function of the forebrain as a "nonspecific arousal mechanism which impinges on lower centers and keeps them operating at high levels of efficiency. Quality changes in behavior after forebrain removal are related to changes in arousal, and the similarity of these changes to those following lesions of the limbic system in mammals is noted" (p. 121). Generally, the functions of the forebrain are still controversial and speculative.

VII. Regeneration

There has been some question regarding the regenerative capacity of the teleost forebrain. Maron (1963) removed the forebrain from 4-day-old *Lebistes reticulatus*, and by the 60th postoperative day the telencephalon did not differ in size or shape from that of the control animals. Segaar (1965) with the stickleback showed that there was some regeneration after lesions to the lateral hemisphere, although the original form was not achieved. If the rostral telencephalon was ablated, there was no regeneration. Bernstein (1967), with goldfish ranging in age from 6 months to 3 years, did not observe any regeneration after removal of all or part of the forebrain or infliction of stab wounds.

There is considerable regeneration after removal of the optic tectum of carp (Kirsche and Kirsche, 1961), although again the original shape and size are not achieved. After spinal cord section (Bernstein, 1964), nerves regenerated to reach their original sites of termination. After cutting the olfactory tract, it was shown behaviorally and histologically that olfactory tracts regenerate in young carp (Westerman and von Baumgarten, 1964). The experiments with regenerating optic nerves to the optic tectum have been used as an experimental model by many investigators (i.e., Attardi and Sperry, 1963; Jacobson and Gaze, 1965; Gaze and

Keating, 1972). Thus the regenerative capacity of the central nervous system of the teleost is dependent on the area of the CNS, the age, and the species.

VIII. Conclusion

The data indicate at this time that the development and organization of the telencephalon of teleosts cannot be accounted for totally on the basis of eversion or as homologous to other vertebrates. The olfactory tracts project to lateral and ventral telencephalic areas, leaving dorsal, central, and medial areas to which only minimal input has been demonstrated with experimental methods. Behavioral studies following ablation imply that the forebrain is involved with a variety of functions, but their exact nature is still obscure. Considerably more anatomical and electrophysiological data must be gathered before more precise answers can be given on the structure and function of the teleostean telencephalon.

IX. References

Ariëns-Kappers, C. U., 1906, The structure of the teleostean and selachian brian, *J. Comp. Neurol.* **16:**1.

Aronson, L. R., 1948, Problems in the behavior and physiology of a species of African mouth breeding fish, *Trans. N.Y. Acad. Sci. Ser. 2* **2:**33.

Aronson, L. R., 1963, The central nervous system of sharks and bony fishes with special reference to sensory and integrative mechanisms, in: *Sharks and Survival* (P. W. Gilbert, ed.), pp. 165–241, Heath, Boston.

Aronson, L. R., and Kaplan, H., 1968, Function of the teleostean forebrain, in: *The Central Nervous System and Fish Behavior* (D. Ingle, ed.), pp. 107–125, University of Chicago Press, Chicago.

Attardi, D. G., and Sperry, R. W., 1963, Preferential selection of central pathways by regenerating optic fibers, *Exp. Neurol.* **7:**46.

Bannister, L. H., 1973, Forebrain structure in *Phoxinus phoxinus,* a teleost of the cyprinid family, *J. Hirnforsch.* **14:**413.

Bernstein, J. J., 1962, Role of the telencephalon in color vision of fish, *Exp. Neurol.* **6:**173.

Bernstein, J. J., 1964, Relation of spinal cord regeneration to age in adult goldfish, *Exp. Neurol.* **9:**161.

Bernstein, J. J., 1967, The regenerative capacity of the telencephalon of the goldfish and rat, *Exp. Neurol.* **17:**44.

Berwein, M., 1941, Beobachtungen and Versuche über das gesellige Leben von Elritzen, *Z. Vgl. Physiol.* **28:**402.

Braford, M. R., and Northcutt, R. G., 1974, Olfactory bulb projections in the bichir, *Polypterus, J. Comp. Neurol.* **156:**165.

Brunner, R. L., Rossis, R. R., Stutz, R. M., and Roth, T. G., 1970, Memory loss following posttrial electrical stimulation of the hippocampus, *Psychon. Sci.* **18:**159.

Chanconie, M., and Clairambault, P., 1975, Développement du télencéphale de *Salmo irideus* Gib., *J. Hirnforsch.* **16:**75.

Crosby, E. C., DeJonge, B. D., Schneider, R. C., 1966, Evidence for some of the trends in the phylogenetic development of the vertebrate telencephalon, in: *Evolution of the Forebrain* (R. Hassler and H. Stephan, eds.), pp. 117–135, George Thieme Verlag, Stuttgart.

Davis, R. E., Kassel, J., and Schwagmeyer, P., 1976, Telencephalic lesions and behavior in the telost *Macropodus opercularis:* Reproduction, startle reaction, and operant behavior in the male, *Behav. Biol.* **18:**165.

Demski, L. S., and Knigge, K. M., 1971, The telencephalon and hypothalamus of the bluegill (*Lepomis macrochirus*): Evoked feeding, aggressive and reproductive behavior with representative frontal section, *J. Comp. Neurol* **143:**1.

Droogleever-Fortuyn, J., 1961, Topographical relations in the telencephalon of the sunfish, *Eupomotis gibbosus, J. Comp. Neurol.* **116:**249.

Fiedler, K., 1967, Ethologische and neuroanatomische Auswirkungen von Vorderhirnexistirpationen bei Meerbrassen (*Diplodus*) and Lippfischen (*Crenilaburs*, Perciformes, Teleostei), *J. Hirnforsch.* **9:**481.

Finger, M., 1975, The distribution of the olfactory tract in the bullhead catfish, *Ictalurus nebulosus, J. Comp. Neurol.* **161:**25.

Friedlander, M. J., 1978, Structure and function of the visual diencephalon of the teleost fish, *Micropterus salmoides,* Ph.D. dissertation, University of Illinois.

Gage, S. P., 1893, The brain of *Diemyctilus viridescens* from larval to adult life and comparisons with the brain of *Amia* and *Petromyzon,* in: *The Wilder Quarter Century Book,* pp. 259–314, Ithaca, N.Y.

Gaze, R. M., and Keating, M. J., 1972, The visual system and "neuronal specificity," *Nature (London)* **237:**375.

Goldstein, K., 1905, Untersuchungen über das Vorderhirn and Zwischenhirn einiger Knochenfische (nebst einigen Beitragen Mittelhirn und Kleinhirn derselben), *Arch. Mikrosk. Anat.* **66:**135.

Hale, E. B., 1956, Social facilitation and forebrain function in maze performance of green sunfish, *Lempomis cyanellus, Physiol. Zool.* **29:**93.

Healey, E. G., 1957, The nervous system, in: *The Physiology of Fishes,* Vol. 2 (M. F. Brown, ed.), pp. 1–119, Academic Press, New York.

Herrick, C. J., 1922, Functional factors in the morphology of the forebrain of fishes, in: *Libro en Honor de D. Santiago Ramón y Cajal,* pp. 143–204, Jiménez y Molina, Madrid.

Herz, M. J., and Peeke, H. V. S., 1971, Impairment of extinction with caudate nucleus stimulation, *Brain Res.* **33:**519.

Holmgren, N., 1922, Points of view concerning forebrain morphology in lower vertebrates, *J. Comp. Neurol.* **34:**391.

Hosch, L., 1936, Untersuchungen über Grosshirnfunktionen der Elritze (*Phoxinus laevis)* und des Gruendlings (Gobio fluviatilis), *Zool. Jahrb. Abt. All. Zool. Physiol. Tiere* **57:**57.

Ito, H., 1973, Normal and experimental studies on synaptic patterns in the carp telencephalon with special reference to the secondary olfactory termination, *J. Hirnforsch.* **14:**237.

Ito, H., and Kishida, R., 1977, Tectal afferent neurons identified by the retrograde HRP method in the carp telencephalon, *Brain Res.* **130:**142.

Ito, H., and Kishida, R., 1978, Telencephalic afferent neurons identified by the retrograde HRP method in the carp diencephalon, *Brain Res.* **149:**211.

Jacobson, M., and Gaze, R. M., 1965, Selection of appropriate tectal connections by regenerating optic nerve fibers in adult goldfish, *Exp. Neurol.* **13:**418.

Johnston, J. B., 1911, The telencephalon of ganoids and teleosts, *J. Comp. Neurol.* **21:**489.

Källén, B., 1947, Some remarks on the subpallial parts of the teleost forebrain, *K. fysiogr. Saellsk, Lund Foerh.* **17:**203.

Källén, B., 1951, Embryological studies on the nuclei and their homologization in the vertebrate forebrain, *Acta Univ. Lund.* **62:**No. 5.

Kaplan, H., and Aronson, L. R., 1967, Effect of forebrain ablation on the performance of a conditioned avoidance response in the teleost fish, *Tilapia h. macrocephala, Anim. Behav.* **15:**436.

Kassel, J., Davis, R. E., and Schwagmeyer, P., 1976, Telencephalic lesions and behavior in the teleost *Macropodus opercularis:* Further analysis of reproductive and operant behavior in the male, *Behav. Biol.* **18:**179.

Kesner, R. P., and Doty, R. W., 1968, Amnesia produced in cats by local seizure activity initiated from the amygdala, *Exp. Neurol.* **21:**58.

Kirsche, W., and Kirsche, K., 1961, Experimentelle Untersuchungen zur Frage der Regeneration und Funktion des Tectum Opticum von *Carassius carassius* L., *Z. Mikrosk. Anat. Forsch.* **67:**140.

Kumakura, S., 1928, Versuche an Goldfischen, denen beide Hemisphären des Grosshirns exstirpirt worden waren, *Nagoya J. Med. Sci.* **3:**19.

Maron, K., 1963, Endbrain regeneration in *Lebistes reticulatus, Folia Biol.* **11:**1.

McIntyre, D. C., 1970, Differential amnesic effect of cortical vs. amygdaloid elicited convulsions in rats, *Physiol. Behav.* **5:**747.

Miller, R. N., 1940, The telencephalic zonal system of the teleost, *Corydora paliatus, J. Comp. Neurol.* **72:**149.

Morgan, G. C., 1974*a*, The early development of the telencephalon of the marine catfish, *Galeichthys felis, J. Hirnforsch.* **15:**427.

Morgan, G. C., 1974*b*, The late embryology and maturation of the telencephalon in the marine catfish, *Galeichthys felis, J. Hirnforsch.* **15:**449.

Morgan, G. C., 1975, The telencephalon of the sea catfish *Galeichthys felis, J. Hirnforsch.* **16:**131.

Nieuwenhuys, R., 1963, The comparative anatomy of the actinopterygian forebrain, *J. Hirnforsch.* **6:**172.

Nieuwenhuys, R., 1967, Comparative anatomy of olfactory centres and tracts, *Prog. Brain Res.* **23:**106.

Nieuwenhuys, R., Bauchot, R., and Arnoult, J., 1969, Le développement du télencéphale d'un poisson osseux primitif, *Polypterus senegalus* Cuvier, *Acta Zool.* **50:**101.

Noble, G. K., 1936, Function of the corpus striatum in the social behavior of fishes, *Anat. Rec.* **64:** Suppl. 34.

Noble, G. K., 1937, Effects of lesions of the corpus striatum on the brooding behavior of cichlid fishes, *Anat. Rec.* **70:**58.

Overmier, J. B., and Gross, D., 1974, Effects of telencephalic ablation upon nest-building and avoidance behaviors in East African mouthbreeding fish, *Tilapia mossambica, Behav. Biol.* **12:**211.

Overmier, J. B., and Savage, G. E., 1974, Effects of telencephalic ablation on trace classical conditioning of heart rate in goldfish, *Exp. Neurol.* **42:**339.

Overmier, J. B., and Starkman, N., 1974, Transfer of control of avoidance behavior in normal and telencephalon ablated goldfish (*Carassius auratus*), *Physiol. Behav.* **12:**605.

Peeke, H. V. S., Peeke, S. C., and Williston, J. S., 1972, Long-term memory deficits for habituation of predatory behavior in the forebrain ablated goldfish (*Carassius auratus*), *Exp. Neurol.* **36:**288.

Peter, R. E., and Gill, V. E., 1975, A stereotaxic atlas and technique for forebrain nuclei of the goldfish, *Carassius auratus, J. Comp. Neurol.* **159:**69.

Peter, R. E., Macey, M. J., and Gill, V. E., 1975, A stereotaxic atlas and technique for forebrain nuclei of the killifish, *Fundulus heteroclitus, J. Comp. Neurol.* **159:**103.

Savage, G. E., 1969, Some preliminary observations on the role of telencephalon in food-reinforced behavior in the goldfish, *Carassius auratus, Anim. Behav.* **17:**363.

Scalia, F. and Ebbesson, S. O. E., 1971, The central projections of the olfactory bulb in a teleost (*Gymnothorax funebris*), *Brain Behav. Evol.* **4:**376.

Schnitzlein, H. N., 1962, The habenula and the dorsal thalamus of some teleosts, *J. Comp. Neurol.* **118:**225.

Schnitzlein, H. N., 1964, Correlation of habit and structure in the fish brain, *Am. Zool.* **4:**21.

Schnitzlein, H. N., 1977, The telencephala of division I of the teleost fishes, *J. Hirnforsch.* **18:**157.

Schnitzlein, H. N., Hamel, E. G., Carey, H. H., Brown, J. W., Hoffman, H. H., Faucette, J. R., and Showers, M. J. C., 1973, The interrelations of the striatum with subcortical areas through the lateral forebrain bundle, *J. Hirnforsch.* **13:**409.

Schwagmeyer, P., Davis, R. E., and Kassel, J., 1977, Telencephalic lesions and behavior in the teleost *Macropodus opercularis* (L.): Effects of telencephalon and olfactory bulb ablation on spawning and foamnest building, *Behav. Biol.* **20:**463.

Segaar, J., 1960. Ethophysiological experiments with male *Gasterosteus aculeatus*, in: *Structure and Function of the Cerebral Cortex* (D. B. Tower and J. P. Shade, eds.), pp. 301–305, Elsevier, Amsterdam.

Segaar, J., 1961, Telencephalon and behavior in *Gasterosteus aculeatus, Behavior* **28:**256.

Segaar, J., 1965, Behavioural aspects of degeneration and regeneration in fish brain: A comparison with higher vertebrates, *Prog. Brain Res.* **14:**143.

Shapiro, S., Schuckman, H., Sussman, D., and Tucker, A. M., 1974, Effects of telencephalic lesions on gill cover response of Siamese fighting fish, *Physiol. Behav.* **13:**749.

Sheldon, R. E., 1912, The olfactory tracts and centers in teleosts, *J. Comp. Neurol.* **22:**177.

Singh, H. R., 1969, Telencephalic nuclear areas in three Indian teleosts, *Acta Anat.* **73:**463.

Ten Cate, J., 1935, Physiologie des Zentralnervensystems der Fische, *Ergeb. Biol.* **11:**335.

Turowski, A., and Danner, H., 1977, Zur Morphologie des Telencephalons von *Salmo irideus* (Teleostei) Golgi-Imprägnationsstudie, *J. Hirnforsch.* **18:**37.

Vanegas, H., and Ebbesson, S. O. E., 1976, Telencephalic projections in two teleost species, *J. Comp. Neurol.* **165:**181.

Westerman, R. A., and von Baumgarten, R., 1964, Regeneration of olfactory paths in carp, *Experienta* **20:**519.

5

Projections of the Teleostean Telencephalon

HORACIO VANEGAS and SVEN O. E. EBBESSON

I. Introduction

It has been hypothesized that the development of the teleostean telencephalon from the rostral end of the neural tube takes place by a process of lateral eversion rather than evagination (cf. Scalia and Ebbesson, 1971). Such a process would thus be a side step in the evolution of the forebrain. However, although the eversion hypothesis has provided a reasonable basis for investigation, the telencephalon of bony fishes remains a source of considerable controversy. Such controversy arises in part from the fact that the structure of the telencephalon is by no means uniform throughout this rich and varied class of vertebrates (cf. Ariëns Kappers *et al.*, 1936), but the disagreements are also due, in an even greater measure, to the fact that the descriptions of fiber connections of telencephalic cell groups in teleosts are based largely on studies of normal material, which are subject to inaccuracies and doubts.

Modern experimental techniques for the study of pathways and terminal synaptic fields have only recently been applied to teleosts. Through the use of these techniques, it has become evident that the large majority of cell groups in the teleostean telencephalon are *not* olfactory in character (Scalia and Ebbesson, 1971), but there is a lack of well-supported knowledge concerning the relationships of such cell groups with those cell groups located in the thalamus, the hypothalamus, and the brainstem. In an initial attempt to disclose some of these relationships, the gross output of the telencephalon was studied in two different types of teleosts by means of Fink–Heimer (1967) techniques. One such type of teleost, *Holocentrus*

HORACIO VANEGAS • Centro de Biofísica y Bioquímica, Instituto Venezolano de Investigaciones Científicas (IVIC), Caracas, Venezuela. SVEN O. E. EBBESSON • Department of Anatomy, Catholic University of Puerto Rico, Ponce, Puerto Rico 00731.

(order Berycomorphi, commonly known as squirrel fish or "candil"), is a coral reef animal. The other type, *Eugerres* (order Percomorphoidea, commonly known as "mojarra"), is a perchlike fish which dwells in brackish waters and littoral lagoons.

In order to study the telencephalic outflow in *Eugerres* and *Holocentrus* the animals were subjected to subtotal ablation of one telencephalic hemisphere and then sacrificed after various survival periods. The degenerating axons originating from the ablated region, as well as their terminals, were selectively impregnated with silver by means of a modified Fink–Heimer (1967) technique [method 7 in Ebbesson (1970)] and then charted on photomacrographs of Nissl-stained sections. The efferent pathways and terminal fields were far more prominent in *Holocentrus* than in *Eugerres,* and are schematically depicted for one example of each type of animal in Figs. 1–21 (see Table I for abbreviations used in figures), where large dots and thin dashes represent axonal degeneration and small dots represent terminal degeneration as defined by Ebbesson (1970). Details regarding experimental procedures and results have been published previously (Vanegas and Ebbesson, 1976).

A few fiber bundles leave the (ablated) telencephalic hemisphere toward the contralateral hemisphere, while a massive group of fibers descends ipsilaterally into the diencephalon and constitutes the four main telencephalic efferent pathways, namely, the telencephalo-tectal (so-called strio-tectal) bundle, the medial forebrain bundle, the lateral forebrain bundle, and the telencephalo-lobar (so-called strio-lobar) bundle (Figs. 4, 5, and 13). Our present knowledge on structure and connections of the teleostean telencephalon, diencephalon, and brainstem is insufficient for an adequate evaluation of homologies between teleosts and other vertebrate classes. Therefore, rather than seeking new names for the efferent pathways, they have been labeled herein according to Meader (1934) and Schnitzlein (1962). It must be emphasized, however, that no adherence is intended to, for example, the "striatal" origin of the strio-tectal or strio-lobar bundles. Whether any of the efferent pathways originate from cell groups homologous to the mammalian striatum or pallium, to the avian archistriatum or ectostriatum, or to portions of the reptilian telencephalon cannot be considered until more detailed studies are completed.

Table I. Abbreviations Used in This Chapter

C	Nucleus corticalis	R	Nucleus rotundus
Cb	Cerebellum	SLB	Strio-lobar bundle
CG	Central gray	STB	Strio-tectal bundle
CIH	Interhemispheric commissure	Tel	Telencephalon
CPO	Postoptic commissure	TeO	Tectum opticum
DMO	Dorsomedial optic nucleus of the thalamus	SM	Stratum marginale
G	Corpus glomerulosum	SO	Stratum opticum
GL	Nucleus geniculatus lateralis ipsum	SFGS	Stratum fibrosum et griseum superficiale
H	Habenula	SGC	Stratum griseum centrale
Hyp	Hypothalamus	SAC	Stratum album centrale
LFB	Lateral forebrain bundle	SPV	Stratum periventriculare
MFB	Medial forebrain bundle	TL	Torus longitudinalis
PT	Pretectal cell groups	TrO	Tractus opticus
PTh	Nucleus prethalamicus	TS	Torus semicircularis

To what extent these fibers are primarily commissural or likewise constitute decussating pathways is not clear at present. They cross the midline on the commissural plate and invade the contralateral hemisphere (Figs. 1, 2, and 10–14). In *Eugerres* this fiber system is rather sparse, but in *Holocentrus* these fibers are clearly seen to course into the contralateral hemisphere and terminate throughout the central mass and, quite abundantly, on the edge of this mass, leaving a rim of degeneration-free tissue just underneath the hemisphere's surface. In spite of the bewildering number of names and homologies proposed (cf. Ariëns Kappers *et al.*,

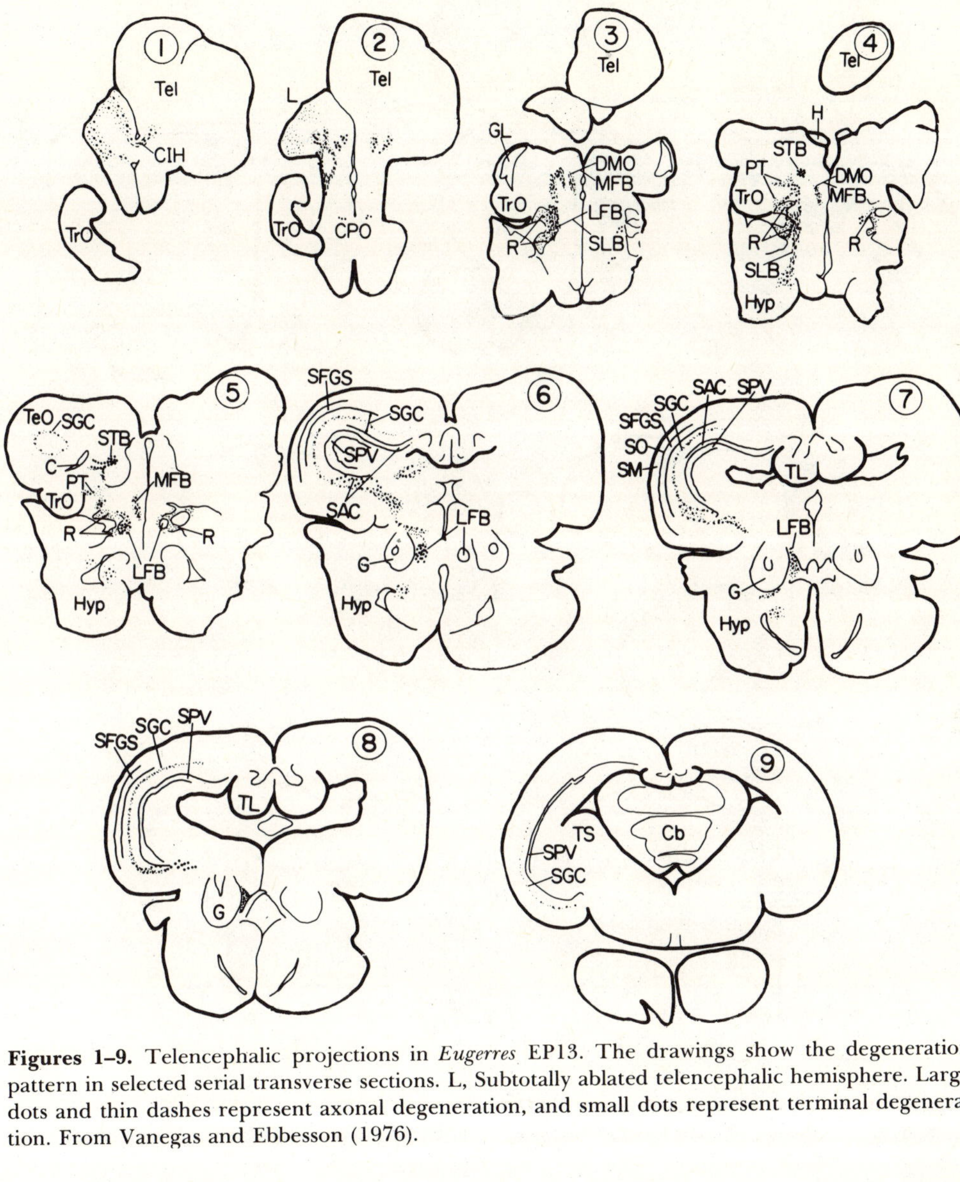

Figures 1–9. Telencephalic projections in *Eugerres* EP13. The drawings show the degeneration pattern in selected serial transverse sections. L, Subtotally ablated telencephalic hemisphere. Large dots and thin dashes represent axonal degeneration, and small dots represent terminal degeneration. From Vanegas and Ebbesson (1976).

1936) for the various telencephalic cell groups (or perhaps because of it), and in view of our lacking knowledge on fiber connections of such cell groups, it is impossible to assess the significance of these commissural connections in terms such as "anterior commissure" and "hippocampal commissure."

III. Projection to Pretectum and Optic Tectum

Among the descending telencephalofugal fibers, those placed most dorsocaudally are destined for pretectal cell groups and for the optic tectum. The so-called

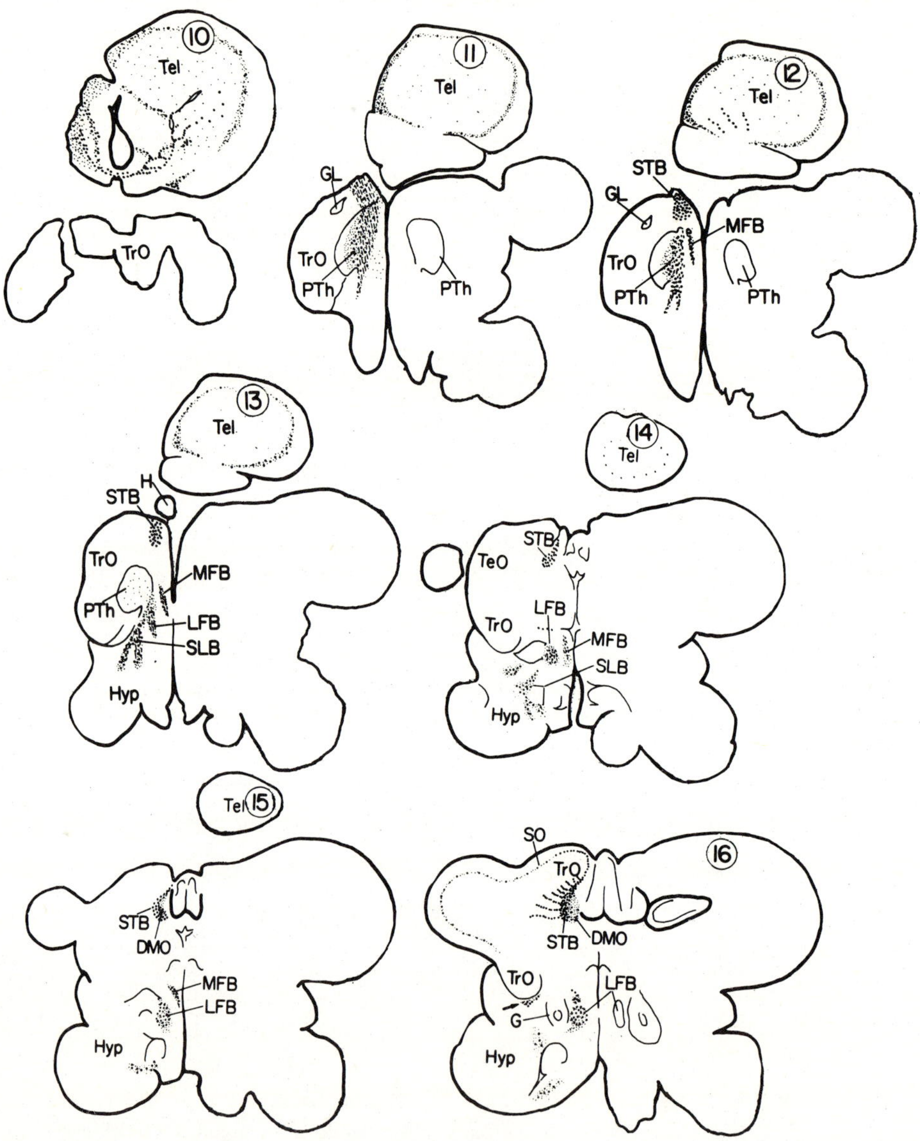

Figures 10–21. Telencephalic projections in *Holocentrus* Ho40. The drawings show the degeneration pattern in selected serial transverse sections. L, Subtotally ablated telencephalic hemisphere. Large

strio-tectal bundle (Figs. 4, 5, and 12–16) carries all telencephalo-tectal fibers in *Holocentrus,* and part of them in *Eugerres,* in which the remainder descend instead (Fig. 3) with the common trunk of the lateral forebrain bundle and strio-lobar bundle (see below). In *Eugerres* telencephalo-tectal fibers are accompanied by (or give rise to; this is not clear) fibers which terminate in several ipsilateral pretectal cell groups (Figs. 4–6). In *Holocentrus* the strio-tectal bundle courses caudalward along the dorsal region of the thalamus, gives off some terminals to the ipsilateral dorsomedial optic nucleus of the thalamus (Figs. 15 and 16; see below), and then fans out as its fibers enter the stratum opticum (SO) and the stratum album centrale (SAC) of the ipsilateral optic tectum (Figs. 16 and 17) (cf. Vanegas *et al.,* 1974;

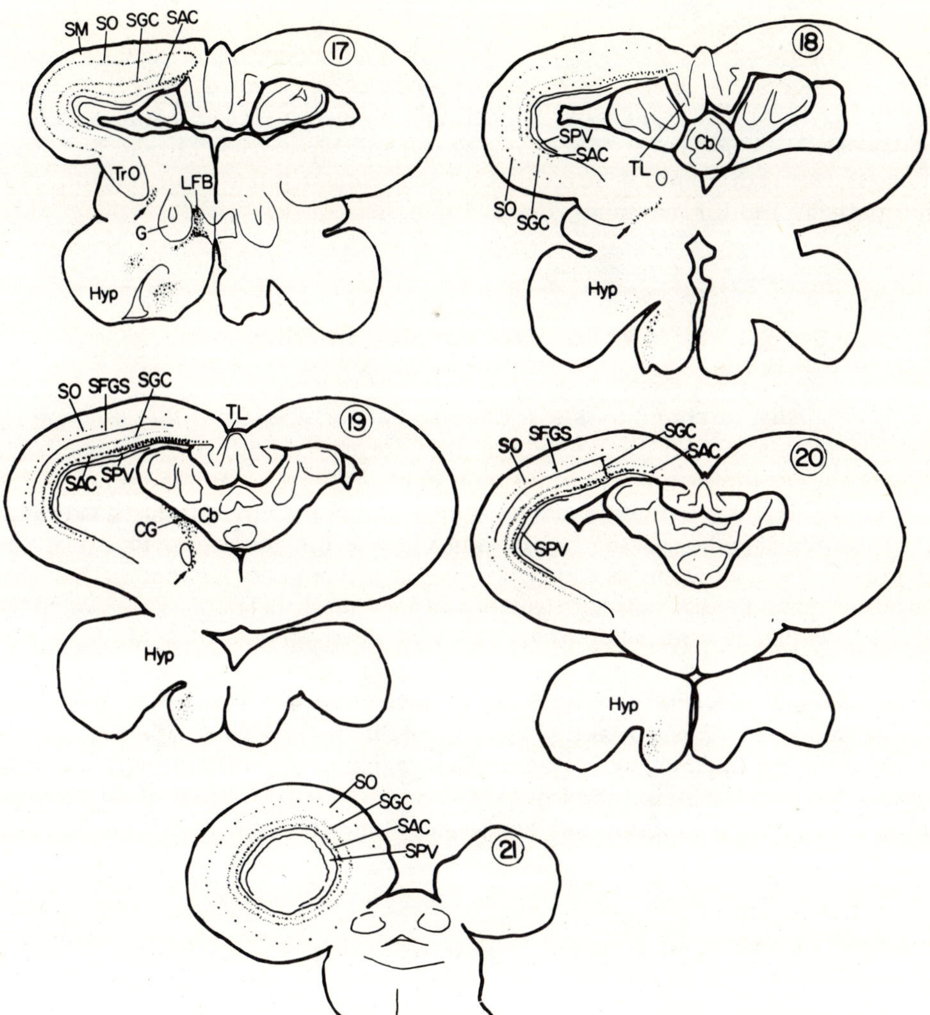

dots and thin dashes represent axonal degeneration, and small dots represent terminal degeneration. From Vanegas and Ebbesson (1976).

Schroeder and Vanegas, 1980). Terminals are given to both these strata, and mostly to the midlevel of the stratum griseum centrale, i.e., the deep boundary of the inner plexiform layer (Figs. 17–21). In *Eugerres* the presence of degenerating fibers or terminals in SO or SAC is uncertain; telencephalo-tectal fibers terminate at the deep boundary of the inner plexiform layer (Figs. 5–9), which is reached by these fibers from the ventrolateral tectal margin, sometimes after a brief course through the SAC (Figs. 5–8).

Termination of telencephalofugal fibers in the deep layers of the optic tectum can probably be considered as a feature common to all vertebrates, since it has been described in elasmobranchs (Ebbesson and Schroeder, 1971), reptiles (Butler and Ebbesson, 1975), birds (Zeier and Karten, 1971), mammals (Lund, 1969; Sterling, 1971), and, presently, teleosts. The projection to stratum opticum in *Holocentrus* is interesting in connection with the finding that, in mammals, there exists a superficial telencephalo-tectal projection which topologically matches the retino-tectal projection (Kawamura *et al.,* 1974). It is noteworthy that telencephalo-tectal terminals at the deep boundary of the inner plexiform layer are located more deeply than retino-tectal terminals and more superficially than tecto-tectal (commissural) terminals (cf. Vanegas, 1975). These spatial relationships also hold true for elasmobranchs (Schroeder and Ebbesson, 1975) and reptiles (Butler and Ebbesson, 1975), and partially also for mammals (Lund, 1969; Sterling, 1971).

IV. Medial Forebrain Bundle

The medial forebrain bundle is a rather slender fiber tract (Figs. 3–5 and 12–15) whose trajectory is reminiscent of the fornix and which probably has no relationship to the medial forebrain bundle of birds and mammals (cf. Zeier and Karten, 1971). It runs caudal-, medial-, and ventralward through the thalamus and ends near the midline at the caudal limits of the ipsilateral hypothalamus while giving terminals all along its course. In *Eugerres,* it supplies terminals (Figs. 3 and 4) to the dorso-medial optic nucleus of the ipsilateral thalamus (Ebbesson, 1972), which is probably equivalent to the nucleus dorsolateralis thalami (Schnitzlein, 1962). This nucleus receives contralateral retinofugal axons via the so-called dorsomedial optic fascicle of Jansen (Vanegas and Ebbesson, 1973) as well as ipsilateral tectofugal axons (Ebbesson and Vanegas, 1976). In *Holocentrus* telencephalofugal input to the dorsomedial optic nucleus is supplied by the strio-tectal bundle (Figs. 15 and 16; see above), but the inputs from retina and optic tectum are similar to those in *Eugerres* (Campbell and Ebbesson, 1969; Ebbesson and Vanegas, 1976).

V. Projection to Nucleus Rotundus or Prethalamicus

The strio-lobar bundle and the lateral forebrain bundle run together as a single, robust fiber tract (SLB/LFB) which descends through the rostral diencephalon, just medial and adjacent to the nucleus rotundus or prethalamicus (Figs.

3 and 11–13). The so-called nucleus prethalamicus of *Holocentrus* (Meader, 1934) is homologous to the so-called nucleus rotundus (but *not* the corpus glomerulosum) of other teleost species (Schnitzlein, 1962), a term also applied here to *Eugerres*. This is a cell mass located between the optic tract and the SLB/LFB trunk (Figs. 3–5, 11-13, 22, and 23). In *Holocentrus* this is a large bean-shaped structure, whereas in *Eugerres* its size is small, and it is divided into dorsal and ventral halves by a fiber

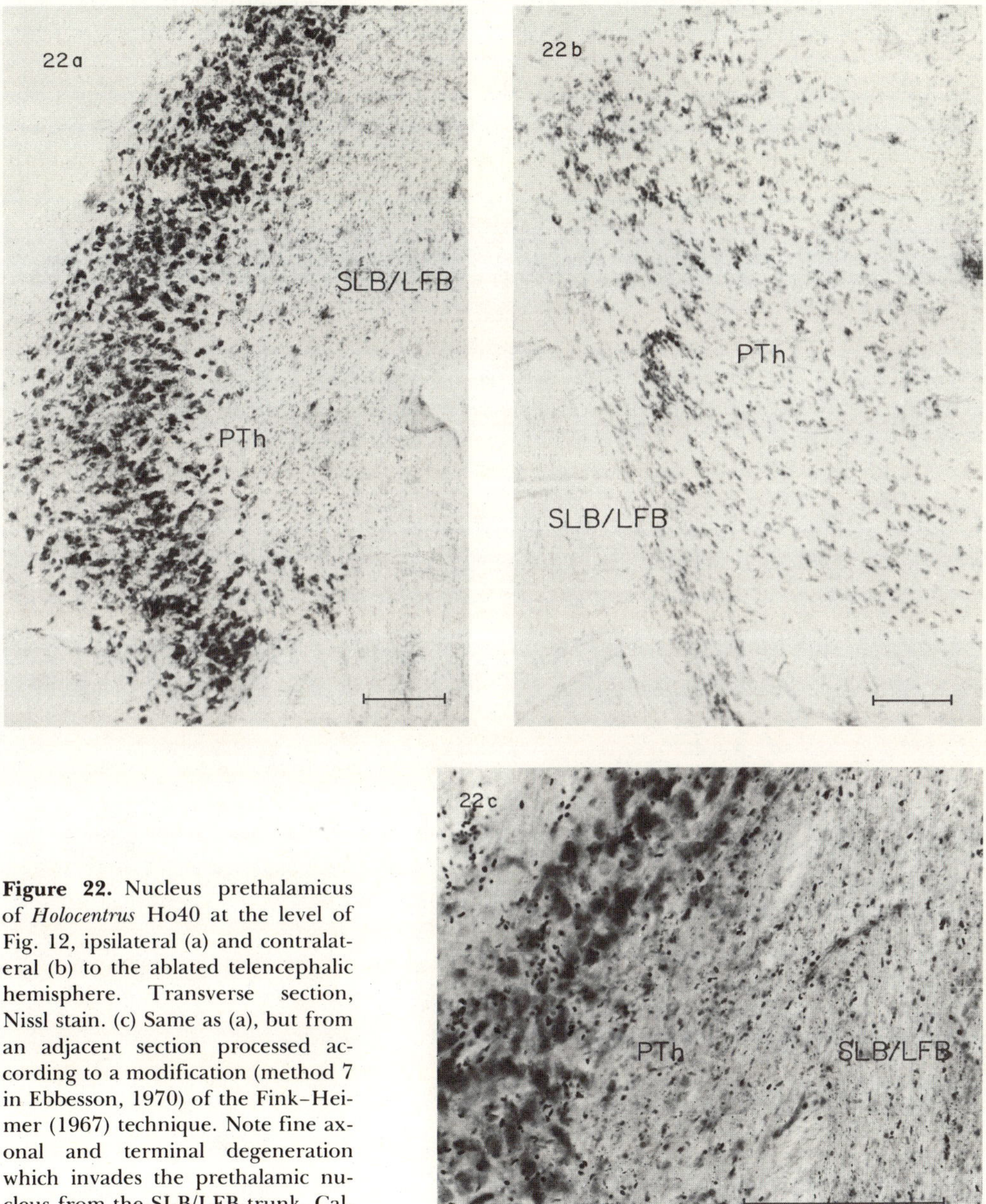

Figure 22. Nucleus prethalamicus of *Holocentrus* Ho40 at the level of Fig. 12, ipsilateral (a) and contralateral (b) to the ablated telencephalic hemisphere. Transverse section, Nissl stain. (c) Same as (a), but from an adjacent section processed according to a modification (method 7 in Ebbesson, 1970) of the Fink–Heimer (1967) technique. Note fine axonal and terminal degeneration which invades the prethalamic nucleus from the SLB/LFB trunk. Calibration line: 100 μm.

tract. In both species, however, the SLB/LFB trunk literally fits into the nucleus's medial concavity. In *Holocentrus* abundant terminals are given by ipsilateral telencephalofugal fibers to the medial, concave region of nucleus prethalamicus (Figs. 11-13 and 22c). The lateral, convex region, on the other hand, has been shown to receive ipsilateral tectofugal fibers (Ebbesson and Vanegas, 1976). It is noteworthy that this lateral region shows considerably increased Nissl-staining properties after ipsilateral telencephalic ablation (Fig. 22a), which suggests a retrograde reaction to the removal of putative target cell groups in telencephalon. In *Eugerres* the termination of telencephalofugal fibers involves the whole nucleus rotundus diffusely (Figs. 3–5), as does also the termination of tectofugal fibers (Ebbesson and Vanegas, 1976). There is, in this species also, a slight increase in the Nissl-staining properties of the nucleus rotundus ipsilateral to the removed telencephalic hemisphere, but the fact that, unlike in *Holocentrus,* the contralateral nucleus rotundus also receives telencephalic fibers (see below) makes it difficult to compare the staining of both sides.

Ebbesson (1972) has proposed the term "central optic nucleus" for the diencephalic cell group which, throughout vertebrate classes, receives no direct input from the retina, possesses a massive tectal input, and projects to telencephalon. The first two of these criteria have been met for nucleus rotundus or prethalamicus (Campbell and Ebbesson, 1969; Vanegas and Ebbesson, 1973; Ebbesson and Vanegas, 1976), and the abovementioned facts suggest that the third criterion would also probably be fulfilled. This would make nucleus rotundus or prethalamicus the teleostean homologue of the reptilian nucleus rotundus, the avian nucleus rotundus, and the mammalian pulvinar or nucleus lateralis posterior thalami (cf. Ebbesson, 1972).

Worthy of mention is the fact that the so-called nucleus geniculatus lateralis (Meader, 1934; Schnitzlein, 1962), which abundantly receives terminals of contralateral retinofugal fibers (Campbell and Ebbesson, 1969; Vanegas and Ebbesson,

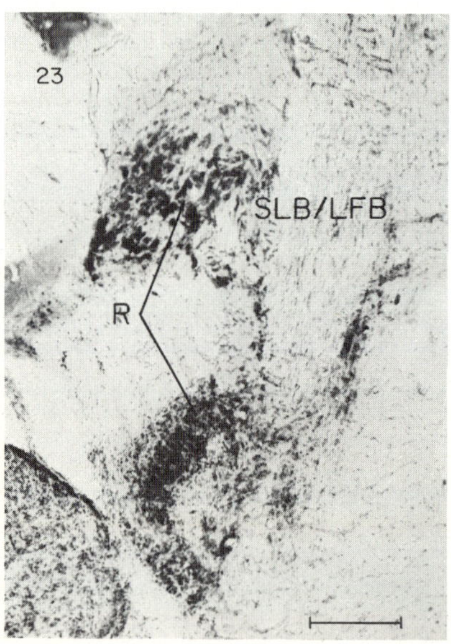

Figure 23. Nucleus rotundus of *Eugerres* EP13, at the level of Fig. 3. Transverse section, Nissl stain. Note that the nucleus has two parts separated by a fiber tract. Calibration line: 100 μm.

1973), showed no degeneration (and no intense Nissl staining) ipsi- or contralaterally after telencephalic ablation, whether in *Holocentrus* or *Eugerres.* In view of this fact, a homology between the mammalian lateral geniculate nucleus and its teleostean homonym seems highly doubtful. It has been suggested (Vanegas and Ebbesson, 1976) that perhaps a retino-geniculo-telencephalic system is lacking in teleosts and that all visual input to the telencephalon might be routed via the optic tectum through the nucleus rotundus or prethalamicus.

VI. Strio-lobar Bundle

Ventromedial to the nucleus rotundus or prethalamicus, the lateral forebrain bundle and the strio-lobar bundle begin to diverge as two separate fiber tracts (Figs. 4, 5, and 13). The latter runs ventral- and slightly caudalward and enters the ipsilateral inferior lobe of the hypothalamus where it turns caudalward, spreads out, and gives numerous terminals (Figs. 4–7 and 13–20).

VII. Lateral Forebrain Bundle

The lateral forebrain bundle is a large fiber tract which runs caudal- and medialward as it gives abundant terminals throughout the ipsilateral hypothalamus (Figs. 5–8 and 13–17). It finally passes just medial to the ipsilateral corpus glomerulosum—to which no terminals are given—and ends on a large cell group located between the corpus glomerulosum and the midline; some terminals are also issued at this level to cell groups located just ventral to the corpus glomerulosum (Figs. 7, 8, and 17).

VIII. Projection to the Central Gray of Brain Stem

In *Holocentrus* the SLB/LFB trunk gives off laterally a small fiber tract (Figs. 16–19, arrow) which remains adjacent to the optic tract, then swings around it while coursing caudal- and medialward, and finally reaches the gray substance at the ipsilateral ventricular floor. Such a distinct projection could not be found in *Eugerres.*

IX. Contralateral Descending Projection

As mentioned earlier, some degenerating terminals were found in the nucleus rotundus contralateral to the resected telencephalic hemisphere of *Eugerres.* The route followed by this contralateral projection was not unequivocally evident, but it might be related to degenerating axons which were consistently seen on the postoptic commissure. No contralateral projections were seen in *Holocentrus.*

X. Final Considerations

As discussed previously, it is at present difficult to make a valid comparison between the efferent system described herein and those telencephalic projections shown to exist in other vertebrate classes. Except for the finding (Ebbesson and Schroeder, 1971) that the telencephalic projections in elasmobranchs are largely contralateral (as also are the thalamotelencephalic pathways in this class), telencephalic projections to diencephalon and brainstem in vertebrates can be considered to be largely ipsilateral, as shown herein for teleosts. When taken together, the efferent pathways of the avian archistriatum (Zeier and Karten, 1971)—namely, the tractus occipito-mesencephalicus (OM) and the tractus occipito-mesencephalicus pars hypothalami (HOM)—cover target areas roughly similar to those reported here for the gross telencephalic projection in teleosts. It is noteworthy, however, that the OM/HOM system does not terminate on the avian nucleus rotundus. This nucleus seems not to be related to the archistriatum but rather to the ectostriatum of birds (Revzin and Karten, 1966), whose homologue was most likely lesioned in the presently described experiments on teleosts (see also Vanegas and Ebbesson, 1976).

In summary, then, although there are some differences between *Eugerres* and *Holocentrus,* the gross telencephalic output in these two types of teleost terminates in the contralateral telencephalic hemisphere and, ipsilaterally, in the nucleus rotundus or prethalamicus (central optic nucleus of the thalamus), in dorsal thalamic cell groups (DMO), in the inferior lobe of the hypothalamus, in the medial hypothalamus as far caudally as a nucleus medial to the corpus glomerulosum (which might be similar to one of Zeier and Karten's "outstanding nuclei" where OM terminates), in pretectal cell groups, in (mostly) the deep layers of the optic tectum, and in the periventricular gray substance of the brain stem.

ACKNOWLEDGMENTS. The work presented herein was partly supported by Grant DF-S1-0313 of the Venezuelan Consejo Nacional de Investigaciones Científicas y Tecnológicas (CONICIT) to H. V., and by National Eye Institute Grant 1 RO1 EY00154 and USPHS-NINDS Career Development Award #1 KO4 NS 46292 to S. O. E. E.

XI. References

Ariëns Kappers, C. U., Huber, G. C., and Crosby, E. C., 1936, reprinted in 1965, *The Comparative Anatomy of the Nervous System of Vertebrates, Including Man,* Hafner, New York.

Butler, A. B., and Ebbesson, S. O. E., 1975, A Golgi study of the optic tectum of the Tegu lizard, *Tupinambis nigropunctatus, J. Morphol.* **146:**215.

Campbell, C. B. G., and Ebbesson, S. O. E., 1969, The optic system of a teleost: *Holocentrus* reexamined, *Brain Behav. Evol.* **2:**415.

Ebbesson, S. O. E., 1970, Selective silver impregnation of degenerating axons and synaptic endings in non-mammalian species, in: *Contemporary Research Methods in Neuroanatomy* (W. J. H. Nauta and S. O. E. Ebbesson, eds.), pp. 132–161, Springer-Verlag, New York.

Ebbesson, S. O. E., 1972, A proposal for a common nomenclature for some optic nuclei in vertebrates and the evidence for a common origin of two such cell groups, *Brain Behav. Evol.* **6:**75.

Ebbesson, S. O. E., and Schroeder, D. M., 1971, Connections of the nurse shark's telencephalon, *Science* **173:**254.

Ebbesson, S. O. E., and Vanegas, H., 1976, Projections of the optic tectum in two teleost species, *J. Comp. Neurol.* **165:**161.

Fink, R. P., and Heimer, L., 1967, Two methods for selective silver impregnation of degenerating axons and their synaptic endings in the central nervous system, *Brain Res.* **4:**369.

Kawamura, S., Sprague, J. M., and Niimi, K., 1974, Corticofugal projections from the visual cortices to the thalamus, pretectum and superior colliculus in the cat, *J. Comp. Neurol.* **158:**339.

Lund, R. D., 1969, Synaptic patterns of the superficial layers of the superior colliculus of the cat, *J. Comp. Neurol.* **135:**179.

Meader, R. G., 1934, The optic system of the teleost, *Holocentrus.* I. The primary optic pathways and the corpus geniculatum complex, *J. Comp. Neurol.* **60:**361.

Revzin, A. M., and Karten H. J., 1966, Rostral projections of the optic tectum and the nucleus rotundus in the pigeon, *Brain Res.* **3:**264.

Scalia, F., and Ebbesson, S. O. E., 1971, The central projection of the olfactory bulb in a teleost (*Gymnothorax funebris), Brain Behav. Evol.* **4:**376.

Schnitzlein, H. N., 1962, The habenula and dorsal thalamus of some teleosts, *J. Comp. Neurol.* **118:**225.

Schroeder, D. M., and Ebbesson, S. O. E., 1975, Cytoarchitecture of the optic tectum in the nurse shark, *J. Comp. Neurol.* **160:**443.

Schroeder, D. M., and Vanegas, H., 1980, Cytoarchitecture of the optic tectum in the teleost *Holocentrus*, in manuscript.

Sterling, P., 1971, Receptive fields and synaptic organization of the superficial gray layer of the cat superior colliculus, *Vision Res.* **11**(Suppl. 3)**:**309.

Vanegas, H., 1975, Cytoarchitecture and connections of the teleostean optic tectum, in: *Vision in Fishes: New Approaches in Research* (M. Ali, ed.), pp. 151–158, Plenum Press, New York.

Vanegas, H., and Ebbesson, S. O. E., 1973, Retinal projections in the perch-like teleost *Eugerres plumieri, J. Comp. Neurol.* **151:**331.

Vanegas, H., and Ebbesson, S. O. E., 1976, Telencephalic projections in two teleost species, *J. Comp. Neurol.* **165:**181.

Vanegas, H., Laufer, M., and Amat, J., 1974, The optic tectum of a perciform teleost. I. General configuration and cytoarchitecture, *J. Comp. Neurol.* **154:**43.

Zeier, H., and Karten, H. J., 1971, The archistriatum of the pigeon: Organization of afferent and efferent connections, *Brain Res.* **31:**313.

6

The Fish Telencephalon and Its Relation to Learning

GEORGE ERIC SAVAGE

I. Introduction

A. Evolutionary Considerations

The study of the mammalian telencephalon, and particularly of its cortex, has given rise to a vast accumulation of knowledge, and yet even at moderately crude levels of analysis its major functions are still poorly understood. This has led to other types of approach to the problems of brain function. One has been the study of the interaction of individual cells, among small neuron populations, an approach exemplified by the study of learning and its neural correlates in *Aplysia* (e.g., see Castellucci *et al.*, 1970; Kupfermann *et al.*, 1970; Pinsker *et al.*, 1970), and another has been the examination of lower vertebrate classes in an attempt to find the roots of the highly evolved brain functions and behaviors seen, for example, in rats and monkeys.

One of the criteria influencing the choice of a suitable group of vertebrates has been its behavioral repertoire. For instance, although various degrees of cortical development are present in amphibians and reptiles (Ariëns Kappers *et al.*, 1936), they are, in general, difficult animals to train. With the exception of birds, fish have proved to be the most useful submammalian animals for a variety of behavioral and physiological studies. They have good color vision (Marks, 1965), they can be easily trained to discriminate color or shape (e.g., see Yager, 1967; Sutherland, 1969), and they can respond to many of the training situations used with mammals

---

GEORGE ERIC SAVAGE • Department of Zoology and Comparative Physiology, Queen Mary College, University of London, London E1 4NS, England.

(e.g., see Bitterman, 1965). Further, their economic importance and suitability for a variety of types of physiological research, ranging from endocrine to biochemical, have led to the formation of a large and useful background of information, which is not available for the next two higher classes of vertebrates, the amphibians and reptiles.

From an anatomical point of view, fish brains are the simplest contemporary vertebrate system. The main sensory inputs are routed to several different termini (vision to the optic tectum, taste to the medulla, smell to the telencephalon), and there is no one integrative area such as the mammalian cortex; indeed, fish have no higher cortex at all, although a rudimentary pyriform cortex is present in lungfish (Schnitzlein and Crosby, 1967). Such homologies of telencephalic structure as can be drawn between fish and mammals relate to basal areas such as the amygdala and hippocampus (Fortuyn, 1961; Schnitzlein, 1964).

To the reasons just outlined for the study of the telencephalon in fish can be added the question put by Edinger and discussed by Sherrington (1906), as to why this region of the brain should have changed so much in the course of vertebrate evolution, as compared with other areas. In the early vertebrates, of which fish represent the simplest yet still much-evolved example, the forebrain was dominated by olfactory, the midbrain by visual, and the hindbrain by acoustico-lateralis and gustatory inputs. It is difficult to see why the telencephalon rather than lower brain areas should have evolved to the dominant role in the higher vertebrates. The suggestion put forward by Edinger and Sherrington was that olfaction must have been the main long-distance sense in the early fish, for the turbid water would have reduced the importance of sight, and gustatory and pressure senses would have been efficient only at relatively short distances. Hence the onus for maintaining contact with prey would be on the forebrain, not on the midbrain, and thus the ability to attend to, and to continue to attend to, new stimuli would reside in this area of brain. As the other senses developed, the control of their use and ultimately their secondary projections would come to lie in the telencephalon.

The study of the fish telencephalon has expanded greatly over the last 15 years, as anatomical, physiological, and behavioral studies have shown that this area of the brain is indeed far from being the simple, purely olfactory area suggested by early studies. Although the behavioral deficits engendered by ablation of the telencephalon are not obvious, the telencephalon has now been implicated in functions ranging from courtship to learning, and it is with these latter aspects of its influence that the present chapter is involved.

B. Anatomy

The major part of this review is concerned with physiological and behavioral aspects of the functioning of the telencephalon, but it is useful to consider briefly some of the anatomical findings that point toward the presence and localization of nonolfactory areas in this part of the fish brain.

The amount of the telencephalon considered to be primarily concerned with olfaction has been a subject of some disagreement, especially in bony fishes. Herrick, writing in 1922, divided the telencephalon into lateral, dorsal, medial, olfactory/somatic, and somatic areas, and he was of the opinion that of these areas only the somatic area had no direct olfactory afference. He considered that the somatic area received thalamic (possibly optic) afferents and sent efferents back to the thalamus. More recently, Nieuwenhuys (1959) working on the telencephalon of the stickleback (*Gasterosteus aculeatus*) has delineated ventral and dorsal areas of the telencephalon as the primary division. The ventral area is mostly concerned with olfaction. The olfactory mucosa connects to the olfactory bulbs by the olfactory nerves. The olfactory bulbs, which may be sessile (as in *Gasterosteus*) or pedunculate and joined to the rest of the brain by olfactory tracts (as in goldfish), connect to the ventral part of the telencephalon. The olfactory tract splits into two portions, the lateral and medial olfactory tracts, and these run through the ventral area. The medial tract sends fibers to several areas; many terminate in the medial part of the ventral area; others cross over in the anterior commissure, which joins the two hemispheres, and terminate in the contralateral medial and posterior part of the ventral area, and there is a true commissure linking the anterior parts of the ventral area. The lateral tract terminates in the posterior part of the ventral area, and also in the region of interface between dorsal and ventral areas. Only fibers of the medial tract, reaching the posterior telencephalon, may ascend to the dorsal part. Nieuwenhuys considers that the ventral area is primarily olfactory but that the olfactory contribution to the dorsal areas is far less than Herrick supposed. Ebbesson and Heimer (1968, 1970) have shown that in the nurse shark (*Ginglymostoma cirratum*) the olfactory projection is primarily to the ventral telencephalon. Ito (1973) working on carp (*Cyprinus carpio*) has demonstrated that following olfactory tract section, degeneration can be observed in the ventral, dorsolateral, and posterior dorsolateral areas of the telencephalon, and Finger (1975) has reported a similar distribution of degeneration following olfactory tract section in the bullhead catfish (*Ictalurus nebulosus*). The dorsal area of the telencephalon is thus generally considered to be largely free of direct olfactory input. Nieuwenhuys (1959) divides it into lateral, dorsal, medial, and magnocellular, or central, areas.

Leading from the telencephalon are two major and three minor tracts (Nieuwenhuys, 1959). The medial forebrain bundle originates in the commissural and postcommissural parts of the medial ventral area, and terminates in the subpreglomerulosus nucleus. This tract presumably carries the major part of the olfactory information leaving the telencephalon. The lateral forebrain bundle is a larger tract and has more complex connections. Its input is from the entire dorsal area of the telencephalon, with the exception of the extreme ventral portion of the lateral area. Some fibers from the medial dorsal area seem to form a true commissure, while others cross and descend in the contralateral lateral forebrain bundle. The tract gives off fibers in the anterior medial and posterior lateral lobes of the hypothalamus, then terminates in the subpreglomerulosus complex, possibly in the preglomerulosus nucleus itself. Two small tracts reach the habenular nucleus in the anterior optic tectum, one from the posterior part of the ventral area and another from the preoptic nucleus just posterior to the anterior commissure. A further tract, containing neurosecretory fibers, links this last nucleus with the ventral hypothalamus and the pituitary.

In view of the potential functional importance of any nonolfactory areas such as those just outlined, it is of considerable interest to know the extent of any ascending connections from the diencephalon and midbrain. Both Johnston (1911) and Sheldon (1912) considered that the lateral forebrain bundle contained ascending fibers, serving to correlate olfactory and gustatory inputs. Dart (1920) studying the telencephalon of *Scyllium* considered that there were fibers ascending from the dorsal thalamus, and possibly from the optic tectum. Herrick (1922) similarly believed that thalamic afferents ran to the somatic area (the central part of the dorsal area). However, despite the use of Golgi preparations by Sheldon (1912) and Nieuwenhuys (1959), it was unclear whether there was any definite basis for these conclusions. More recently, however, studies by Schroeder and Ebbesson (1974) using Nauta–Gygax and Fink–Heimer stains have demonstrated degeneration within the telencephalon following diencephalic and mesencephalic lesions. Diencephalic lesions cause degeneration in pathways leading to the central nucleus. Both ipsilateral and contralateral degeneration is found following unilateral thalamic lesions, presumably relating to the ipsilateral and contralateral distribution of the lateral forebrain bundle described above. The contralateral projection is to a central area of the more dorsal telencephalon, and the ipsilateral projection runs somewhat lateral to this, with some fibers running to the ventral telencephalon. Since thalamic afferents from the spinal cord and optic system had previously been demonstrated (Ebbesson *et al.,* 1972), Schroeder and Ebbesson (1974) considered it at least possible that there could be projection of such information to the telencephalon. Physiological evidence for ascending functions is discussed below.

Contemporary anatomical studies of the fish telencephalon thus show that older ideas of a purely olfactory function were too simple, and this chapter focuses on some other aspects of its functioning now appearing (see also Chapter 7 in this volume). The majority of studies have been of the effects of lesions of the telencephalon, but electrical studies are also showing that there are interesting nonolfactory processes in this area of brain.

II. Ablation of the Telencephalon

A. General Effects

Ten Cate (1935) cites Desmoulins (1825) as having been the first to remove the telencephalon from a variety of teleost fish. No obvious changes in posture or locomotion were noted. Similar results were reported by other workers using elasmobranchs (e.g., Loeb, 1891; Bethe, 1899; Polimanti, 1911; Rizzolo, 1929) and teleosts (e.g., Vulpian, 1866; Reisinger, 1915; Meader, 1939). Although some early workers such as Ferrier (1876) and Polimanti (1912) reported various deficits such as persistent swimming and lack of feeding, most of these were probably due either to excessive lesions extending into the diencephalon or to the formation of clots lying on the surface of the optic tectum, the resulting pressure causing forced rolling, pitching, and yawing. No such results have been found in more recent experiments where operative technique has been better, and histological controls have been adequate; indeed, careful observation of telencephalon-ablated and sham-operated fish swimming in a tank fails to distinguish between the animals.

Janzen (1933) carefully examined the posture and movement of both bilaterally and unilaterally lesioned fish, and found these to be quite normal. Even when such lesioned animals were unilaterally blinded, only a very transient tendency to swim to the intact side was observed, as compared with the normal animals, and this vanished in 1 hr. Removal of fins produced no greater deficits than in normal fish.

Work by various authors indicates that there may be ephemeral postoperative deficits, relating to feeding (Janzen, 1933), shoaling (Kumakura, 1927) and conditioning (Bernstein, 1962). These will be discussed below. Such deficits have vanished completely by 1–2 days after operation.

1. Olfactory Functions

Steiner (1888) noted that when he removed the telencephalon from *Scyliorhinus* and *Squalius* both fish had to rely on vision to detect food, and that the former animal, which normally relies on smell for detecting food, was greatly affected in its ability to catch prey.

Parker (1910, 1911, 1922) first suggested that a distinction could be drawn between smell and taste in fish. Using *Ameiurus* and *Fundulus* species, he found that the animals could discriminate between worms and inert substances such as cotton wool, when these were concealed in identical porous bags. However, if the olfactory tracts were cut, the ability to make such a distinction was abolished. Strieck (1925), using blinded minnows (*Phoxinus* species), found that they could be trained differentially to go to cotton wool balls previously dipped in solutions of musk or skatol, considered to be olfactory stimuli, and that removal of the telencephalon caused the ability to discriminate to vanish. However, when animals were trained to differentiate glucose and quinine, considered to be gustatory stimuli, ablation of the telencephalon had no effect on the retention of this ability. These experiments indicate both the importance of the telencephalon for olfaction and its unimportance in the retention of one type of nonolfactory task.

2. Feeding

In view of the feeding method of the cyprinids such as the goldfish (*Carassius auratus*), a species widely used in telencephalon research, it is perhaps not surprising that there are no reports of any persistent changes in feeding following the operation. Normally, the animals browse on detritus on the bottom of the tank and test the edibility of this by taste rather than smell. Janzen (1933) noted transient postoperative changes in telencephalon-ablated goldfish, in that their first reaction to food falling through the water was 1–2 hr after operation. However, when the falling food reached the bottom of the tank, it was ignored, and only on the second day after operation did fish eat food lying there. Troschicheva (1974), examining bullheads (Cottidae) and cod (*Gadus*), noted a similar effect, that the food-obtaining behavior of operated fish was similar to that of normal fish a minimum of 2 hr after operation, and a maximum of 1 day was needed for all fish to recover.

Examining the amount of food consumed, Janzen (1933) fed *Chironomus* larvae to normal and ablated goldfish, and found that the number eaten was comparable in the two groups. Savage (1969*b*) examined a number of aspects of feeding, using goldfish. Using a chamber similar to that designed by Meesters (1940), he trained fish to swim to a screen, fixed to which were two holders containing food, and timed runs to the food once asymptotic levels of performance had been attained. Ablated fish were, if anything, faster than normal fish. Averaging the first, second, etc., trial each day over 5 days, the mean times on trials 1 and 10 were not different in either group; thus there was no evidence of satiation as gauged by speed of running, a common measure of motivation (e.g., see Crespi, 1944). Another test of motivation is to interpose a noxious stimulus (usually shock) between the animal and its food, and to see how much of this stimulus the animal will endure to reach food (e.g., see Jenkins *et al.,* 1926). Applying this to the situation just outlined, Savage found that the voltage at which fish would no longer run was lower in operated than in normal fish, but not significantly so. When animals were given 10 trials at the highest voltage at which they would swim to the food, no cessation of running occurred in the operated animals due to reduced motivation as feeding proceeded, and the reaction times observed were similar to those of the normal fish. Finally, a longer-term automatic experiment showed that the rates of feeding of normal and operated fish were equal, and that gains in weight over this period were similar. Thus many of the likely simple food-related deficits appear to be absent following telencephalic ablation. There have been no quantitative observations on other species, but in general there are no reports of feeding deficits. Hosch (1936) examined feeding in operated specimens of *Gobio* and *Phoxinus,* and found no differences in feeding behavior, although no quantitative observations were made as to the amount of food taken.

Since food-seeking behavior is apparently normal following removal of the telencephalon, few studies of the effects of ablation on other behavior have used control fish with olfactory tract section. One of the earlier investigations of social behavior, that of Berwein (1941), did utilize such controls. She observed that in minnows the time taken for a newcomer to be accepted into a shoal was shorter for ablated fish than for both olfactory tract-sectioned and normal animals, and that the last two groups showed similar acceptance times. Habituation to a new environment, where individuals were transferred into an unfamiliar tank, was more rapid in ablated than in tract-sectioned and normal fish, when activity and feeding were used as criteria. However, as will be shown below (Section V), recent mammalian studies would lead to caution against a too-rapid discounting of possible olfactory influences on behavior unrelated to feeding.

3. Duration of Effect

A number of authors have demonstrated transient behavioral deficits following the removal of the telencephalon, which differ from the long-lasting phenomena that form the subject of this discussion, and such short-term deficits are conveniently discussed here. Mention has been made of Janzen's (1933) observation that goldfish show no feeding responses for 1–2 hr after operation, and then only to snap at food dropping through the water, and that they will seek food on the bottom of the tank only after 1–2 days. Kumakura (1927) noted that the removal of the telencephalon in goldfish caused a reduction in activity and that when the animals swam they did not form shoals. Over a period of up to 14 days the fish gradually associated, until they shoaled once more. Bernstein (1962) found that telencephalon-ablated goldfish, classically conditioned to red/green discrimination, using cardiac deceleration as an index, showed responses based on the brightness and not the color of the stimuli. However, if a 4-hr period was left between operation and training, the ability to perform a color discrimination was fully restored. Thus no change had occurred in the retention of the problem, but apparently telencephalic ablation had temporarily disrupted color vision. [The interpretation of these findings is difficult, for in mammals most behavioral recovery following brain lesion takes weeks rather than hours (e.g., see Eidelberg and Stein, 1974) and, as will be shown below, the majority of deficits associated with telencephalic ablation show no improvement with time, in the absence of training.]

Whatever the source of the major deficits following removal of the telencephalon, there appears to be little recovery. Regeneration may occur in the olfactory tract of carp (Westerman, 1965), but Bernstein (1967) found that following bilateral or unilateral removal of the goldfish telencephalon, no regeneration appeared in brains examined up to 2 years later. Even small transections or stab wounds resulted in only columnar epithelium and some glial cells being formed; there was no true new nervous tissue. Thus there is no evidence for any structural recovery from the ablation or lesions discussed here, as far as goldfish are concerned. However, other species have been shown to regenerate, and some care is thus needed in analyzing behavioral results in these fish. Marón (1963) has shown that complete regeneration of the guppy (*Lebistes reticulatus*) telencephalon can occur in 3–4 months. Following complete removal of the telencephalon, the anterior diencephalon becomes covered with a stratified epithelium, which forms two vesicles, and these thicken into the two halves of the telencephalon. Segaar (1965) using the stickleback (*Gasterosteus aculeatus*) found that deficits occurred in the social behavior of the animal following various telencephalic lesions. However, after 1 month, some fish began to manifest reduced or altered deficits, and this was found to correlate with some degree of anatomical recovery. Damage to the anterior telencephalon was not repaired, but laterally and posterior-laterally lesioned fish showed considerable degrees of regeneration.

No measurable behavioral recovery occurs in goldfish following ablation, since Hainsworth *et al.* (1967) examined active avoidance in normal and ablated fish, and found the same acquisition deficits if the ablated fish were trained 1 day or 56 days after operation. Two other groups of fish were trained, then the telencephalon was removed and the animals were retrained 1 day or 56 days after the operation. The postoperative avoidance deficit was of the same magnitude in the two groups, and the improvement in performance was at the same rate.

Since removal of the telencephalon involves the cutting of afferents to, or the actual removal of, the preoptic nucleus, it has been a possibility that the behavioral deficit observed following telencephalon ablation might be primarily hormonal rather than neural. The immediacy of the behavioral effects and their persistence unchanged over a period of months, taken together with their specificity, make this unlikely.

4. Spontaneous Reactions

A behavioral distinction between normal and operated fish is possible, even without considering olfaction or learning, as was shown by Janzen (1933) in goldfish. Vulpian (1866) had reported that removal of the telencephalon of carp (*Cyprinus carpio*) reduced the activity of operated fish; that although movements once initiated were apparently normal, it appeared to be more difficult to elicit movements in operated than in normal fish. Janzen, examining this aspect of behavior in greater detail, characterized two faculties in fish, spontaneity and initiative; the former he considered to involve self-generated movements, the second the ability to respond to environmental change. Telencephalon-ablated fish lacked the latter but not the former.

Janzen observed the rate of opercular movement in five confined and habituated fish before and after removal of the telencephalon. In all five fish, while the mean ventilatory rate remained the same, spontaneous changes in rate, as determined by the differences between maxima and minima observed over 30-sec periods, decreased following the operation. Similar observations on four fish before and after operation showed that the variation in the rate of horizontal eye movements was different under constant external conditions, the operated fish again seeming less variable, although the mean figures were similar.

In tests of optomotor reactions Janzen found that the operated fish showed stronger responses than normal animals and were apparently less able to "break away" from the rotating stripes. Unilateral ablation of the telencephalon produced optomotor responses of a fixity intermediate between that of normal fish and bilaterally ablated fish, but there was no correlation between the direction of stripe rotation, any turning bias shown by the fish, and the side of the telencephalon removed. However, although the removal of the telencephalon appears to change the level of responsiveness of a fish, the effect of unilateral removal cannot be assessed since the optokinetic effect was visible to both eyes and hence projected to both sides of the brain. Thus any lateralization of effect of one side of the telencephalon is unlikely to have been demonstrated by this method.

Although these previous observations could be interpreted as due to changes in the level of readiness to respond to stimuli, it is difficult to explain Janzen's next experiment in this way. He placed fish individually in an aquarium, across which was a line of vertical bars at regular intervals. Normal fish would swim through this array, even if the bar separation was decreased from 4 cm to 1.8 cm. The bilaterally ablated fish, on the other hand, would swim between the wider bars rather more than would normal fish but would hardly ever swim between the narrower ones.

Janzen also examined the tendency of goldfish to seek out familiar conditions. Fish were placed individually in a start box, from which they could pass into one of two similar chambers by moving left or right. The brightness of each of the three chambers could be made "light" or "dark" by gray paper. Taking the sum of the results, 77% of normal and 84% of lesioned fish would seek out the same brightness level as in the start box, irrespective of side preference, so there was a slightly greater tendency in the lesioned fish to adhere to previous stimulus patterns.

Hosch (1936), using minnows (*Phoxinus laevis*) and gobies (*Gobio fluviatilis*), observed similar decreases in variability of behavior. He observed that not only did the rate of eye movement in *Gobio* become less variable following operation but also the mean number of such movements decreased. Similarly, optomotor responses in *Phoxinus* were more developed in the lesioned fish, which seemed unable to ignore the stripes. He conducted an experiment which was almost the reverse of Janzen's brightness preference one; gobies (*Gobio fluviatilis*) were allowed to swim in an aquarium whose floor was covered with squares of different brightness. While in the intact condition, they maintained a fairly definite preference for dark grays; following operation, no real preference was seen, with the fish distributed over every brightness. Thus as far as spontaneous behavior is concerned, it appears that removal of the telencephalon reduces the tendency of the animal to change its response to stimuli, as evidenced by a lowering of variability of eye and respiratory movements, and by an increase in fixity of behavior, as seen in optokinetic situations. The preference tests again show fixity if the preference has been previously "forced" but a lack of preference if no such previous experience has been presented. Such failures could be due to an inability to modify existing behavior patterns, or an attentional failure, and further evidence for and discussion of these possibilities will be presented later.

5. Arousability and Fear

Janzen (1933) observed that his operated goldfish were far less hesitant in moving into new situations than were normal fish, and Hosch (1936) noted that his operated animals could sometimes completely ignore a stimulus such as a bang on the side of the tank while at other times they would overreact as compared with normal animals and swim wildly round the tank. [Karamian *et al.* (1967) similarly found that operated fish were less likely to seek shelter from startling stimuli.] Hosch also found that, when placed in a "hide" in the corner of a new tank, most of the lesioned fish would leave it immediately whereas unoperated fish would remain there for long periods. In unpublished experiments conducted by the present author, using an escape problem like that used by Ingle (1965*a*), it was found that operated goldfish would escape almost immediately or not at all whereas normal fish were more consistent, with all their escape times well between these extremes. Ingle (1965*a*), however, noted that when normal goldfish were placed in a confined space, they would soon swim through a hole in the wall to escape into a larger tank. Lesioned fish, on the other hand, would tend to remain in the original tank. Hosch (1936) also reported that telencephalon-ablated fish were far less active than normal fish, and experiments by Karamian (1956) showed that following ablation of the telencephalon of a variety of teleost and elasmobranch fish, including goldfish, carp, skates, and dogfish, the animals showed lessened activity, and when they were disturbed the swimming induced died away much more quickly than in normal fish. This has more recently been confirmed in the author's laboratory using photocells to measure the activity (Savage, 1968*a*) and by Overmier and Curnow (1969).

Such observations have led to the suggestions that the operated fish are less arousable (Aronson, 1968), unusually fearless (Hosch, 1936), or, alternatively, so fearful that they do not react unless the stimulus is extreme (Regestein, 1968).

Convenient indices of arousal are decreases in the ventilatory rate and heart rate (Otis *et al.*, 1957), and studies of the unconditioned responses of goldfish to novel stimuli have shown that the magnitude and duration of these changes are comparable in normal and operated animals (Savage, 1969*b*; Overmier and Savage, 1974).

Recent investigations by the present author have examined various types of arousal response in goldfish kept in the dark. When presented with 10-sec periods of light every 2 min, telencephalon-ablated fish showed the same magnitude of bradycardia, and took the same number of trials to habituate this response, as did operated control and olfactory tract-sectioned animals. Control and operated animals again showed equivalent responses when the intertrial interval was lengthened to 30 min, or if the level of ambient light was increased. Other tests examined the ability to switch attention. For instance, if a novel stimulus was presented to one eye, the bradycardiac response was developed. If a second novel stimulus was presented to the contralateral eye 10 sec later, while the original stimulus was still present, a second bradycardia was seen. If a stimulus was bobbed continually in front of one eye, novel stimuli elicited cardiac deceleration when presented to the other eye. These responses all occurred in telencephalon-ablated fish, and such observations tend to argue against such operated animals being less arousable, or less able to switch attention.

Laming (1976) has demonstrated that three parameters, heart rate, respiration rate, and electromyogram amplitude, show significantly different changes when a fish is aroused as opposed to frightened, as assessed by observation of the animal's behavior. Since these changes are rarely observed in ablated fish on presentation of novel stimuli, it is unlikely that excessive fear is a reason for lack of reactivity. Lack of a fear response is argued against by the fact that operated fish condition classically using fear-inducing unconditioned stimuli such as electric shock.

Telencephalon-ablated animals do seem to show lessened reactivity, at least in constant conditions, since the rates of eye and gill movement have been shown to be less variable and the activity of the whole animal to be considerably decreased. However, since simple measurements of arousal yield no differences between normal and ablated fish, any arousal hypothesis must not be too sweeping.

B. Habituation

Relatively little work has been done on the waning of innate responses in the absence of reinforcement in fish, and still less on any participation by the telencephalon. Two studies in this field have, however, suggested that there is some telencephalic involvement. Peeke *et al.* (1972) allowed goldfish to feed on brine shrimps, and, when this habit was established, placed the prey in glass containers. The fish were given daily sessions of 10 min exposure to this situation, and the rate of decrease in number of bites was measured. The ablated fish showed a significantly slower overall rate of habituation than the normal fish, but during each day they appeared to habituate as fast as the latter. It was concluded that the animals could learn in the short term but that transfer to long-term storage had been impaired. Shapiro *et al.* (1974) found that the rate of gill erection to a mirror image was lower in ablated than in normal Siamese fighting fish (*Betta splendens*). When the rate at which such a response habituated was measured over a period of 20 days, it was found that there was a significantly greater rate of habituation in the normal than in the lesioned fish. Both these studies suggest the same sort of perseveration seen in earlier parts of the discussion.

C. Classical Conditioning

1. Simple Conditioned Responses

The initial work on classically conditioned (Pavlovian) responses was that of Karamian (1956) and Baru (cited by Karamian). Baru used 10-sec presentations of light or sound as the conditioned stimulus (CS) and shock as the unconditioned stimulus (UCS). She examined responses in a variety of fish including lampreys, dogfish, skates, the beluga (*Huso huso*), the stellate sturgeon (*Acipenser stellatus*), and various teleosts including carp. In the beluga, a "weak" conditioned response was observed in approximately 80 trials. Bilateral removal of the telencephalon did not prevent subsequent acquisition of responses, nor did it interfere with the retention of previously trained responses. Kholodov (1960) showed that telencephalic ablation did not affect the ability of fish to condition aversively using sound or magnetic field as conditioned stimuli (method not specified) but that light associations were "unstable."

Overmier and Curnow (1969) examined the acquisition of conditioned responses in normal and ablated goldfish using spaced trials (10 per day). Overall activity was used as an index of conditioning, and animals were trained using 10 sec light followed by shock. The response magnitude of the sham-operated and ablated fish increased to the same activity level over 10 days of training, and there were no statistical differences between the groups.

In addition, pseudoconditioning trials were carried out, in case the "learned" responses seen in either the normal or the lesioned fish were due to spurious arousal due to shocking. Randomly spaced presentations of light and shock gave no responses like those obtained with contiguous CS and UCS. In the light of previous observations on activity changes in ablated fish, it is of interest that Overmier and Curnow noted that responses to light alone (which they called "sensitization" but was merely habituation) caused responses in normal fish which were greater than those of the ablates. They attributed this to the fact that, as they demonstrated, the ablated fish were in any case significantly less spontaneously active than the normal fish. In the light of this activity difference, mentioned by other workers, it is all the more significant that no classical conditioning deficit was observed. No simple arousal deficit hypothesis could cover these results.

2. Trace Conditioned Responses

One possibility remaining with regard to classical conditioning is that telencephalic involvement is important only when there is a temporal delay between CS offset and UCS onset. Such a hypothesis has been suggested for certain aspects of instrumental conditioning and was investigated by Overmier and Savage (1974). Goldfish were conditioned using light and shock, with a 5-sec CS, then a 5-sec gap before the shock, and heart rate changes were used as an index of response. Acquisition rates were similar in normal and ablated fish, and controls for pseudoconditioning also gave similar lack of acquisition in normal and ablated animals.

Since these last experiments were conducted under massed-training conditions, and in view of the suspected importance of massed vs. spaced conditioning in avoidance studies, to be discussed below, Farr and Savage (1978) have recently examined trace conditioning using extended (10-sec) trace intervals and spaced training. Ablated fish and olfactory tract-sectioned fish used gave statistically similar results. In addition, 15-sec trace intervals, with massed training, gave equal acquisition in the two groups. Extinction of the trace conditioned response, both under spaced and massed trial conditions, was statistically similar in normal and ablated fish. Thus an explanation of telencephalic function based on memory-trace decay seems unlikely.

3. Differential Conditioned Responses

Karamian (1956) cites an experiment by Baru in which she elaborated differential negatively reinforced classical responses in a carp, following bilateral removal of the telencephalon. Although the stimuli used were not specified, Karamian stated that the rate of acquisition of such a differential response was similar in normal and operated animals.

Bernstein (1961*a,b,* 1962) used goldfish and measured cardiac deceleration as an index of conditioning. Fish were trained differentially to respond to one of the pair red/green and not to the other using brightness controls similar to those used by McCleary and Bernstein (1959). Most animals were trained with equal brightnesses of the colors, as judged by human eye, and were then tested with pairs which differed markedly in brightness, that is, light green/dark red in one test, dark green/light red in another. Bernstein (1961*a*) initially found that, following training, while the normal fish generalized to color and did not respond to gray stimuli, the operated fish apparently responded to brightness and gave differential responses to the gray stimuli. Later, Bernstein (1961*b*) confirmed that prior telencephalon ablation had no effect on differential brightness discrimination or on the ability to generalize to other brightness problems. More recently, Bernstein (1962) showed that the ability to form a color discrimination and the ability to achieve interocular transfer of this reappeared 4 hr after operation. With regard to possible lateralization of telencephalic function, it is of interest that unilateral ablation temporarily abolished the ability to condition differentially to color via the eye contralateral to the damage but not via the ipsilateral eye.

However, so far as lesion studies are concerned, the telencephalon is not involved in classical conditioning in any permanent way.

4. Positive Conditioning

An obvious gap in our knowledge of the relation between the telencephalon and classical conditioning is that no experiments have been conducted using positive reinforcement. The reason is methodological, in that it is difficult to administer food to fish under the same controlled conditions as shock can be administered. Perhaps it may be possible to use odor or taste introduced into the water flowing over a clamped animal. Alternatively, since, as Campbell (1968) has demonstrated, goldfish will actually *seek* very mild electrical stimulation of the body surface, this may be positively reinforcing to a clamped animal. Direct stimulation of the fish brain can be positively reinforcing, as will be discussed below, but such stimulation may well affect things other than reinforcement and hence be difficult to interpret. Only when less ambiguous methods of positive reinforcement are available will it be possible to see if the generalizations made here apply to all classical conditioning.

D. Avoidance Problems

1. Simple Avoidance

a. Learning. Much of the recent behavioral work on the telencephalon has centered on the study of active avoidance, since it became apparent to several workers that, if the lesion impaired some functions such as speed of decision, avoidance tasks would be ideal for demonstrating this. Aronson and Kaplan (1965; Kaplan and Aronson, 1967) examined instrumental avoidance learning in *Tilapia macrocephala*. Animals were placed in aquaria divided into two halves and were trained to swim through a 4-cm-diameter hole in the dividing partition, when an overhead light came on, to avoid shock. A two-way shuttlebox system was used, with animals being trained to leave whichever box they were in at the beginning of a trial. Of five fish operated on and then trained, four were examined for several months before they performed avoidances, and even then their performances were erratic. Hainsworth *et al.* (1967) and Savage (1968*a,* 1969*a*) used goldfish in similar light avoidance situations, involving one-way avoidance, the fish being returned to the same start box at the beginning of each trial. Both reported considerable acquisition deficits for a 15-sec CS-UCS interval, for example, a 40–50% asymptote of avoidance as compared to a normal 90–100%. These deficits lasted during training over 200 and 250 trials, respectively, and there appeared to be no complete recovery. Neither study reported the variability of response noted by Aronson. More recently, Overmier and Gross (1974) have shown that ablation of the telencephalon in *Tilapia mossambica* causes the same sort of two-way avoidance acquisition deficits as reported for *T. macrocephala* by Aronson.

Savage (1968*a,* 1969*b*) examined the responses of naive operated fish when trained using 400-Hz sound as CS and a 5-sec CS-UCS interval. Exactly the same type of deficit was found as for light, so that the deficit generalized to at least two sensory modalities.

Thus the acquisition deficit is seen in both one- and two-way avoidance situations, and although it is possible to draw anatomical homologies between the mammalian hippocampus and part of the telencephalon (e.g., see Schnitzlein, 1964) there are no such behavioral differences between the two types of avoidance as have been found in hippocampally lesioned rats (Olton and Isaacson, 1968).

Dewsbury and Bernstein (1969) have clained that the avoidance deficit is a product of the type of box used. Using a shuttlebox with no barrier between start and goal boxes, and a 10-sec CS-UCS interval, they reported that naive ablated goldfish acquired a light avoidance as fast as did normal animals. When a 4-sec CS-UCS period was used, and a central barrier was placed between the two boxes, acquisition was poor in the ablated fish. Using the same arrangement, but a 10-sec CS-UCS interval, no deficit was seen in the operates. This is not in agreement with results reported by Savage (1969*a*) using shorter and longer intervals than 10-sec, who found a consistent deficit; and it seems likely that, as suggested above, time is not an important variable but that the type of box may be. The absence of a barrier in the initial experiment leads to a possibility that the situation is not a true avoidance one, since the animals may show a classically conditioned arousal and movement, sufficient to initiate undirected swimming. The use of some differential response might help to clear up this ambiguity. Since the rate of spontaneous crossings increased markedly during training in the "easy" situation, it is possible that sensitization was operating.

(Finally, despite the apparent ease with which the naive ablated animals learned the 10-sec "no door" problem, removal of the telencephalon from previously trained fish still caused a significant deficit, even though a considerable degree of improvement did occur, and such a finding is not explained by an "ease of performance" hypothesis.)

b. Retention. Aronson and Kaplan (1963; Kaplan and Aronson, 1967) using

Tilapia macrocephala removed the telencephalon from fish trained with the schedule described above. Following operation, animals which were previously avoiding consistently ceased to do so, and maintained only a low avoidance level despite several hundred further trials. Aronson (1968) also examined the retention of avoidance when a 500-Hz tone was used as CS and obtained similar results. Hainsworth *et al.* (1967) and Savage (1968*a*, 1969*a*) found a similar postoperative deficit in goldfish trained to avoid light with a 15-sec CS-UCS interval. Avoidances dropped from 90–100% to 10–15% and reached a maximum of 40–50% over 100–150 trials. Savage (1969*a*, comparing postoperative performances of naive and previously trained fish, concluded that despite the deficit in the latter group, when compared with the controls, they were nevertheless superior to the naive fish in number of avoidances, and thus there was some evidence for retention. Such retention could not be detected in other ways, however, for when photocells were placed beneath the start boxes no conditioned startle response was seen, as was observed in normal animals at an early stage of training.

Similar results were obtained for animals trained to avoid sound, in *Tilapia* by Aronson (1968) and in goldfish by Savage (1969*a*).

c. Olfaction. Herrick (1948) had suggested that the telencephalon might provide an unspecific facilitation of the activities of lower brain areas and that hence it was possible that a major cause of the avoidance deficit observed was lack of olfactory input to the telencephalon causing decreased facilitation of such areas.

A number of investigators thus examined the possibility that the deficit in avoidance was due in some way to loss of olfaction. Savage (1969*a*) trained animals following bilateral olfactory tract section and found their acquisition of the avoidance response comparable with that of unoperated fish, while Kaplan and Aronson (1967) trained fish before and after this operation and found no postoperative deficit. Thus olfactory involvement can be ruled out as far as aversive deficits are concerned, but controls of this sort have rarely been performed in studies of appetitive conditioning, so some caution is still needed in interpreting these results.

d. Escape Behavior. Although these studies show a considerable measure of agreement with regard to the avoidances made by lesioned fish operated before and after training, there are discrepancies in the findings on escape times, that is, the time taken to move from the start to the goal box once the CS-UCS interval has elapsed, and a shock been given. Despite almost identical procedures of administering shocks for up to 1 min after CS onset, one group of workers (Hainsworth *et al.,* 1967; Savage, 1968*a*, 1969*a*; Overmier and Gross, 1974) reported no differences in escape latency between normal and operated fish, whereas Kaplan and Aronson (1967) found increases from 2–5 sec preoperatively to near their maximum allowed time of 30 sec postoperatively.

This is possibly due to the fact that the training apparatus used by Aronson was much larger relative to the size of the fish than were those used by the other workers; hence the latter fish had less (no) possibility of facing in the wrong direction when the CS was presented. Kaplan and Aronson (1967) noted that, when operated, their fish ceased to maintain "efficient intertrial habits such as waiting at the hole," and this presumably accounted for some at least of the increased escape time and the variability of this, since fish would have had to swim to the hole area from other points of the start box. Since it will be shown below that telencephalic ablation can affect maze performance, it is possible that a large avoidance box introduces parameters other than are usually found in such situations.

e. Thresholds. A possibility remained that telencephalic removal affected the speed of response, or raised sensory thresholds, and this led Savage (1969*a*) to conduct experiments using 5- and 15-sec avoidance intervals and then a much smaller light stimulus than before. Aronson and Kaplan (1963, 1965) had used a 2.5-sec CS-UCS interval, and Hainsworth *et al.* (1967) and Savage (1969*a*) a 15-sec interval. If the speed of decision-making had been affected by the lesion, intermediate trial times should have produced intermediate results, but the use of a 5-sec interval for light avoidance (Savage, 1969*a*) produced results far more similar to those for the longer than the shorter interval, so there was no reason to suppose that a low CS-UCS interval prevented learning by ablated fish. Similarly, the use of a much smaller stimulus intensity (Savage, 1969*a*) produced only the "normal" deficit, and not the total failure that might have been expected if sensory thresholds had been raised.

f. Sensitivity to Shock. The evidence for noninvolvement of the telencephalon in classical conditioning, cited above, would tend to render unlikely any possibility that avoidance deficits could be due to lack of effect of the shock. Nevertheless, even if the classical component of the avoidance response could be acquired, the shock could still be inadequate in promoting the instrumental component. The rapid escapes shown by fish in the smaller avoidance boxes would argue against this, and Savage (1969*b*) showed that the magnitude of response to inescapable shocks, given at the same rate and number as during avoidance training, increased in the same way in normal and lesioned fish. It appeared that there could be a failure to transfer between the classical and instrumental aspects of avoidance behavior.

g. Transfer. Such transfer between classical and avoidance conditioning has, however, been demonstrated by Overmier and Starkman (1974). Goldfish were trained to avoid a tone. then differentially trained classically using color. Next, the colored stimuli were used as avoidance cues, and both normal and ablated fish transferred at equal and correct levels of avoidance provided that regular "priming" trials with the tone were provided. Thus the fear induced by classical conditioning could be used to induce avoidance, and therefore this could not be the cause of the avoidance deficit.

h. Trial Spacing. Work by Ingle (1965*a*) has questioned whether any deficit exists in naive ablated animals learning avoidance. He found perfectly normal rates of acquisition using goldfish in apparatus similar to that used by Hainsworth *et al.* (1967) and Savage (1969*a*). However, Ingle massed his training into 1 day, whereas the latter workers spaced their trials at 20 and 10 each day, respectively. Subsequent work by Savage (1968*b*) suggested that the spacing of trials was an important variable; with 10 trials each day naive lesioned fish learned poorly, whereas at 30 trials each day they performed as well as normals. (Normal fish showed the usual phenomenon of decreased speed of learning as trials were massed.) This was interpreted as meaning that the lesioned animal more rapidly loses the excitation or arousal needed to maintain attention but that if this is heightened by repeated trials, normal or near-normal performance results. Although similar results have been reported by one group of workers using appetitive techniques (see below), there appears to be little difference between the acquisition rates of the fish used by Savage (1969*a*) and by Hainsworth *et al.* (1967), using 10 and 20 trials per day, respectively, although Savage (1968*b*) showed such a difference for 10-, 20-, and 30-trial groups. Similarly, Kaplan and Aronson (1967) report that massed trials produced worse results than spaced trials in normal *Tilapia* but similar postoperative results. (However, the lack of daily training makes interpretation of these results difficult.) Thus the massed trial effect and its interpretation are matters of some uncertainty at the moment.

2. Differential Avoidance

In view of the established lack of telencephalic ablation effect on discriminatory conditioned responses, it might have been expected that in differential avoidance there would be a failure to avoid the aversive stimulus but no failure not to avoid the neutral stimulus. However, Savage (1969*a*) found that the results for learning such a differential discrimination with symmetrical reinforcement closely paralleled those for simple avoidance, in that the total number of avoidances was reduced compared with normal fish but the accuracy of discrimination was also seriously impaired. Animals trained then lesioned showed the same types of deficit. In view of this latter result, it seemed likely that there had been a failure of reinforcement addressing under instrumental conditions, causing effective extinction of correct responding. Savage suggested that the delay between CS offset and reaching the goal box was too long for the rapidly forgetting lesioned fish, which could not then consolidate such information. He used a trace avoidance paradigm to test this (Savage, 1968*b*) in which a door was opened between two boxes and fish had to avoid or not depending on the presence of a 500-Hz tone prior to the door's opening. Normal fish could achieve better than chance level performances, whereas the lesioned fish could not. Because the overall avoidance levels of the two groups were made more nearly equal by this technique, the suggestion of some form of short-term failure was supported in that the presence or absence of the cue had apparently been forgotten.

3. Partial Lesions and Commissure Sections

Little work has been done on any aspect of behavior and partial telencephalic lesions, and, in view of the likelihood that the telencephalon is involved in several types of process, experiments of this nature may prove valuable, especially when linked to effective "split-brain" preparations. Although the behavioral methods used to assess these lesions vary, experiments are so few that they are most conveniently considered here.

a. Partial Lesions. As noted earlier, Janzen was first to report behavioral effects of unilateral telencephalic removal, in 1933. No abnormalities of posture or locomotion were seen, nor was there any effect on feeding reactions. Optomotor reactions were intermediate in intensity between those of bilaterally ablated fish and those of normal fish, but there was no relation between the side of brain damaged and any turning preference. Hosch (1936) failed to detect any difference between normal and unilaterally damaged *Phoxinis laevis* in a similar situation. Janzen also observed an intermediacy of behavior, compared with that of lesioned and unlesioned fish, when animals were allowed to swim through a curtain of vertical wires. When fish were given a choice in a side-preference box, unilateral ablation resulted in a clear bias of turning preference toward the intact side, the mean figures for eight fish being 73%:27%, as opposed to 51%:49% for normal fish and 47%:53% for bilaterally ablated fish. Such results suggested that there was a lateralized effect of the remaining telencephalic hemisphere, but, as stated above, since both eyes were analyzing each problem, any reduced efficiency on the lesioned side, via the contralateral eye, would be masked by compensation by the other side, except perhaps in a T-maze choice situation. The most obvious way to examine for such effects would be to train via one eye at a time.

Using electrolytic lesions, Savage (1969*a*) studied the effect of unilateral lateral and central area lesions on the acquisition of vertical/horizontal rectangle discriminative avoidance by unilaterally trained goldfish. It was found that central area lesions could impair discrimination, although the avoidance level was normal, when animals were trained to the eye contralateral to the lesion, but if they were trained to the eye ipsilateral to the lesion, both avoidance and discrimination were unimpaired. (The optic tracts in fish exhibit complete crossing over; thus the projection to one side of the optic tectum is completely from the contralateral eye.) If the lateral area was damaged, however, avoidance became reduced, with variable effects on accuracy of discrimination. Again, this deficit appeared to be confined to the training side contralateral to the lesion. Thus a possible duality and lateralization of function were revealed, and such possible localization bears further investigation.

b. Commissures and Transfer. It is now well documented that fish show high levels of interocular transfer of responses to shape discrimination problems, provided that these problems are not too difficult (e.g., see Savage, 1979). The routes for such transfer of information are becoming clearer, but of the multiplicity of commissures in the teleost brain, none has as yet attained the functional precedence of the corpus callosum of the mammals (e.g., see Myers, 1965). Mark (1966) has implicated the tectal commissure in interhemispheric transfer of both approach and avoidance tasks, but Yeo and Savage (1975) have shown that differential cardiac conditioning will transfer perfectly in fish with this commissure sectioned, as have Ingle and Campbell (1977) using differential avoidance. Possibly this discrepancy in results is explained by difficulties experienced by the tectally split fish in transferring some motor components of the task. McCleary (1960) and Shapiro (1965) have both shown that the successful demonstration of transfer is dependent either on an easy problem or on careful pretraining of both eyes on the motor aspects of the paradigm. If the tectal commissure is involved to some degree in the transfer of motor information relating to an imperfectly learned task, then splits of this commissure may appear to impede transfer of responses to a discrimination.

Other potential transfer routes are the posterior commissure and the series of postoptic commissures. Both Yeo and Savage (1976) and Ingle and Campbell (1977) have shown that fish with sections of the posterior commissure can transfer discriminations but that section of the "postoptic" commissures causes transfer failure. In particular, Yeo and Savage have implicated the horizontal or the horizontal and minor commissures in this deficit. At present, it is not possible to specify which of these commissures is the route of transfer.

Ingle and Campbell (1977) have also demonstrated the nonimportance of the anterior commissure of the telencephalon. Savage (1969*a*) split this and found that the level of avoidance fell on the as-yet-untrained side and the accuracy of discrimination fell to chance level. Fish took approximately 40 trials to reach their pre-transfer level of accuracy. Possibly this discrepancy in results lies in the fact that the latter work was done with spaced trials, that of Ingle with massed trials. Taken with the effects of unilateral lesions described above, such a result suggests that the influence of each telencephalic hemisphere is lateralized, but further work is needed to clarify the situation.

In view of the considerable commissural and decussating connection between nonolfactory as well as olfactory parts of the telencephalon, some degree of transfer might be expected, but the situation is as yet unclear. Bianki (1972) used differential approach and avoidance problems on *Carassius auratus, C. carassius, Cyprinus carpio,* and *Acipenser ruthenus.* He found that section of the anterior commissure did not interfere with discrimination of visual or auditory problems, although the method of presentation of these is unclear, but that an olfactory discrimination was slightly disturbed. However, since, as will be seen below, normal simple approach problems are not interfered with by ablation, section of the commissure might not be expected to interfere with retention; and, since it is not clear as to what extent any avoidance training was unilateral, it remains to be seen how the operation affects transfer of these types of discrimination. Bianki indicated that section of the tectal commissure (which may well have also damaged the posterior commissure) interfered with visual and auditory problems, but insufficient detail was given, and in any case tectal splits may have motor consequences, as seen above.

4. Passive Avoidances

As Overmier has pointed out, tests of active avoidance confuse learning and avoidance, in that giving a telencephalon-ablated fish an active avoidance problem is giving the animal something which biases it not to learn. Thus in passive avoidance problems the bias is in favor of the operated fish, since animals have to learn not to move.

Overmier and Flood (1969) made one of the very few studies of passive avoidance, training fish to swim from start to goal box, then to cease to do this to avoid being shocked on entering the goal box. Operated fish were inferior in learning passive avoidance. Their established lack of activity cannot explain this result, and it is more easily explained in terms of an inability to reverse previous preferences, a tendency noted before. Further, Overmier and Flood found that not only was the day-to-day performance of the operates lower than that of normals but also the trial-to-trial performance was poorer. They supposed that part at least of the explanation of the performance could be due to short-term memory decay. There are, however, some hesitations as to regarding this situation as a typical passive avoidance one. Although the incentive to enter the goal box was partly a positive one, in that food was present, there were also negative incentives to *leave* the start box, in that the depth of water in that box was shallow (about 1 inch) and that in the goal box twice this depth. In addition, at the initiation of each trial a bubbling aerator was placed in the start box, and this has been used as negative reinforcement, notably by the Russian school (e.g, see chapters by Voronin and Kholodov and by Prazdnikova in Pavlovskii, 1964). Thus the initial situation may have resembled a mixture of avoidance and approach with a further component of avoidance then added, which makes interpretation difficult.

As mentioned above, the amount of food consumed, the rate of conversion, and the motivation to feed, whether measured by the electric current needed to deter feeding or by the speed of moving to feed, are all comparable in normal and ablated fish (Savage, 1969*b*). Thus, although the telencephalon is undoubtedly involved with smell, deficits in food-reinforced behavior due to abnormalities in feeding are not to be expected.

1. Simple Approach Tasks

Scharrer (1928) was the first to investigate any relation between positively reinforced learning and the telencephalon, in the course of work on the pineal body. He used blinded fish, trained to feed when a light was presented overhead. The fish soon showed swimming movements to the light alone, and this response remained when the telencephalon was removed.

Flood and Overmier (1971) have shown, however, that in a simple runway task, ablated fish are inferior to normal or olfactory tract-sectioned animals, at least when trained using spaced trials (10 trials per session). However, when trials were massed (30 per session) the performance of the ablated fish resembled that of the normal and tract-sectioned animals. Flood and Overmier interpreted this as evidence for a short-term memory failure in the ablated fish, as had been suggested earlier to explain the same phenomenon in avoidance learning. Once the fish had acquired the runway task, their asymptotic performances were similar irrespective of operation or trial spacing. In extinction, there were differences between the two operated groups and the normal fish, and this difference was attributed to lack of olfaction. This is one of the few cases reported in which section of the olfactory tracts has caused a deficit comparable to that caused by telencephalon ablation, and it suggests that such controls are urgently needed in the types of experiment discussed in this section.

Telencephalon-ablated fish also experience difficulties in learning operant tasks. Savage (1969*b*) used a photocell instead of a bar-press and observed the rate at which such a task was spontaneously acquired by fish, with "priming" food placed over the cell on the day before the start of training. The ablated fish were slow to acquire the task, but once they had learned it they performed at the same rate as normal fish.

When the initial ("exploratory") portion of the cumulative response curve for the two groups was examined, considerable similarity was noted, and the subsequent divergence of the traces was explained by supposing a failure to associate light-beam interruption with feeding. It was suggested that the "priming" food caused the same amount of exploratory activity in both groups but that the lesioned fish could not associate temporally and spatially separate events such as interruption of the beam and presentation of food, and hence would extinguish the response to the photocell. When normal animals were "primed" and then left with an inoperative feeder, the cumulative curve of beam interruptions was similar to that of the fed ablated fish.

Similar findings have been reported by Aronson and Herberman (1960). Specimens of *Tilapia* were trained to push a paddle, when introduced into the tank, to obtain food, and then sham, olfactory tract, and telencephalic operations were performed. Subsequently, only the last group showed deficits, their response latency increasing and varying considerably. Kholodov (1960), training carp (*Cyprinus carpio*) to snap at a bead in response to red light in order to obtain food, found no difference in acquisition times between normal and operated animals. In an extension of this experiment, Kholodov appears to have achieved a type of secondary conditioning (one of the few reports of this in fish; e.g., see Sanders, 1940), and the potential importance of any investigation of this sort is considerable, since one hypothesis of forebrain function gives it a role in the processing of secondary reinforcement data. Kholodov took a fish trained on the response to the red light, and presented a green light following the red. The fish responded to the green light with a bite at the bead, although prior association with red light was the only "reinforcer" available. Removal of the telencephalon did not interfere with the response to these stimuli.

2. Discriminatory Approach Tasks

Janzen (1933), Nolte (1933), and Hosch (1936) all examined the effects of prior telencephalic ablation on the acquisition of simultaneous visual discrimination tasks, reinforced by food. Janzen (1933) trained goldfish with a red/blue color discrimination (without brightness controls, however) and made allowances for possible olfactory or gustatory cueing. Although the operated fish were marginally poorer over the middle part of discrimination training (a commonly observed phenomenon), their asymptotes, and the time taken to reach these, were identical. Janzen observed that the operated fish were "less sure" in their choice and somewhat slower than the intact animals. Nolte (1933) examined the discriminative ability of both minnows (*Phoxinus laevis*) and sticklebacks (*Gasterosteus aculeatus*). He found that both species with partial or total telencephalic ablation were able to learn color discriminations or to retain them following ablation. The shapes of generalization gradients obtained before and after operation were identical. Other animals were trained with a vertical/horizontal problem and showed no postoperative deficits. Hosch (1936) used a star/circle discrimination with normal and operated minnows and found equal rates of acquisition.

Berwein (1941) trained lesioned minnows with a sequential temperature discrimination and found that acquisition rates were greater in the normal fish. Since virtually all other approach tasks have used simultaneous discrimination, such a deficit bears further investigation.

Kholodov (1960) reported little impairment in ablated fish trained on a red/green discrimination. Malyukova (1964), using a method similar to that used by Kholodov (1960) involving responding to presented shapes by snapping at beads, has examined the effects of localized electrolytic lesions on the retention of a triple discrimination involving a circle, a triangle, and a cross. Following lesion, fish swam and fed normally but tended to avoid both shapes and beads, and if they responded to these the level of accuracy was impaired.

More recently, Aronson and Herberman (as reported by Aronson, 1968) used the paddle-pushing response described above, and trained *Tilapia* to discriminate between vertical and horizontal stripes. They reported that following ablation of the telencephalon the response latencies rose, the actual number of responses decreased, and the accuracy of discrimination varied from 50% to 100% from day to day. In view of the known inability of these fish to cope with the response itself following lesion, as mentioned above, it is difficult to assess the meaning of this apparent discriminative failure.

Graeber *et al.* (1972) have shown that the operation can affect the learning of differential visual approach tasks in the nurse shark (*Ginglymostoma cirratum*). This is one of the few studies to demonstrate failure of operated animals in a simple approach discrimination. The animals were trained to go to black/white shapes, then to vertical/horizontal stripes. Fish with the telencephalon ablated showed an inability to learn the contrast problem, although their response latencies were low. The animals could easily learn a position (i.e., go left) habit. Only lesions in the posterior telencephalon caused this deficit. Animals trained, then operated on, were unable to improve on their immediate postoperative deficit. In view of the inability of animals to perform the visual discrimination, and yet their ability to perform the side-seeking task, Graeber and his co-workers concluded that the lesion had interfered with the possible visual projection already discussed from an anatomical viewpoint whose physiological aspect is to be discussed below. However, in view of the lack of effect of the lesion on similar tasks reported here, and the known side persistence of lesioned fish (see below), an alternative explanation is given by another experiment. Savage and Swingland (1969) showed that operated goldfish could learn a vertical/horizontal problem as well as could control fish, but that, if a delay was introduced between response and reward, extinction of accuracy of response, but not of the response itself, occurred. They argued that the memory trace of the shape was erased too quickly, following the response, in the telencephalon-ablated fish, so that reinforcement, when it arrived, was ineffective in causing maintenance of a learned shape preference. Thus extinction toward random preference would occur. Since the method used involved the animals swimming away from the shapes to obtain the food, it is not clear whether delay of reinforcement or delay following removal of the stimulus was the effective factor. Nevertheless, comparing this and the situation used by Graeber *et al.* (1972), similarities become apparent, in that the sharks used by Graeber had to swim under and past the discrimination stimuli before being rewarded. This corresponds exactly to the delay situation used by Savage and provides an alternative explanation of the deficits seen. However, since little is known of many aspects of elasmobranch behavior and brain function, and in view of the possible greater visual representation in the cartilaginous than in the bony fish telencephalon, tests of conventional approach with immediate reinforcement tasks are needed to clarify this point. In bony fish at least, visual discrimination is unimpaired by prior telencephalic ablation, and as yet only delay treatment has exposed any deficit.

3. Mazes

Mazes constitute a special case of approach learning in that the reward is concealed, and not obvious, as it is in the discrimination situations just outlined.

Hosch (1936) trained minnows to take food from a holder on one side of the tank, and, when a side preference was well established, reversed it. Operated and normal fish were similar in their success in the reversal of this task, although other authors, using more conventional spatial problems, do not concur.

Zunini (1954) found that minnows (*Phoxinus laevis*) could learn to find their way into a glass jar for food, a test devised by Russell (1931), or could learn some of the mazes devised by Beniuc (1938). Once the fish were trained, he removed the telencephalon from some animals, and these showed large increases in the times taken to run the mazes. Naive lesioned animals were similarly slow to learn the mazes.

Hale (1956) trained normal and telencephalon-ablated goldfish to swim from one box to another to obtain food. Operated fish took longer to learn the task, and their asymptotic times were far greater than those of normal fish. When Hale removed the telencephalon from trained fish, their reaction times rose to equal those of trained ablated fish; thus there was evidence for retention following lesion. Another experiment concerned with the social facilitation of this task showed that groups of three normal fish learned the maze far faster than single fish. The same effect was seen in operated fish, demonstrating a failure in one aspect of learning and a lack of deficit in another.

Warren (1961) also reported an inferiority of ablated fish in mazes, using the paradise fish (*Macropodus opercularis*). Out of 12 mazes used, the operates were superior in one, equal in five, and inferior in six. When trained in a T maze, the operated fish were not inferior in learning the original problem or in alternate reversals (i.e., going in the original direction). They were, however, inferior in learning the reversals which involved going in the opposite direction to that trained initially. This suggested that inhibition of previously learned responses was a problem in ablated fish. This tendency of ablated fish to retain the originally trained task was also investigated by Ingle (1965*b*) using his continuous Y maze, in which fish turn at the end of each maze arm, then return along it. Using the punishment of colliding with a glass door, he trained his animals to turn in the same direction on each trial, and found that the ablated fish performed better than the normal fish, and that even if animals were trained to alternate, the operated fish were the equal of the normal animals. Frank *et al.* (1972) have also examined this problem, using goldfish in a Y maze, but with positive rather than negative reinforcement. Using olfactory tract-sectioned controls, they found that reversals were more difficult for the ablated fish, although to latency differences were observed. Ablated fish persisted in previously trained behavior. An inability to correct wrong choices in a maze may form at least part of the reason for failure in such situations, although, of course, delay of reward, which also operates in a maze, could well be another factor impairing the performance of operated fish.

III. Electrical Recording from the Telencephalon

A. Olfaction

As when considering the results of ablation studies, it is convenient to review briefly some of the major physiological findings on the olfactory working of the telencephalon, for such considerations help to circumscribe the remaining nonolfactory functions.

A considerable amount of work has been done on the functions of the olfactory bulb, and it has become apparent that much information processing occurs there, before the telencephalon proper is reached. Hara and Gorbman (1967), using goldfish, found resting bulbar electroencephalogram (EEG) frequencies of 14–16 Hz, of amplitudes ranging from 70 to 100 μV. When a 0.06 M NaCl solution was applied to the nares (Oshima and Gorbman, 1966), high-amplitude waves were generated, at frequencies of 10–15 Hz. These lasted for 1–2 sec and were followed by lower-amplitude waves of 4–8 Hz, for a short period, then still lower-amplitude waves of 9–13 Hz, which lasted 40–120 sec. The evoked response in the olfactory bulb increased linearly with the concentration of NaCl used (Hara and Gorbman, 1967).

The importance of the olfactory bulbs, as opposed to the telencephalon proper, in the analysis of olfactory stimuli is becoming apparent. Satou (1974) analyzed the frequencies and power distribution of potentials evoked in the olfactory nerve, bulb, and telencephalon of the Himé salmon (*Oncorhynchus nerka*) and showed that changes in spectrum, representing analysis of odor, occurred between the nerve and bulb, but not between the bulb and telencephalon. Hara *et al.* (1973), using rainbow trout (*Salmo gairdneri*), showed that a typical change occurred in the EEG of the olfactory bulb, when the olfactory epithelium was chemically stimulated. The normal 2–6 Hz rhythm changed to 7–11 Hz. The EEG was then analyzed for power and frequency against time, and the power spectra proved to be specific to the chemical used, so that again it seemed likely that much olfactory analysis was occurring in the olfactory bulb, before information was relayed to the olfactory areas of the telencephalon.

Such an ability of the olfactory system to analyze fine differences of smell is apparently the basis of homing in some species of fish, especially salmon. Hara *et al.* (1965) demonstrated that the bulbar EEG of salmon showed changes to home-stream water but to no others. However, as Hara (1970) has pointed out, such a reaction could be due to the presence of olfactory cues from other salmon, and Oshima *et al.* (1969) have shown that the presentation of non-home-stream water to a fish can for a period cause an EEG response similar to that for the home stream. Dizon *et al.* (1973) examined this problem in the cohoe salmon (*Oncorhynchus kisutch*) and concluded that the presence of other salmon in the water doubled the home-stream EEG response.

Thus it appears that much olfactory analysis is accomplished by the olfactory bulbs, and that telencephalic olfactory involvement is more limited than previously thought. The extent of such involvement has been investigated by experiments in which the olfactory bulbs have been disconnected from the rest of the telencephalon, by cutting of the olfactory tracts, which is an easy operation in animals like goldfish, where the bulbs are pedunculate rather than sessile. It has been known for some time that there are efferent as well as afferent fibers in the olfactory tracts (e.g., see Nieuwenhuys, 1967) and some aspects of the mode of function of such fibers are shown by this operation. Using animals sectioned between the midbrain and hindbrain, Oshima and Gorbman (1966) found that section of the olfactory tract reduced the type of NaCl-induced bulbar response described above, eliminating the secondary responses and reducing the size of the primary one. In subsequent work using intact fish, Hara and Gorbman (1967) found that section of the olfactory tracts enhanced the bulbar response to NaCl, and by finer sectioning they were able to demonstrate that the centrifugal influence was in this case carried by the medial olfactory tract. Döving (1966) and Döving and Hyvärinen (1969) examined the spontaneous firing rates of neurons in the olfactory bulb and showed that their rates could be changed by stimulation of either the ipsilateral or the contralateral olfactory tract. Hara and Gorbman (1967) also reported that the stimulation of one olfactory bulb caused depression of EEG activity in the contralateral bulb. This inhibition could be reduced by electrical stimulation of the anterior commissure, which has been shown to contain commissural fibers joining the two anterior olfactory areas (Nieuwenhuys, 1959).

Although much olfactory analysis occurs before the telencephalon, nevertheless there is an olfactory projection, whose terminations are detectable by physiological as well as anatomical means. For instance, Döving and Gemne (1965) have shown that there are three major components in the compound action potential of the burbot (*Lota lota*), corresponding to varying conduction rates, and it is possible that the slowest bundle of fibers may supply the hypophysis. Kandel (1964), using goldfish, found that the neurosecretory cells of the preoptic nucleus were driven by olfactory tract stimulation and that stimulation of the pituitary caused antidromic impulses to reach this nucleus. Such a system would occupy only the ventral parts of the telencephalon, and since neurohypophyseal hormones have shown to be involved with ionic regulation (Maetz and Juien, 1961) such a direct connection between the NaCl-sensitive nares and the appropriate hormones is not surprising.

Oshima and Gorbman (1966) found in goldfish that perfusion of the nares by NaCl solutions gave a maximal response at depths of 1000–1500 μm, in the medial part of the hemisphere. This corresponds to the medial ventral area, which anatomical considerations have already implicated as a primarily olfactory region.

Bruckmoser and Dieringer (1973) examined evoked responses and their distribution in *Scylliorhinus* and *Torpedo* following electrical stimulation of the mucosa or of the olfactory bulbs. Responses in *Scylliorhinus* were distorted by the presence of large secondary olfactory potentials, which spread over the surface of the telencephalon, but in *Torpedo,* where such spread was not observed, the secondary olfactory response was restricted to the anterior primary olfactory projection area, and only small evoked potentials were recorded from posterior parts of the telencephalon.

Devitsina (1973) working on burbot (*Lota lota*) and pike (*Esox lucius*) stimulated the olfactory nerve electrically and found that evoked potentials were of a considerable size in the bulb, less in the anterior telencephalon, and small in the dorsal telencephalon midway from front to rear.

Even if there is no direct olfactory afference to the dorsal telencephalon, this does not imply a lack of connections in the reverse direction, for Hara and Gorbman (1967) showed that while electrical stimulation of the anterior telencephalon did not markedly depress bulbar EEG activity, stimulation of the posterior dorsal areas had a much greater effect on the bulb ipsilateral to the stimulation. Further ascending influences, traveling through the telencephalon, were shown by Döving and Gemne (1966) in the burbot (*Lota lota*), where second-order olfactory neurons showed a decrease in spontaneous firing following touches to the skin.

B. Ascending Influences

In higher vertebrates the highest projections of all the major sensory systems reach the enlarged dorsal areas of the telencephalon, but there has been considerable disagreement, on both anatomical and physiological grounds, as to the existence of such projections in fish. As was outlined in the preceding part of this section, physiological evidence shows that much of the telencephalon, especially the anterior portion, is devoted to olfaction, but there is increasing anatomical evidence of ascending fibers from the diencephalon and possibly from the mesencephalon. Much of the neurophysiological work has centered on whether such ascending fibers cause changes in the EEG and whether such changes represent specific projections of one sensory modality such as vision.

1. EEG Arousal

Early electroencephalographic work showed that even if there was no direct projection of such specific sensory information to the telencephalon, the presentation of stimuli could change the overall electrical activity of the area, giving rise to an arousal of the EEG. Enger (1957) observed that in free-swimming unanesthetized cod (*Gadus callarias*), an 8–13 Hz rhythm dominated the telencephalon, appearing in spindles of 0.5–5 sec duration. This rhythm was interspersed with lower-frequency activity (4–6 Hz) and apparently derived from or correlated with a similar 8–13 Hz rhythm in the optic tectum, for it never occurred in the absence of the tectal rhythm. This 8–13 Hz "alpha" activity was seen primarily in resting fish, especially in the dark. A 4–6 Hz rhythm was observed in the telencephalon under both dark and light conditions. (When nembutal anesthesia was applied, the 8–13 Hz rhythm came to dominate the brain, and higher frequencies were absent. Under deeper anesthesia, this rhythm faded out, and the brain became dominated by slow wave activity, at a maximum in the telencephalon.) When photic stimulation was presented, an arousal reaction of the EEG was seen, in both telencephalon and mesencephalon, with an increase of the basic rhythm to 18–32 Hz. No such reaction was seen in the medulla. After photic stimulation ceased, the 8–13 Hz rhythm returned in 1–2 min. Under slight anesthesia, the change caused was slighter, with frequencies of 14–18 Hz being seen.

Schadé and Weiler (1959) and Schadé (1959) made similar types of observations on the goldfish (*Carassius auratus*). They reported a 4–8 Hz rhythm in the telencephalon of a resting fish in the dark that changed to a 9–14 Hz rhythm as the ambient light increased. A 35–40 Hz rhythm was sometimes observed. Anesthesia with urethane caused the higher frequencies to vanish. On photic stimulation, 18–24 Hz rhythms were seen in the tectum and less reliably in the telencephalon, but no such reaction was recorded in response to single flashes.

Godet *et al.* (1964) demonstrated that in the lungfish (*Protopterus annectens*) there was an arousal reaction of the telencephalic EEG in response to olfactory stimuli, and this could last for 1 min. The reaction was absent in cocooned animals undergoing estivation. More recently, Laming (1976) has shown that arousal reactions in goldfish caused by visual and auditory stimuli, measured by cardiac and respiratory responses, are accompanied by definite EEG changes in both the optic tectum and the telencephalon. The amplitude of the EEG falls, while its frequency rises.

Maliukina and Vornovitski (1966), using two species of carp (*Cyprinus carpio* and *Carassius carassius*), found telencephalic EEGs of 4–7 Hz, interspersed with 12–25 Hz rhythms. They found that cutting between the telencephalon and tectum caused a decrease in activity of the tectum, indicating a possible telencephalic facilitatory effect on that area. Zagorulko (1965) reported that removal of the telencephalon in carp reduced the size of tectal light-evoked potentials. This result again supports the idea that the telencephalon may influence the magnitude of responses at lower levels in the brain.

The available evidence thus suggests that the electrical activity of the telencephalon is modifiable by changes in nonolfactory sensory inflow and that a variety of types of sensory input are capable of initiating such changes.

2. Specific Sensory Afference

Since a number of anatomical studies, notably those of Ebbesson, have shown tracts ascending from the thalamus to the telencephalon, there are firm grounds for suggesting that the diencephalon and more posterior brain areas may project foward. The arousal pattern of the EEG set up in the telencephalon by the various sensory stimulations used might be due to nonspecific action of the recticular formation, or to an actual projection of specific sensory afferents into the telencephalon, whose activation would in turn set up an arousal EEG there. A direct sensory projection should enable discrete evoked potentials to be observed in response to single stimuli, and the presence of such evoked potentials indicating specific sensory afference has been the subject of some disagreement.

Russian workers have reported evoked telencephalic potentials in response to visual, auditory, and tactile stimuli (Voronin and Guselnikov, 1959; Voronin *et al.*, 1968) and to visual stimuli (Maliukina and Flerova, 1960). Maliukina and Vornovitski (1966) observed visual evoked potentials in the telencephalon of *Carassius carassius* and *Cyprinus carpio.* The latency of the tectal evoked potential was 40–45 msec, and a telencephalic potential was recorded with a latency of 50–65 msec. A response was also reported in the telencephalon ipsilateral to the eye stimulated, with a latency of 55–70 msec. Section of the brain between the telencephalon and tectum contralateral to the stimulated eye abolished the telencephalic potential, whereas a similar ipsilateral section did not. More recently, Veselkin and Kovačević (1973) examined a series of elasmobranchs including *Raja, Torpedo,* and *Scyllium* and reported that visual evoked potentials were seen in the posterior telencephalon. The potential was a negative one when recorded on the surface, but inverted at a depth of 500 μm in *Scyllium,* indicating an origin between these points. The latency of a negative wave, seen in the tectum, in response to visual stimulation, was anything from 4–5 msec (*Raja*) to 10–15 msec (*Torpedo*). The extreme values for the latency of such a projection in the telencephalon were 40–180 msec. In *Dasyatis* multiunit discharges were observed in response to flashes of light, and these correlated with the initial peak of the evoked potential. All these responses were localized in the dorsal area of the posterior telencephalon, and the visual evoked potential in the telencephalon was reported as being extremely susceptible to "fatigue" on repeated stimulation. Distruction of the tectum did not abolish the telencephalic evoked potential, so the input route was considered to be via the thalamus. Stimulation of the thalamus in *Dasyatis* produced telencephalic evoked potentials with a latency of 30–40 msec, and electrical stimulation of the dorsal surface of the animal caused telencephalic potentials, with a long latency of 100–200 msec. Karamian *et al.* (1973) have given evidence that dorsal column stimulation of the spinal cord in the lamprey (*Lampetra fluviatilis*) causes telencephalic evoked potentials, so somatic sensory information may project to this area.

Cohen *et al.* (1973) have also claimed the existence of a visual projection, in the telencephalon of the shark (*Ginglymostoma cirratum*), in the central telencephalic area. Platt *et al.* (1974) have reported that various types of input in some elasmobranchs, primarily *Torpedo* and *Scyliorhinus,* can cause specific evoked potentials in the telencephalon. Stimulating the maxillary nerve, they found that telencephalic evoked potentials of variable latency could be recorded, and similar evoked potentials were recorded in response to electric field changes in the water surrounding the fish.

There is thus a considerable body of evidence showing not only the presence of undifferentiated EEG arousal following various types of sensory stimulation but also the presence of evoked potentials associated with such reactions. However, an extensive series of experiments by Karamian *et al.* (1966) leads to caution with regard to acceptance of the presence of visual evoked potentials. No visual evoked potentials were observed in *Lampetra* or *Raja,* although such responses were seen in *Rana* and *Varanus.* [Enger (1957) and Schadé and Weiler (1959) reported an absence of visual evoked potentials in bony fish.] Likewise, Veselkin (1964), cited by Veselkin and Kovačević (1973), reported an absence of visual evoked potentials in *Raja* and *Dasyatis,* and Guselnikov *et al.* (1964) considered that telencephalic evoked potentials derived mainly from the leakages of the massive tectal potential generated close by. The optic tectum is a considerable generator of such potentials, and it may be difficult to differentiate any true telencephalic potentials from potentials originating in the tectum, except by latency differences of the sort reported by Veselkin and Kovačević (1973). Telencephalic visual projections in various higher vertebrates have been reported by Karamian *et al.* (1966), in turtles (*Emys*) by Guselnikov *et al.* (1974), and in the frog (*Rana*) by Gruberg and Ambros (1974). More definite conclusions will be possible when more is known of the unit activity of the telencephalon.

Finally, it should be mentioned that there are as yet no studies on the neurophysiological correlates of learning in fish. Work of this sort is needed and should help to resolve some of the questions as to whether the telencephalon plays a tonic or a phasic role in learning, and if the latter at precisely what stage of acquisition its presence is most necessary. Such knowledge could place most useful limitations on the rather diffuse theories of function discussed below.

IV. Electrical Stimulation of the Telencephalon

A. Effects on General Behavior and on Feeding

It was noted by early workers, including Ferrier (1876), that stimulation of both the elasmobranch and the teleost telencephalon gave rise to eye movements, movements of fins, and even movements of the lateral musculature. No later work has confirmed this (e.g., see Chauchard and Chauchard, 1927), and such observations were almost certainly due to the spread of excessive stimulation current to areas such as the optic tectum and the motor nuclei of the thalamus.

Grimm (1960) found that electrical stimulation of the olfactory tracts could initiate complete feeding performances in goldfish but that stimulation of the telencephalon was not so effective in doing this; however, no details of the telencephalic sites and responses were given. Fiedler (1964, 1967) reported that telencephalic stimulation in *Crenilabrus* and *Lepomis* produced feeding and some yawning and anterior/posterior movements which did not fit into any obvious pattern of behavior. Demski and Knigge (1971), using the bluegill sunfish (*Lepomis macrochirus*), observed feeding to be elicited in response to stimulation of hypothalamic sites and of the ventromedial telencephalon. Savage (1971), using goldfish, found that stimulation of the anterior parts of the telencephalon gave rise to feeding movements but that these movements could not be elicited from the posterior and lateral areas. He concluded that the feeding responses were likely to be a result of spurious olfactory sensory stimulation and not a result of a change in feeding motivation, since, as has been see, telencephalon-ablated fish feed normally. Savage and Roberts (1975) have also shown that food-sated fish will show feeding responses only if the posterior hypothalamus is stimulated and that stimulation of the anterior hypothalamic areas, through which the forebrain bundles pass, does not induce feeding in these animals. Since the majority of reports just mentioned did not specify the feeding regimes used, it is possible that the sole cause of feeding behavior elicited was an olfactory cue rather than a motivational change. Savage (1971) also observed that stimulation of posterior/lateral areas of the telencephalon gave rise to various undirected behaviors which he grouped together under "arousal reactions" since they resembled the responses of fish when the sides of the tank were hit gently.

In addition to such an obvious function as feeding, there have been other types of behavioral observation more related to the social behavior of fish. Demski and Knigge (1971) examining the bluegill (*Lepomis macrochirus*) observed that nest building was evoked by stimulation of the central part of the dorsal telencephalon, whereas stimulation near the habenula (which has connections with the telencephalon) caused inhibition of aggression and facilitation of courtship. Clark *et al.* (1960) reported that stimulation of the telencephalon in catfish could produce movement of the barbels and that such movements were very repeatable. Nevertheless, the telencephalon is not involved in all such behavior, since Demski and Gerald (1972) found that sound production in the toadfish (*Opsanus beta*) could not be elicited by telencephalic stimulation.

At a different level of function, Ingle (personal communication) has observed that telencephalic stimulation affects heart rate, and Wright (1978) has examined this systematically. Decreases of heart rate in resting fish are a sign of arousal or fear, and it was found that similar decelerations were caused by electrical stimulation of sites in the posterior but not the anterior telencephalon. The lowest thresholds were found in the central part of the telencephalon, and in free-swimming implanted fish the threshold to elicit such cardiac deceleration coincided with the threshold to produce the behavioral signs of arousal, such as orientation movements. The effect of telencephalon stimulation on heart rate was found to be extremely anesthetic sensitive; even under 1:10,000 MS222 anesthesia fish showed no response, whereas other brain areas such as the hypothalamus and medulla gave cardiac effects even when the fish was under 1:2000 MS222. It is interesting that Segura (1969) has reported that telencephalic stimulation in the toad (*Bufo* sp.) causes bradycardiac responses, and sometimes independent changes of blood pressure. Unfortunately, there are no observations as to the behavioral effects of such stimulation.

B. Reinforcement Effects

Both Boyd and Gardner (1962) and Savage (1971) have examined the behavior of implanted goldfish for reinforcement effects, using similar techniques of reversal of end-preference in a tank. Boyd and Gardner reported on one telencephalic area found to be negatively reinforcing and one tectal area found to be positively reinforcing, although the interpretation of the tectal result is difficult in view of the many functions of the area. Savage examined a number of telencephalic sites and found that, apart from anterior olfactory areas, where stimulation caused an increase in preference for the stimulated area of the tank, most telencephalic areas were negatively reinforcing, the greatest effect being in the lateral areas. Examining the threshold currents needed to produce either arousal or a negatively reinforcing effect, he concluded that the central area of the telencephalon had a lower threshold for arousal and the lateral area a lower threshold for negative reinforcement. Thus there may be at least two nonolfactory functions, located in adjacent areas of the telencephalon.

C. Effects on Other Brain Areas

Hallowitz *et al.* (1971) have provided evidence that part of the telencephalon may influence the activity of other areas of the brain. They stimulated the telencephalon of the sunfish *Lepomis macrochirus* and *L. gibbosus* and showed that the rate of firing of units in the parvocellular area of the preoptic nucleus was affected. These units had a rate of spontaneous firing of one per several seconds, and stimulation raised this to at least one per second. Stimulation of either the ipsilateral or the contralateral telencephalon gave this result. On the ipsilateral side, stimulation of dorsolateral areas, whether in anterior, middle, or posterior parts of the telencephalon, gave greater facilitation than did stimulation in the central dorsal area. Larger cells were found in the preoptic nucleus, which were thought to be those described as neurosecretory by Kandel (1964), and stimulation of the telencephalon inhibited firing of these. The preoptic area is known to be involved in endocrine function, and since stimulation of the olfactory trace causes depletion of granule content in this nucleus in the goldfish (Peter and Gorbman, 1968) and lesion to the nucleus abolishes the ability to respond to arginine vasotocin by spawning in *Fundulus* (Macey *et al.*, 1974), such results show modulation of an established pathway within the telencephalon but not any influence on other lower areas of the brain. It will be interesting to see if the activity of such lower brain areas is also affected by telencephalic stimulation. The only work of this sort is that of Zagorulko (1965), who found that stimulation of the telencephalon in carp inhibited tectal visual evoked potentials. Such modulation, if confirmed, is of the greatest importance to theories of forebrain function.

D. Effects on Learning

There have been few studies on the effects of telencephalic stimulation on learning, since there are obvious difficulties in allowing for the interference of such factors as feeding and reinforcement mentioned above. However, Malyukova (1964) has reported that low-current telencephalic stimulation in goldfish interferes with the retention of a food-reinforced simultaneous visual discrimination. Animals were trained to discriminate a circle, a triangle, and a cross, and to signal by pulling a bead near the appropriate shape to obtain a food reward. A common pattern was seen in the four fish used: as the current was increased, first there was no effect, then "aversive" reactions occurred, and finally "automatic motor reactions" were seen. The aversive reactions would seem to indicate negative reinforcement as described above, and the motor reactions are likely to have been due to current spread. However, three of the fish, which had previously shown 100% responses to the circle, showed near chance-level responses at currents below those giving negative reactions. A similar result was seen when Malyukova examined the effects of different frequencies of stimulation. It was also reported that during stimulation fish would seek the negative shapes but that as little as 10 sec after the cessation of stimulation they would respond correctly to the positive shape. With higher currents there was an immediate avoidance of all three shapes, and it could be 20 min to 3 hr before stable responses were observed again. Many of these results can be explained by assuming that the animals were in a conflict situation between potentially positive stimuli and negative stimulation. Since no controls were done on the effect of stimulation on the bead response alone, no conclusions can be drawn as to the effects of telencephalic stimulation on retention.

Wright (1978) made an attempt to find whether or not the telencephalon was involved in classical conditioning, using electrical stimulation of the brain. Goldfish were cardiac conditioned using light as the CS and a variety of UCSs. Some fish were trained using a shock applied to the side of the body (B); some were trained using telencephalic stimulation (T); some were trained using both (BT); some were trained using cerebellar stimulation (C) (this was also found to be negatively reinforcing); some were trained using both body and cerebellar stimulation (BC). The rationale was that using paired UCSs the effects would be additive if both stimuli were merely negatively reinforcing but subtractive if other processing was also involved. All groups learned the task equally well, but groups T and BT extinguished the conditioned response very much faster than the others. Since groups C and BC were statistically similar to group B, brain stimulation *per se* was not the cause of failure, but, more specifically, the deficit was associated with stimulation of the telencephalon. Controls for sensitization showed that reinforcement alone delivered by way of either the telencephalon or the body wall caused no subsequent responses to light alone. Further tests showed that in free-swimming fish the intensities of stimulation used in telencephalic and body wall stimulation produced equal amounts of aversion. Although such findings are suggestive of interference with retention, and to some extent parallel observations on the effects of hippocampal stimulation, such as those of Zornetzer *et al.* (1973), much more work is needed on stimulation effects on the learning of other types of problem and on the time course of such interference.

V. Theories of Telencephalic Function

A. Introduction

Because of the relative paucity of information relating to the fish telencephalon, it is difficult to make definite statements as to its functions. Any theories about such functions have to rely heavily on evidence supplied by lesion studies of what the telencephalon does not do and are hampered by a considerable degree of ignorance of organization at other brain levels. In addition, much of the work reported here has centered on the learning ability of ablated animals, and there is far less known about the retention of various problems learned before ablation. Further, there is an embarrassing lack of physiological evidence relating to telencephalic function, so any ideas presented here are likely to be of naive simplicity compared with similar hypotheses relating to the lower areas of the mammalian telencephalon.

In view of the marked division of the fish telencephalon into olfactory and nonolfactory areas, and of the relative lack of effect on behavior of olfactory tract section as opposed to telencephalic removal, it is possible to make a distinction between olfactory and nonolfactory functions but difficult to specify the latter. It seems increasingly likely that, although various theories can explain some of the facts, none can encompass them all, and that more precise behavioral and lesion work will delineate functional areas within the large areas of telencephalon currently grouped together as "nonolfactory." Considering that the fish telencephalon contains areas possibly homologous with the olfactory cortex, hippocampus, septum, and amygdala of mammals (e.g., see Schnitzlein, 1964), the hazards of considering it as a single functional entity are obvious.

Several major hypotheses have been presented, citing failures of arousal, of ability to change responses, of memory consolidation, and of secondary reinforcement as consequences of telencephalon removal, and these will now be discussed.

B. Arousal

As has been seen above, there are few obvious behavioral deficits engendered by telencephalic ablation, and the majority of such deficits are to be seen in social rather than individual contexts (e.g., see Segaar, 1965). Nevertheless, many of the early workers reported generalized behavioral deficits which may loosely be grouped as changes in responsiveness. Most theories seeking to explain the learning and retention deficits described here have done so by reference to mechanisms primarily associated with learning, yet a deficit in responsiveness would explain much of the data reviewed here. Although a number of workers have suggested such an idea, its most consistent proponent has been Aronson (e.g., see Aronson, 1968). Taking as a basis the facts that, as seen throughout this review, telencephalic ablation rarely abolishes but more typically reduces learned behavior and that a similar occurrence is seen in instinctive situations (Noble, 1936; Aronson, 1948), he argues that the influence of the forebrain is that of nonspecific facilitation, due to arousal.

Evidence that would implicate the telencephalon in arousal is not consistent. There are no reports of lower speeds of performance in appetitive or aversive situations or of lower CS-UCS intervals impeding the performance of lesioned animals. Measurements of decreased heart and ventilatory rates, associated with reactions to novel stimuli, show no differences. Classical conditioning, with shock reinforcement, leads to normal acquisition, and the response to shock itself is normal. Feeding responses and rates are normal.

Conversely, arousal EEGs have been reported in the telencephalon, and even though these are generally associated with similar mesencephalic patterns they do show some possible involvement of the telencephalon in arousal. Sensory information of at least one type is apparently routed to this area, as evidenced by the presence of visual evoked potentials, which are presumably able to initiate arousal in the telencephalon. Stimulation of the telencephalon produces arousal, and on the basis of lesion studies it is known that operated animals are less spontaneously active than normal animals and less likely to explore new environments. Such decreases in behavior might be explicable on the basis of an olfactory input nonspecifically arousing the telencephalon, but the few studies of olfactory tract-sectioned fish have shown that their behavior is not usually subject to the group of deficits normally associated with telencephalic ablation. (This last possibility is discussed below.)

These conflicting pieces of evidence show that a simple arousal deficit is unlikely to explain telencephalic function. In any case, "arousal" is an imprecise term, capable of a number of interpretations. Andrew (1974) has pointed out that while variations of response within a single modality have sometimes been cited as arousal changes, more usually the term is associated with changes in general rather than specific behavior. Changes in a specific behavior are unlikely to be the source of the deficits observed here, which extend across instinctive and learned behavior and aversive and appetitive conditioning. It might be possible to make such a case for a simple failure in motor responsiveness, were it not for the fact that approach and escape speeds are normal, despite decreases in spontaneous locomotion. The most obvious source of a general arousal deficit would be the destruction of an area similar in function to the reticular formation of mammals (Moruzzi and Magoun, 1949). Damage to this in mammals causes severe if sometimes temporary behavioral deficits, generally listed under "lack of arousal," and causes the EEG to resemble that of sleep (Lindsley *et al.,* 1950). Such a generalized failure cannot explain the data presented here, since certain types of learning such as classical conditioning and simultaneous visual discrimination are hardly affected by the lesion. Further, anatomical homologies and what little physiological evidence there is (e.g., see Piddington, 1971) suggest that there is a mesencephalic reticular formation in fish, which would not be directly affected by telencephalic removal. However, if it is possible to discount one type of arousal, there is evidence that arousal is in no way a unitary process. Routtenberg (1968) has proposed two types of arousal in mammals, arousal I being reticular and concerned primarily with drive and output, arousal II being limbic and concerned with input such as reinforcement, which would explain the wide representation of positive self-stimulation sites in the area (Olds, 1958). (Such a possibility of reinforcement processing is discussed below.)

In the context of types of arousal, considerable caution is needed in discounting the effects of removal of the olfactory sense. Although the majority of experiments reviewed above, in which tract section alone was performed, showed no difference between these and unoperated animals, the study of Frank *et al.* (1972) did detect a difference. Further, Cain (1974) examined the results of damage to the mammalian olfactory bulb and concluded that the effects are far more extensive than a mere loss of smell. Among the effects reviewed are reduction of sexual behavior, aggression, social contact, and grooming, and changes in activity and learning. Learning deficits have been observed in passive avoidance, mazes, and classical conditioning, but not in two-way avoidance. There are some obvious parallels with the deficits reported in fish in the present review. Cain suggests that the olfactory system affects the limbic system and that the removal of olfactory afference influences the arousal system (Routtenberg's type II) at the limbic level. As will be seen below, it is possible to combine some current ideas and to assume that arousal contingent on certain types of reinforcement is lacking and hence no associations can be formed. In the present context, therefore, any arousal deficits might be due to the removal of an organizing area in the telencephalon or to the lack of olfactory influence at a lower level, although, of course, any limbic analogues are within the telencephalon.

Suggestions could be made that the telencephalon affects the level of sensory inflow, as does the reticular formation (Granit, 1955). However, the most delicate tests of discrimination conducted on fish—those of Nolte (1933)—failed to show any differences in pre- and postoperative color generalization gradients. Most other tests have used conspicuously different stimuli, and little is known of any performance over any similar discriminative range relating to shape or orientation.

Hebb (1949) related arousal to the ∩-shaped curve of strength of arousal vs. performance; thus at low and high levels of arousal performance would be poor. A shift in the position of such a curve would result in a changed level of performance. A shift of responsiveness of this sort could explain many of the deficits seen in fish, such as postoperative "forgetting" of previously trained avoidance, but could not explain why, with a CS, UCS, and CS/UCS interval identical to that used in avoidance training, a classically conditioned response should be retained. Few studies have attempted to investigate this possibility by variation of CS or UCS intensity, but one study by the present author (Savage, 1969*a*) in which the CS intensity was considerably reduced failed to demonstrate either further reduction or an improvement in the avoidance of ablated animals. A similar (unpublished) study of UCS intensity variations gave the same results.

Nor can the type of arousal characterized as activation (Moruzzi, 1969) explain the data reviewed here. In this model, the level of arousal determines not necessarily the intensity of responses but the type of such responses. Although the studies of learning reported here have generally been concerned with very limited aspects of behavior, and might have failed to detect such shifts, the ethological studies have reported changes not in type but in intensity of behavior. Further, the wide range of deficits found makes it unlikely that the same shift in activation could explain them all.

One obvious meaning of the term "arousal" is that described by Sokolov (1963) as the orienting reaction or OR. In this theory, neuronal models are formed in the brain, and incoming data are compared to these. Failure to find a match induces a complex of responses (including cortical arousal) mediated by the reticular formation, characterized as an OR. Following re-presentation of the stimulus, a model of it is formed, and the OR is no longer elicited; thus habituation is said to have occurred. Few observations of this sort have been made on fish, but the few which have show that the cardiac component of the OR is present and habituates as well in normal as in ablated fish. Autonomic responses have been as yet little studied in fish, and, as Hinde (1970) has pointed out, there are dangers in assuming that changes seen during "arousal" will covary, or are part of a single process, so caution is needed in ruling out failure of an OR as the cause of deficit. At present, the indices of arousal in fish are probably so insensitive that they are incapable of measuring any but the most dramatic shifts. For example, Laming (1976) has found that in normal fish cardiac, respiratory, and skeletal muscle changes are all extremely variable during the first presentation of a novel stimulus, even in highly controlled conditions, and that the rates of habituation of such responses is again very different in different individuals.

Such evidence as there is does not support the idea that the telencephalon is involved in any of the generalized activities discussed above under arousal. In discussing these possibilities, the idea of facilitation has been ignored, and since it forms part of Aronson's hypothesis it needs to be dealt with here. The action of the telencephalon is seen as being nonspecific, the area having its effects by exerting a tonic influence on lower brain centers, thus increasing their speed and efficiency of action. It has just been shown that models of such facilitation acting by changing levels of arousal are unlikely, but since it is well known that, at a unit level, heterosynaptic facilitation may be involved in learning (Castellucci *et al.*, 1970) such facilitation of preferred pathways might be caused by the area. Thus levels of arousal might remain normal, but the ability to process information might be reduced. The drawback of such a model is that its predictive power is limited; for instance, telencephalon-ablated fish are capable of retaining learned information relating to approaching shapes, but not that relating to which shape to respond to, in a delay situation; it is difficult to see why one should be forgotten and not the other. Similarly, stimuli processed perfectly under classical conditioning are apparently not properly processed under avoidance conditions. Further, if facilitation is necessary for learning, why should there be such an enormous deficit in animals trained and then lesioned?

The only direct physiological test of the hypothesis is that of Hallowitz *et al.* (1971), but this tested the influence of the telencephalon on itself, rather than on other brain areas. The observations of Zagorulko (1965) and of Maluikina and Vornovitski (1966), that section between telencephalon and diencephalon causes decrease of the tectal EEG, and of Zagorulko (1965), that stimulation of the telencephalon reduces visual evoked potentials, are suggestive of facilitation, but more observations are needed, involving stimulation, before the physiological basis of facilitation can be considered proven. Facilitation may be a mechanism by which the telencephalon can act, but at present it is to vague a concept to be of predictive value.

The discussion so far has tended to discount arousal failure as a possibility in explaining why telencephalic lesions have such a severe effect on so many types of behavior. However, to say that an animal is aroused is not to say that it can utilize that arousal properly. Pribram and McGuinness (1975) have outlined three processes involved in attention control, arousal, activation, and effort. The first of these has been discussed above. Activation is seen here (in a sense different from that discussed above due to Moruzzi) as a readiness to respond, such a readiness being associated (in mammals at least) with contingent negative variation (CNV), although, of course, CNV can be associated with other expectancy phenomena such as the awaiting of the results of action (Weinberg, 1972). Since all the failures yet detected in fish relate to paradigms involving movement of the animal, it is possible that they could be explained by a failure in response readiness of this sort. However, since some appetitive tasks have been found in which no deficits have been observed, the explanation could not be of such simplicity. A related suggestion is that, since the major telencephalic deficits are in instrumental learning, the failure is due to an inability to change response patterns (e.g., see Flood *et al.,* 1976). Simultaneous visual discrimination tasks would not be affected by a deficit of this sort, since no differential responses are required, merely approach. Such an inability would show up most clearly in reversal studies, and, indeed, as has been seen above, maze studies have demonstrated such a reversal deficit. The demonstration of a passive avoidance deficit fits in with this suggestion. Extinction should be slower in the lesioned fish, but this has not been observed in avoidance studies. On this hypothesis, the introduction of delays between stimulus or response and reinforcement should have no effect as compared with the behavior of normal fish, and this is not so. A further expectation, as yet untested, is that a successive (go/no-go) visual discrimination, with immediate reinforcement, should be more impaired in lesioned than in normal fish. Further, unless some sort of arousal dependency is assumed, the supposed inability of lesioned fish to modify behavior patterns does not explain the massed/spaced trial phenomenon.

C. Attention and Consolidation

Effort, as defined by Pribram and McGuinness (1975), is the linking of arousal and activation to produce a meaningful response. Hippocampal lesions in monkeys, for instance, can lead to habituation of overt behavioral responses to distracting stimuli, but not to decrease of distraction as measured by success in discrimination (Douglas and Pribram, 1969). An attentional failure of this sort might explain fish telencephalic deficits. By analogy, arousal habituation, as measured by the cardiac OR, is normal, yet the ability to maintain attention may not be. Distraction could explain why avoidance tasks are poorly learned, and why delay has such a drastic effect on many tasks. It would also explain postoperative failures. It would not, seemingly, explain why no classical deficits have been observed in simple or differential conditioning. However, the situation in which classical conditioning is conducted differs from all other learning situations in its absolute constancy. Thus, although trace paradigms have been used, the lack of deficit could be explained by lack of anything to distract the animal. [The mammalian frontal lobe deficit in delay situations (Malmo, 1942; French and Harlow, 1955) provides a parallel.] The lack of deficit in simultaneous visual approach tasks would possibly be due to the animal orienting to and swimming toward the shapes, thus effectively maintaining its attention on them. In either case, delayed response or distraction methods should show up this type of deficit in a variety of paradigms.

Savage (1968*a*) suggested that an attentional failure of this sort would also lead to a short-term memory consolidation deficit in telencephalon-ablated fish. Thus, even if an association could be made, the lack of telencephalic involvement would cause rapid discarding and hence poor retention. The suggestion of the short/long-term memory hypothesis (see John, 1967, for an excellent discussion) is that initially memory information is stored as a labile, transitory form, and that by a process of consolidation it becomes less amenable to destruction. It was suggested, for example, that in the avoidance situation, reinforcement associated with avoiding the CS would come some time after CS termination and thus be ineffective in training the animal. Even if animals proved capable of learning under such conditions, lack of telencephalic mediation of short-term memory would cause retention failure. If attention decayed in this fashion, then massed training should allow a greater measure of attention and concomitant consolidation, and hence retention. This was proved to be the case in both aversive and appetitive situations. In a habituation situation, Peeke *et al.* (1972) have shown that lesioned fish can learn during a session but forget between sessions. Other evidence supportive of this suggestion is that delays between CS and UCS have been shown to interfere with performance in aversive and appetitive tasks, although not in classical conditioning. A possible explanation for this discrepancy has been outlined above.

One prediction of an hypothesis of this sort is that in avoidance the postoperative performance of previously trained fish should resemble an extinction curve for normal animals, since the established associations should be gradually eliminated by the delay inability just outlined. All workers have reported a postoperative performance which is minimal, and which improves. In fact, all hypotheses dealing with specific failures in information processing suffer from this drawback: that in predicting acquisition deficits they do not predict the total and immediate avoidance deficit seen postoperatively in trained fish. Whether some arousal failure corresponds with an attentional one is unclear, for lesioning following training has received little attention from other than avoidance studies, Nolte's (1933) results remaining one of the few reports on approach tasks, apart from some extremely general comments in the Russian literature.

Any failure of attention showing as inability to form short-term associations should be revealed by the classical tests of delayed responses. Although delayed rewards in both positive and negative situations have been used, there have been delays not only between response and reward but also between CS termination and reward, and this has led to uncertainty as to which is the important delay (Flood *et al.,* 1976). Unfortunately, it is difficult to provide a delayed response situation similar to that used with mammals, and the only report of delayed responses (Schiller, 1948) used a situation in which fish were out of sight of the stimuli for a period while detouring to reach food. Such a paradigm will, however, provide a good test of a short-term retention failure in the operated fish.

Further, no experiments at all have been conducted with the use of distracting stimuli. If attention is impaired, then acquisition and retention, even of classical paradigms, will be affected. This paradigm provides a critical test of the present hypothesis. Perhaps a vigilance task is the best way of assessing attention—that is, the continual presentation of a series of signals, only a few of which are significant (Mackworth, 1969, 1970). The physiological correlates of a loss of attention may show up in changes in the EEG, and there is preliminary evidence for a reduction in the tectal EEG following telencephalic ablation, indicating a possible telencephalic influence on input. In this context, it is interesting that Bannister (1973), in an anatomical study of the telencephalon of the minnow (*Phoxinus phoxinus)*, has outlined a possible circuit which includes the dorsolateral and central areas of the telencephalon and the glomerulosus complex of the diencephalon. Such re-exciting chains may form the anatomical basis of the attention mechanism discussed here.

Lastly, if an attentional failure extends into memory consolidation, then the phenomenon of learning within but not between sessions, as reported by Peeke *et al.* (1972), is worth further investigation. Work using electroconvulsive shock (ECS) (Davis *et al.,* 1965) and protein synthesis inhibitors (Agranoff *et al.,* 1966) as well as analysis of RNAs during training (Shashoua, 1970, 1972) has suggested that in goldfish, as in other vertebrates examined, consolidation occurs in the period 60–120 min after training. The varying of intersession intervals below and above this period will lead, if the hypothesis is correct, to better long-term retention below the period and poorer above, as learned information fails to consolidate without the stimulus of further training.

Recent work has made it less likely that a general memory decay deficit can explain the effects seen following removal of the telencephalon, for classical conditioning of fish using long (15-sec) trace intervals has yielded no difference between control and experimental fish (Farr and Savage, 1978). Despite the fact that the trace period was one of darkness and as such least likely retroactively to destroy the CS trace, such evidence militates against the simple short-term memory failure hypothesis. It is more likely that any such decay is of a specific type of information, as outlined in the next section.

D. Secondary Reinforcement Processing

A final major hypothesis is one due to Overmier (Flood *et al.,* 1976) and utilizes the two-process theory of learning first suggested by Mowrer (1947) and discussed more recently in work by Rescorla and Solomon (1967) and Gray (1975). This theory suggests that operant responses are acquired in two stages, an initial classical conditioning stage followed by instrumental learning. In view of the total lack of effect of telencephalic ablations on learning and retention of simple and discriminative classical paradigms, there can be little doubt that the first stage of learning is not affected. Failure must lie in the transfer of such information to the phase of instrumental learning. The two-process theory considers such transfer as being due initially to the emotional/motivating signals generated by the CS, initiating the instrumental response, and secondarily to such a response being perpetuated by the reinforcement derived by CS termination. That is, in the case of avoidance, CS termination terminates the conditioned fear state, and in this it is positively reinforcing.

Overmier and Starkman (1974) have shown that if goldfish are classically trained with a color discrimination, and then trained on avoidance of a tone, avoidance trials using the classical stimuli give correct (if low-level) avoidances. Thus the conditioned motivational state induced by the classically trained CS is usable in the avoidance situation, and it has been suggested that second-order reinforcement utilization is impaired by the lesion.

Flood *et al.* (1976) consider that deficits in avoidance learning are explicable by the failure of CS termination on avoidance to cause appropriate reinforcement. Similarly, delay deficits can be explained by assumed disruption of secondary reinforcers, associated with the CS, whose presence is necessary to maintain temporal connection between the CS (or response to the CS) and reinforcement.

Results obtained by Farr (Farr and Savage, 1978) indicate some support for this hypothesis. Olfactory tract-sectioned control and telencephalon-ablated fish were trained classically using light, and two other groups (control and ablated) were pseudoconditioned. Following acquisition by the classical conditioning groups, all fish were given preference tests in a T maze. Once such preferences were established, turns to the preferred side were "rewarded" by presentations of the same light CS that had been used during the classical training. Control animals reversed their preference, whereas classically trained lesioned fish and both the pseudoconditioning groups did not. This suggests that the control fish utilized secondary reinforcement from the CS to terminate the old preference, whereas the ablated fish did not. The fact that these differences were manifested under a massed training regime is additional evidence that a basic difference between the control and operated animals has been detected, for, as has been seen, in appetitive and avoidance paradigms previously used, massing trials has generally resulted in similar behavior in the two groups.

However, even if this last hypothesis proves able to encompass most of the learning deficits observed, it is difficult to use it to explain why, once fish have been trained, the removal of the telencephalon causes such massive avoidance deficits. If secondary reinforcers have been used to establish the habit in a normal animal, then removal of the ability to utilize them should cause progressive extinction of responses postoperatively, not the total immediate deficit observed, nor should there be relearning of the magnitude seen. There may be some interaction of reinforcement and attention deficits.

E. Conclusions and Prospects

It has become increasingly apparent that the several hypotheses relating to telencephalic function are incomplete and that none of them can encompass all the types of deficits seen following ablation of the area. It seems likely that a combination of certain aspects of each is more near the truth than any one alone, and it is perhaps naive to suppose otherwise. This final discussion of hypotheses has deliberately ignored the scanty evidence available on the effects of partial telencephalic lesions, yet it is surely here that future work will clarify the position. To take one study, that of Segaar and Nieuwenhuys (1963), on the social behavior of the three-spined stickleback (*Gasterosteus aculeatus*), there is plenty of evidence for localization of function. For instance, bilateral removal of the anterior olfactory area or of the lateral dorsal area lowered aggression but had less effect on sexual or parental behaviors. Bilateral damage to the rear dorsomedial area, on the other hand, "leveled out" all three behaviors, so that the normal fluctuations corresponding with the breeding cycle were not seen. When electrolytic lesions were used, tiny bilateral damages in the dorsomedial area could cause different and gross aberrations of behavior, dissimilar to those seen by Schönherr (1955) using total ablation. Work of this sort, applied to learning situations, is necessary before function can be localized and defined, for total ablation, a crude tool, has perhaps gone as far as it can in providing pointers to the workings of the telencephalon.

It has often been pointed out (e.g., see Segaar, 1965; Aronson, 1968) that anatomical homologies would link the fish telencephalon with the limbic system of higher vertebrates, since no true cortical structures are present. Indeed, such considerations prompted recent studies on avoidance in fish by a number of groups of workers. However, although behavioral parallels can be drawn between various types of limbic deficit and total telencephalic deficits, the mammalian deficits generally pertain to one part of the system and do not attempt to explain the whole. The telencephalic structures representing the limbic system are normally thought of as being the amygdala, hippocampus, septum, and cingulate and entorhinal cortices. These areas have been implicated in a variety of functions ranging from unspecific facilitation (Gloor, 1960) to social dominance (Rosvold *et al.*, 1954), response inhibition (Zucker and McCleary, 1964), attention (Grastyan *et al.*, 1959), short-term memory processing (Uretsky and McCleary, 1969), and reinforcement processing (Richardson, 1973). The current position in fish telencephalon research is attempting to fit a similar (if more restricted) series of putative functions into one hypothesis embracing a comparatively large and heterogeneous area. What little information there is suggests that reinforcement and attention capabilities may be dissociable, and until work has moved toward greater attempts to localize function, to define deficits due to lesions before and after training, and to perform the wealth of controls seen in mammalian studies, hypotheses will remain embarrassingly vague. Nevertheless, better examination of such a relatively simple system promise a speedier analysis of the basic processes involved in learning and memory than may be possible in higher and more complex vertebrates.

VI. References

Agranoff, B. W., Davis, R. E., and Brink, J. J., 1966, Chemical studies on memory fixation in goldfish, *Brain Res.* **1**:303.

Andrew, R. J., 1974, Arousal and the causation of behaviour, *Behaviour* **51**:135.

Ariëns Kappers, C. U., Huber, G. C., and Crosby, E. C., 1936, *The Comparative Anatomy of the Nervous System of Vertebrates*, Macmillan, New York.

Aronson, L. R., 1948, Problems in the behavior and physiology of a species of african mouthbreeding fish (*Tilapia macrocephala*), *Tr. N.Y. Acad. Sci. Ser. 2* **2**:33.

Aronson, L. R., 1968, Function of the teleostean forebrain, in: *The Central Nervous System and Fish Behavior* (D. J. Ingle, ed.), pp. 107–125, University of Chicago Press, Chicago.

Aronson, L. R., and Herberman, R., 1960, Persistence of a conditioned response in the cichlid fish *Tilapia macrocephala* after forebrain and cerebellar ablations, *Anat. Rec.* **138**:332.

Aronson, L. R., and Kaplan, H., 1963, Forebrain function in avoidance conditioning, *Am. Zool.* **3**:483.

Aronson, L. R., and Kaplan, H., 1965, Effect of forebrain ablation on the acquisition of a conditioned avoidance response in the teleost fish *Tilapia macrocephala, Am. Zool.* **5**:654.

Bannister, L. H., 1973, Forebrain structure in *Phoxinus phoxinus,* a teleost of the cyprinid family, *J. Hirnforsch.* **14**:413.

Beniuc, M., 1938, The roundabout path of the fighting fish (*Betta splendens*), *Proc. Zool. Soc. London* **108**:403.

Bernstein, J. J., 1961*a*, Loss of hue discrimination in forebrain-ablated fish, *Exp. Neurol.* **3**:1.

Bernstein, J. J., 1961*b*, Brightness discrimination following forebrain ablation in fish, *Exp. Neurol.* **3**:297.

Bernstein, J. J., 1962, Role of the telencephalon in color vision in fish, *Exp. Neurol.* **6**:173.

Bernstein, J. J., 1967, The regenerative capacity of the telencephalon of the goldfish and the rat, *Exp. Neurol.* **17**:44.

Berwein, M., 1941, Beobachtungen und Versuche über das gesellige Leben von Elritzen, *Z. Vergl. Physiol.* **28**:402.

Bethe, A., 1899, Die Locomotion des Haifisches (*Scyllium*) und ihre Beziehungen zu den einzelnen Gehirntheilen und zum Labyrinth, *Pflügers Arch.* **76**:70.

Bianki, V. L., 1972, The hypothesis on the origin factors of the forebrain paired structure in the phylogenesis of the vertebrates, in: *Cerebral Interhemispheric Relations* (J. Černáček and F. Podivinský, eds.), pp. 29–42, Publishing house of the Slovak Academy of Sciences, Bratislava.

Bitterman, M. E., 1965, The evolution of intelligence, *Sci. Am.* **212(1)**:92.

Boyd, E. S., and Gardner, L. C., 1962, Positive and negative reinforcement from intracranial stimulation of a teleost, *Science* **136**:648.

Bruckmoser, P., and Dieringer, N., 1973, Evoked potentials in the primary and secondary projection areas of the forebrain in elasmobranchs, *J. Comp. Physiol.* **87**:65.

Cain, D. P., 1974, The role of the olfactory bulb in limbic mechanisms, *Psychol. Rev.* **10**:654.

Campbell, H. J., 1968, Peripheral self-stimulation as reward, *Nature (London)* **218**:104.

Castellucci, V., Pinsker, H., Kupfermann, I., and Kandel, E. R., 1970, Neuronal mechanisms of habituation and dishabituation of the gill-withdrawal reflex in *Aplysia, Science* **167**:1745.

Chauchard, A., and Chauchard, B., 1927, Recherches sur les localisations cérébrales chez les poissons, *C. R. Soc. Biol.* **184**:696.

Clark, S. L., Chung, M. Y., Shine, L., and Clark, M. R., 1960, Responses in free swimming fishes to electrical stimulation of the cerebellum, *Am. J. Anat.* **106**:121.

Cohen, D. H., Duff, T. A., and Ebbesson, S. O. E., 1973, Electrophysiological identification of a visual area in shark telencephalon, *Science* **182**:492.

Crespi, L. P., 1944, Amount of reinforcement and level of performance, *Psychol. Rev.* **51**:341.

Dart, R. A., 1920, A contribution to the morphology of the corpus striatum, *J. Anat.* **55**:1.

Davis, R. E., Bright, P. J., and Agranoff, B. W., 1965, Effect of ECS and puromycin on memory in fish, *J. Comp. Physiol. Psychol.* **60**:162.

Demski, L. S., and Gerald, J. W., 1972, Sound production evoked by electrical stimulation of the brain in toadfish (*Opsanus beta*), *Anim. Behav.* **20**:507.

Demski, L. S., and Knigge, K. M., 1971, The telencephalon and hypothalamus of the bluegill (*Lepomis macrochirus*): Evoked feeding, aggressive and reproductive behavior with representative frontal sections, *J. Comp. Neurol.* **143**:1.

Desmoulins, A., 1825, *Anatomie des Systèmes Nerveux des Animaux Vertébrés Appliqué à la Physiologie et à la Zoologie,* Méquignon-Marvis, Paris.

Devitsina, G. V., 1973, On certain morphological and functional properties of the olfactory bulb of pike and burbot, *Vestnik Moskovsk. Univ.* **1**:10.

Dewsbury, D. A., and Bernstein, J. J., 1969, Role of the telencephalon in performance of conditioned avoidance responses by goldfish, *Exp. Neurol.* **23**:445.

Dizon, A. E., Horrall, R. M., and Hasler, A. D., 1973, Olfactory electroencephalographic responses of homing Coho salmon, *Oncorhynchus kisutch,* to water conditioned by conspecifics, *U.S. Natl. Marine Fish. Serv. Fish. Bull.* **71**:893.

Douglas, R. J., and Pribram, K. H., 1969, Distraction and habituation in monkeys with limbic lesions, *J. Comp. Physiol. Psychol.* **69**:473.

Döving, K. B., 1966, Efferent influence upon the activity of single neurons in the olfactory bulb of the burbot, *J. Neurophysiol.* **29**:675.

Döving, K. B., and Gemne, G., 1965, Electrophysiological and histological properties of the olfactory tract of the burbot (*Lota lota* L.), *J. Neurophysiol.* **28**:139.

Döving, K. B., and Gemne, G., 1966, An electrophysiological study of the efferent olfactory system in the burbot, *J. Neurophysiol.* **29**:665.

Döving, K. B., and Hyvärinen, J., 1969, Afferent and efferent influences on the activity pattern of single olfactory neurons, *Acta Physiol. Scand.* **75**:111.

Ebbesson, S. O. E., and Heimer, L., 1968, Olfactory bulb projections in two species of sharks (*Galeocerdo cuvieri* and *Ginglymostoma cirratum*), *Anat. Rec.* **160**:469.

Ebbesson, S. O. E., and Heimer, L., 1970, Projections of the olfactory tract fibres in the nurse shark (*Ginglymostoma cirratum*), *Brain Res.* **17**:47.

Ebbesson, S. O. E., Jane, J. A., and Schroeder, D. M., 1972, A general overview of major interspecific variations in thalamic organisation, *Brain Behav. Evol.* **6:**92.

Eidelberg, E., and Stein, D. G., 1974, Functional recovery after lesions of the nervous system, *Neurosci. Res. Prog. Bull.* **12:**191.

Enger, P. S., 1957, The electroencephalogram of the codfish (*Gadus callarias*), *Acta Physiol. Scand.* **39:**55.

Farr, E. J., and Savage, G. E., 1978, First- and second-order conditioning in the goldfish and their relation to the telencephalon, *Behav. Biol.* **22:**50.

Ferrier, D., 1876, *The Functions of the Brain,* Smith-Elder, London.

Fiedler, K., 1964, Versuche zur Neuroethologie von Lippfischen und Sonnenbarschen, *Verh. Deutsch. Zool. Gesell. Kiel.* **28:**569.

Fiedler, K., 1967, Verhaltenswirksame Strukturen in Fischgehirn, *Verh. Deutsch. Zool. Gesell. Heidelberg* **31:**602.

Finger, T. E., 1975, The distribution of the olfactory tracts in the bullhead catfish, *Ictalurus nebulosus, J. Comp. Neurol.* **161:**125.

Flood, N. B., and Overmier, J. B., 1971, Effects of telencephalic and olfactory lesions on appetitive learning in goldfish, *Physiol. Behav.* **6:**35.

Flood, N. B., Overmier, J. B., and Savage, G. E., 1976, Teleost telencephalon and learning: An interpretive review of data and hypotheses, *Physiol. Behav.* **16:**783.

Fortuyn, J. D., 1961, Topographical relations in the telencephalon of the sunfish, *Eupomotis gibbosus, J. Comp. Neurol.* **116:**249.

Frank, A. H., Flood, N. B., and Overmier, J. B., 1972, Reversal learning in forebrain ablated and olfactory tract sectioned teleost, *Carassius auratus, Psychon. Sci.* **26:**149.

French, G. M., and Harlow, H. F., 1955, Locomotor reaction decrement in normal and brain-damaged monkeys, *J. Comp. Physiol. Psychol.* **48:**496.

Gloor, P., 1960, The amygdala, in: *Handbook of Physiology,* Sect. 1, Vol. 2: *Neurophysiology* (J. Field, H. Magoun, and V. Hall, eds.), pp. 1395–1420, American Physiological Society, Washington, D.C.

Godet, R., Bert, J., and Collomb, H., 1964, Apparition de la réaction d'éveil télencéphalique chez *Protopterus annectens* et cycle biologique, *C. R. Soc. Biol.* **158:**146.

Graeber, R. C., Schroeder, D. M., Jane, J. A., and Ebbesson, S. O. E., 1972, The importance of telencephalic structures in visual discrimination learning in nurse sharks, *Proc. Soc. Neurosci. 2nd Annu. Meet.,* pp. 8–11.

Granit, R., 1955, Centrifugal and antidromic effects on ganglion cells of the retina, *J. Neurophysiol.* **18:**388.

Grastyán, E., Lissak, K., Madarasz, I., and Donhoffer, H., 1959, Hippocampal electrical activity during the development of conditioned reflexes, *EEG Clin. Neurophysiol.* **11:**409.

Gray, J. A., 1975, *Elements of a Two-Process Theory of Learning,* Academic Press, New York.

Grimm, R. J., 1960, Feeding behavior and electrical stimulation of the brain of *Carassius auratus, Science* **131:**162.

Gruberg, E. R., and Ambros, V. R., 1974, A forebrain visual projection in the frog (*Rana pipiens*), *Exp. Neurol.* **44:**187.

Guselnikov, V. I., Onufrieva, M. I., and Supin, A. Y., 1964, Projection of visual, olfactory and lateral line receptors in the fish brain, *Fiziol. Zh. SSSR im. L. M. Sechenov* **50:**1104.

Guselnikov, V. I., Pivovarov, A. S., and Tsitolovsky, L. E., 1974, Synaptic processes in the neurones of the forebrain general cortex of the turtle to visual stimulation, *Zhurnal Vyssh. Nerv. Devatel. I. P. Pavlova* **24:**800.

Hainsworth, F. R., Overmier, J. B., and Snowdon, C. T., 1967, Specific and permanent deficits in instrumental avoidance responding following forebrain ablation in the goldfish, *J. Comp. Physiol. Psychol.* **63:**111.

Hale, E. B., 1956, Social facilitation and forebrain function in maze performance of green sunfish, *Lepomis cyanellus, Physiol. Zool.* **29:**93.

Hallowitz, R. A., Woodward, D. J., and Demski, L. S., 1971, Forebrain activation of single units in preoptic area of sunfish, *Comp. Biochem. Physiol.* **40A:**733.

Hara, T. J., 1970, An electrophysiological basis for olfactory discrimination in homing salmon: A review, *J. Fish. Res. Bd. Can.* **27:**565.

Hara, T. J., and Gorbman, A., 1967, Electrophysiological studies of the olfactory system of the goldfish, *Carassius auratus* L. 1. Modification of the electrical activity of the olfactory bulb by other central nervous structures, *Comp. Biochem. Physiol.* **21:**185.

Hara, T. J., Ueda, K., and Gorbman, A., 1965, Electroencephalographic studies of homing salmon, *Science* **149:**884.

Hara, T. J., Freese, M., and Scott, K. R., 1973, Spectral analysis of olfactory bulbar responses in rainbow trout, *Jpn. J. Physiol.* **23:**325.

Hebb, D. O., 1949, *The Organization of Behavior,* Wiley, New York.

Herrick, C. J., 1922, Functional factors in the morphology of the forebrain of fishes, *Libro en Honor de S. Ramón y Cajal* **1:**143.

Herrick, C. J., 1948, *The Brain of the Tiger Salamander,* University of Chicago Press, Chicago.

Hinde, R. A., 1970, *Animal Behaviour,* 2nd ed., McGraw-Hill, New York.

Hosch, L., 1936, Untersuchungen über Grosshirnfunktion der Elritze (*Phoxinus laevis*) und des Grundlings (*Gobio fluviatilis*), *Zool. Jahrb. Abt. Zool. Physiol.* **57:**57.

Ingle, D. J., 1965*a*, Behavioral effects of forebrain lesions in goldfish, *Proc. 73rd Am. Psychol. Assoc.,* p. 143.

Ingle, D. J., 1965*b*, The use of the fish in neuropsychology, *Persp. Biol. Med.* **8:**241.

Ingle, D. J., and Campbell, A., 1977, Interocular transfer of visual discriminations in goldfish after selective commissure lesions, *J. Comp. Physiol. Psychol.* **91:**327.

Ito, H., 1973, Normal and experimental studies on synaptic patterns in the carp telencephalon, with special reference to the secondary olfactory termination, *J. Hirnforsch.* **14:**237.

Janzen, W., 1933, Untersuchungen über Grosshirnfunktion des Goldfisches (*Carassius auratus*), *Zool. Jahrb. Abt. Zool. Physiol.* **52:**591.

Jenkins, T. N., Warner, L. H., and Warden, C. J., 1926, Standard apparatus for the study of animal motivation, *J. Comp. Psychol.* **6:**361.

John, E. R., 1967, *Mechanisms of Memory,* Academic Press, New York.

Johnston, J. B., 1911, The telencephalon of selachians, *J. Comp. Neurol.* **21:**1.

Kandel, E. R., 1964, Electrical properties of hypothalamic neuroendocrine cells, *J. Gen. Physiol.* **47:**691.

Kaplan, H., and Aronson, L. R., 1967, Effect of forebrain ablation on the performance of a conditional avoidance response in the teleost fish, *Tilapia macrocephala, Anim. Behav.* **15:**438.

Karamian, A. I., 1956, *Evolution of the Function of the Cerebellum and Cerebral Hemispheres,* Megdiz, Leningrad (transl. by Israel Program for Scientific Translations, Jerusalem, 1962).

Karamian, A. I., Veselkin, N. P., Belekhova, M. G., and Zagorulko, T. M., 1966, Electrophysiological characteristics of tectal and thalamo-cortical divisions of the visual system in lower vertebrates, *J. Comp. Neurol.* **127:**559.

Karamian, A. I., Malyukova, I. V., and Sergeev, B. F., 1967, The participation of the forebrain of bony fish in the creation of complicated conditioned reflexes and general behavioural reactions, in: *Behaviour and Reception of Fishes,* pp. 109–114, Ichthyological Committee of the Ministry of Fisheries, Nauka, Moscow.

Karamian, A. I., Agayan, A. L., and Veselkin, N. P., 1973, The evoked potentials in various regions of the brain of lamprey during stimulation of the dorsal column of the spinal cord, *Biol. Zh. Armenii* **26:**56.

Kholodov, Y. A., 1960, Simple and complex food-obtaining conditioned reflexes in normal fish and in fish after removal of the forebrain, *Zh. Vyssh. Nerv. Devatel. I. P. Pavlova* **5:**201.

Kumakura, S., 1927, Versuche an Goldfischen, denen beide Hemisphären des Grosshirns extirpiert worden waren, *Nagoga J. Med. Sci.* **3:**19.

Kupfermann, I., Castellucci, V., Pinsker, H., and Kandel, E. R., 1970, Neuronal correlates of habituation and dishabituation of the gill-withdrawl reflex in *Aplysia, Science* **167:**1743.

Laming, P. R., 1976, Physiological aspects of arousal in the goldfish, *Carassius auratus,* Ph.D. thesis, University of London.

Lindsley, D. B., Schreiner, L. H., Knowles, W. B., and Magoun, H. W., 1950, Behavioral and EEG changes following chronic brain stem lesions in the cat, *EEG Clin. Neurophysiol.* **2:**483.

Loeb, J., 1891, Über den Anteil des Hörnerven an den nach Gehirnverletzung auftretenden Zwangsbewegungen, Zwangslagen und assoziierten Stellungsänderungen der Bulbi und Extremitäten, *Pflügers Arch.* **50:**66.

Macey, M. J., Pickford, G. E., and Peter, R. E., 1974, Forebrain localization of the spawning reflex response to exogenous neurohypophysial hormones in the killifish, *Fundulus heteroclitus, J. Exp. Zool.* **190:**269.

Mackworth, J. F., 1969, *Vigilance and Habituation,* Penguin Books, Harmondsworth, U.K.

Mackworth, J. F., 1970, *Vigilance and Attention,* Penguin Books, Harmondsworth, U. K.

Maetz, J., and Juien, M., 1961, Action of neurohypophyseal hormones on the sodium fluxes of a freshwater teleost, *Nature (London)* **189:**152.

Malmo, R. B., 1942, Interference factors in delayed response in monkeys after removal of frontal lobes, *J. Neurophysiol.* **5:**295.

Maluikina, G. A., and Flerova, G. N., 1960, New data on the functions of the fore-brain in teleosts, *Zh. Obshchei Biol.* **21:**381.

Maluikina, G. A., and Vornovitski, E. G., 1966, Some problems of physiology of visual analysers, *Vopr. Ikhtiol.* **6:**140.

Malyukova, I. V., 1964, Effect of electrical stimulation and partial coagulation of the forebrain (prosencephalon) and valvula cerebelli on the food-obtaining conditional reflexes in fishes, *Zh. Vyssh. Nerv. Devatel. I. P. Pavlova* **14:**895.

Mark, R. F., 1966, The tectal commissure and interocular transfer of pattern discrimination in cichlid fish, *Exp. Neurol.* **16:**215.

Marks, W. B., 1965, Visual pigments of single goldfish cones, *J. Physiol. (London)* **178:**14.

Marón, K., 1963, Endbrain regeneration in *Lebistes reticulatus, Folia Biol.* **11:**1.

McCleary, R. A., 1960, Type of response as a factor in interocular transfer in fish, *J. Comp. Physiol. Psychol.* **53:**311.

McCleary, R. A., and Bernstein, J. J., 1959, A unique method for control of brightness cues in study of color vision in fish, *Physiol. Zool.* **32:**284.

Meader, R. G., 1939, Notes on the functions of the forebrain in teleosts, *Zoologica* **24:**11.

Meesters, A., 1940, Über die Organization des Gesichtsfeldes der Fische, *Z. Tierpsychol.* **4:**84.

Moruzzi, G., 1969, Sleep and instinctive behaviour, *Arch. Ital. Biol.* **107:**175.

Moruzzi, G., and Magoun, E. W., 1949, Brain-stem reticular formation and activation of the EEG, *EEG Clin. Neurophysiol.* **1:**455.

Mowrer, O. H., 1947, On the dual nature of learning—A re-interpretation of "conditioning" and "problem-solving," *Harvard Educ. Rev.* **17:**102.

Myers, R. E., 1965, The neocortical commissures and interhemispheric transmission of information, in: *Functions of the Corpus Callosum* (G. Ettlinger, ed.), pp. 1–17, CIBA Foundation Study Group 20, Churchill, London.

Nieuwenhuys, R., 1959, The structure of the telencephalon of the teleost *Gasterosteus aculeatus, Proc. Kon. Ned. Akad. Wetensch. Amsterdam Ser. C* **62:**341.

Nieuwenhuys, R., 1967, Comparative anatomy of olfactory centres and tracts, *Prog. Brain Res.* **23:**1.

Noble, G. K., 1936, The function of the corpus striatum in the social behavior of fishes, *Anat. Rec.* **64:**34 (Suppl.3).

Nolte, W., 1933, Experimentelle Untersuchungen zum Problem der Lokalisation des Assoziationsvermögens im Fischgehirn, *Z. Vergl. Physiol.* **18:**255.

Olds, J., 1958, Self-stimulation experiments and differentiated reward systems, in: *Reticular Formation of the Brain* (H. H. Jasper, L. D. Proctor, R. S. Knighton, W. C. Noshay, and R. T. Costello, eds.), pp. 671–687, Little, Brown, Boston.

Olton, D. S., and Isaacson, R. L., 1968, Hippocampal lesions and active avoidance, *Physiol. Behav.* **3:**719.

Oshima, K., and Gorbman, A., 1966, Olfactory responses in the forebrain of goldfish and their modification by thyroxine treatment, *Gen. Comp. Endocrinol.* **7:**398.

Oshima, K., Hahn, W. E., and Gorbman, A., 1969, Olfactory discrimination of natural waters by salmon, *J. Fish. Res. Bd. Can.* **26:**2111.

Otis, L. S., Cerf, J. A., and Thomas, G. J., 1957, Conditioned inhibition of respiration and heart rate in the goldfish, *Science* **126:**263.

Overmier, J. B., and Curnow, P. F., 1969, Classical conditioning, pseudoconditioning, and sensitization in "normal" and forebrainless goldfish, *J. Comp. Physiol. Psychol.* **68:**193.

Overmier, J. B., and Flood, N. B., 1969, Passive avoidance in forebrain ablated teleost fish, *Carassius auratus, Physiol Behav.* **4:**791.

Overmier, J. B., and Gross, D., 1974, Effects of telencephalic ablation upon nest-building and avoidance behaviors in East African mouthbreeding fish, *Tilapia mossambica, Behav. Biol.* **12:**211.

Overmier, J. B., and Savage, G. E., 1974, Effects of telencephalic ablation on trace classical conditioning of heart rate in goldfish, *Exp. Neurol.* **42:**339.

Overmier, J. B., and Starkman, N., 1974, Transfer of control of avoidance behavior in normal and telencephalon ablated goldfish (*Carassius auratus*), *Physiol. Behav.* **12:**605.

Parker, G. H., 1910, Olfactory reactions in fishes, *J. Exp. Zool.* **8:**535.

Parker, G. H., 1911, The olfactory reactions of the common Killifish, *Fundulus heteroclitus* (Linn.), *J. Exp. Zool.* **10:**1.

Parker, G. H., 1922, *Smell, Taste, and Allied Senses in the Vertebrates,* Lippincott, Philadelphia.

Pavlovskii, E. N., 1964, *Techniques for the Investigation of Fish Physiology,* Israel Program for Scientific Translations, Jerusalem.

Peeke, H. V., Peeke, S. C., and Williston, J. S., 1972, Long-term memory deficits for habituation of predatory behavior in forebrain ablated goldfish (*Carassius auratus*), *Exp. Neurol.* **36:**288.

Peter, R. E., and Gorbman, A., 1968, Some afferent pathways to the preoptic nucleus of the goldfish, *Neuroendocrinology* **3:**229.

Piddington, R. W., 1971, Central control of auditory input in the goldfish. 1. Effect of shocks to the midbrain, *J. Exp. Biol.* **55:**569.

Pinsker, H., Kupfermann, I., Castellucci, V., and Kandel, E. R., 1970, Habituation and dishabituation of the gill-withdrawl reflex in *Aplysia, Science* **167:**1740.

Platt, C. J., Bullock, T. H., Czéh, G., Kovačević, N., Konjević, Dj., and Gojković, M., 1974, Comparison of electroreceptor, mechanoreceptor, and optic evoked potentials in the brain of some rays and sharks, *J. Comp. Physiol.* **95:**323.

Polimanti, O., 1911, Contributi alla fisiologia del sistema nervoso centrale e del movimento dei pesci. I. Selacoidei, *Zool. Jahrb. Abt. Zool. Physiol.* **30:**473.

Polimanti, O., 1912, Contributi alla fisiologia del sistema nervoso centrale e del movimento dei pesci. III. Teleosti. *Zool. Jahrb. Abt. Zool. Physiol.* **32:**367.

Pribram, K. H., and McGuinness, D., 1975, Arousal, activation and effort in the control of attention, *Psychol. Rev.* **82:**116.

Regestein, Q. R., 1968, Some monocular emotional effects of unilateral hypothalamic lesions in goldfish, in: *The Central Nervous System and Fish Behavior* (D. J. Ingle, ed.), pp. 139–144, University of Chicago Press, Chicago.

Reisinger, L., 1915, Die zentrale Lokalisation des Gleichgewichtssinnes der Fische, *Biol. Zentr.* **36:**472.

Rescorla, R. A., and Solomon, R. S., 1967, Two-process learning theory: Relationships between Pavlovian conditioning and instrumental learning, *Psychol. Rev.* **74:**151.

Richardson, J. S., 1973, The amygdala: historical and functional analysis, *Acta Neurobiol. Exp.* **33:**623.

Rizzolo, A., 1929, A study of equilibrium in the smooth dogfish (*Galeus canis* Mitchill) after removal of different parts of the brain, *Biol. Bull.* **57:**245.

Rosvold, H. E., Mirsky, A. F., and Pribram, K. H., 1954, Influence of amygdalectomy on social behavior in monkeys, *J. Comp. Physiol. Psychol.* **47:**173.

Routtenberg, A., 1968, The two-arousal hypothesis: Reticular formation and limbic system, *Psychol. Rev.* **75:**51.

Russell, E. S., 1931, Detour experiments with sticklebacks (*Gasterosteus aculeatus*), *J. Exp. Biol.* **8:**393.

Sanders, F. K., 1940, Second-order olfactory and visual learning in the optic tectum of the goldfish, *J. Exp. Biol.* **17:**416.

Satou, M., 1974, Electrical responses at various levels of the olfactory pathway in Himé salmon, *Oncorhynchus nerka, Jpn. J. Physiol.* **24:**389.

Savage, G. E., 1968*a*, Function of the forebrain in the memory system of fish, in: *The Central Nervous System and Fish Behavior* (D. J. Ingle, ed.), pp. 127–138, University of Chicago Press, Chicago.

Savage, G. E., 1968*b*, Temporal factors in avoidance learning in normal and forebrainless goldfish (*Carassius auratus*), *Nature (London)* **218:** 1168.

Savage, G. E., 1969*a*, Telencephalic lesions and avoidance behaviour in the goldfish *(Carassius auratus), Anim. Behav.* **17:**362.

Savage, G. E., 1969*b*, Some preliminary observations on the role of the telencephalon in food-reinforced behaviour in the goldfish, *Carassius auratus, Anim. Behav.* **17:**760.

Savage, G. E., 1971, Behavioural effects of electrical stimulation of the telencephalon of the goldfish, *Carassius auratus, Anim. Behav.* **19:**661.

Savage, G. E., 1979, Interocular transfer and commissure function in lower vertebrates, with special reference to fish, in: *Structure and Function of the Cerebral Commissures* (I. S. Russell, M. W. van Hof, and G. Berlucchi, eds.), p. 34, Macmillan, New York.

Savage, G. E., and Roberts, M. G., 1975, Behavioral effects of electrical stimulations of the hypothalamus of the goldfish (*Carassius auratus*), *Brain Behav. Evol.* **12:**42.

Savage, G. E., and Swingland, I. R., 1969, Postively reinforced behaviour and the forebrain in goldfish, *Nature (London)* **221:**878.

Schadé, J. P., 1959, Bilateral synchrony and arousal in EEG of fish, *EEG Clin. Neurophysiol.* **11:**613.

Schadé, J. P., and Weiler, I. J., 1959, Electroencephalographic patterns of the goldfish (*Carassius auratus*), *J. Exp. Biol.* **36:**435.

Scharrer, E., 1928, Die Lichtempfindlichkeit blinder Elritzen, *Z. Vergl. Physiol.* **7:**1.

Schiller, P. H., 1948, Delayed responses in minnows, *J. Comp. Physiol. Psychol.* **41:**233.

Schnitzlein, H. N., 1964, Correlation of habit and structure in the fish brain, *Am. Zool.* **4:** 21.

Schnitzlein, H. N., and Crosby, E. C., 1967, The telencephalon of the lungfish, *Protopterus*, *J. Hirnforsch.* **9:**105.

Schönherr, J., 1955, Über die Abhängigkeit der Instinkthandlungen vom Vorderhirn und Zwischenhirn (Epiphyse) bei *Gasterosteus aculeatus* L., *Zool. Jahrb. Abt. Zool. Physiol.* **65:**357.

Schroeder, D. M., and Ebbesson, S. O. E., 1974, Non-olfactory telencephalic afferents in the Nurse shark (*Ginglymostoma cirratum*), *Brain Behav. Evol.* **9:**121.

Segaar, J., 1965, Behavioural aspects of degeneration and regeneration in fish brain, *Prog. Brain Res.* **14:**143.

Segaar, J., and Nieuwenhuys, R., 1963, New etho-physiological experiments with male *Gasterosteus aculeatus*, *Anim. Behav.* **11:**331.

Segura, E. T., 1969, Effect of forebrain stimulation on blood pressure, heart rate, and ST-T complex in toads, *Am. J. Physiol.* **217:**1149.

Shapiro, S. M., 1965, Interocular transfer of pattern discrimination in the goldfish, *Am. J. Physiol.* **78:**21.

Shapiro, S. M., Schuckman, H., Sussman, D., and Tucker, A. M., 1974, Effect of telencephalic lesions on the gill cover response of Siamese fighting fish, *Physiol. Behav.* **13:**749.

Shashoua, V. E., 1970, RNA metabolism in goldfish brain during acquisition of new behavioral patterns, *Proc. Natl. Acad. Sci. USA* **65:**160.

Shashoua, V. E., 1972, A multistage transduction model for information processing in the nervous system, *Int. J. Neurosci.* **3:**299.

Sheldon, R. E., 1912, The olfactory tracts and centers in teleosts, *J. Comp. Neurol.* **22:**177.

Sherrington, C. S., 1906, *The Integrative Action of the Nervous System*, Yale University Press, New Haven (reprinted 1961).

Sokolov, E. N., 1963, *Perception and the Conditioned Reflex*, Pergamon Press, Oxford.

Steiner, J., 1888, Die Fische, in: *Die Functionen des Zentralnervensystems und ihre Phlogenese*, Abt. 2., Vieweg und Sohn, Braunschweig.

Strieck, K., 1925, Untersuchungen über den Geruchs- und den Geschmackssinn der Elritze, *Z. Vergl. Physiol.* **2:**122.

Sutherland, N. S., 1969, Shape discrimination in the rat, octopus and goldfish: A comparative study, *J. Comp. Physiol. Psychol.* **67:**160.

Ten Cate, J., 1935, Physiologie des Zentralnervensystems der Fische, *Ergebn. Biol.* **11:**335.

Troschicheva, P. V., 1974, The role of the forebrain in visual reception and food reflexes of two species of bullheads (Cottidae) from the Baerents Sea, *Vopr. Ikhtiol. AN SSSR* **14:**903.

Uretsky, E., and McCleary, R. A., 1969, Effect of hippocampal isolation on retention, *J. Comp. Physiol. Psychol.* **68:**1.

Veselkin, N. P., and Kovačević, N., 1973, Non-olfactory afferent projections of the telencephalon of elasmobranchii, *J. Evol. Biochem. Physiol.* **9:**585.

Voronin, L. G., and Guselnikov, V. I., 1959, Some comparative physiological data on the biological reactions of the brain, *Zh. Vyssh. Nerv. Devatel. I. P. Pavlova* **9:**398.

Voronin, L. G., Guselnikov, K. G., Guselnikov, V. I., and Supin, A. J., 1968, On the problem of the evolution of the vertebrate afferent systems, *Prog. Brain Res.* **22:**541.

Vulpian, A., 1866, *Leçons sur la Physiologie Générale et Comparée du Système Nerveux*, Germer-Baillière, Paris.

Warren, J. M., 1961, The effect of telencephalic injuries on learning by paradise fish, *Macropodus opercularis*, *J. Comp. Physiol Psychol.* **54:**130.

Weinberg, H., 1972, The contingent negative variation: Its relation to feedback and expectant attention, *Neuropsychology* **10:**299.

Westerman, R. A., 1965, Specificity in regeneration of optic and olfactory pathways in teleost fish, in: *Studies in Physiology* (D. R. Curtis and A. K. McIntyre, eds.), pp. 263–269, Springer, Berlin.

Wright, D. E., 1978, Effects of electrical stimulation of the brain of the goldfish, *Carassius auratus,* Ph.D. thesis, University of London.

Yager, D., 1967, Behavioral measures and theoretical analysis of spectral sensitivity and spectral saturation in the goldfish, *Carassius auratus, Vision Res.* **7:**707.

Yeo, C. H., and Savage, G. E., 1975, The tectal commissure and interocular transfer of a shape discrimination in the goldfish, *Exp. Neurol.* **49:**291.

Yeo, C. H., and Savage, G. E., 1976, Mesencephalic and diencephalic commissures and interocular transfer in the goldfish, *Exp. Neurol.* **53:**51.

Zagorulko, T. M., 1965, Interaction between the forebrain and visual centres of the midbrain in teleosts and amphibians, *Zh. Evol. Biokhim. Fiziol.* **1:**449.

Zornetzer, S. F., Chronister, R. B., and Ross, B., 1973, The hippocampus and retrograde amnesia: Localization of some positive and negative memory disruptive sites, *Behav. Biol.* **8:**507.

Zucker, I., and McCleary, R. A., 1964, Perseveration in septal cats, *Psychon. Sci.* **1:**387.

Zunini, G., 1954, Researches on fish's learning, *Arch. Neerl. Zool.* **10:**127(Suppl.2).

7

Telencephalon and Behavior in Teleost Fish

A Neuroethological Approach

JAN P. C. de BRUIN

I. Introduction

A. Ethological Introduction

In his ethological analysis of fish behavior Baerends (1971) distinguishes between behavioral functions associated with the maintenance of the body and those associated with the maintenance of the species. The first category encompasses respiration, locomotion, feeding, schooling, and defense against predators. Nesting behavior, courtship, fertilization, parental care, and agonistic behavior are functions of the second category.

This chapter will deal with the behavioral functions of the second category, and some data will be presented on feeding and schooling behavior. The telencephalon of teleost fish does not seem to be involved in respiration or locomotion, and no data are available on telencephalic functions involving defense against predators. The role of the telencephalon in learning and memory is described in Chapter 6 of this volume.

JAN P. C. de BRUIN • Netherlands Central Institute for Brain Research, IJdijk 28, Amsterdam, The Netherlands.

B. Neuroanatomical Introduction

1. Telencephalic Areas

The telencephalon of teleost fish is a remarkable neural structure. In the nineteenth century scientists had discovered that the telencephalon could be entirely removed without resulting in clear behavioral changes. In 1888 the German anatomist Steiner remarked that the forebrain of bony fish is "eine Form *ohne* Inhalt" (Nieuwenhuys, 1960). However, a simple neuroanatomical view of its connections with the olfactory epithelium via the olfactory bulbs precludes denial of an olfactory function. If Steiner's remark had been true, this chapter would have been a very short one. Its bulk suggests that the teleost telencephalon is not only "eine Form *mit* Inhalt" but also more than just an olfactory brain part.

Another reason why the telencephalon can be considered a remarkable structure is its ontogenetic development. Unlike the forebrain of other vertebrate classes, in which the development of the telencephalon is characterized by an invagination of the ventricles, the teleost forebrain shows a process of eversion, by which the ventricles assume a T shape. This results in a completely different arrangement of the periventricular neuroblasts. In consequence, the outgrowth and migration of nerve cells are not centrifugal but rather centripetal.

This fundamental difference in ontogenetic development caused considerable confusion in the terminology of the fish telencephalon, clearly illustrated in Fig. 1, in which two terminologies are juxtaposed.

On the one hand there is the classical terminology based on the names of telencephalic structures as they are commonly used in the description of the mammalian telencephalon. In this description a basic division of six telencephalic areas

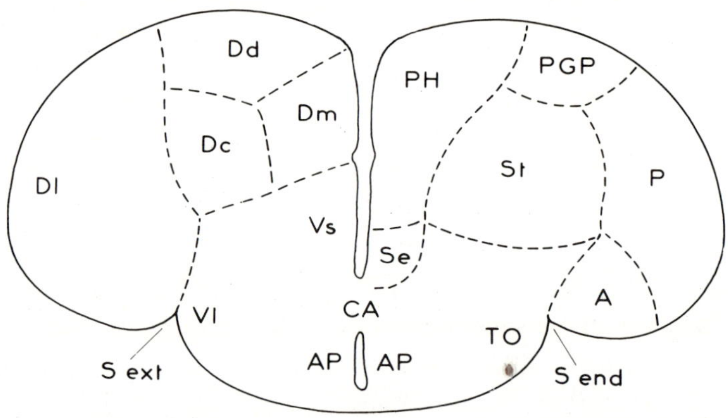

Figure 1. Schematic cross section through the telencephalon of a perciform teleost (*Betta splendens*) at the level of the anterior commissure. The left hemisphere is labeled according to Nieuwenhuys (1960, 1963), the right hemisphere, slightly modified, according to the classical nomenclature of Droogleever-Fortuyn (1961) and Schnitzlein (1968). A, Amygdala; AP, area praeoptica; CA, commissura anterior; Dc, area dorsalis pars centralis; Dd, area dorsalis pars dorsalis; Dm, area dorsalis pars medialis; Dl, area dorsalis pars lateralis; P, pyriform area; PH, primordial hippocampal formation; PGP, primordial general pallium; Se, septal area; S. end, sulcus endorhinalis; S ext, sulcus externus; St, striatum; TO, olfactory tubercle; VL, area ventralis pars lateralis; Vs, area ventralis pars supracommissuralis.

is proposed for all vertebrate classes (Crosby *et al.*, 1966). For the teleost telencephalon they are (Schnitzlein, 1968) primordial hippocampal formation (dorsomedial), septal nuclei (ventromedial), olfactory tubercle (ventral), pyriform area, basolateral amygdala and corticomedial amygdala (dorsolateral), primordial general pallium (dorsal), and striatum (central). Both pallium and striatum show a minor degree of development in fish compared to that in other vertebrate classes.

On the other hand there is the terminology proposed by Nieuwenhuys (1959, 1960, 1963). He divides the telencephalon of teleost fish into two major regions: an area dorsalis telencephali and an area ventralis telencephali. Both areas may be subdivided based on cytoarchitectonic differences. The dorsal area is subdivisible into a lateral, a dorsal, a medial, and a central part, and, depending on the species studied, further subdivisions are possible. The ventral area is subdivisible into a dorsal, a lateral, and a ventral part, and in the region of the commissura anterior into a supracommissural and a postcommissural part.

Synonyms in the description of telencephalic areas are numerous, and the reader may study the lists of synonyms presented by Nieuwenhuys (1963) or Peter and Gill (1975) to obtain an idea of the pluriformity of telencephalic terminology. In this survey the nomenclature of Nieuwenhuys will be used.

2. Telencephalic Fiber Connections

A number of fiber tracts connect the telencephalon with either the olfactory bulbs or the more caudally located parts of the brain. The medial and lateral olfactory tracts (tractus olfactorius medialis and tractus olfactorius lateralis), both arising from the olfactory bulb, reach the ventral telencephalic area and the caudoventral portion of the dorsal telencephalic area, respectively.

Three fiber tracts pass through the telencephalic peduncles toward diencephalic centers. The medial forebrain bundle (fasciculus medialis telencephali) largely originates in the supracommissural and postcommissural parts of the ventral telencephalic area to terminate mainly in the dorsal part of the hypothalamus. The lateral forebrain bundle (fasciculus lateralis telencephali) is by far the largest telencephalic fiber tract of the teleost telencephalon. Its fibers derive from most parts of the dorsal telencephalic area and terminate in the ventral part of the diencephalon, notably in the nucleus rotundus and adjacent nuclei, and in the inferior lobes of the hypothalamus. The third fiber tract is the stria medullaris, which forms the connection between forebrain nuclei and the epithalamic area (nuclei habenulae). In teleost fish this connection is mainly formed by the tractus taeniae, originating in the caudoventral portion of the dorsal area. The stria also includes the fiber tracts which connect the area praeoptica with the habenular region (Nieuwenhuys, 1960, 1963). Some studies have indicated that besides these telencephalic–diencephalic connections (limited to the prosencephalon), the telencephalon in several fish groups also has direct connections with the tectum mesencephali (e.g., Holmgren, 1920; Fiedler, 1967*a*) and the tegmentum mesencephali (Beccari, 1943).

The two telencephalic hemispheres are interconnected by the anterior commissure, in which, among others, the medial olfactory tract and the lateral forebrain bundle decussate. In some teleosts another telencephalic commissure is found, situated dorsocaudal to the anterior commissure. Although this commissure is sometimes considerably larger than the anterior commissure (e.g., in *Betta splendens*, de Bruin, 1977), only a few fibers seem to cross here. Detailed studies in teleosts, dealing with the question as to what extent the fibers contained in the forebrain bundles are ascendent or descendent, are lacking. However, various authors give tentative hypotheses based on histological (Golgi-stained or degeneration preparations) or stimulation studies (Johnston, 1911; Holmgren, 1920; Nieuwenhuys, 1959, 1963; Fiedler, 1967*a,b*). It seems likely that there is a greater proportion of ascending fibers in the lateral forebrain bundle than in the medial forebrain bundle.

Studies in other nonmammalian vertebrates have provided more experimental evidence. Ebbesson and Schroeder (1971) and Schroeder and Ebbesson (1974) have studied the nonolfactory telencephalic connections of an elasmobranch fish, the nurse shark (*Ginglymostoma cirratum*). Using degeneration staining techniques, they demonstrated that the lateral forebrain bundle (tractus pallii according to their terminology) primarily contains descending fibers from the telencephalon to the thalamus, epithalamus, hypothalamus, tectum mesencephali, and brain stem as well as ascending fibers from, e.g., the thalamus.

Studies in American frogs (*Rana* sp.) show the major telencephalic efferent fiber bundles to be the medial and lateral forebrain bundles, having their terminals in the diencephalon (dorsal and ventral thalamus, hypothalamus) and the tegmentum mesencephali (Halpern, 1972). Kicliter and Northcutt (1975) demonstrated that the main afferent pathways to the telencephalon of *Rana* sp. are the medial and lateral forebrain bundles, arising not only from diencephalic areas but also from levels caudal to the isthmus of the mesencephalon. It seems that more experimental data are necessary, especially in teleost fish, to determine to which degree the medial and lateral forebrain bundles contain descending and ascending fibers.*

II. Methods of Studying Telencephalic Functions

A. Ablation and Specialized Lesions

Ablation of the telencephalon is usually performed by cutting either the olfactory nerves (in species with sessile olfactory bulbs) or the olfactory tracts (in species with nonsessile olfactory bulbs). The telencephalon is then separated from the diencephalon by transsecting the peduncles, which in large part consist of the lateral and medial forebrain bundles. The telencephalon is now devoid of its neural connections and can be carefully removed by suction. Depending on the extent of its anterior extension, a portion of the preoptic area is removed as well.

Various researchers have also studied the behavioral changes following ablation or localized electrolytic lesions (coagulations) of, predominantly, the dorsal telencephalic and the preoptic areas. Since the fish skull, unlike that of mammals, does

* In a recent degeneration study involving the removal of one telencephalic hemisphere, Vanegas and Ebbesson (1976) witnessed telencephalic projections in the optic tectum, the nucleus rotundus complex, and the caudal parts and inferior lobes of the hypothalamus.

not provide any external landmarks useful in determining the precise location of a lesion site, it is necessary to use those visible landmarks provided by the brain itself, e.g., the commissura posterior (Peter and Gill, 1975) or the epiphysis cerebri (de Bruin, 1977). Special stereotaxic apparatus for use in fish studies have been described in the literature (Peter, 1970; Vanegas and Quezada, 1974; Peter and Gill, 1975).

When data are unavailable on the possible behavioral (or other) functions of a neural structure, a classical and direct approach is the removal of this structure and an investigation of the subsequent behavioral changes. Total ablation studies, complemented with specialized lesion experiments, have presented conclusive evidence regarding the behavioral functions of the teleost telencephalon. One must be aware, however, of the limitations involved in interpreting behavioral changes resulting from lesions of the telencephalon. A change in a specific behavioral system may also result from nonspecific disturbances in attention, motivation, general activity, or sensorimotor capacities. The study of possible changes in other behavioral systems might help to clarify the specificity of the lesion.

A direct correlation between the ablation of a central nervous structure and the subsequent behavioral changes provides us with another interpretational problem. Lesions not only destroy the cell bodies of a particular brain region but also may interrupt fiber tracts. Thus a behavioral change could also arise from another brain region deafferented by the interruption of a fiber tract. Moreover, mammalian studies have shown that brain lesions may alter the level of biogenic amines in other brain parts (Thompson, 1971), while changes in hormonal levels in fish following telencephalic lesions have been suggested (Fielder, 1967*a*). These limitations must be kept in mind when interpreting behavioral changes resulting from brain lesions.

B. Stimulation and Recording

Two other techniques often used in brain and behavior studies—stimulation of and recording from the brains of freely moving animals—have been used in few fish studies. One of the reasons is that most fish species examined in ethological studies are of such a small size that considerable technical problems must be overcome. Examples, however, may be found in the studies of Fiedler (1964, 1966, 1967*b*) and Demski *et al.* (Demski, 1973; Demski and Knigge, 1971; Demski and Gerald, 1974; Demski *et al.*, 1975*a*), who succeeded in electrically stimulating and/or recording from telencephalic and other brain areas in free-swimming fish and were able to relate their electrical data to the behavior of the fish.

Demski and Knigge (1971) describe their preparations as follows:

> a small hole was made in the skull [of the bluegill, *Lepomis macrochirus*] and two stainless steel screws were fixed in the nasal bones. Up to four monopolar electrodes were placed with reference to visual landmarks on the dorsal surface of the brain. Following insertion of the electrodes, the cranial opening was filled with gelfoam and covered with spray-on wound dressing. Acrylic cement was then applied in several coats to the electrodes, screws and exposed areas of the skull.

Stimulation was provided by the conventional stimulators commonly used in avian and mammalian stimulation studies. A bare wire was used as the indifferent electrode and placed in the water of the test aquarium.

Electrical stimulation has the clear advantage of enabling a functional analysis of miniscule portions of an "intact" central nervous system. It can be applied repeatedly when the investigator chooses, thus permitting a greater diversity in environmental factors, choice of stimulus animals, and group composition. Many axons are stimulated simultaneously, the direction of the current being both orthodromic and antidromic. Therefore, electrical stimulation must be considered a nonphysiological stimulus, since it distorts the normal functional pattern of the affected neural elements.

Since the direction of the current follows the normal anatomical pathways of conduction, electrical recordings hardly interfere with the normal functioning of the nervous system and are, physiologically, less disruptive for the organism. Although the data obtained from electrical recordings of brain activity can be correlated with the animal's behavior, this method does not permit an investigation of the causal relationship.

C. Histological Control

The test animals are sacrificed following postoperative behavioral tests, the brains are exposed, and, when ablations have been done, the extent of the damage to the brain can be examined macroscopically. It is, however, necessary to extend this macroscopic examination with a detailed histological survey. Consequently, the brain is carefully extirpated, fixed, embedded, serially sectioned, and stained. Most investigators choose staining methods which show both cell bodies and fibers (e.g., the techniques described by Bodian, Klüver Barrera, and Marchi). Localizations are often determined by the Prussian blue method, identifying the iron ions resulting from stimulation, in combination with cell body staining techniques. Details of these various procedures have been given by Segaar (1965), Fiedler (1967*a*), and Demski and Knigge (1971).

The next step is to demarcate the damaged area and to plot the precise location of the electrode site. Descriptive stereotaxic atlases, such as exist for many mammalian species, were not available until recently for the fish brain. Peter and coworkers now have published detailed stereotaxic atlases for the telencephalon of two fish species, the goldfish (*Carassius auratus*) (Peter and Gill, 1975) and the killifish (*Fundulus heteroclitus*) (Peter *et al.*, 1975). These atlases are based on the labeling of all forebrain nuclei in cross sections 0.1 mm apart. A grid was drawn over each cross section with lines 0.2 mm apart, thus permitting a very accurate description of location and size of the lesion or electrode placement.

In their studies of the three-spined stickleback (*Gasterosteus aculeatus*), Segaar and Nieuwenhuys (1963) followed a somewhat different method to describe the exact locations of their telencephalic lesions. The more prominent telencephalic nuclear masses of the stickleback were mapped out, proceeding from the ventromedial to the ventrolateral side of the forebrain along its ventricle surface. Such maps facilitate a description as to what extent each telencephalic nucleus is removed or damaged.

III. Behavioral Changes following Ablation and Specialized Lesions of the Telencephalon

A. Introduction

Interest in the functions of the forebrain of both teleost and elasmobranch fishes began as early as the first half of the nineteenth century, when various researchers extirpated the telencephalon. The results of these experiments and those performed before 1930 illustrated that the telencephalon of fish was important only with regard to olfactory functions. No changes could be found in equilibrium, locomotion, vision, and general behavior of the experimental animals following telencephalon ablation. Whenever other than olfactory behavioral changes were found, they were attributed to damage of other brain areas, or, in the case of stimulation studies, to the involvement of other brain areas than the telencephalon proper. Many of these experiments have been summarized by Ten Cate (1935) and Segaar (1965) and therefore will not be further dealt with in this review.

Janzen (1932/1933) was one of the first researchers to present conclusive evidence that the telencephalon of fish should be looked at as more than just an olfactory brain area, when he proved that regulatory and associative functions must be attributed to the telencephalon as well. These functions had been thought to be restricted to more caudally located areas of the fish brain. Janzen distinguished between "spontaneous s.s." and "initiative" properties in the behavior of the goldfish he studied. While no noticeable changes occurred in the spontaneity of the behavior following telencephalon ablation, a considerable decrease in the initiative of the forebrainless goldfish was evident. In one of his experiments Janzen used a set of narrow iron bars through which the fish could swim between two identical compartments of the tank. While normal fish swam frequently through even the closest bars without touching them, forebrainless fish swam through the bars only when they were placed wide apart. While Janzen's study provided evidence for an associative function of the telencephalon, Wrede (1932) showed that the telencephalon of the minnow *Phoxinus laevis* (Atheriniformes, Cyprinodontidae)* had integrative properties as well. Telencephalon-ablated minnows, unable to smell, also failed to discriminate between certain taste stimuli which normally occur in combination with odor stimuli. Wrede argued that the telencephalon was not only an olfactory center but also of considerable importance in the integration of olfactory and gustatory stimuli.

Both Ten Cate (1935) and Segaar (1965) have summarized many studies on the role of the telencephalon in schooling behavior in a variety of fish species: goldfish, gudgeons, minnows (Atheriniformes, Cyprinodontidae), bogues (Perciformes, Sparidae), and cichlids (Perciformes, Cichlidae). In general, telencephalon-ablated fish are less likely to form schools.

* Whenever a fish species is mentioned in the text for the first time, its classification is given; the division in orders is according to Greenwood *et al.* (1966), the division in families is according to Jordan (1963).

B. Nesting Behavior

Various detailed studies of the three-spined stickleback, *Gasterosteus aculeatus* (Gasterosteiformes, Gasterosteidae), provided an ethological basis for both Schönherr's (1955) and Segaar's (1956, 1965) ethophysiological investigations on the functions of the forebrain in reproductive behavior. As a brief ethological introduction, it may be mentioned that the male, after establishing a territory, builds a tunnel-shaped nest in the substratum, which he defends by charging and biting other rival males. Male courtship characteristically consists of the zig-zag dance by which he both attracts a female and leads her to the entrance of the nest. The female creeps through the nest, deposits the eggs, and is followed by the male, who fertilizes the clutch. The male ventilates the eggs by assuming an oblique position, head pointed downward, in front of the nest entrance and directing a water current through the nest. This behavior is called fanning and is commonly used as a measure of the level of male parental behavior. Both Schönherr and Segaar demonstrated quite clearly that telencephalic lesions may result in drastic changes in nestbuilding behavior. Whereas the olfactory bulbs do not seem to be involved, extensive lesions, in which both the rostral and lateral portions of the telencephalon are removed, do not abolish any of the separate parameters characteristic of nestbuilding, except creeping through, the behavioral act by which the tunnel in the nest is made. Thus the nest remains flat and the female cannot creep through to spawn.

Total telencephalon removal has a considerable effect on the taxis component of nestbuilding. Although the operated males perform the separate digging movements, these are not restricted to one particular place on the sandy bottom of the tank but occur at various places, resulting in many pits but not in a consistent nest. Therefore, both types of operation prevent a successful reproductive cycle.

Studies on telencephalon removal and nestbuilding behavior in the Siamese fighting fish, *Betta splendens* (Perciformes, Osphronemidae), confirmed the findings of Segaar. This species builds a floating nest, consisting of air bubbles surrounded with mucus. Following telencephalon removal, however, air bubbles may be found over the entire water surface in the tank and the separate nestbuilding acts do not result in a cohesive nest (de Bruin, 1977).

Other studies on forebrain function and nest building were performed by Overmier and Gross (1974) in the cichlid fish *Tilapia mossambica,* a species which like the three-spined stickleback builds a nest prior to active courtship behavior. Nestbuilding was quantitatively expressed in the amount of substratum cleared of gravel by nest-digging activities. Thus a clean and smooth nest area resulted on which the eggs could be deposited. The authors did not mention a loss of orientation in nestbuilding behavior following telencephalon removal. However, the surface of the nest area was considerably smaller when compared with preoperative control measurements.

As a possible explanation of the persistance of the taxis component in Overmier and Gross's experiments, one may argue that, considering the size of the fish used, their tanks were relatively smaller than those used by Segaar. The much smaller sticklebacks used by the latter author were housed in somewhat larger tanks. Segaar mentions that in small tanks telencephalon-ablated sticklebacks may dig one single pit, be it of enormous size, vs. a postoperative decrease of pit size as described by

Overmier and Gross. Although the latter authors postulate that their results are in agreement with those of Segaar, the agreement, in our opinion, does not extend beyond the fact that the forebrain clearly plays a role in nestbuilding. In *Tilapia mossambica* nestbuilding quantitatively decreased, whereas in *Gasterosteus aculeatus* it was greatly exaggerated.

C. Sexual and Parental Behavior

The conclusion resulting from the many experiments reported before 1930, that reproductive behavior in fish was unaffected by telencephalon ablation, was further disputed by the studies of Noble (1936, 1937; Noble and Borne, 1941), working at the American Museum of Natural History. He studied the telencephalic functions with regard to aggressive behavior and various components of reproductive behavior (courtship and sexual behavior). The experimental animals were representative species from three fish families: *Lebistes reticulatus, Xiphophorus bimaculatus* and *Xiphophorus helleri* (Atheriniformes, Cyprinodontidae), *Hemichromis bimaculatus* and *Tilapia macrocephala* (Perciformes, Cichlidae), and *Betta splendens* (Perciformes, Osphronemidae). The results of these studies can hardly be summarized more concisely than they were when originally published in the Supplements of the *Anatomical Record.* Many data of the quite extensive studies are, however, missing, such as those on the exact location and extent of the ablations, their histological controls, and a more detailed description of the behavioral changes following telencephalic operations. Moreover, one wonders which delimitations Noble had in mind when he mentioned that his ablations involved the "corpus striatum" and the "posterior tubercle." Is the naming of the "striatum" by Noble (1936) concordant with the demarcation presented in Fig. 1? In that case, according to Nieuwenhuys's (1963) terminology it is synonymous with the central part of the dorsal telencephalic area only. However, one wonders whether Noble really meant such a restricted area of the telencephalon. Which part of the forebrain Noble (1936) had in mind when discussing the function of the "posterior tubercle" is even more obscure. This is probably a part of the ventral telencephalic area, situated caudal to the anterior commissure, and including part of the preoptic area as well.

Some of Noble's statements are of great interest with regard to later research. His remark that "part of the posterior tubercle is required for the movements of egg laying and fertilization [in cichlid fish]" (Noble, 1936) is in concordance with the study of Macey *et al.* (1974), who clearly demonstrated the importance of the preoptic area for the spawning behavior in the killifish, *Fundulus heteroclitus* (Atheriniformes, Cyprinodontidae).

Another statement from the same publication that "some deficiencies following [other] lesions tend to disappear on successive layings" is in agreement with the results of Segaar's (1962, 1965) elaborate studies of the three-spined stickleback. This author also found that deficiencies in reproductive behavior disappeared during the course of successive reproductive cycles, and he showed that this could very well result from regenerative processes in the fish telencephalon.

Noble's findings regarding sexual behavior can be summarized by stating that in *Hemichromis bimaculatus* telencephalic lesions led to a lack of coordination and synchronization. In cyprinodont species (*Lebistes reticulatus* and *Xiphophorus helleri*), showing a less complex mating behavior (series of stereotyped components in which the female is the passive partner), normal mating behavior was inhibited but not prevented. The data on *Betta splendens* were somewhat contradictory; in the 1936 abstract the same conclusion was reached for both *Betta splendens* and *Lebistes reticulatus,* i.e., near complete ablation of the forebrain inhibited but did not prevent normal mating behavior. In the 1941 abstract, however, it was mentioned that in *Betta splendens* all sexual behavior was eliminated when most of the forebrain was removed.

In spite of the incompleteness of Noble's publications, they form a stimulus for many later studies on the role of the telencephalon in reproductive and aggressive behavior in a variety of fish species.

Aronson and co-workers, working in the same Institute as Noble, were among the first to continue his experiments. Following a description of the mating and spawning behavior of the mouthbreeding cichlid fish (*Tilapia macrocephala*), Aron son (1948) also gave the results of some neurological experiments dealing with changes in the reproductive behavior resulting from ablation of one or both telencephalic hemispheres. Whereas early courtship patterns appeared to be unaffected, the behavioral patterns immediately related to the actual spawning were clearly impaired. Hemidecerebrates showed a slight degree and decerebrates a marked degree of disturbance in reproductive behavioral patterns. Aronson submitted as a tentative conclusion that the forebrain does not integrate any of these behavioral patterns but rather facilitates the functioning of other parts of the brain which more precisely control these activities. Such a conclusion is in agreement with mammalian studies in which the cerebral cortex is considered a facilitator of sexual activities.

Further studies on mating behavior were performed by Kamrin and Aronson (1954), using a poeciliid fish species, the male platyfish (*Xiphophorus maculatus*). Nine behavioral parameters were chosen, all belonging to reproductive behavior *s.l.* Operations consisted of ablations of various portions of the forebrain. Postoperative behavioral changes were characterized by a decrease in frequency in eight of the nine parameters; copulation was absent in most experimental animals but persisted in a few at a lower frequency. In contrast, gonopodial swinging, a behavioral parameter characteristic of the initial stage of male courtship and performed at some distance from the female, did not decrease in frequency, but in some animals even showed an increase. Although Kamrin and Aronson performed operations in which only parts of the telencephalon were removed, they offered no data on possible correlations between changes in reproductive behavior and the location of those small ablations. Their conclusions regarding forebrain functions are the same as those of Aronson (1948): In the cichlid and poeciliid fish studied the forebrain facilitates the activities of lower parts of the brain. They suggest that this function is related, in particular, to visually directed processes. Kamrin and Aronson, moreover, argue that similar functions of the forebrain in sexual behavior are postulated for both birds and mammals.

Aronson's later studies were mainly concerned with forebrain functions and various learning processes in fish. They are dealt with in more detail in Chapter 6 in this volume. The results of studies on social behavior and learning, together with some electrophysiological and neuropharmacological evidence, have led Aronson to postulate the *arousal hypothesis.* The forebrain of bony fishes does not participate directly in the organization of behavior but must be regarded as a nonspecific, facilitative regulator of lower brain mechanism: such a system can function independently of olfaction (Aronson and Kaplan, 1968; Aronson, 1970). The results of other studies show that the arousal hypothesis is not always sufficient to encompass telencephalic functions.

In his studies on the effects of lesions in the parietal and other regions in another poeciliid fish, the guppy (*Lebistes reticulatus*), Pflugfelder (1954) remarked on the behavioral changes following total telencephalon removal. Although Pflugfelder observed neither courtship nor mating in the operated males, he writes that reproduction is not affected by this operation. The reader may be reminded of Kamrin and Aronson's findings that, in the related species *Xiphophorus maculatus,* a decrease occurred in the frequency of the sexual acts with the exception of the courtship behavioral pattern gonopodial swinging. Moreover, these authors observed copulation in a few males, even in a male in which the forebrain was completely ablated, except for small remnants of the preoptic area.

In their ethophysiological investigations of the three-spined stickleback (*Gasterosteus aculeatus*) Schönherr (1955) and Segaar (1956) dealt with forebrain functions and reproductive behavior. Although forebrainless males, while exhibiting a decreased motivation, reacted to responsive females with the zig-zag dance, they were unable to lead the females to a localized place in the tank. The same is true for fanning behavior, which occurs as "displaced" fanning in various localities in the tank.

In his successive studies, Segaar (1961, 1962, 1965) paid considerable attention to localized, smaller ablations and coagulations of the dorsal telencephalic area and their impact on three groups of behavioral components. These groups of components ("systems") were studied not only in a qualitative but also in a quantitative way by measuring the frequency of bites directed at an opponent in a glass cylinder (aggression), by counting the number of zig-zags the male performed when courting a responsive female in a glass cylinder (sex), and by measuring the duration of the fanning behavior at the nest entrance (parental behavior). These measurements were taken on a daily basis during the whole reproductive cycle, which averages 7 days between fertilization of the eggs and hatching. Besides the postoperative changes in the above-mentioned parameters of the separate behavioral systems, Segaar laid great emphasis on the balance between these systems, the aggression–sex–parental pattern. During the course of a normal reproductive cycle the sexual "drive" gradually decreases, whereas the parental "drive" increases, reaching its maximum at the time of hatching. Changes in the aggressive drive during the reproductive cycle are less pronounced: there is a slight increase during the first few days, followed by a decrease; the lowest values are reached at hatching time, then the aggression of the male increases.

Segaar's findings on the influence of partial ablations of the dorsal telencephalic area on the aggression–sex–parental pattern may be summarized as follows: After bilateral ablation of either the frontal or the lateral portion of the telencephalic hemispheres, the parental care was high and the sexual drive of short duration compared to the preoperative pattern. Bilateral ablation of the mediocaudal part of the dorsal portions of the telencephalic hemispheres had an opposite effect: parental care was low and sexual motivation remained high. The effects of these operations on aggression are contrary to those on parental behavior, the former leading to a decrease and the latter to an increase in aggression (Table I).

Very small lesions in the dorsomediocaudal area of the telencephalon did not appear to alter aggressive and sexual behavior, their influence being restricted to parental behavior. With small bilateral lesions placed in the medial telencephalon close to the sulcus ypsiloniformis, parental care remained low. When similar lesions were placed more caudal and closer to the midline, parental care was normal until the middle of the reproductive cycle, when a second wave of parental activity occurred, exceeding its normal level. A high in parental care during the whole of the reproductive cycle was reached when bilateral lesions were placed either in the extreme medial part of the mediocaudal area or in the dorsomedial area, approximately halfway along the length of the hemispheres (Table 1).

It will be clear that Aronson's arousal hypothesis is insufficient to encompass these properties of telencephalic functioning. Segaar (1965) uses three terms for the description of the function of the fish telencephalon: "facilitation," "inhibition," and "integration." Facilitation is involved in the telencephalic control of both sexual and aggressive behavior. For nestbuilding the telencephalon exerts integrative functions as well, whereas telencephalic inhibition centers were witnessed with respect to parental behavior.

Data from both mammalian and avian studies as well as preliminary data from

Table I. Behavioral Changes during the Reproductive Cycle of the Three-Spined Stickleback (*Gasterosteus aculeatus*) following Small Telencephalic Ablations or Coagulations[a]

	Between fertilization of the eggs and hatching		
	Aggressive behavior	Sexual behavior	Parental behavior
1. 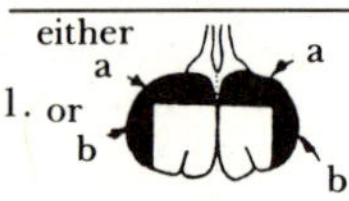	Low	Brief	High
2. 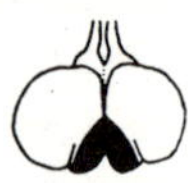	High	Continual	Low
3. 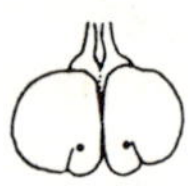	Normal	Normal	Low
4. 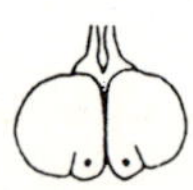	Normal	Normal	Normal during first half of cycle; high during second half of cycle
5. 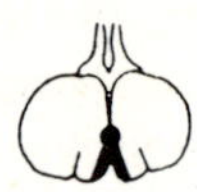	Normal	Normal	High

[a] After Segaar (1965).

fish studies suggested that the preoptic area plays an important role in the regulation of reproductive behavior. This function of the preoptic area in fish has been further investigated by Peter and co-workers. Although their studies mainly concentrate on the hypothalamic and preoptic control of the activity of various organs (e.g., the thyroid gland and the gonads), these authors have also studied preoptic and telencephalic functions with regard to behavior.

In a lesion study Macey *et al.* (1974) determined which area of the brain was responsible for the spawning reflex response in the killifish, *Fundulus heteroclitus* (Atheriniformes, Cyprinodontidae). This behavior consists of an S-shaped flexure of the body with additional characteristic quivering movements, and flattening of the anal and dorsal fins. The lesions were stereotaxically placed in various diencephalic and telencephalic areas. Following the operation the fish were tested for their ability to respond to exogenous neurohypophyseal hormones (either synthetic arginin vasotocin or hog posterior pituitary suspension) injected intraperitonially. The telencephalic lesion sites examined were the dorsal telencephalic area, mainly its central nucleus, and the preoptic area. It appeared that lesions in the dorsal telencephalic area did not abolish the spawning response, nor did this response disappear following lesions in such diencephalic areas as the habenular region, the nucleus lateralis tuberis, and the nucleus posterior tuberis. Lesions in the preoptic area, however, had drastic effects: a complete disappearance of the response as well as of the behavior associated with natural spawning activities. The authors argue that the preoptic area has a dual function. On the one hand its neurosecretory cells are considered the source of the hormone that elicits the spawning behavior, while on the other hand this area is thought to detect the hormone and integrate input from other brain regions, in such a way integrating reproductive behavior (cf. Demski and Knigge, 1971; Hallowitz *et al.*, 1971).

D. Aggressive Behavior

Aggressive behavior in fish is most often associated with the defense of a territory, either for food or for reproduction, or with the establishment and maintenance of a hierarchy. Even fish species which normally live in schools without any noticeable aggressive interactions will show aggressive acts during the reproductive period. Aggression includes such elements as attack (butting, biting, snapping at the opponent, and chasing him away), threat (erection of the gill covers, spreading of fins, undulating movements of the body, tail beating), flight (swimming away from the opponent), and submissive behavior (characterized by a decrease of body coloration, a folding of the fins, and certain body postures, mostly with the head turned upward). It has become customarily to use the term "agonistic behavior" to include elements of attack, threat, and flight. Noble and Borne (1941) were the first to provide data on telencephalon and aggression. They found that aggressive behavior in *Hemichromis bimaculatus, Betta splendens,* and *Xiphophorus helleri* persisted even after a complete ablation of the forebrain. However, the normal fighting patterns appeared to be considerably modified. The authors concluded that, following forebrain removal, an integration of aggressive behavior was not possible.

These data on the functioning of the forebrain with regard to aggressive behavior were further elaborated by Hale (1956), who studied its possible mediative role in aggressive behavior in the (American) sunfish, *Lepomis cyanellus* (Perciformes, Centrarchidae). Previous behavioral studies of this species had provided an ethological basis for Hale's neurological experiments. The aggressive behavior of this species falls into four categories: fighting, driving within social hierarchies, territorial defense, and defense of the nest.

Removal of either the olfactory bulbs or of a telencephalic hemisphere did not significantly alter aggressive behavior compared with that of control fish. Bilateral lesions of the dorsal telencephalic area (including its central nucleus) reduced fighting behavior. This decrease was more pronounced when the precommissural parts of the ventral telencephalic areas were invaded as well (nomenclature adapted to Nieuwenhuys, 1960, 1963). Removal of the ventral telencephalic area, leaving the dorsal telencephalic area intact—an extremely difficult operation—also resulted in a considerable decrease of aggression. Fighting behavior was almost completely eliminated if the total forebrain was removed, i.e., if the area preoptica was also ablated as far caudad as the midpoint of the optic chiasma. Hale was unable to observe any reproductive behavior in the two telencephalon-ablated males that had shown reproductive behavior (nestbuilding and courtship) prior to the operation. He summarized his findings by stating that the main difference between operated and unoperated fish lay in the initiation of aggression: the larger the area of the forebrain removed, the more difficult it became to elicit aggressive behavior in both males and females. However, once fighting behavior was elicited, the pattern was normal in all respects. These conclusions are basically in agreement with those of Aronson (1948) and Kamrin and Aronson (1954) in their studies on forebrain functioning and reproductive behavior in cichlid and poeciliid fish species.

In the three-spined stickleback (*Gasterosteus aculeatus*) aggression in forebrainless males is considerably reduced without a loss of any of the separate components (Segaar, 1965). The approach of a forebrainless male toward an opponent entering its territory is usually much slower, and when the opponent does not immediately retreat the ensuing fight lacks the vigor of fights between "normal," territorial males.

Partial ablations can either increase or decrease the level of aggression during the period between the fertilization and hatching of the eggs. Ablation of either the frontal or the lateral portions of the telencephalic hemispheres results in a decrease of the biting frequency and a mediocaudal ablation in an increase.

Fiedler studied the behavior of various perciform fish species and their neural and hormonal regulation systems. His neuroethological studies concentrated on three groups of fish, wrasses of the genus *Crenilabrus* (Perciformes, Labridae), breams of the genus *Diplodus* (Perciformes, Sparidae), and sunfish of the genus *Lepomis* (Perciformes, Centrarchidae). In his degeneration studies Fiedler (1966, 1967*a*, 1969) described the effects of total telencephalon ablation and of smaller coagulations on aggression, also presenting a few results of these effects on the intensity of male courtship. Both in *Crenilabrus* and in *Diplodus* forebrain removal resulted in a decrease of aggression, the intensity of fights between males being measured as the number of bites and pushes against a somewhat smaller conspecific test fish. In *Crenilabrus* the aggression dropped with about 60% compared to preoperative levels, whereas in *Diplodus* the decrease was only about 20%. Fiedler attributes these differences partly to species differences in wound healing (in *Cren-*

ilabrus wound healing is a much slower process than in *Diplodus*) and partly to neuroanatomical differences in the position of the preoptic area (in *Crenilabrus* the nucleus praeopticus pars magnocellularis has a much more rostralward extension than in *Diplodus*). Thus telencephalon extirpation in *Crenilabrus* resulted in the removal of a much larger portion of the preoptic area than in *Diplodus*. Other observations of Fiedler, based on postoperative histological controls, showed that the degree to which the preoptic area was removed accounted for differences in aggression. The larger the part of the preoptic area removed, the lower the fighting tendency appeared to be. Fiedler presumed that this effect was caused by interruption of the preoptico-hypophyseal tract, thus disturbing the hypothalamo-hypophyseal system.

Smaller lesions in various telencephalic areas may either decrease or increase the fighting tendency of *Crenilabrus tinca* as demonstrated by Fiedler in his 1966 paper. An increase in aggression (Fiedler terms it "inhibition") was found following coagulation of either the anterior commissure, the frontal part of the telencephalon, or, to a lesser degree, the dorsal nucleus of the dorsal telencephalic area. Coagulation of the frontal part of the telencephalon also increased male courtship behavior.

In *Diplodus annularis* small coagulations in similar areas always resulted in a smaller or larger decrease in the intensity of the intermale fights, depending on the location of the coagulation. Fiedler argued that the decrease of aggression was largest when the connections between the olfactory bulbs and the diencephalon via the medial forebrain bundles were interrupted and when the greatest number of degenerated fibers were found in the region of the diencephalic nucleus rotundus complex. Fiedler's findings of an inhibiting role of the telencephalon with regard to aggression and courtship behavior are of great interest, especially since the majority of previous researchers attributed only facilitatory properties to the telencephalon. However, Fiedler's findings were based on only a few individuals and a few preoperative observations. These studies most certainly require replications with larger numbers.

The Siamese fighting fish (*Betta splendens*) is known for its differentiated and highly ritualized aggressive and sexual behavior. The preliminary studies on telencephalon and behavior in this species (Noble and Borne, 1941) were followed by studies of Shapiro *et al.* (1974) and de Bruin (1973, 1977), both dealing with changes in aggressive behavior following telencephalic lesions. Shapiro *et al.* (1974) compared the behavior of telencephalic-lesioned and sham-operated fish toward live conspecific stimuli and the mirror image. The size of the lesions varied from a minimal extent of 30% to a near-total ablation of the telencephalic hemispheres. Their findings were basically in agreement with Noble and Borne's observations that "there is a decrease in response frequency but no diminution of response strength once a response is elicited." The behavioral response on which they based their results was the erection of the gill covers, shown by a male *Betta* during approach and during frontal display. Both frequency and duration of gill cover erection were taken as a measure of response strength. The frequency of responses to both a live *Betta* stimulus and the mirror image was lower in the operated fish than in the control fish. Telencephalon removal, however, did not alter the duration of the response. The differences in response rate to mirror and *Betta* stimuli were about equal to those of the control group. However, there was distinct habituation of the response during the 20 daily mirror confrontations. This habituation was highest in the control group, whereas the lesioned group exhibited a slighter and more irregular waning of the response, with an increase in response rate on days 9 and 10, thus suggesting that a sensitization might have occurred (cf. the dual-process theory of habituation of Groves and Thompson, 1970).

The frequency of gill cover erections was lower in animals with minimal telencephalon removal than in those with maximal telencephalon removal. However, the behavioral data presented are only suggestive of such a difference. Moreover, histological data presented by these authors are only preliminary, and it would be especially interesting to know the extent of damage to the preoptic nucleus and its impact on differences in the rate of gill cover erections.

Further studies on telencephalon and behavior in *Betta splendens* were conducted by de Bruin (1973, 1977). The starting point for this study was Noble and Borne's (1941) observation of a decrease in aggression following telencephalon removal and Segaar's (1965) description of differential telencephalic functions regarding aggressive, sexual, and parental behavior of the three-spined stickleback. The results of this investigation will be published shortly, so a short summary will be presented here.

The aggressive behavior of a male *Betta splendens* can be studied in terms of the responses either toward another male or toward its own mirror image. The latter method provides a more standardized experimental test situation without disturbing interferences of the stimulus male on the behavioral response of the test male. Aggressive responses toward an opponent or the mirror image can be divided into three major components. During *frontal display* the opponent is faced, the gill covers are protruded, and butting, thrusting, and biting movements are directed at the opponent. During *lateral display* the fish assumes a broadside position with full fin erection and performs various types of undulating body and fin movements including tail beating. Bouts of frontal and lateral display alternate with *withdrawal:* the fish retreats from the stimulus with rapid, undulating movements. Such a retreat is usually of short duration and is soon followed by an approach with gill cover erection.

Telencephalon removal results in a decrease in aggression, but not in its disappearance. The degree to which aggression drops also depends on the degree of damage to the preoptic area: the smaller the remaining preoptic area, the larger the impairment of aggressive behavior. Such a postoperative change of aggressive behavior is revealed as a change in pattern of its major components. The frequency, and to a smaller degree also the duration of the frontal display, diminishes, while its characteristic parameters, butting and biting, decrease in frequency or disappear from the display altogether. A real attack is lacking, and the aggressive display is exclusively a threat display. If the decrease of aggression is moderate (e.g., when the preoptic area has been left intact), the lateral display may increase in duration and is accompanied by an increase in frequency of a parameter such as tail beating, accentuating the lateral threat properties of the display. A large decrease in aggression (e.g., if both telencephalic hemispheres and a large part of the preoptic area have been removed) changes the balance among the three components altogether. Bouts of frontal and lateral display are of short duration and alternate with long periods of withdrawal.

Localized smaller lesions in the dorsal telencephalic area have further differentiated these findings. Depending on location and size of the lesion, aggressive behavior may either increase or decrease. An increase in aggression is characterized by a higher frequency of frontal display accompanied by a higher number of butting and biting movements. Withdrawal behavior may completely disappear, the aggressive display then consisting of an alternation between frontal and lateral display.

The finding of both facilitative and inhibitive properties in telencephalic functioning with regard to aggressive behavior supports the ideas of Segaar (1965). Moreover, Fiedler (1966) also mentions some preliminary results indicating an increase in aggression in *Crenilabrus* following small coagulations of telencephalic areas. Apparently, the telencephalon also has an inhibitory role in various kinds of behavior.

IV. Behavioral Observations during Stimulation of and Recording from the Telencephalon

A. Nesting Behavior

Although various lesion studies have indicated the importance of the telencephalon for nestbuilding in teleost fish (Segaar, 1956, 1965; Overmier and Gross, 1974; de Bruin, 1977), only Demski and Knigge's (1971) study presents complementary evidence from stimulation experiments. They described how normal nestbuilding in freely moving sunfish (*Lepomis macrochirus* and *L. cyanellus*) was evoked by stimulation of telencephalic sites. Particular reference is made to the central part of the dorsal telencephalic area (Dc in Fig. 1), and they describe the behavioral repertoire evoked by stimulation of this area as circling a particular spot on the bottom, followed by body undulations in which the caudal fin was swept across the gravel on the bottom of the tank. Separate sweeping movements could be evoked by stimulation of the area caudal to the anterior commissure, the adjacent preoptic area, and the hypothalamus.

B. Sexual and Parental Behavior

Demski *et al.* (1975*a*) studied forebrain functioning and reproductive behavior by mapping the neural pathway involved in the release of sperm. In the green sunfish (*Lepomis cyanellus*) they stimulated various brain areas and used seminal discharge, usually preceded by anal fin erection, as the adequate response. They showed that the neural part of the sperm release system extends from the preoptic area to the spinal cord, passing through the hypothalamus, the "tegmentum and basal nuclei of the midbrain," and the medulla. Sperm release could be evoked not only from the preoptic area but also from the adjacent ventral telencephalic areas, both postcommissural and precommissural, as well as from the forebrain bundles, situated lateral and dorsolateral to the preoptic region. In an interpretation of their results the authors emphasized the similarities of this pathway in the green sunfish to data on brain areas in representatives of other vertebrate classes from which electrical stimulation evoked seminal discharge or other aspects of spawning or copulatory behavior.

Judging from these comparative data, Demski and co-workers presumed that the preoptic area contains neurons that are sensitive to hormones playing a role in reproduction. Activation of the reproductive system by various external stimuli may be decreased by these hormones. The role of the preoptic area in courtship behavior was illustrated by Demski and Knigge (1971). Courtship behavior, consisting of rapid swimming to a female and circling her, was evoked in the sunfish when electrodes were placed in the caudal portion of the preoptic area.

Hallowitz *et al.* (1971) examined the interrelationship of the dorsal telencephalic area and the preoptic area. In anesthesized and immobilized sunfish various areas of the dorsal telencephalon, known for their function with regard to behavioral responses, were stimulated and the responses from the preoptic area, presumably its parvocellular elements, were recorded. The results demonstrated that these forebrain areas exert an excitatory influence on the preoptic–anterior hypothalamic area.

In comparing their results with similar studies in mammals, the authors mentioned that, besides facilitation, they noted inhibiting influences of telencephalic stimulation on preoptic-hypothalamic units. Their observation not only indicates a similarity between fish and mammals but also supports both Segaar's and Fiedler's results of telencephalic inhibitory influences on behavior. The authors also substantiated Segaar's observation that a specific telencephalic area was involved in the control of specific behavioral components. It appeared that many preoptic–anterior hypothalamic units could be activated only by a particular combination of stimuli from dorsal telencephalic areas.

Prolactin, an adenohypophyseal hormone, is known for its role in reproductive behavior. Parental behavior and nestbuilding are stimulated by the administration of low doses of prolactin (Fiedler, 1970). In order to determine the possible function of the telencephalon in detecting differences in the prolactin level, Fiedler and Blüm (1972) recorded the activity of forebrain neurons in anesthetized and immobilized fish following intramuscular injections of prolactin. These studies form a link between their ethoanatomical and ethoëndocrinological investigations. The pars dorsalis of the dorsal telencephalic area appeared to be especially sensitive to change of the blood prolactin level. Following intramuscular injection of prolactin the neuronal activity of this brain area increased, first showing positive prepotentials and then trains of spikes of high frequency and also high amplitude. This phenomenon was very clear with low doses of prolactin whereas higher doses had an inhibitive effect on the activation of this forebrain area. In *Astronotus ocellatus* (Perciformes, Cichlidae) the activating doses of prolactin were 0.2–0.3 IU per gram of body weight and the inhibiting doses 0.5–0.8 IU, whereas in *Lepomis gibbosus* these doses were somewhat lower.

Based on the latency times between the injection of prolactin and the onset of forebrain activity, the authors suggested that the hormone receptor units were not localized within the telencephalon proper, but in hypothalamic centers. Moreover, an injection of prolactin directly into the forebrain did not elicit such changes in the activity of forebrain neurons as resulted from intramuscular injections of this hormone.

Besides their lesion and recording studies in anesthetized and immobilized fish, Fiedler and co-workers performed brain stimulation and recording experiments in free-swimming fish of the species *Crenilabrus tinca, C. quinquemaculatus,* and *Lepomis gibbosus* (Fiedler, 1964, 1967*b*). They studied quite a variety of areas in the telencephalon, the diencephalon, the mesencephalon, and the cerebellum. Stimulation of the telencephalon may evoke various behavioral patterns. Besides separate responses such as butting and biting, which may belong to either aggressive or feeding systems, Fiedler observed series of behavioral acts, starting with appetitive behavior and ending with consummatory acts, such as feeding behavior: searching the bottom, taking up sand, chewing, and spitting out. When retreating ("Zurückweichen") was evoked by stimulation, snapping ("Zuschnappen") quite often occurred during the period following stimulation, a rebound phenomenon.

It is interesting, from a behavioral point of view, that stimulation in the region of the anterior commissure resulted in snapping and retreating. This balance changed in favor of retreating at a higher stimulus intensity. Similar findings were reported by Von Holst and Von Saint Paul (1960) in their stimulation studies in the domestic chicken.

In a summary of his stimulation results Fiedler lists the separate behavioral parameters and the stimulation sites from which they could be evoked. Both "charging at" ("Vorwärtsstossen") and "retreating" ("Zurückweichen") could be elicited from telencephalon, diencephalon, mesencephalon, and cerebellum. Telencephalic sites from which "charging at" could be elicited proved to be the area dorsalis pars dorsalis, the area dorsalis pars medialis, the area dorsalis pars dorsolateralis, and the bulbus olfactorius. Retreating could be elicited from the area dorsalis pars dorsalis, the commissura anterior, and the tractus olfactorius medialis. These findings provoke more questions than Fiedler's study can answer. Is the fact that a single behavioral parameter can be elicited from so many areas indicative of a high degree of plasticity or of a manyfold representation of control areas, or are all those areas part of one and the same neural circuit?

In his 1964 paper Fiedler presented some findings on registration of brain activity in freely moving fish *Crenilabrus tinca* and *Lepomis gibbosus.* When the electrode was placed in the tegmentum mesencephali near the posterior commissure, Fiedler was able to record positive potentials during butting movements directed toward a smaller fish. Cathodic stimulation via the same electrode resulted in butting, *in vacuo* snapping, and yawning, conformable to the recordings from the same area. In *Lepomis gibbosus* an electrode was placed in the anterior commissure, and recordings were made during the approach to a brine shrimp (*Artemia*), showing bursts of spikes. The subsequent snapping, chewing, and swallowing of the prey were accompanied by slow diphasic action potentials. Stimulation via the same electrode resulted in a complete sequence of feeding behavior: searching, snapping, spitting out, and also retreating. Snapping and retreating are the extremes of a single behavioral system, the balance between these acts depending on the stimulus intensity; an increase of the stimulus changes the balance toward more frequent retreating.

In their stimulation studies with freely moving sunfish (*Lepomis macrochirus* and *L. cyanellus*) Demski and Knigge (1971) evoked both feeding and aggressive behavior by stimulation of the hypothalamus in the area of the nucleus rotundus complex and in the area surrounding the lateral recess of the inferior hypothalamic lobe. Stimulation of some sites of these areas resulted in a complete feeding response, which included searching the surface, searching the bottom, snapping up prey, chewing and swallowing and/or snapping up gravel or debris, and spitting out, while other sites elicited only isolated components, e.g., snapping. These responses quite frequently alternated with aggressive behavior—chasing or biting another bluegill, or biting at the mirror image. Weak or inconsistent aggressive responses could also be elicited from more frontal electrode sites, namely the diencephalic habenular region and the dorsal part of the ventral telencephalic area.

It is interesting from a behavioral point of view that the authors describe aggressive afterresponses following courtship behavior which was evoked by stimulation in the preoptic region. They suggest that the preoptic area may be involved in the regulation of aggressive activity normally associated with reproduction.

In a comparative study Demski (1973) stimulated similar hypothalamic regions in the mouthbreeding cichlid fish *Tilapia heudelotti macrocephala.* Feeding and aggressive responses could be evoked from areas similar to those in the examined sunfish (Demski and Knigge, 1971), namely the area surrounding the lateral recess of the third ventricle. Demski was unable to distinguish between separate anatomical substrates for feeding and aggression. Thus the type of behavior evoked by stimulation also depended on the internal state of the animal (e.g., experience) and on external, environmental conditions (e.g., the presence of a rival male or food). Stimulation studies, both in birds (Von Holst and Von Saint Paul, 1960) and in mammals (Valenstein *et al.,* 1970), have emphasized the importance of these internal and external conditions for the response evoked.

Based on the location of the electrode sites from which feeding and aggressive behavior could be evoked, Demski (1973) suggested that the medial forebrain bundle be considered the fiber tract which mediates both types of behavior. This idea is supported by the results of Grimm (1960), who, in goldfish, evoked feeding behavior by stimulation of the olfactory tracts; these tracts project to the ventral telencephalic area, in which the medial forebrain bundle originates (cf. Section I.B.2).

Without denying the importance of the medial forebrain bundle, the role of the lateral forebrain bundle in the mediation of aggressive behavior should not be underestimated. Various portions of the dorsal telencephalic area are reported to have a function in the regulation of aggressive and other types of behavior. The bulk of the fiber connections of the dorsal telencephalic area with other brain areas are formed by the lateral forebrain bundle (cf. Section I.B.2).

More recently Demski *et al.* (1975*b*) have extended their behavioral work with a detailed histological and electron microscopic description of the structure of the hypothalamic lobes, which, judging from their previous studies, should be considered an important control region for both feeding and aggressive behavior. These modes of behavior could be evoked only from a restricted area in the inferior lobes present around the lateral recess, and not from the more laterally and ventrolaterally situated nucleus diffusus lobi lateralis, a sizable nucleus extending over the entire length of the large inferior hypothalamic lobes. The reason why this nucleus does not seem to be directly involved in feeding and aggression remains unclear. It is either lacking or poorly developed in some other nonmammalian vertebrate groups such as the cyclostomes, elasmobranchs, and other nonteleostean fish. It is interesting to note that in the goldfish Baumgarten and Braak (1967) found the cells surrounding this lateral recess, contrary to the nucleus diffusus, to contain a high level of catecholamines, probably norepinephrine. The preoptic area is innervated by a large number of catecholaminergic fibers, originating from the cells around the lateral recess. While the role of the nucleus diffusus remains unclear, these neuropharmacological facts support neuroethological data pointing to an important relationship between the preoptic area and the hypothalamus.

D. Arousal and Reward

Olds and Milner (1954) discovered a positive reinforcement in modes of behavior when certain areas of the brain of the rat were stimulated. This led to similar research in other vertebrate groups, including fish. Boyd and Gardner (1962) demonstrated that such areas were also present in the brain of the goldfish (*Carassius auratus*). Side preference tests, in which the animal received a stimulus via an electrode placed in the brain, were a part of their experimental procedure. The stimulus was supposed to have positive reinforcing properties if the fish chose the same side of the tank where it had received the stimulus. Negative reinforcing properties would result in an avoidance of that side of the tank. Based on the schematic representation of the electrode placements (Fig. 2 in Boyd and Gardner's paper), it may be concluded that stimulation of the frontal and dorsal parts of the dorsal telencephalic area has either neutral or aversive (negative reinforcing) effects. A positive reinforcement was found if the electrode was placed in the optic tectum.

Although Boyd and Gardner's preliminary observation of the existence of both positively and negatively rewarding areas in the brain of the goldfish indicated a similarity in normally functioning reward systems in both mammals (e.g., rats) and fish (goldfish), it remains unclear why electrode placements in the telencephalon of the goldfish failed to show such positive reinforcing properties. Various authors investigating self-stimulation stressed that the reward system could arouse behavior. In the rat, reward sites along the medial forebrain bundle gave arousal reactions following electrical stimulation (Rolls, 1975).

This contradiction has been investigated by Savage (1971), who electrically stimulated the telencephalon of goldfish and observed the ensuing behavioral effects. In general, stimulation resulted in arousal reactions (i.e., rapid extensions of the fins and tail flaps), their thresholds depending on the location of the electrode. Savage also studied the rewarding properties of these sites, but he could find no positive correlation between a low threshold and the degree of the reward—neither positive, nor negative, nor neutral. Two of the 11 electrode placements, one in the frontal part of the ventral telencephalic area and one in the medial part of the dorsal telencephalic area, resulted in positive reinforcing properties, the remaining nine being either negative (aversive) or neutral. One may conclude, judging from both of these studies, that there is no direct neuroanatomical correlation between the telencephalic arousal system and the telencephalic reward system. This subject is further dealt with in Chapter 6 in this volume.

V. Regenerative Aspects

Although regeneration in the adult central nervous system of teleosts is not so rapid and so successful as in amphibians, various authors reported regeneration of the cerebellum, the tectum opticum, and the telencephalon of teleost fish. Kirsche (1965) compiled data on central nervous system regeneration in teleosts. He stressed that only if the ependymal matrix zones of neuroblasts and glioblasts were left undamaged during the ablation did regeneration occur.

Regeneration has been witnessed in the tectum opticum of the crucian carp (*Carassius carassius* L.) (Kirsche and Kirsche, 1961) and the goldfish (*Carassius gibelio auratus* Bloch) (Pflugfelder, 1965), in the telencephalon of the guppy (*Lebistes reticulatus*) (Maroń, 1963) and the stickleback (*Gasterosteus aculeatus*) (Segaar, 1962, 1965), and, following a small ablation, in the cerebellum of the goldfish (*Carassius gibelio auratus* Bloch) (Pflugfelder, 1965).

Kirsche's (1961) and Segaar's (1962, 1965) observations are of great interest from a behavioral point of view. Kirsche described how a unilateral ablation of the tectum opticum is followed by severe locomotor disturbances which gradually disappear during the regeneration of the tectum opticum. Bilateral ablation of the lateral portions of the telencephalon (area dorsalis pars lateralis) of the stickleback (Segaar, 1962) resulted in changes in parental and sexual behavior (cf. Section III.C). These postoperative changes gradually disappeared during successive reproductive cycles and proved to be synchronous with the regeneration of the lateral telencephalic lobes. New neurons assumed the original laminated structure of the hemisphere.

However, other studies on the regenerative capacity of the telencephalon in goldfish failed to show a regenerative outgrowth of neuroblasts and glioblasts. Bernstein (1967) performed various types of telencephalic lesions in the goldfish (*Carassius auratus*), including removal of the lateral portions, which is comparable to the abovementioned telencephalic operation of the stickleback (Segaar, 1962). While Bernstein was unable to observe an outgrowth of new nerve cells, he did notice the formation of "cysts, partially or completely lined with pseudostratified columnar epithelial cells." Pflugfelder (1965), studying reparative and regenerative processes in the brain of the goldfish (*Carassius gibelio auratus* Bloch), was unable to find regenerative processes in the telencephalon at all. Small telencephalic coagulations were "repaired" through "Narbengewebe," the cysts probably being formed by glial cells.

It is difficult to compare Segaar's (1962) telencephalic lesions in the stickleback with Pflugfelder's (1965) and Bernstein's (1967) in their crucian carp and goldfish. Pflugfelder does not give an exact demarcation of his lesion sites, and it must be emphasized that Segaar found regeneration only following ablations of the lateral portions of the telencephalon (area dorsalis pars lateralis). Although Bernstein's operations consisted of removal of the lateral portions of the telencephalon, he terms this region "pars medialis, area dorsalis," which, in Segaar's terminology, is the region bordering the medial part of the ventricle. Although both Pflugfelder's and Bernstein's results strongly suggest that, unlike in the guppy and the stickleback, telencephalic regeneration does not occur in the goldfish, it should be kept in mind that the similarity of the ablated areas is quite uncertain.

Segaar (1965) discusses the regeneration of neurons in terms of a plasticity of the fish brain in response to environmental factors. This plasticity, from a phylogenetic point of view, may account for the great variation in the structure and function of the teleost telencephalon (Meader, 1939).

VI. Concluding Remarks

Until approximately 1930, the telencephalon of teleost fish was considered an olfactory brain part. Its function with regard to general behavioral aspects was not accepted, although some experimental results did indeed suggest such functions (review in Ten Cate, 1935).

However, many experiments performed in the 1930s and during the following decades quite clearly indicated the importance of the telencephalon for "initiative," schooling, learning, and reproductive and aggressive behavior. It is of historic interest that parallel to the development and rise of the science of ethology functions regarding the regulation of social behavior were attributed to the teleost telencephalon (Noble, 1936, 1937; Noble and Borne, 1941; Aronson, 1948). The behavioral functions of the telencephalon were synthesized in the arousal hypothesis (Aronson, 1970), which considers the telencephalon a "nonspecific activating regulator of lower brain mechanisms."

Although Aronson's arousal hypothesis fits many experimental results from both learning and "innate" behavior studies, it is insufficient to encompass those results indicative of inhibitive and integrative properties of telencephalic functioning. Moreover, many experiments suggested that specific telencephalic areas influence specific types of behavior (Segaar, 1965; Fiedler, 1966; Hallowitz *et al.*, 1971, Demski and Knigge, 1971; de Bruin, 1973, 1977). More experimental data from various teleosts will be needed before these results can be integrated into a general theory.

At present, most authors compare the teleost telencephalon with the (mammalian) limbic system, because of the similarity of their behavioral functions (Segaar, 1965; Aronson, 1970). Some anatomists extend this view also to neuroanatomical homologies, as is reflected in studies of Droogleever-Fortuyn (1961) and Schnitzlein (1968) (see also Section I.B).

The previous hypothesis of an important role of the hypothalamus in feeding and aggressive behavior has been experimentally supported by Demski's studies. This hypothesis partly arose from comparisons with other vertebrate groups in which such functions were demonstrated and partly from studies which showed that social behavior (aggression and reproduction) changed but did not disappear following telencephalon removal.

Other experiments have shown that the preoptic area also fulfills an important role in the regulation of reproductive, aggressive, and feeding behavior. As to aggressive behavior, this was apparent from lesion studies in which either small or extensive damage of this area resulted in a smaller or a greater decrease in the postoperative level of aggression (Fiedler, 1969; de Bruin, 1977). Stimulation studies (Demski and Knigge, 1971) support this finding. The role of the preoptic area in reproductive behavior was shown in a lesion study by Macey *et al.* (1974) and in stimulation studies by Demski and Knigge (1971) and Demski *et al.* (1975*a*).

The lack of an adequate application of anatomical knowledge and specific techniques has proved to be a severe handicap for behavioral studies on teleost forebrain functioning. Many students of behavior investigating brain functions of teleost fish did not give adequate histological data on ablations and lesions. Strikingly, many have started research programs to fill this gap, either on their own or in cooperation with neuroanatomists. Examples may be found in the collaboration between Segaar and Nieuwenhuys (1963), the latter providing the map of the stickleback forebrain needed for plotting the location and extent of coagulations and ablations. Demski described the sunfish telencephalon during and following his stimulation studies (Demski and Knigge, 1971), and provided a detailed histological study of the hypothalamus, the substratum from which both feeding and aggressive behavior could be evoked (Demski *et al.*, 1975*b*). Recently, Peter and coworkers have prepared detailed stereotaxic atlasses of the forebrains of the two fish species which they used in their neuroendocrinological and behavioral studies, the goldfish (*Carassius auratus*) (Peter and Gill, 1975) and the killifish (*Fundulus heteroclitus*) (Peter *et al.*, 1975). These authors also developed a stereotaxic apparatus to be used for precise electrode placement in the telencephalon and the diencephalon. It is to be hoped that the use of these stereotaxic techniques and atlasses will further stimulate collaboration among students of the behavior, neuroanatomy, neurophysiology, and neuroendocrinology of fish in clarifying the functions of the forebrain.

ACKNOWLEDGMENTS. The author is indebted to Prof. Dr. J. Ariëns Kappers and Dr. J. Segaar for their critical comments and valuable suggestions, and to Mrs. S. Lust-Bosboom for her typing of the manuscript.

VII. References

Aronson, L. R., 1948, Problems in the behavior and physiology of a species of African mouthbreeding fish, *Trans. N.Y. Acad. Sci.* **2**:33.

Aronson, L. R., 1970, Functional evolution of the forebrain in lower vertebrates, in: *Development and Evolution of Behavior* (L. R. Aronson, E. Tobach, D. S. Lehrman, and J. S. Rosenblatt, eds.), pp. 75–107, Freeman, San Francisco.

Aronson, L. R., and Kaplan, H., 1968, Functions of the teleostean forebrain, in: *The Central Nervous System and Fish Behavior* (D. Ingle, ed.), pp. 107–125, University of Chicago Press, Chicago.

Baerends, G. P., 1971, The ethological analysis of fish behavior, in: *Fish Physiology* (W. S. Hoar and D. J. Randall, eds.), pp. 279–370, Academic Press, New York.

Baumgarten, H. G., and Braak, H., 1967, Catecholamine im Hypothalamus vom Goldfisch (*Carassius auratus*), *Z. Zellforsch.* **80**:246.

Beccari, N., 1943, *Neurologia comparata, Anatomo-Funzionale dei Vertebrati, compreso l'uomo,* Sansoni Edizioni Scientifiche, Firenze.

Bernstein, J. J., 1967, The regenerative capacity of the telencephalon of the goldfish and rat, *Exp. Neurol.* **17**:44.

Bernstein, J. J., 1970, Anatomy and physiology of the central nervous system, in: *Fish Physiology,* Vol. IV (W. S. Hoar and D. J. Randall, eds.), pp. 1–90, Academic Press, New York.

Boyd, E. S., and Gardner, L. C., 1962, Positive and negative reinforcement from intracranial stimulation of a teleost, *Science* **136**:648.

Crosby, E. C., de Jonge, B. R., and Schneider, R. C., 1966, Evidence for some of the trends in the phylogenetic development of the vertebrate telencephalon, in: *Evolution of the Forebrain* (R. Hassler and H. Stephan, eds.), pp. 117–135, Thieme Verlag, Stuttgart.

de Bruin, J. P. C., 1973, Aggression in the Siamese fighting fish (*Betta splendens* Regan), its measurements and its telencephalic regulation, *Abstr. XIIIth Int. Ethol. Conf.*, August 14–22, Washington, D.C.

de Bruin, J. P. C., 1977, Telencephalic functions in the behaviour of the Siamese fighting fish, *Betta splendens* Regan (*Pisces, Anabantidae*), thesis, University of Amsterdam.

Demski, L. S., 1973, Feeding and aggressive behavior evoked by hypothalamic stimulation in a cichlid fish, *Comp. Biochem. Physiol.* **44A:**685.

Demski, L. S., and Gerald, J. W., 1974, Sound production and other behavioral effects of midbrain stimulation in free-swimming toadfish, *Opsanus beta, Brain Behav. Evol.* **9:**41.

Demski, L. S., and Knigge, K. M., 1971, The telencephalon and hypothalamus of the bluegill (*Lepomis macrochirus*): Evoked feeding, aggressive and reproductive behavior with representative frontal sections, *J. Comp. Neurol.* **143:**1.

Demski, L. S., Bauer, D. H., and Gerald, J. W., 1975*a*, Sperm release evoked by electrical stimulation of the fish brain: A functional-anatomical study, *J. Exp. Zool.* **191:**215.

Demski, L. S., Evan, A. P., and Saland, L. C., 1975*b*, The structure of the inferior lobe of the teleost hypothalamus, *J. Comp. Neurol.* **161:**483.

Droogleever-Fortuyn, J., 1961, Topographical relations in the telencephalon of the sunfish, *Eupomotis gibbosus, J. Comp. Neurol.* **116:**249.

Ebbesson, S. O. E., and Schroeder, D. M., 1971, Connections of the nurse shark's telencephalon, *Science* **173:**524.

Fiedler, K., 1964, Versuche zur Neuroethologie von Lippfischen und Sonnenbarschen, *Verh. Dtsch. Zool. Ges. Kiel* **28:**569.

Fiedler, K., 1966, Degenerationen und Verhaltenseffekte nach Elektrokoagulationen im Gehirn von Fischen (Diplodus, Crenilabrus-Perciformes), *Verh. Dtsch. Zool. Ges. Göttingen* **30:**351.

Fiedler, K., 1967*a*, Ethologische und neuroanatomische Auswirkungen von Vorderhirnexstirpationen bei Meerbrassen (*Diplodus*) und Lippfischen (*Crenilabrus,* Perciformes, Teleostei), *J. Hirnforsch.* **9:**481.

Fiedler, K., 1967*b*, Verhaltenswirksame Strukturen im Fischgehirn, *Verh. Dtsch. Zool. Ges. Heidelberg* **31:**602.

Fiedler, K., 1969, Neuronale Steuerung des Verhaltens bei Fischen, *Umsch. Wiss. Tech.* **69:**807.

Fiedler, K., 1970, Hormonale Steuerung des Verhaltens von Fischen, *Umsch. Wiss. Tech.* **70:**508.

Fiedler, K., and Blüm, V., 1972, Prolactin-sensitive neurons in the forebrain of some fishes, *Experientia* **28:**1384.

Greenwood, P. H., Rosen, D. E., Weitzman, S. H., and Myers, G. S., 1966, Phyletic studies of telostean fishes, with a provisional classification of living forms, *Bull. Am. Mus. Nat. Hist.* **131:**339.

Grimm, R. J., 1960, Feeding behavior and electrical stimulation of the brain in *Carassius auratus, Science* **131:**161.

Groves, P. M., and Thompson, R. F., 1970, Habituation: A dual-process theory, *Psychol. Rev.* **77:**419.

Hale, E. B., 1956, Effects of forebrain lesions on the aggressive behavior of green sunfish, *Lepomis cyanellus, Physiol. Zool.* **29:**107.

Hallowitz, R. A., Woodward, D. J., and Demski, L. S., 1971, Forebrain activation of single units in preoptic area of sunfish, *Comp. Biochem. Physiol.* **40A:**733.

Halpern, M., 1972, Some connections of the telencephalon of the frog, *Rana pipiens, Brain Behav. Evol.* **6:**42.

Holmgren, N., 1920, Zur Anatomie und Histologie des Vorder- und Zwischenhirns der Knochenfische, *Acta Zool.* **1:**137.

Janzen, W., 1932/1933, Untersuchungen über Grosshirnfunktionen des Goldfisches (*Carassius auratus*), *Zool. Jahrb. Abt. Allg. Zool. Physiol. Tiere* **52:**591.

Johnston, J. B., 1911, The telencephalon of ganoids and teleosts, *J. Comp. Neurol.* **21:**489.

Jordan, D. S., 1963, *The Genera of Fishes and a Classification of Fishes,* Stanford University Press, Stanford, Calif.

Kamrin, R. P., and Aronson, L. R., 1954, The effects of forebrain lesions on mating behavior in the male platyfish, *Xiphophorus maculatus, Zoologica* **39:**133.

Kicliter, E., and Northcutt, R. G., 1975, Ascending afferents to the telencephalon of ranid frogs: An anterograde degeneration study, *J. Comp. Neurol.* **161:**239.

Kirsche, W., 1965, Regenerative Vorgänge im Gehirn und Rückenmark, *Ergeb. Anat. Entwicklungsgesch.* **38:**143.

Kirsche, W., and Kirsche, K., 1961, Experimentelle Untersuchungen zur Frage der Regeneration und Funktion des Tectum opticum von *Carassius carassius* L., *Z. Mikrosk-Anat. Forsch.* **67:**140.

Macey, M. J., Pickford, G. E., and Peter, R. E., 1974, Forebrain localization of the spawning reflex response to exogenous neurohypophyseal hormones in the Killifish, *Fundulus heteroclitus, J. Exp. Zool.* **190:**269.

Maroń, K., 1963, Endbrain regeneration in *Lebistes reticulatus, Folia Biol.* **11:**3.

Meader, R. E., 1939, The forebrain of bony fishes, *Proc. K. Ned. Akad. Wet. Ser. C* **42:**657.

Nieuwenhuys, R., 1959, The structure of the telencephalon of the teleost *Gasterosteus aculatus, Proc. K. Ned. Akad. Wet. Ser. C* **62:**341.

Nieuwenhuys, R., 1960, *Het Telencephalon der Actinopterygii,* Acad. Proefschrift, Amsterdam.

Nieuwenhuys, R., 1963, The comparative anatomy of the actinopterygian forebrain, *J. Hirnforsch.* **6:**171.

Noble, G. K., 1936, The function of the corpus striatum in the social behavior of fishes, *Anat. Rec.* **64:**34.

Noble, G. K. 1937, Effect of lesions of the corpus striatum on the brooding behavior of cichlid fishes, *Anat. Rec.* **70:**58.

Noble, G. K., and Borne, R., 1941, The effect of forebrain lesions on the sexual and fighting behavior of *Betta splendens* and other fishes, *Anat. Rec.* **79:**49.

Olds, J., and Milner, P., 1954, Positive reinforcement produced by electrical stimulation of septal area and other regions of the rat brain, *J. Comp. Psychol.* **47:**419.

Overmier, J. B., and Gross, D., 1974, Effects of telencephalic ablation upon nest building and avoidance behaviors in East African mouthbreeding fish, *Tilapia mossambica, Behav. Biol.* **12:**211.

Peter, R. E., 1970, Hypothalamic control of thyroid gland activity and gonadal activity in the goldfish, *Gen. Comp. Endocrinol.* **14:**334.

Peter, R. E., 1973, Neuroendocrinology of teleosts, *Am. Zool.* **13:**743.

Peter, R. E., and Gill, V. E., 1975, A stereotaxic atlas and technique for forebrain nuclei of the goldfish, *Carassius auratus, J. Comp. Neurol.* **159:**69.

Peter, R. E., Macey, M. J., and Gill, V. E., 1975, A stereotaxic atlas and technique for forebrain nuclei of the killifish, *Fundulus heteroclitus, J. Comp. Neurol.* **159:**103.

Pflugfelder, O., 1954, Wirkungen partieller Zerstörungen der Parietalregion von *Lebistes reticulatus, Roux' Arch. Entwicklungsmech.* **147:**42.

Pflugfelder, O., 1965, Reparative und regenerative Prozesse nach partieller Zerstörung von Fischgehirnen, *Zool. Jahrb. Physiol.* **71:**301.

Rolls, E. T., 1975, *The Brain and Reward,* Pergamon Press, Oxford.

Savage, G. E., 1971, Behavioural effects of electrical stimulation of the telencephalon of the goldfish, *Carassius auratus, Anim. Behav.* **19:**661.

Schnitzlein, H. N., 1968, Introductory remarks on the telencephalon of fish, in: *The Central Nervous System and Fish Behavior* (D. Ingle, ed.), pp. 97–100, University of Chicago Press, Chicago.

Schönherr, J., 1955, Über die Abhängigkeit der Instinkthandlungen von Vorderhirn und Zwischenhirn (Epiphyse) bei *Gasterosteus aculeatus* L., *Zool. Jahrb. Abt. Allg. Zool. Physiol. Tiere* **65:**357.

Schroeder, D. M., and Ebbesson, S. O. E., 1974, Nonolfactory telencephalic afferents in the nurse shark (*Ginglymostoma cirratum*), *Brain Behav. Evol.* **9:**121.

Segaar, J., 1956, Brain and instinct with *Gasterosteus aculeatus, Proc. K. Ned. Akad. Wet. Proc. C* **59:**738.

Segaar, J., 1961, Telencephalon and behaviour in *Gasterosteus aculeatus, Behaviour* **18:**256.

Segaar, J., 1962, Die Funktion des Vorderhirns in Bezug auf das angeborene Verhalten des dreidornigen Stichlingsmännchen (*Gasterosteus aculeatus* L.)—Zugleich ein Beitrag über Neuronenregeneration im Fischgehirn, *Acta Morphol. Neerl. Scand.* **5:**49.

Segaar, J., 1965, Behavioural aspects of degeneration and regeneration in fish brain: A comparison with higher vertebrates, *Prog. Brain Res.* **14:**143.

Segaar, J., and Nieuwenhuys, R., 1963, New etho-physiological experiments with male *Gasterosteus aculeatus,* with anatomical comment, *Anim. Behav.* **11:**331.

Shapiro, S., Schuckman, H., Sussman, D., and Tucker, A. M., 1974, Effects of telencephalic lesions on the gill cover response of Siamese fighting fish, *Physiol. Behav.* **13:**749.

Ten Cate, J., 1935, Physiologie des Zentralnervensystems der Fische, *Ergeb. Biol.* **11:**335.

Thompson, T., 1971, Introducing subcortical lesions by electrolytic methods, in: *Methods in Psychobiology,* Vol. I (R. D. Myers, ed.), pp. 131–155, Academic Press, London.

Valenstein, E. S., Cox, V. C., and Kakolewski, J. W., 1970, Reexamination of the role of the hypothalamus in motivation, *Psychol. Rev.* **77:**16.

Vanegas, H., and Ebbesson, S. O. E., 1976, Telencephalic projections in two teleost species, *J. Comp. Neurol.* **165:**181.

Vanegas, H., and Quezada, A., 1974, A rigid setup for microelectrode research in fish, *Physiol. Behav.* **12:**137.

Von Holst, E., and Von Saint Paul, U., 1960, Vom Wirkungsgefüge der Triebe, *Naturwissenschaften* **47:**409.

Wrede, W. L., 1932, Versuche über den Artduft der Elritzen, *Z. Vergl. Physiol.* **17:**510.

8

Organization of the Amphibian Telencephalon

R. GLENN NORTHCUTT and EARL KICLITER

I. Introduction

A. The Amphibia

Living amphibians comprise three different groups or orders: Anura (frogs and toads, approximately 2600 species), Urodela (salamanders, approximately 300 species), and Apoda (caecilians, approximately 150 species). Each group is clearly separated from the others by extensive structural variation, and each is characterized by a distinct life style. These three orders are easily distinguished from their earliest appearance in the fossil record, but they also share a number of unique characters which suggest common ancestry. These characters include teeth with a weak, uncalcified segment between the base and crown (pedicellate teeth) and similarities in the middle ear bones and vertebral–skull articulation. Parsons and Williams (1963) concluded from these characters that modern amphibians represent a monophyletic group, the Lissamphibia. Most workers employ this tenable model of amphibian affinities; however, additional data are needed to accept this hypothesis (Thomson, 1968; Estes and Reig, 1973), particularly for the apodans.

A notable exception to the monophyletic hypothesis of Parsons and Williams is proposed by Jarvik (1960). Jarvik's interpretation of living Amphibia is based on comparisons of snouts and limbs of living and fossil amphibians and two groups of

R. GLENN NORTHCUTT • Division of Biological Sciences, University of Michigan, Ann Arbor, Michigan 48109. EARL KICLITER • Department of Anatomy and Laboratory of Neurobiology, Division of Biological Sciences, University of Puerto Rico School of Medicine, San Juan, Puerto Rico 00901.

fossil rhipidistians. These crossopterygian fishes are generally believed to have given rise to amphibians. Jarvik argues that urodeles arose from one group of rhipidistians (the porolepiforms) whereas anurans arose from a different group (the osteolepiforms). Jarvik did not consider apodans in his analysis, but his hypothesis would indicate at least a diphyletic origin for modern amphibians, which would, therefore, not constitute a natural taxonomic group. Jarvik's hypothesis is not widely supported, but it has generated a great deal of interest (e.g., see Ørvig, 1968).

Living amphibians constitute a remnant of a once dominant vertebrate group that gave rise to the first really successful terrestrial vertebrates, the reptiles. Modern amphibians clearly differ in many ways from the ancestral labyrinthodont amphibians that gave rise to reptiles, and living amphibians should not be considered ancestral to reptiles (Romer, 1966; Hecht, 1969). However, modern amphibians likely evolved from labyrinthodonts (Estes and Reig, 1973) and retain a number of ancestral characters as they exhibit a simpler level of organization than other tetrapods. Examination of the nervous systems of living amphibians not only will result in a better understanding of the organization and function of the amphibian nervous system, but also will allow us to identify traits held in common with other anamniotes, thus affording us a more complete picture of vertebrate brain evolution.

B. The Amphibian Telencephalon—Primitive or Degenerate?

C. J. Herrick (1948), in the preface of his now classic treatment of the brain of the tiger salamander, argued that the brain of salamanders was primitive and relatively unspecialized, and that it represented the level of brain organization from which subsequent vertebrate brains evolved. Herrick's assumption that the brains of salamanders are among the simplest of those of living vertebrates has been justified by repeated observations. However, we have also become aware that the various salamander families commonly exhibit paedomorphic traits such as retention of external gills, loss or reduction of limbs, and loss or reduction of the dermal skeleton (DeBeer, 1958; Hecht, 1969; Wake, 1966).

Modern amphibians differ in many ways from Paleozoic amphibians, particularly regarding loss or reduction of much of the dermal skeleton and, in many cases, retention of larval traits. This realization has led us to assume that modern amphibians are degenerate labyrinthodonts and, therefore, that all their traits must be secondarily simplified. This facile assumption ignores the concept of mosaic evolution. All morphological traits of an organism are not under the same selective pressures at the same intensities; thus different traits evolve at different rates. Reduction in the dermal skeleton and changes in head shape are clear adaptations to feeding and buccal breathing in many modern amphibians (Gans, 1970) and appear to be reflected by only minor changes in the central nervous system. Thus each trait or, more likely, collections of traits must be analyzed to determine whether they are primitive or specialized. One cannot assume because some traits are primitive or specialized that *all* traits in a given taxon have an identical history.

How then do we determine if modern amphibian brains, specifically their telencephalons, are primitive or degenerate without benefit of a fossil record? No single criterion permits determination of primitive and specialized states. However, a number of criteria are applicable. Individual character states frequently form series whose trends from primitive to specialized can be recognized—for example, vertebrate limb evolution and ear ossicle evolution are classic cases. Frequently the most common character state in a group of taxa being examined is assumed to have evolved very early in the group and thus to be primitive for the group. However, this assumption can lead to erroneous conclusions unless the character state also occurs outside the category being analyzed. For example, all placental mammals possess a corpus callosum; therefore, this would be the presumed primitive state for mammals. However, marsupials and monotremes do not possess a callosum. So it is highly unlikely that the presence of a corpus callosum represents the primitive mammalian condition; it is far more likely that a callosum evolved early in the placental radiation and rapidly became the common (successful) trait.

In this chapter we will present evidence suggesting that (1) telencephalic trends can be recognized among tetrapods and two other anamniote radiations; (2) the pattern of telencephalic organization exhibited by amphibians is not unique to them but may also characterize primitive ray-finned fishes and elasmobranchs; (3) the distribution of this pattern among several widely different classes of anamniote vertebrates argues that the amphibian telencephalon does exhibit a pattern of organization that may have characterized the telencephalon of primitive amphibians.

II. Species Studied

The species used in this study are listed in Table I. No significant differences were evident among the ranids or among the bufonids. The anurans sampled represent relatively primitive taxa (*Ascaphus* and *Xenopus*) and advanced taxa from three different families (*Bufo, Hyla,* and *Rana*). Quantitative differences clearly

Table I. Species Studied

Class Amphibia
Subclass Lissamphibia
Order Anura
Ascaphus truei
Bufo americanus
Bufo marinus
Hyla crucifer
Rana catesbeiana
Rana pipiens
Rana temporaria
Xenopus laevis
Order Urodela
Ambystoma tigrinum
Amphiuma means
Cryptobranchus alleganiensis
Necturus maculosus
Order Apoda
Ichthyophis glutinosus
Nectocaecilia haydee

exist among these families, but the telencephalon exhibits remarkable uniformity in regional differentiation. For example, the medial pallium of all anurans exhibits a thickened medial pallium with migrated cells, in contrast to remaining parts of the pallium, and this condition is diagnostic of the order, regardless of family.

The salamanders studied include taxa from four different families and represent both terrestrial and permanently aquatic salamanders.

Similarly, the apodans examined include two different families representing both aquatic and terrestrial forms. *Ichthyophis* is a terrestrial burrowing form whose reproduction is oviparous. The eggs are deposited on land; larvae undergo a free-swimming aquatic stage. *Nectocaecilia* is a permanently aquatic form inhabiting streams and ponds.

While the present sample of amphibians is extremely small, it suggests that significant quantitative differences do exist among orders and among families. A thorough systematic examination of amphibian nervous systems would no doubt yield significant insights into their evolutionary adaptations and would elucidate their troubled taxonomy.

III. Normal Morphology

The telencephalon of amphibians consists of paired, evaginated cerebral hemispheres and olfactory bulbs (Fig. 1) and an unevaginated portion called the telencephalon medium. The telencephalon medium (present but unlabeled in Figs. 6, 9B, 10A, and 12A–C) is formed rostrally by the lamina terminalis, through which pass the anterior and pallial commissures and the periventricular preoptic nucleus and recess. More laterally, the telencephalon medium contains the forebrain bundles, anterior entopeduncular nucleus, and caudal portions of the amygdala complex.

The cerebral hemispheres join the telencephalon medium at the level of the interventricular foramen (Figs. 9 and 12A). The cerebral ventricles contain a choroid plexus formed by a rostral extension of the plexus of the roof of the telencephalon medium. The hemispheres are essentially tubular and are capped rostrally by the olfactory bulbs, which form as secondary evaginations of the hemispheres. Thus the bulbs are hollow and contain rostral extensions of the lateral ventricles [Figs. 2, 8A (slitlike in this case), and 11A].

The telencephalon of amphibians has been the subject of numerous anatomical investigations (Anura: Herrick, 1910, 1925, 1933; Ramón y Cajal, 1922; Söderburg, 1922; Röthig, 1926; Ariëns Kappers *et al.,* 1936; Hoffman, 1963, 1966; Howell and Hoffman, 1966; Clairambault, 1967, 1968, 1969, 1976; Clairambault and Derer, 1968; Baroz *et al.,* 1969; Clairambault and Capanna, 1970; Lascano *et al.,* 1971; Hoffmann, 1973; Northcutt, 1974; Northcutt and Royce, 1975; Parent, 1975; Kicliter and Ebbesson, 1976; Scalia, 1976*a,b*; Urodela: Fish, 1895; Herrick, 1925, 1933, 1948; Kreht, 1931; Thireau *et al.,* 1973; Thireau, 1976; Kokoros and Northcutt, 1977; Apoda: Kuhlenbeck, 1922, 1953; Olivecrona, 1964; Kuhlenbeck *et al.,* 1967). These contributions will not be individually reviewed; rather, we will describe the telencephalic cellular groups in a representative of each amphibian order and comment on significant differences characterizing the telencephalon of frogs, salamanders, and apodans. The nomenclature employed is that of Northcutt (1974) and Kicliter and Ebbesson (1976) with minor modification.

The telencephalon of amphibians exhibits less variation than that of any other vertebrate class; the same cellular groups can be recognized in all amphibian orders, with few exceptions. We will first describe the anuran condition utilizing the bullfrog, *Rana catesbeiana,* then comment on the condition in salamanders—illustrating the tiger salamander, *Ambystoma tigrinum*—and the apodan *Ichthyophis glutinosus.*

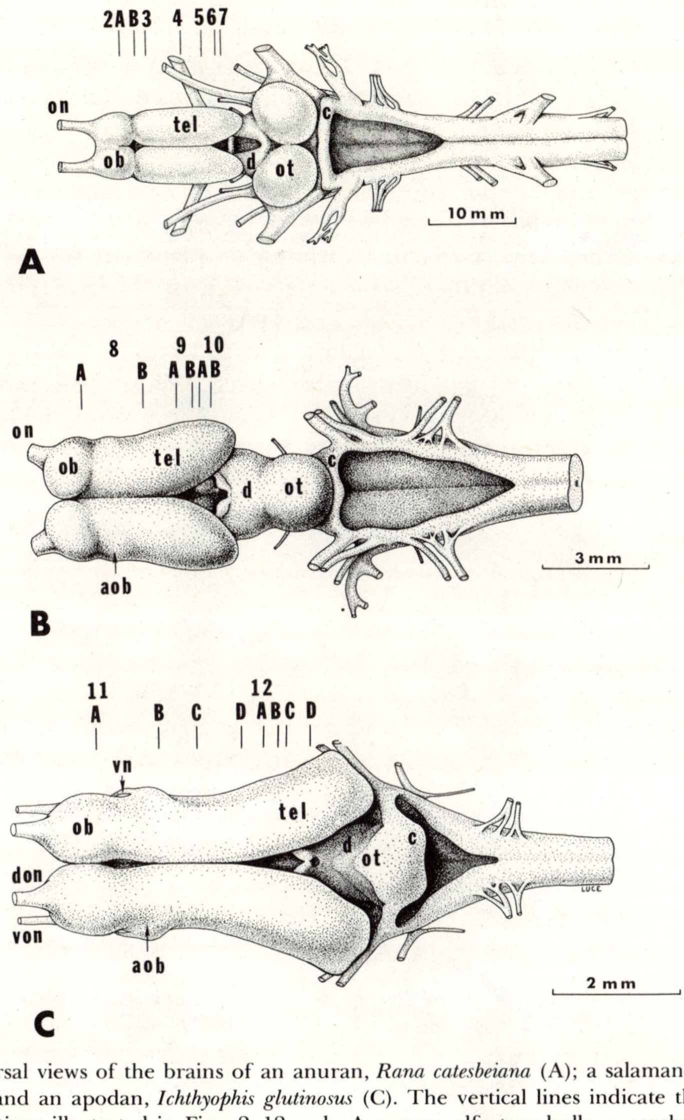

Figure 1. Dorsal views of the brains of an anuran, *Rana catesbeiana* (A); a salamander, *Ambystoma tigrinum* (B); and an apodan, *Ichthyophis glutinosus* (C). The vertical lines indicate the level of the transverse sections illustrated in Figs. 2–12. aob, Accessory olfactory bulb; c, cerebellum; d, diencephalon; don, dorsal ramus of the olfactory nerve; ob, olfactory bulb; on, olfactory nerve; ot, optic tectum; tel, telencephalic hemisphere; von, ventral ramus of the olfactory nerve; vn, vomeronasal nerve.

A. Olfactory Bulbs

The olfactory bulbs evaginate from the rostral telencephalic wall and secondarily form main and accessory bulbs. The accessory bulb is a specialized thickening of the caudal ventrolateral wall of the main bulb and thus does not possess a ventricle (Figs. 1, 3, and 11B). In *Rana* the anterior, ventral, and anterolateral surfaces of the olfactory bulb are covered by the implantation cone of the olfactory nerve. The implantation cone is that area of the bulb where axons of the olfactory nerve diverge and terminate on the surface of the bulb forming terminal glomeruli (gl in Figs. 2, 8A, and 11A). In some salamanders (e.g., *Cryptobranchus*) and apodans the olfactory nerve consists of distinct dorsal and ventral divisions (Fig. 1C), which enter the cranial cavity as separate rami. The dorsal ramus distributes to the rostral pole and dorsal surface of the bulb and the ventral ramus to the ventral and lateral surfaces. When the olfactory nerve is composed of separate rami, the vomeronasal nerve is closely associated with the ventral ramus.

The olfactory bulbs of all amphibians consist of concentric laminae in the following centripetal order: (1) olfactory nerve fibers and glomerular layer, (2) external cellular layer composed of small granule and larger mitral cells, (3) extragranular plexiform layer composed of secondary olfactory fibers, (4) internal granule layer, and (5) ependyma (Figs. 2, 8A, and 11A).

The glomeruli are spherical aggregates formed by the olfactory nerve axon terminals and dendrites of the deeper mitral cells. Mitral cells possess several dendrites, and a single mitral neuron sends dendrites to several glomeruli. Axons of the mitral cells enter the extragranular plexiform layer and constitute the secondary olfactory pathways leaving the olfactory bulb.

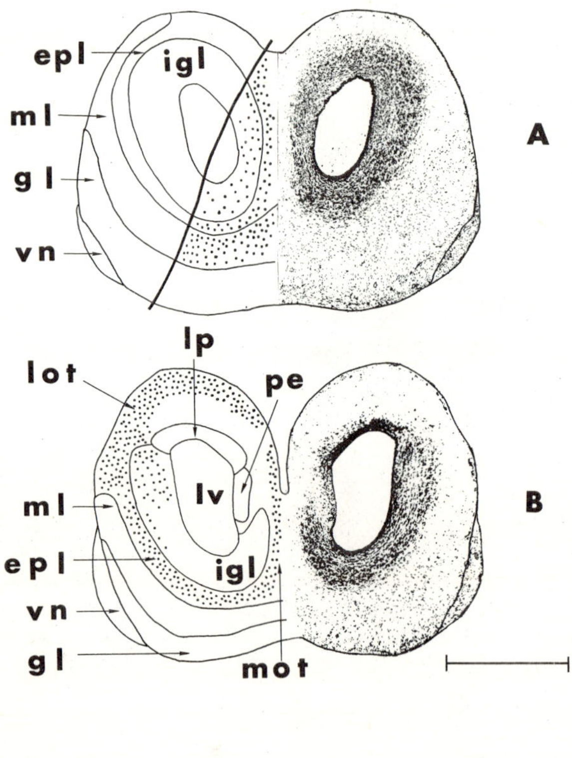

Figure 2. Transverse sections through middle (A) and caudal (B) levels of the main olfactory bulb in the bullfrog. A Nissl preparation is shown on the right, and the contralateral side is drawn on the left. The heavy line running obliquely in the left half of A marks the medial extent of a main olfactory bulb lesion. Degenerated fibers and preterminal degeneration are represented by stippling in Figs. 2–7. epl, Extragranular plexiform layer; gl, glomerular layer; igl, internal granule layer; lot, lateral olfactory tract; lp, lateral pallium; ml, mitral or external cellular layer; mot, medial olfactory tract; pe, postolfactory eminence; vn, vomeronasal nerve. Bar scale equals 1 mm. Figure after Northcutt and Royce (1975).

The internal granule layer lies deep to the mitral cell layer and forms the most conspicuous cellular layer of the olfactory bulb. The granule cells possess no axons, but their dendritelike processes radiate toward the glomerular layer, where they arborize in the extragranular plexiform layer or among the mitral cells. Some of their processes reach the glomerular layer, but they have not been observed to end within the glomeruli (Nieuwenhuys, 1967).

The internal granule layer continues farther caudally than the other bulbar laminae and is replaced first dorsally by the telencephalic pallial areas, then ventrally by the subpallial areas (Figs. 2–4 and 11B). The transition from internal granule layer to hemispheric areas is sudden and morphologically distinct, as there are a decrease in the cellular packing density and a marked increase in the diameter of the hemispheric pallial neurons. Many studies (Kuhlenbeck, 1922; Herrick, 1948; Hoffman, 1963) report a zone of relatively "undifferentiated" cells—the anterior olfactory nucleus—interposed between the bulbar formations and the hemispheric areas. This nucleus supposedly constitutes a secondary olfactory target, which, in turn, projects to most telencephalic areas distributing tertiary olfactory projections. The area usually labeled anterior olfactory nucleus in amphibians is, in fact, the caudal internal granule layer of the olfactory bulb, and experimental studies have failed to reveal such tertiary projections (Scalia *et al.*, 1968; Northcutt and Royce, 1975). Thus there appears no justification for recognizing such a nucleus or zone in amphibians.

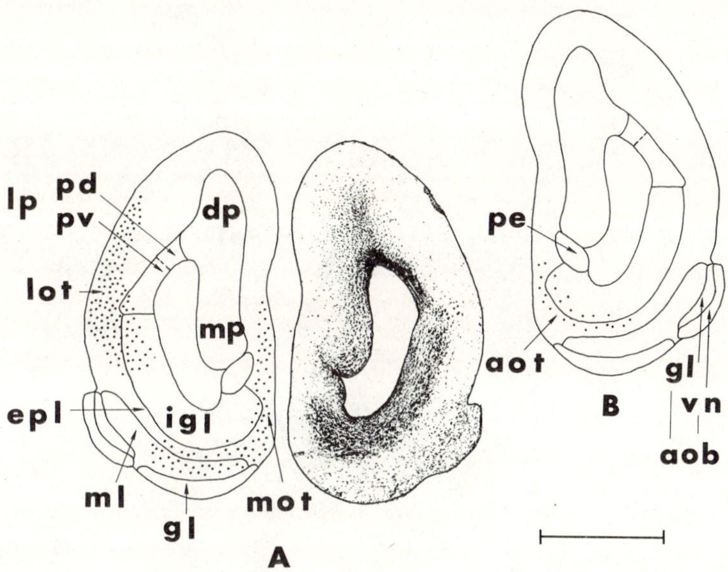

Figure 3. Transverse sections through the rostral pole of the telencephalon in the bullfrog at the level of the accessory olfactory bulb (A). Nissl-stained section on right. Left hemisphere shows degeneration after main olfactory bulb lesion. B: Line drawing of the contralateral hemisphere at the same telencephalic level as the Nissl preparation illustrating the position of the crossed secondary olfactory pathways. aob, Accessory olfactory bulb; aot, anterior olfacto-habenular tract; dp, dorsal pallium; epl, extragranular plexiform layer; gl, glomerular layer; igl, internal granule layer; lot, lateral olfactory tract; lp, lateral pallium; ml, mitral layer; mot, medial olfactory tract; mp, medial pallium; pd, pars dorsalis of lateral pallium; pe, postolfactory eminence; pv, pars ventralis of lateral pallium; vn, vomeronasal nerve. Bar scale equals 1 mm. Figure after Northcutt and Royce (1975).

The accessory olfactory bulb occupies the ventrolateral caudal wall of the main olfactory bulb and is characterized by the same neural laminae as the main bulb (Figs. 3 and 11B). The accessory olfactory bulb is actually a specialized region of the main olfactory bulb and is the sole recipient of vomeronasal nerve terminals. The vomeronasal nerve arises from a specialized ventromedial portion (vomeronasal organ) of the olfactory organ (see Section IV.A) as a specialization of the olfactory system associated with the origin of land vertebrates.

B. Pallium

Four pallial or roof telencephalic regions can be recognized in amphibians: dorsal, lateral, and medial pallial sheets, and a pars lateralis of the amygdala. The pallium replaces the internal granule layer of the olfactory bulb rostrally, and the pallial boundary is marked by a sharp increase in neuronal size.

1. Medial Pallium

The medial pallium (archipallium of Ariëns Kappers *et al.,* 1936; primordium hippocampi of Herrick, 1933) occupies the dorsomedial hemispheric wall (Figs. 3–

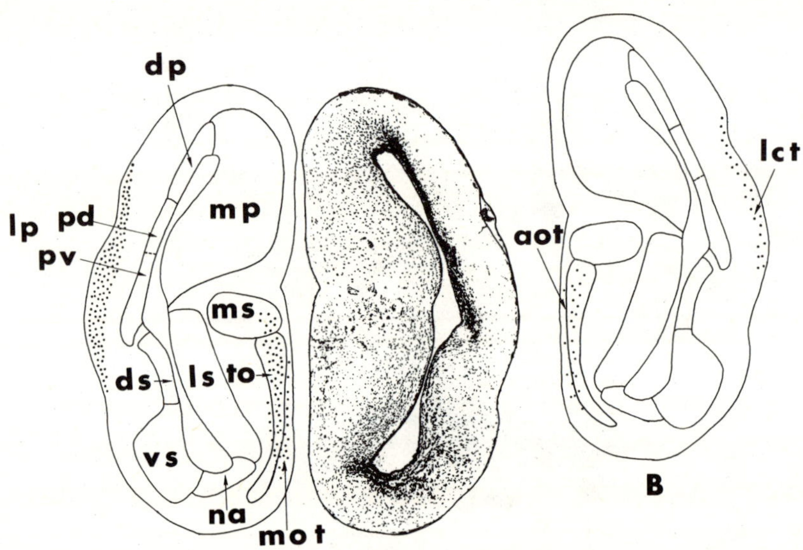

Figure 4. Transverse sections through a midtelencephalic level in the bullfrog. A: Position of the ipsilateral secondary olfactory pathways. B: Position of the crossed secondary pathways at the same telencephalic level. This level marks the most caudal extent of the ipsilateral medial olfactory tract. aot, Anterior olfacto-habenular tract; dp, dorsal pallium; ds, dorsal striatum; lct, lateral cortico-habenular tract; lp, lateral pallium; ls, lateral septum; mot, medial olfactory tract; mp, medial pallium; ms, medial septum; na, nucleus accumbens; pd, pars dorsalis of lateral pallium; pv, pars ventralis of lateral pallium; to, olfactory tubercle; vs, ventral striatum. Bar scale equals 1 mm. Figure after Northcutt and Royce (1975).

12), a position comparable to that of mammalian hippocampus—thus the original basis for its proposed homology. In anurans the medial pallium is separated from the ventrally located septum by a cell-poor zone, the zona limitans medialis. The dorsal boundary of the medial pallium is less distinct, as its cells gradually condense and grade into the dorsal pallial formation (Figs. 3–12).

The medial pallium of anurans differs distinctly from the remaining pallial areas by its hypertrophy (its wall is at least twice as thick as the remaining pallium) and pronounced cell migrations (e.g., Fig. 4). Hoffman (1963) divided the medial pallium into dorsal and dorsomedial divisions. These divisions are difficult to identify in Nissl-stained sections, but they are easily distinguished in Golgi preparations (Kicliter and Ebbesson, 1976).

Two principal cell types characterize the dorsal division of the medial pallium in *Rana* (Hoffman, 1963; Kicliter and Ebbesson, 1976): flask-shaped cells with three to five dendrites projecting toward the meningeal surface and stellate cells whose dendrites ramify in all directions.

The dorsomedial division is highly developed at midhemispheric levels and disappears just caudal to the pallial commissure. The principal cell type is a pyramidal neuron, somewhat larger than the flask-shaped cells, with dendrites oriented medially and laterally.

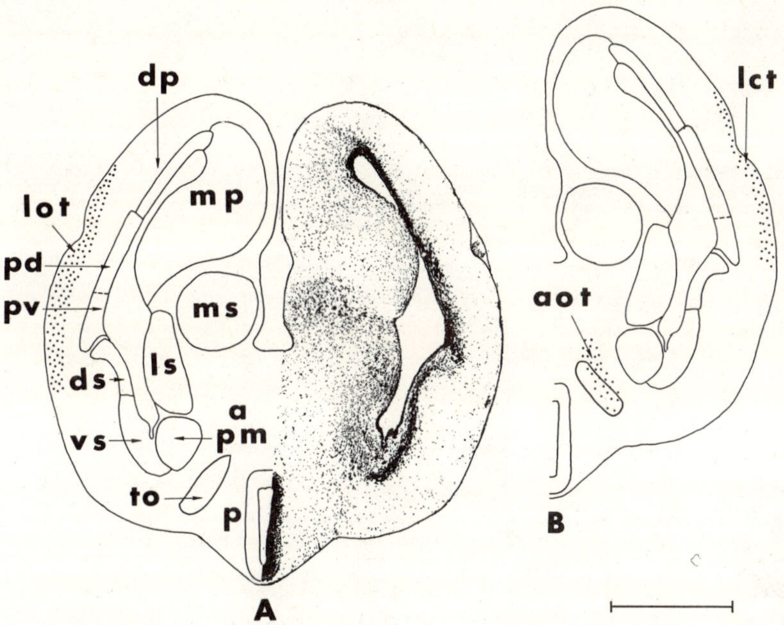

Figure 5. Transverse section at the level of the rostral telencephalon medium in the bullfrog. A: Caudal continuation of the ipsilateral lateral olfactory tract. B: Course of the crossed secondary pathways at the corresponding contralateral hemispheric level. aot, Anterior olfacto-habenular tract; apm, amygdala, pars medialis; dp, dorsal pallium; ds, dorsal striatum; lct, lateral cortico-habenular tract; lot, lateral olfactory tract; ls, lateral septum; mp, medial pallium; ms, medial septum; p, periventricular preoptic nucleus; pd, pars dorsalis of lateral pallium; pv, pars ventralis of lateral pallium; to, olfactory tubercle; vs, ventral striatum. Bar scale equals 1 mm. Figure after Northcutt and Royce (1975).

Four fiber systems are known to be associated with the medial cortex of anurans: (1) dorsal association tract, (2) precommissural fornix, (3) pallial commissure, and (4) anterior thalamic tract. Lesions of the lateral pallium (Kokoros, 1973; Scalia, 1976*a*) give rise to a pathway that projects over the hemispheric roof—as the dorsal association bundle—terminating in the medial pallium. Lesions of the medial pallium give rise to a descending tract—the precommissural fornix—which terminates among the septal nuclei and also passes rostrally to terminate in the postolfactory eminence (Figs. 2 and 3) (Halpern, 1972; Kokoros, 1973). A postcommissural fornix—a projection from the medial pallium to the hypothalamus—has not been reported in *Rana* (Halpern, 1972) but does exist in *Bufo* (Kokoros, 1973). Lesions or injections of horseradish peroxidase in the medial pallium reveal projections to the contralateral medial pallium via the pallial commissure (Fig. 6) (Kokoros, 1973; Scalia, 1976*a*). In addition to receiving olfactory projections rostrally (see Section IV.B), the medial pallium receives an ascending thalamic projection from an anterior portion of the dorsal thalamus (Scalia and Colman, 1975; Kicliter, 1979). This thalamic region receives both visual (Scalia and Gregory, 1970) and hypothalamic (Neary and Wilczynski, 1977*a*) inputs which converge in the medial pallium.

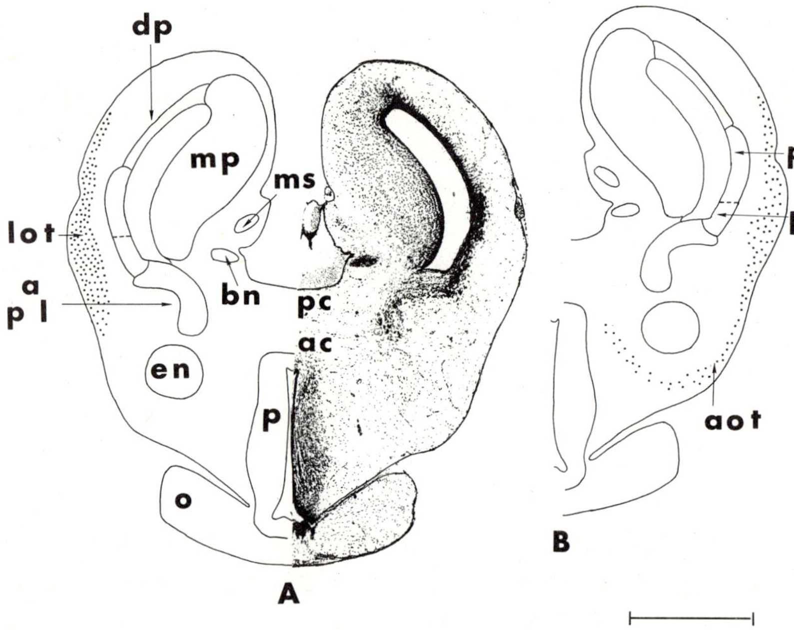

Figure 6. Transverse sections at a telencephalic level immediately caudal to the level of the interventricular foramina in the bullfrog. A: Position of the ipsilateral lateral olfactory tract at a level immediately rostral to the entry of the decussating fibers into the stria medullaris. B: Comparable level in the contralateral hemisphere where the crossed secondary olfactory fibers skirt the forebrain bundles and the preoptic area occupies a medial hemispheric position. ac, Anterior commissure; aot, anterior olfacto-habenular tract; apl, amygdala, pars lateralis; bn, bed nucleus of the pallial commissure; dp, dorsal pallium; en, anterior entopeduncular nucleus; lot, lateral olfactory tract; mp, medial pallium; ms, medial septum; o, optic nerve; p, periventricular preoptic nucleus; pc, pallial commissure; pd, pars dorsalis of lateral pallium; pv, pars ventralis of lateral pallium. Bar scale equals 1 mm. Figure after Northcutt and Royce (1975).

In salamanders and apodans the medial pallial wall is thicker than the remaining pallial wall (Figs. 8–12). Dorsal and dorsomedial divisions of the medial pallium also occur in representatives of these orders as in anurans. Whereas salamanders also possess a medial pallium characterized by migrated cells, apodans possess almost no cell migrations in this pallial division (Figs. 11 and 12). The medial pallial wall, however, is thickened, and rostrally a distinct sulcus (Fig. 11D) is produced by inward folding of the medial wall. While cell migration does not occur in the medial pallium of apodans, the wall has obviously expanded. The medial pallium is clearly the largest single pallial element and extends far caudally to caudal diencephalic levels (Figs. 1C and 12D).

There are no experimental telencephalic studies on apodans, and only preliminary data exist for *Ambystoma* (Kokoros and Northcutt, 1977). However, commissural and pre- and postcommissural fornix pathways in *Ambystoma* are indicated by the overall pattern of pallial efferents reported.

2. Dorsal Pallium

The anuran dorsal pallium begins just dorsal and caudal to the most rostral extent of the medial pallium (Fig. 3). Söderberg (1922) first identified the dorsal pallium in anurans as a small crescent of cells, some 300 μm in cross-sectional diameter, between the lateral and medial pallia. Subsequent workers have generally retained this terminology (Herrick, 1933; Hoffman, 1963). However, this area is

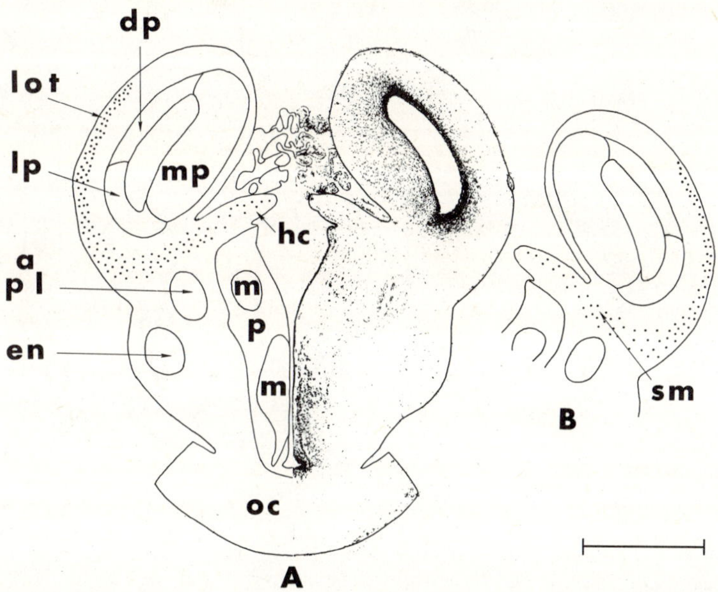

Figure 7. Transverse sections at the level of the caudal hemispheric pole in the bullfrog. A: Entry of the ipsilateral olfactory pathway into the stria medullaris. B: Comparable level in the contralateral hemisphere and the distribution of the crossed secondary olfactory fibers. apl, Amygdala, pars lateralis; dp, dorsal pallium; en, anterior entopeduncular nucleus; hc, habenular commissure; lot, lateral olfactory tract; lp, lateral pallium; m, pars magnocellularis of the periventricular preoptic nucleus; mp, medial pallium; oc, optic chiasm; p, periventricular preoptic nucleus; sm, stria medullaris. Bar scale equals 1 mm. Figure after Northcutt and Royce (1975).

only a transitional region in anurans; if a dorsal pallial formation is recognized, it should include the more lateral field (Northcutt, 1974). This is clearly the case in salamanders, where traditionally the more lateral field is included as dorsal pallium (Herrick, 1948). We have employed this broader concept of dorsal pallium, and the anuran dorsal pallium is defined here as a densely packed periventricular plate of neurons, bordered medially by a scattered transitional zone and laterally by a thinner, more densely packed concave plate of cells representing the lateral pallium (Figs. 3–7). Thus the dorsal pallium, as defined here, includes what has previously been termed the pars dorsalis of the lateral pallium (Hoffman, 1963).

The dorsal pallium of *Rana* likely receives olfactory fibers along its most rostral extent, and may receive input from the lateral pallium via the dorsal association tract en route to the medial pallium. Thalamic projections are known to reach the dorsal pallium and appear to project via the medial forebrain bundle (Kicliter and

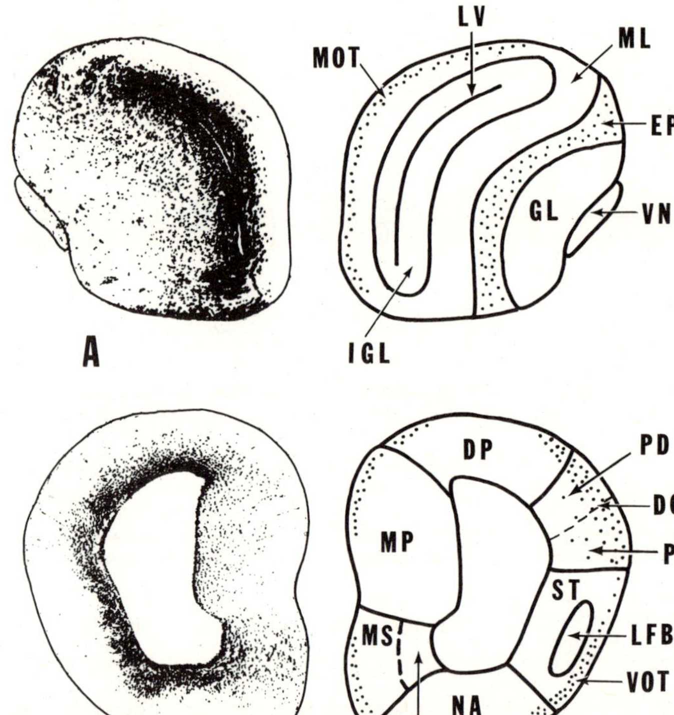

Figure 8. Transverse sections through the caudal olfactory bulb (A) and rostral telencephalic hemisphere (B) of the tiger salamander. Stippling represents the course of the secondary degenerating olfactory fibers following partial ablation of the olfactory bulb. DOT, Dorsolateral olfactory tract; DP, dorsal pallium; EPL, extragranular plexiform layer; GL, glomerular layer; IGL, internal granule layer; LFB, lateral forebrain bundle; LS, lateral septum; LV, lateral ventricle; ML, mitral layer; MOT, medial olfactory tract; MP, medial pallium; MS, medial septum; PD, pars dorsalis of lateral pallium; PV, pars ventralis of lateral pallium; NA, nucleus accumbens; ST, striatum; VN, vomeronasal nerve; VOT, ventrolateral olfactory tract. Bar scale equals 0.5 mm.

Northcutt, 1975). The nature of the information conveyed by this tract is presently unknown, but the dorsal pallium of *Rana* is characterized by short-latency, visually evoked potentials (Northcutt, unpublished observations), and the dorsal pallium may represent a third visual area within the amphibian telencephalon.

Dorsal pallial lesions in *Bufo* (Kokoros, 1973) do not reveal interhemispheric connections, nor does the dorsal pallium appear to possess projections that exit the telencephalon. The dorsal pallium in *Bufo* appears to project to the lateral and medial pallia. However, lesions would also have interrupted the dorsal association tract, crossing in the molecular layer of the dorsal pallium; thus autoradiographic experiments are needed to confirm this projection.

Dorsal pallial fields can be recognized in salamanders and apodans (Figs. 8–12), and there are no notable differences among amphibian orders. There are no experimental studies on connections of the dorsal pallium in salamanders and apodans.

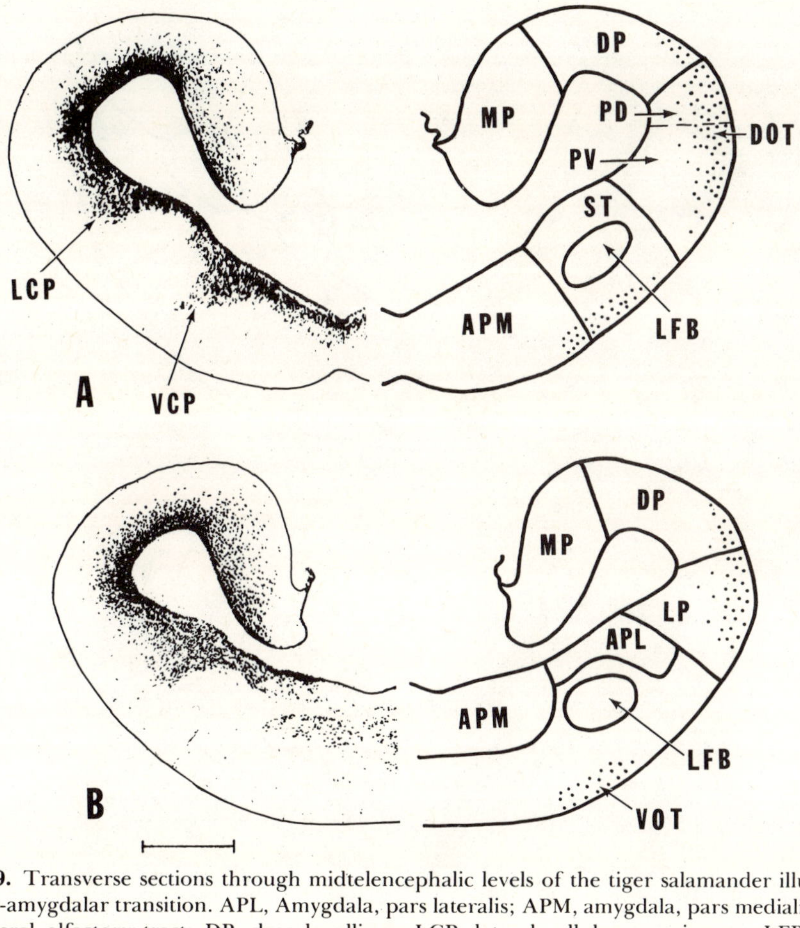

Figure 9. Transverse sections through midtelencephalic levels of the tiger salamander illustrating the strio-amygdalar transition. APL, Amygdala, pars lateralis; APM, amygdala, pars medialis; DOT, dorsolateral olfactory tract; DP, dorsal pallium; LCP, lateral cellular prominence; LFB, lateral forebrain bundle; LP, lateral pallium; MP, medial pallium; PD, pars dorsalis of lateral pallium; PV, pars ventralis of lateral pallium; ST, striatum; VCP, ventral cellular prominence; VOT, ventrolateral olfactory tract. Bar scale equals 0.5 mm.

3. The Lateral Pallium

The anuran lateral pallium (nucleus olfactorius dorsolateralis of Herrick, 1948; paleopallium of Ariëns Kappers *et al.*, 1936; primordial piriform of Hoffman, 1963) is the most rostrally occurring pallial component (Fig. 2B). The portion of the pallium recognized here as the lateral pallium corresponds to the pars ventralis of the lateral pallium of Northcutt (1974). Two divisions of this cell group can be recognized—a pars dorsalis and a pars ventralis (Figs. 3–6). Rostrally the pars dorsalis can be distinguished from the dorsal pallium by the concave, more compact nature of its periventricular cell plate (Fig. 3). The cells of pars ventralis are more scattered, and the cell plate is thicker (Figs. 3–6). The dominant cell type is a neuron with a spherical or flask-shaped cell body and two or three apical dendrites radiating toward the meningeal surface (Kicliter and Ebbesson, 1976).

Both pars dorsalis and pars ventralis receive olfactory projections via the lateral olfactory tract, which occupies the outer half of the molecular layer of the lateral pallium (Figs. 4–7).

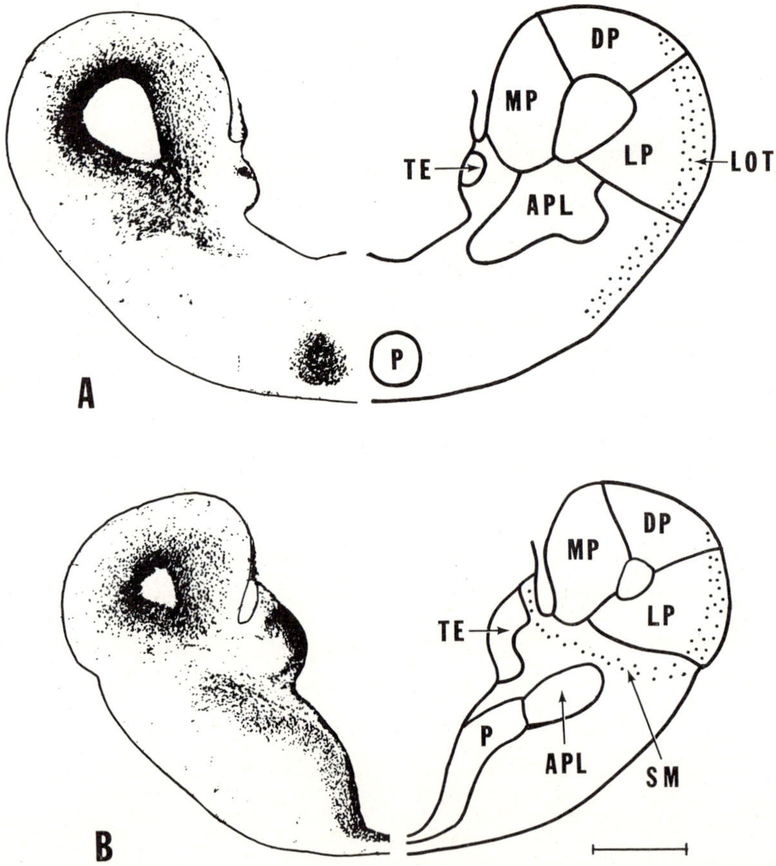

Figure 10. Transverse sections through caudal telencephalic levels in the tiger salamander. APL, Amygdala, pars lateralis; DP, dorsal pallium; LOT, lateral olfactory tract; LP, lateral pallium; MP, medial pallium; P, periventricular preoptic nucleus; SM, stria medullaris; TE, thalamic eminence. Bar scale equals 0.5 mm.

The most ventral portion of the lateral pallium is characterized by a ventrolaterally directed tip, termed the lateral prominence by Herrick (1948) or the superimposed portion of the lateral pallium by Hoffman (1963). This lateral prominence can be followed from the level of the accessory olfactory bulb (Fig. 3) to the posterior hemisphere, where it is incorporated into the pars lateralis of the amygdala (Fig. 6). The efferent pathway of the accessory olfactory bulb (the accessory olfactory tract, Fig. 13) courses along the lateral edge of the length of the lateral prominence. The lateral prominence likely receives input from this tract. Neary and Wilczynski (1977*a*) noted that the lateral prominence also receives a hypothalamic input, as does the pars lateralis of the amygdala, which is closely associated with the lateral prominence. Further study may well reveal that the lateral prominence is a portion of the amygdala rather than a division of the lateral pallium.

The lateral pallium of salamanders and apodans is well developed (Figs. 8–12), and dorsal and ventral divisions can easily be recognized in *Ambystoma* (Figs.

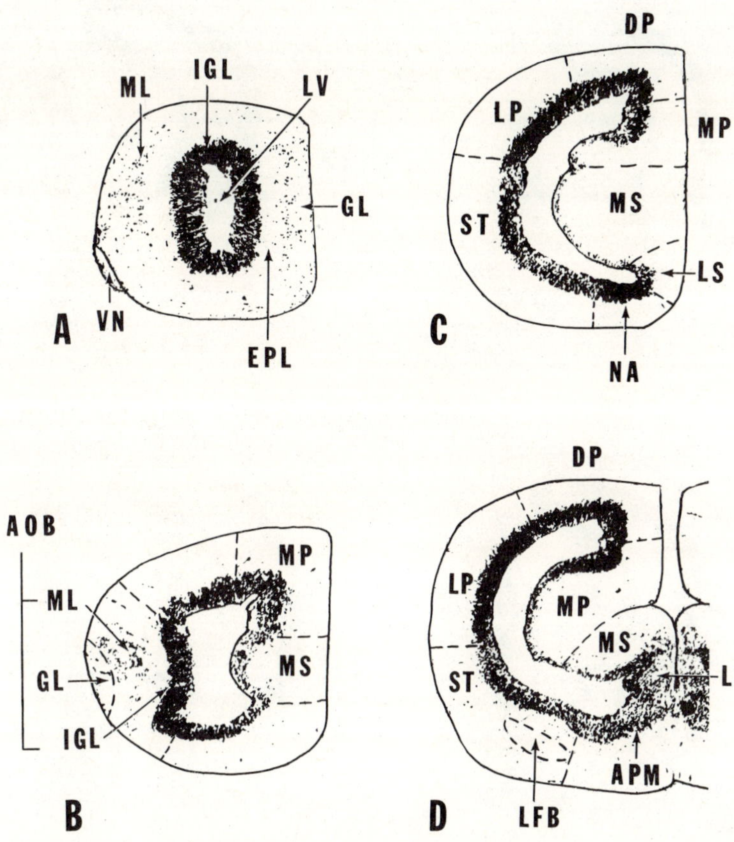

Figure 11. Transverse sections through the rostral telencephalon of an apodan, *Ichthyophis*. AOB, Accessory olfactory bulb; APM, amygdala, pars medialis; DP, dorsal pallium; EPL, extragranular plexiform layer; GL, glomerular layer; IGL, internal granule layer; LFB, lateral forebrain bundle; LP, lateral pallium; LS, lateral septum; LV, lateral ventricle; ML, mitral layer; MP, medial pallium; MS, medial septum; NA, nucleus accumbens; ST, striatum; VN, vomeronasal nerve. Bar scale equals 0.5 mm.

8B and 9). A pronounced lateral prominence exists in *Ambystoma* (Fig. 9A) but is not nearly so well developed in *Ichthyophis* (Fig. 12).

4. Pars Lateralis of the Amygdala

There are two very different views in the neuroanatomical literature regarding the organization and evolution of the vertebrate amygdala. Herrick (1921, 1948) argued that the amygdala is a single cell mass—located in the caudal ventrolateral wall of the cerebral hemispheres—and is a caudal continuation of the striatum, a subpallial cell group. On the other hand, Källén (1951*a*) argued that the amygdala is not a unitary cell mass but rather consists of both pallial and subpallial divisions. In mammals the pallial amygdala (corticomedial division) is a ventromedial contin-

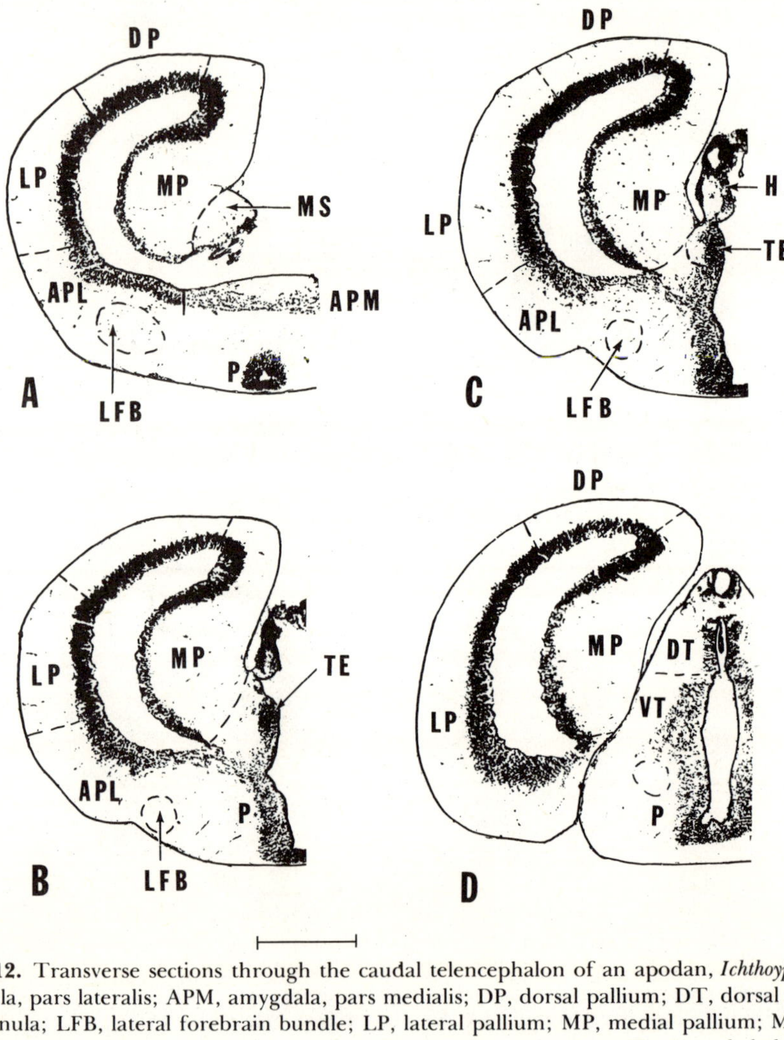

Figure 12. Transverse sections through the caudal telencephalon of an apodan, *Ichthoyphis*. APL, Amygdala, pars lateralis; APM, amygdala, pars medialis; DP, dorsal pallium; DT, dorsal thalamus; H, habenula; LFB, lateral forebrain bundle; LP, lateral pallium; MP, medial pallium; MS, medial septum; P, periventricular preoptic nucleus; TE, thalamic eminence; VT, ventral thalamus. Bar scale equals 0.5 mm.

uation of the pyriform cortex, and a portion of the corticomedial amygdala receives the sole projections of the accessory olfactory bulb (Winans and Scalia, 1970). The corticomedial amygdala of mammals lies in contact, but is not continuous, with the basolateral division of the amygdala. The two divisions are also characterized by different histochemical and connectional properties (Hall, 1972).

A similar pattern characterizes the amygdala of amphibians. Based on histochemical (Northcutt, 1974) and connectional (Scalia, 1972; Northcutt and Royce, 1975; Neary and Wilczynski, 1977*a*) data, two distinct cellular nuclei of pallial and subpallial origin can be identified.

The pars lateralis of the amygdala can first be recognized as an elongation of

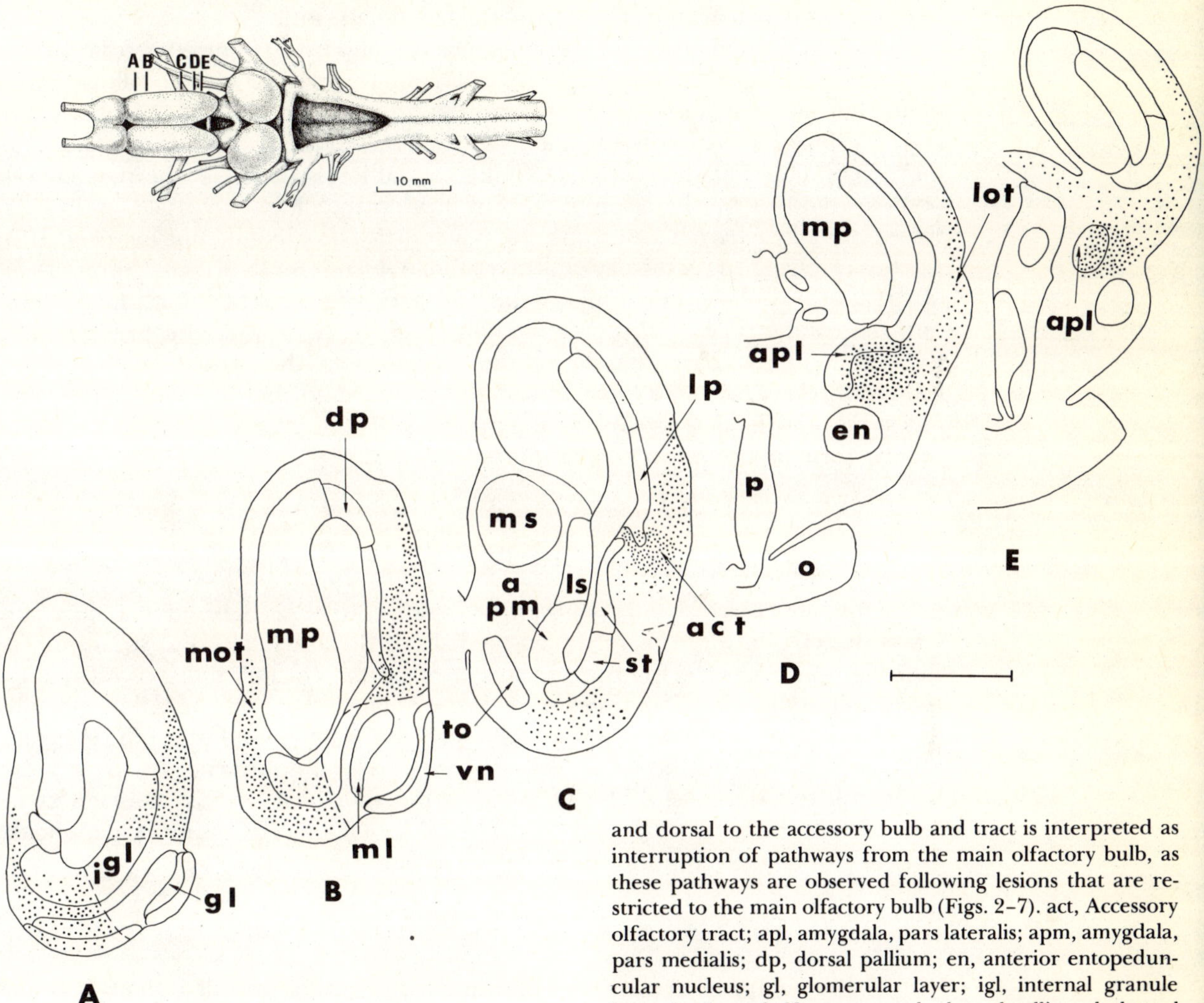

Figure 13. Transverse sections through the left telencephalic hemisphere of a bullfrog illustrating the course and termination of the accessory olfactory tract. The dashed line in A, B, and C marks the boundary of the lesion involving the left accessory bulb. The charted degeneration ventral and dorsal to the accessory bulb and tract is interpreted as interruption of pathways from the main olfactory bulb, as these pathways are observed following lesions that are restricted to the main olfactory bulb (Figs. 2–7). act, Accessory olfactory tract; apl, amygdala, pars lateralis; apm, amygdala, pars medialis; dp, dorsal pallium; en, anterior entopeduncular nucleus; gl, glomerular layer; igl, internal granule layer; lot, lateral olfactory tract; lp, lateral pallium; ls, lateral septum; ml, mitral layer; mot, medial olfactory tract; mp, medial pallium; ms, medial septum; o, optic nerve; p, periventricular preoptic nucleus; st, striatum; to, olfactory tubercle; vn, vomeronasal nerve. Bar scale equals 1 mm. Figure after Northcutt and Royce (1975).

the lateral pallium (lateral cellular prominence) in *Rana* (Fig. 4). Caudal to the level of the interventricular foramen (Fig. 6), the pars lateralis expands to form a C-shaped nucleus, displacing ventrolaterally the dwindling striatum whose caudal continuation is recognized as the anterior entopeduncular-nucleus (Fig. 6). More caudally the pars lateralis becomes oval in shape (Fig. 7) and even further caudally fuses with the periventricular grey of the preoptic area.

Dendrites of pars lateralis cells are directed ventrolaterally into a neuropil which is the terminal target of the accessory olfactory tract. Neary and Wilczynski (1977*a*) reported that pars lateralis in *Rana* also receives projections from the hypothalamus. Halpern (1972) reported that the pars lateralis in *Rana* projects to the dorsal and ventral thalamus, and Scalia (1976*a*) reported projections to the hypothalamus (see Section IV.B.3 for further discussion).

A distinct pars lateralis of the amygdala can also be recognized in salamanders and apodans (Figs. 9, 10, and 12). In salamanders a distinct lateral cellular prominence can be seen dorsal to the striatum at an interventricular hemispheric level (Fig. 9). This plate rapidly expands ventromedially, as in anurans, replacing the more ventrally located striatum. At more caudal levels (Fig. 10), the pars lateralis occupies most of the hemispheric wall ventral to the lateral ventricle, and can be traced caudally where it fuses with the periventricular preoptic nucleus (Fig. 10B). Lesions involving the accessory olfactory bulb in *Ambystoma* (Northcutt, unpublished observations) reveal degeneration in an accessory olfactory tract that can be traced into the caudal pole of the pars lateralis where it fuses with the preoptic area. Expansion of the pars lateralis of the amygdala in the caudal hemisphere of *Ichthyophis* (Fig. 12A–C) occurs in a manner similar to that in other amphibians, but is more difficult to follow as the apodans do not possess so distinct a lateral cellular prominence as do salamanders and anurans.

C. Subpallium

Four subpallial or basal telencephalic regions can be recognized in amphibians: septal nuclei, olfactory tubercle, pars medialis of the amygdala, and striatum. The subpallium replaces the internal granule layer of the olfactory bulb rostrally, but at levels well beyond the first appearance of the pallium (Fig. 4). The bulbo-subpallial transition is more gradual than the bulbo-pallial transition, and, since the subpallial cells are smaller than the pallial cells, the most rostral occurrence of the striatum is difficult to distinguish. The majority of the subpallial nuclei terminate at the laminal terminalis (Fig. 5). Only the medial septal nucleus and entopeduncular nucleus can be traced more caudally (Figs. 6 and 7).

1. Septal Nuclei

The septal nuclei occupy the ventromedial hemispheric wall and are bounded dorsally by the medial pallium and the zona limitans medialis (Figs. 4–6). Ventrally the septal area is continuous, without a cell-free break, with other cellular formations. The septal wall has traditionally been divided into lateral and medial nuclei; however, four additional cellular groups occupy the same area: the postolfactory eminence (Figs. 2 and 3), the bed nucleus of the pallial commissure (Fig. 6), the olfactory tubercle (Figs. 4 and 5) and the pars mediális of the amygdala (Fig. 5). Only the postolfactory eminence and the bed nucleus of the pallial commissure will be discussed under the heading of septal nuclei.

The postolfactory eminence is the most rostrally located subpallial nucleus in *Rana* (Fig. 2), and it rapidly disappears at more caudal levels as the remaining subpallial nuclei arise (Fig. 4). The postolfactory eminence likely receives olfactory input via the medial olfactory tract, as well as projections from the medial pallium (Halpern, 1972). Nothing is presently known regarding its efferent connections, but its position and afferents suggest that it should be considered a rostral septal nucleus.

A distinct postolfactory eminence has not been recognized in salamanders (Herrick, 1948), but a dense cellular plate—labeled septum by Herrick—occupies a topographical position comparable to that of the eminence in *Rana.* This rostral septal area in *Ambystoma* also receives direct olfactory projections and may be homologous to the anuran postolfactory eminence.

Septal organization in apodans is so unique among amphibians that it is almost impossible to homologize apodan septal nuclei without experimental data. Apodans, unlike other amphibians, possess a rostral septal area several times the size of the medial pallium (Fig. 11B,C). At its first appearance, the septal area bulging into the ventricle could be mistaken for the medial pallium (Fig. 11B). However, further caudally a more dorsal elevation begins to develop and represents the medial pallium (Fig. 11C). The septal elevation gradually shrinks in size and continues caudally, adjacent to the medial pallium (Fig. 12A), as does the septal area in anurans (Figs. 5 and 6).

The most rostral portion of the apodan septal elevation (Fig. 11B) may be homologous to the postolfactory eminence of anurans or may represent only a rostral portion of the medial septal nucleus. Experimental studies are needed to resolve this question.

In anurans two cell groups—the lateral and medial septal nuclei—occupy the bulk of the ventromedial hemispheric wall caudal to the postolfactory eminence (Figs. 4–6). The lateral septal nucleus occupies a periventricular position and ends caudally at the lamina terminalis. It is bounded ventrally by the pars medialis of the amygdala (Fig. 5), which gradually replaces the lateral septal nucleus at more caudal levels.

The medial septal nucleus appears rostrally as a migrated spherical nucleus and expands rapidly at midhemispheric levels (Fig. 5), where it appears laminated due to the passage of medial forebrain bundle fibers. At more caudal levels it lies dorsal to the interventricular foramen and continues only slightly more caudally (Fig. 6).

Neurons of the lateral and medial septal nuclei possess multiple dendrites that project predominantly medially to aborize among the fibers of the medial forebrain bundle. These dendrites probably also synapse with fibers of the medial olfactory tract (Fig. 4).

The septal nuclei of *Rana* receive bilateral pathways from the brain stem (Kicliter and Northcutt, 1975)—possibly homologous to mammalian ascending noradrenergic pathways—and from the hypothalamus (Neary and Wilczynski, 1977*a*) and the medial pallium (Halpern, 1972). Lesions of the septum reveal a descending pathway in the medial forebrain bundle reaching ventral thalamic, preoptic, and hypothalamic areas (Halpern, 1972). Additional studies are needed to determine if thalamic nuclei project to the septum. However, the septal nuclei are clearly a focal point for converging sensory information, and they likely represent a major source of telencephalic efferents affecting lower brain centers.

Lateral and medial septal nuclei have been recognized in salamanders and apodans (Figs. 8, 11, and 12) but are not nearly so well developed as in anurans. The rostral and ventromedial telencephalic wall in salamanders is likely homologous to the anuran septum, but it is presently impossible to decide if they possess the same nuclei. A similar problem exists in apodans due to the extreme hypertrophy of the septal wall and absence of the extensive cell migrations that characterize the medial septal nucleus in anurans.

The bed nucleus of the pallial commissure can also be included as part of the septal area. The bed nucleus begins anteriorly as a spherical, densely packed, small-celled nucleus located ventral to the medial septal nucleus at a caudal hemispheric level (Fig. 6). As the bed nucleus is traced caudally, it acquires a larger cell population and fuses with the dorsolateral edge of the periventricular preoptic nucleus (Fig. 7). The bed nucleus possesses reciprocal connections with the medial pallium (Kicliter, 1979).

A similar nucleus occupies the same topographical position in salamanders and apodans and is termed the thalamic eminence (Figs. 10 and 12). While this nucleus is much larger than the anuran bed nucleus, the thalamic eminence also appears first at caudal hemispheric levels and is traced caudally, where it occupies the dorsal third of the diencephalic wall rostral to the appearance of the dorsal thalamic nuclei (Figs. 10B and 12B,C).

2. Olfactory Tubercle

The cell group labeled olfactory tubercle in *Rana* (Figs. 4 and 5) was first termed this by Herrick (1910) and Söderberg (1922). Hoffman (1963) termed the same cell group the nucleus of the diagonal band of Broca, as did Kicliter and Ebbesson (1976). Scalia *et al.* (1968) followed the usage of Röthig (1912) and included this cell group as part of the medial septal nucleus, as did Northcutt and Royce (1975) in their description of the olfactory projections in *Rana*. At present there is scant evidence to support the validity of any one of these terms in regard to possible homologies with other vertebrates. Kicliter and Ebbesson (1976) describe this cell group as arising ventral to the internal granule layer at caudal olfactory bulb levels, where it rapidly expands medially and dorsally to occupy a superficial position in the ventromedial telencephalic wall (Fig. 4). At more caudal levels it divides into dorsal and ventral components, which disappear at midhemispheric levels, the ventral component extending more caudally than the dorsal component (Fig. 5). This nucleus likely receives olfactory input, as terminals of the medial olfactory tract are seen among the cell bodies of the nucleus (Figs. 4 and 5). Nothing is known regarding its efferents.

The "olfactory tubercle" of anurans is most likely homologous to either the olfactory tubercle or the nucleus of the diagonal band of amniotes. It may, however, be a field homologue of both nuclei. Olfactory projections to the nucleus of the diagonal band were not seen in experimental studies of the lagomorph *Oryctolagus* (Broadwell, 1975) or in *Tupaia* (Skeen and Hall, 1977).

The olfactory tubercle of amniotes arises embryonically as a migrated cell group of the ventral basal matrix, as does the anuran "olfactory tubercle" (Söderberg, 1922; Källén, 1951*b*). At present it seems reasonable to retain Herrick's designation of this anuran cell group as olfactory tubercle, considering its receipt of olfactory projections and its probable embryonic origin in the ventral subpallium. A similar migrated cell group has not been identified in salamanders or apodans.

3. Pars Medialis of the Amygdala

The anuran pars medialis of the amygdala is first seen rostrally as a more densely packed nucleus ventral to the lateral septal nucleus and immediately rostral to the lamina terminalis (Fig. 5). The pars medialis rapidly enlarges as it is traced caudally, replacing the lateral septal nucleus as it forms a distinct ridge in the floor of the lateral ventricle. It fuses across the midline with the contralateral pars medialis, forming a C-shaped complex whose body lies in the lamina terminalis with its arms directed rostrally beneath the lateral septal nucleus. Hoffman (1963) described the rostral half of this nucleus as a caudal continuation of his nucleus accumbens and the commissural half as his bed nucleus of the anterior commissure.

Few data exist on the connections of the amphibian pars medialis. It probably does not receive olfactory input in anurans, but a hypothalamic input has been reported (Neary and Wilczynski, 1977*a*), and reciprocal connections with the septal nuclei also appear to exist (see Section VI.B).

A distinct pars medialis exists in salamanders and apodans, and the pars medialis of *Ambystoma*—unlike that of anurans—probably receives olfactory input via the ventrolateral olfactory tract (Fig. 9).

4. The Striatum

The anuran lateral subpallial wall consists of a tier of nuclei: a lateral striatum proper, and a medial nucleus accumbens adjacent to the septal nuclei (Figs. 4 and 5). At rostral levels, the lateral striatum consists of a pars dorsalis and pars ventralis distinguished by differences in packing density and degree of cell migration (Figs. 4 and 5). The pars dorsalis can be traced caudally to the level of the lamina terminalis. At this level it is impossible to determine if the cell group disappears or merges ventrally with the pars ventralis. The pars ventralis can be followed more caudally, where it moves ventrolaterally into the lateral forebrain bundle and is termed the anterior entopeduncular nucleus (Figs. 6 and 7).

The more medially located nucleus accumbens arises immediately caudal to the accessory olfactory bulb, replacing the internal granule layer of the olfactory bulb. It occupies a subependymal position in the floor of the lateral ventricle (Fig. 4), and in Nissl stains its cells stain more darkly than adjacent populations. Nucleus accumbens can be traced to the level of the lamina terminalis, where it disappears.

The striatum contains large multipolar cells whose dendrites radiate into the lateral striatal neuropil and small cells whose short dendrites form less extensive arbors in the lateral neuropil.

The lateral forebrain bundle forms a comma-shaped profile in the lateral neuropil of the striatum, and lesions of the midbrain tegmentum reveal an ascending projection that terminates in the neuropil of the striatum, forming a shell around the striatal neuropil (Rubinson and Colman, 1972). Parent (1975) reported a similar shell of catecholamine terminals in the striatal neuropil. This pathway may be homologous to the ascending nigrostriatal pathway of amniotes. Lesions of the middle dorsal thalamic area in *Rana* reveal ascending pathways that end in the striatum (Gruberg and Ambros, 1974; Kicliter and Northcutt, 1975). The middle dorsal thalamic zone receives tectal and auditory input but no direct retinal projections (Rubinson, 1968; Lázár, 1969; Neary, 1974).

In *Rana* lesions of the lateral striatum reveal descending projections via the lateral forebrain bundle to the midbrain tegmentum and to a lateral cell group in the isthmus ventral to nucleus isthmi (Halpern, 1972). These projections are strikingly similar to the projections of the mammalian striatum via the strio-nigral and ansa lenticularis pathways, and they strongly suggest that the anuran striatum is homologous to the amniote striatum.

Salamanders and apodans possess striatal divisions (Figs. 8–12) similar to those of anurans, and *Ambystoma* appears to possess striatal projections similar to those of anurans (Kokoros and Northcutt, 1977). There is one major difference between the striatal afferents in *Ambystoma* and *Rana*. The striatum in *Ambystoma* appears to receive a much heavier olfactory input than in *Rana*, via a ventrolateral olfactory tract (Figs. 8 and 9) that does not appear to exist in *Rana*.

IV. Organization of the Olfactory System

A. Olfactory Organs

Most amphibians possess two separate chemoreceptor organs within each nasal cavity. These are an olfactory organ and a vomeronasal or Jacobson's organ (Fig. 13). Each gives rise to a distinct nerve, and each terminates in a separate bulbar region of the telencephalon. The olfactory complex is always larger than the vomeronasal complex, which is absent in some aquatic salamanders (e.g., *Necturus* and *Proteus*).

The nasal cavity of amphibians opens rostrally at the external naris and caudally at the choana; thus the nasal cavity communicates directly with the oral cavity. The nasal cavity typically consists of three chambers or recesses: the superior (principal) chamber, the middle chamber, and the inferior chamber (Fig. 14; McCotter, 1917; Scalia, 1976*a*). In anurans the principal chamber is ovoid, and its floor reveals an elevated ridge termed the olfactory eminence. The external naris opens into the rostrodorsal roof of the principal chamber, and the choana forms an opening in the caudal ventrolateral floor of the principal chamber lateral to the olfactory eminence (Fig. 14B). The roof, medial wall, and rostral pole of the principal chamber are covered by a thick sensory epithelium that gives rise to the dorsal division of the olfactory nerve, whereas the sensory epithelium of the olfactory eminence gives rise to the ventral division of the olfactory nerve. The two sensory epithelial patches of the principal chamber are not continuous but are separated by a thinner nonsensory epithelium.

The middle nasal chamber (Fig. 14A) lies below the rostral floor of the principal chamber and communicates with both the principal and inferior chambers.

The walls of the middle nasal chamber contain no sensory epithelia and thus do not give rise to any part of the olfactory nerve.

The inferior chamber is rectangular and as long as the principal chamber, but it is much narrower in its dorsoventral axis (Fig. 14). A rostromedial diverticulum or duct exists in most anurans and ends blindly rostral and ventral to the principal chamber. The walls of this medially directed duct form the thickened sensory epithelium termed the vomeronasal or Jacobson's organ (Fig. 14A). The vomeron asal epithelium gives rise to the vomeronasal nerve, thus forming the most medial component of sensory fibers leaving the nasal cavity. The vomeronasal nerve is closely associated with fascicles of the olfactory nerve until it reaches the rostral pole of the olfactory bulb, where it moves ventrolaterally to course along the outer edge of the olfactory bulb and terminate more caudally in the laterally located accessory olfactory bulb (Figs. 2, 3, 8A, and 11A,B).

The remaining portion of the inferior chamber—some 90% of its surface—does not contain sensory epithelium but forms an extensive lateral or maxillary recess that communicates with the principal chamber via the choana (Fig. 14B).

In most anurans the vomeronasal organ is a rostromedial diverticulum of the inferior nasal chamber. However, in salamanders and the anuran *Bombina* the

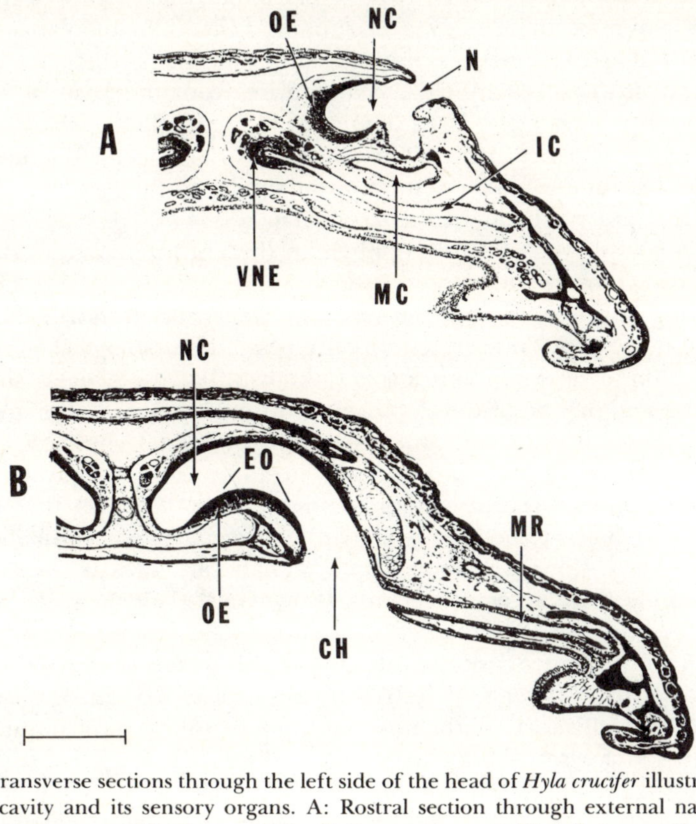

Figure 14. Transverse sections through the left side of the head of *Hyla crucifer* illustrating anatomy of the nasal cavity and its sensory organs. A: Rostral section through external naris. B: Caudal section through choana. CH, Choana; EO, olfactory eminence; IC, inferior nasal chamber; MC, middle nasal chamber; MR, maxillary recess; N, external naris; NC, nasal cavity; OE, olfactory sensory epithelia; VNE, vomeronasal sensory epithelium. Bar scale equals 0.5 mm.

vomeronasal diverticulum occupies a rostrolateral position. Differences in adult topography might suggest that vomeronasal organs are not homologous among different amphibians. However, the vomeronasal organ always arises embryonically from a ventromedial segment of the amphibian olfactory anlage (Medvedeva, 1968) and axons of the vomeronasal organ always terminate in a caudal ventrolateral accessory olfactory bulb. Thus it is likely that vomeronasal organs of different amphibians are homologous despite mediolateral variation in adult position.

In reptiles (except *Sphenodon*) the vomeronasal organ does not communicate with the nasal cavity but opens directly into the oral cavity (Parsons, 1970). Thus chemical stimuli must be introduced through the mouth for the vomeronasal organ to be stimulated. The situation is not so clear in amphibians. Chemical stimuli could reach the vomeronasal epithelium by passing through the external naris and principal and middle nasal chambers, or from the oral cavity via the lateral recess of the inferior nasal chamber (Fig. 14). At present we do not know what class(es) of chemical stimuli excites the vomeronasal organ in amphibians, the route of delivery, or the biological significance of the stimuli.

The sensory epithelia of the anuran olfactory and vomeronasal organs consist of a thickened pseudostratified columnar epithelium formed by three distinct cell classes: sensory bipolar cells, supporting cells, and basal cells (Graziadei, 1971; Graziadei and Metcalf, 1971; Scalia, 1976*a*). The superficial surface of the olfactory epithelium is a mosaic of sensory and support cells. The bipolar sensory cells possess superficial apical processes that extend beyond the surface of the olfactory epithelium and are covered by cilia. Axons arise from the base of the sensory bipolar cells and penetrate the basal lamina of the epithelium, where they collect as fascicles of the olfactory nerve. The third class, basal cells, do not reach the surface of the olfactory epithelium and appear similar to the basal elements of the nonsensory respiratory mucosa of the nasal chambers.

The basal cells of the olfactory epithelium undergo mitosis and differentiate into new bipolar sensory neurons (Graziadei and DeHan, 1973). This process occurs following surgical trauma, but also appears to occur normally, thus suggesting that the receptors possess a short life span. The biological significance of olfactory receptor turnover in anurans is unknown, but the process suggests that new classes of receptors might develop during different stages in the life history of the organism. Food preferences and other environmental chemical clues differ during developmental stages—or seasonally in anurans—and may be correlated with changes in olfactory receptor populations.

The vomeronasal epithelium is similar to the olfactory epithelium, but its bipolar sensory cells possess microvilli rather than cilia. Nor is the vomeronasal epithelium supplied by accessory glands (Bowman's glands) as is the olfactory epithelium.

The neurophysiology of anuran olfactory receptors has been reviewed recently by Gesteland (1976). A potential (electro-olfactogram, EOG) can be recorded from the surface of the olfactory epithelium in response to odorous stimulation. The EOG peaks in about 1 sec, then falls exponentially over a few seconds following a brief, rapidly fluctuating vapor stimulus (Ottoson, 1956). The amplitude of the EOG is a power function of the amount of odorous material reaching the mucosa per unit time when the mucosa is exposed to a brief stimulus. Substances with low water solubilities evoke EOGs with prolonged falling phase time constants (Ottoson,

1956), and different regions of the epithelium vary in their responsiveness to different odors (Daval *et al.,* 1970; Mustaparta, 1971). Thus receptors responsive to certain classes of substances may be spatially segregated within the olfactory epithelium.

Single-cell responses of the olfactory receptors are complex and are not simply related to the properties of the stimulus substances (Gesteland, 1976). At present the coding of stimulus quality and its receptor mechanism(s) are unknown.

B. Olfactory Projections

Amphibian olfactory bulbs are goblet-shaped structures that form the rostral poles of the cerebral hemispheres (Fig. 1). The accessory olfactory bulb, when present, is a small hemispherical elevation located more posteriorly on the ventrolateral hemispheric wall (Fig. 1). Each bulbar formation is supplied by its own nerve—the olfactory bulbs by the olfactory nerves and the accessory olfactory bulbs by the vomeronasal nerves (Fig. 1). In anurans the olfactory bulbs are fused at the midline through a region termed the interbulbar adhesion. This adhesion marks a continuation of the glomerular and mitral cell layers ventrally, but each bulb retains distinct extragranular plexiform and internal granule layers (Fig. 2). Although it would seem possible that each olfactory nerve projects to both bulbs because of the adhesion, experimental transection of single olfactory nerves in *Rana* (Northcutt and Royce, 1975) reveals that each olfactory nerve projects only to the ipsilateral olfactory bulb.

1. Projections of the Olfactory Bulb

Among anurans, secondary olfactory projections have been experimentally demonstrated only in *Rana pipiens* (Scalia *et al.,* 1968) and *Rana catesbeiana* (Northcutt and Royce, 1975).

Olfactory bulb lesions not involving the accessory olfactory bulb result in degenerating fibers in the extragranular plexiform layer of the caudal bulb which collect to form the medial and lateral olfactory tracts (Fig. 2). Ipsilaterally, degenerating fibers in the medial olfactory tract can be traced to the level of the lamina terminalis (Figs. 3 and 4). The medial olfactory tract projects within the nuclear boundaries of the medial septal nucleus and the olfactory tubercle.

Rostrally, degenerating fibers are seen in the extragranular plexiform and internal granule layers streaming dorsally and laterally to form the lateral olfactory tract (Fig. 2B). This tract continues adding fibers at its ventrolateral edge until it reaches the level of the accessory olfactory bulb (Fig. 3A). As the lateral olfactory tract moves caudally, it spreads over the lateral surface of the hemisphere but is confined to the outer molecular zones of the dorsal striatum, the lateral pallium, and the ventral half of the dorsal pallium (Figs. 3–7). The lateral olfactory tract runs the entire length of the cerebral hemisphere and can be traced into the caudal hemispheric pole (Fig. 7).

At the level of the telencephalon medium (Fig. 6), fibers in the ventral edge of the ipsilateral lateral olfactory tract turn medially, after skirting the pars lateralis of the amygdala, and enter the stria medullaris (Fig. 7). These fibers cross in the habenular commissure and enter the contralateral stria medullaris and lateral olfactory tract (Fig. 7).

Crossed olfactory projections have been reported for both *Rana pipiens* (Scalia *et al.,* 1968) and *Rana catesbeiana* (Northcutt and Royce, 1975), but reports of their extent do not agree. In *R. pipiens* the crossed fibers were traced to the external plexiform region of the pars lateralis of the amygdala, and this relationship was considered evidence for an olfactory bulb projection to the contralateral amygdala (Scalia *et al.,* 1968). However, Northcutt and Royce (1975) reported more extensive crossed projections in *R. catesbeiana;* two separate crossed pathways were described in bullfrogs. A lateral pathway—identified by Herrick (1948) as the lateral cortico-habenular tract—was traced rostrally beyond a midtelencephalic level (Fig. 4B). A second pathway was traced ventrally and medially around the forebrain bundles (Fig. 6B), where it skirts the preoptic area (Fig. 5B), then passes rostrally in a position comparable to the ipsilateral medial olfactory tract (Fig. 4B). This crossed medial component passes rostrally into the internal granule and extragranular plexiform layers of the caudal olfactory bulb (Fig. 3B) and corresponds to the anterior olfacto-habenular tract of Herrick (1921).

Two factors limit precise identification of secondary olfactory targets: the uniformly fine nature of degenerating particles precludes accurate distinction between degenerating axons and terminals at light microscopic levels; and much of the degeneration appears outside the nuclear boundaries, suggesting that most terminals are of an axo-dendritic nature. Conclusions regarding secondary olfactory fiber targets are thus based on density of particles, proximity of degenerating particles to cell groups, and termination of the degenerating pathways in specific targets beyond which the pathways can not be traced.

The ipsilateral medial olfactory tract probably projects to the rostral ventromedial portion of the medial pallium, the postolfactory eminence, the rostral lateral septum, and the olfactory tubercle (Figs. 3 and 4).

The ipsilateral lateral olfactory tract probably projects to the dorsal striatum, the lateral pallium, and the ventral half of the dorsal pallium, as this pathway courses through the outer half of the molecular zones of all these neural populations (Figs. 3–7). Crossed secondary olfactory pathways to the contralateral hemisphere also appear to exist. A crossed lateral pathway, the lateral cortico-habenular tract, may terminate in the ventral portion of the dorsal pallium, the lateral pallium, and a restricted portion of the dorsal striatum. A crossed medial pathway, the anterior olfacto-habenular tract, terminates in the internal granule layer of the olfactory bulb and could form connections with the preoptic area, septal nuclei, and olfactory tubercle, through which it passes on its way to the olfactory bulb.

There are no experimental studies on secondary olfactory projections in apodans, and only a brief account of the olfactory projections for a single salamander, *Ambystoma tigrinum,* has been reported (Royce and Northcutt, 1969). A more detailed account of secondary olfactory projections in *Ambystoma* is illustrated in Figs. 8–10. Olfactory bulb lesions, sparing the more caudally situated accessory olfactory bulb, reveal degenerating fibers in the caudal olfactory bulb, collecting medially just beneath the bulbar surface and laterally in the extragranular plexiform layer (Fig. 8A). The degenerating medial fibers form a medial olfactory tract that distributes to the rostral ipsilateral dorsal pallium, medial pallium, and septal nuclear region (Fig. 8B). The medial olfactory tract is confined to the rostral cerebral hemisphere and does not reach so far caudally as the lamina terminalis. Thus projections of the medial olfactory tract of *Ambystoma* are remarkably similar to those of the medial tract of *Rana*.

In *Ambystoma* the lateral olfactory tract forms in the lateral extragranular layer, courses caudally, then divides into dorsolateral and ventrolateral tracts as it flows dorsal and ventral to the accessory olfactory bulb (Figs. 8B and 9). These two divisions of the lateral olfactory tract remain separate throughout most of their caudal course, sparing a dorsal segment of the striatum (Figs. 8B and 9A). More caudally (Fig. 10A), the dorsolateral and ventrolateral tracts merge, extend into the caudal lateral hemispheric pole, and enter the stria medullaris (Fig. 10B), where they cross in the habenular commissure and distribute in the contralateral dorsolateral and ventrolateral olfactory tracts. Degenerating fibers in these crossed tracts were not traced to rostral telencephalic levels.

The projection pattern of the lateral olfactory tracts in *Ambystoma* and *Rana* show certain similarities, but the lateral tract in *Ambystoma* is far more extensive and likely involves additional targets. The course of the dorsolateral olfactory tract in *Ambystoma* closely resembles the course of the lateral olfactory tract in *Rana* in that it likely distributes to the ventral half of the dorsal pallium, the lateral pallium, and a dorsal portion of the striatum (Figs. 3–10). The ventrolateral olfactory tract in *Ambystoma* likely distributes to the ventral striatum and the pars medialis of the amygdala (Figs. 8–10). A comparable olfactory tract does not appear to exist in ranids.

2. Projections of the Accessory Olfactory Bulb

The accessory olfactory bulb projections in amphibians have been experimentally determined in *Rana pipiens* (Scalia, 1972) and *Rana catesbeiana* (Northcutt and Royce, 1975). Lesions of the accessory olfactory bulb (Fig. 13) not only destroy the accessory olfactory bulb but also interrupt secondary olfactory pathways arising in the internal granule and extragranular plexiform layers of the main olfactory bulb. However, comparison of the chartings of an accessory olfactory bulb lesion (Fig. 13) and an olfactory bulb lesion (Figs. 2–7) reveals the existence of a new degenerating pathway that collects lateral to the strio-pallial boundary (act in Fig. 13C). This pathway courses caudally to terminate in the ipsilateral pars lateralis of the amygdala (Fig. 13D,E). Herrick (1921) first described this pathway but believed that it terminated on only a dorsolateral portion of the amygdala. However, experimental studies reveal that the entire rostrocaudal extent of the pars lateralis of the amygdala receives this projection. The pathway from the accessory olfactory bulb corresponds in part to the ventrolateral tract of Herrick (1921) and is here termed the accessory olfactory tract.

3. Further Connections of the Telencephalic Olfactory Areas

There are few experimental studies on efferent connections of the cerebral hemispheres in amphibians (*Ambystoma*: Kokoros and Northcutt, 1977; *Bufo*: Kokoros, 1973; *Rana*: Halpern *et al.*, 1968; Halpern, 1972; Scalia, 1976*a*), and all these studies involved large lesions of the cerebral hemispheres. Thus data on precise projections of many individual telencephalic areas are presently unavailable.

Lesions, or injections of [^{3}H]proline into the pars lateralis of the amygdala in *Rana,* reveal the existence of an amygdalo-hypothalamic tract (Scalia, 1976*a*). Hypothalamic projections to the deep layers of the optic tectum and to the tegmentum have recently been reported in *Rana* (Neary and Wilczynski, 1977*a*). Thus one olfactory channel from the vomeronasal organ to tectal and tegmental levels might be mediated via accessory olfactory bulb–hypothalamo-tectal or -tegmental pathways.

Halpern (1972) reported that the pars lateralis of the amygdala in *Rana* also projects to the posterocentral and posterolateral thalamic nuclei. A caudal portion of the posterolateral nucleus is also known to receive retinal and tectal inputs (Rubinson, 1968; Scalia and Gregory, 1970) and to project to the optic tectum (Wilczynski and Northcutt, 1977). Lesions of the caudal posterolateral nucleus in anurans profoundly affect tectal unit habituation and receptive field size (Ingle, 1973) and stimulus approach or avoidance behavior (Ewert, 1970). These results suggest that olfactory information might alter prey approach and predator avoidance behaviors via a second olfactory channel from the vomeronasal organ to tectum via an amygdalo-posterolateral nuclear pathway.

Experimental analyses of the lateral pallium in *Bufo* (Kokoros, 1973) and *Rana* (Scalia, 1976*a*) have not revealed a hypothalamic pathway as exists in mammals. Instead, the lateral pallium projects to the medial pallium via the dorsal association tract. Medial pallial projections to the septum and hypothalamus have been reported in *Bufo marinus* (Kokoros, 1973) and probably exist in *Ambystoma tigrinum* (Kokoros and Northcutt, 1977). If further studies do not reveal additional lateral pallial projections, olfactory influences on nontelencephalic centers must be mediated by septal or medial pallial pathways.

Our present information regarding higher-order olfactory pathways is still very incomplete, but sufficient data exist to suggest that vomeronasal and olfactory chemoreception is conveyed by distinctly separate pathways—at least within the telencephalon—and that at least three or four fairly distinct olfactory channels may exert chemoceptive influences on the pretectum, tectum, hypothalamus, and tegmentum.

C. Olfactory Mediated Behaviors

The role of olfaction in amphibian behavior is not well documented, because of a paucity of field studies and the difficulty of designing operant conditioning paradigms to test learning and discrimination abilities in amphibians.

Olfactory cues are likely utilized by several species of *Bufo* and *Pseudacris* in returning to home ponds for reproduction (Grubb, 1973*a,b*). These animals exhibit a preference for the odor of water from their home ponds, as opposed to that of foreign ponds. Experimentally induced anosmia in several species of *Bufo* and *Rana* hinders orientation to breeding sites (Oldham, 1967; Tracy and Dole, 1969).

Olfactory cues are also used in feeding sequences. Tadpoles recognize certain food odors and demonstrate preferences (Risser, 1914). *Rana pipiens* discriminates more rapidly between noxious and nonnoxious prey objects with both olfactory and visual cues than with either type of cue exclusively (Sternthal, 1974). *Bufo* will pursue large stimuli, that are normally avoided, when such stimuli are presented in conjunction with a familiar prey odor (Ewert, 1970).

These studies demonstrate the significance of olfactory cues in behavioral categories such as prey approach and avoidance, orientation, and migration. However, we have little idea of the specific nature of the chemical cues, the site of stimulation (whether olfactory organ or vomeronasal organ), or the central pathways utilized in mediating these behaviors.

V. Ascending Telencephalic Afferents

Amphibian telencephalons receive at least visual, auditory, and somatosensory information via systems of fibers which ascend from the diencephalon and more caudal levels of the brainstem. This statement requires some qualification, as most data are for *Rana*; other amphibian genera remain to be studied. Nonetheless, a major achievement of comparative neurological studies over the past 20 years has been to establish that these ascending systems appear as important as olfaction in amphibian telencephalic functions (for review, see Kicliter and Ebbesson, 1976). Undoubtedly, amphibian telencephalons receive ascending information other than that most easily characterized as sensory; yet sensory systems have drawn the greatest attention. There are at least two reasons for this. First, comparative neurologists are interested in comparisons, and telencephalic sensory systems in amphibians are, or appear to be, most easily compared with telencephalic organization in other vertebrate classes. Second, investigations of sensory systems have produced striking results more quickly than those of systems less easily characterized.

It has been known for many years that two large fiber bundles—the medial and lateral forebrain bundles—connect the telencephalon with more caudal regions of amphibian brains (Haslam, 1889; Rubaschkin, 1903; Ramón y Cajal, 1922; Herrick, 1925, 1948; Röthig, 1926; Hoffman, 1963; Schnitzlein *et al.*, 1973). The study of normal material suggested that these bundles conveyed axons of cells located in the thalamus and brainstem to ventral regions of the hemispheres. The medial forebrain bundle was generally believed to relate the septum and medial pallium on the medial wall of the hemisphere with the preoptic area and hypothalamus. The lateral forebrain bundle was reported to connect the striatum on the ventrolateral wall of the hemisphere with the dorsal thalamus through a dorsal peduncle, and with the ventral thalamus, hypothalamus, and mesencephalic tegmentum through a ventral peduncle.

Some refinement of these conclusions is possible as a result of investigations over the past decade using experimental neuroanatomical techniques. Thus the origins and terminations of the forebrain bundles are now known more completely. While many details of the ascending telencephalic connections are still not fully appreciated, we can review the advances that have been made.

A. Anterograde Degeneration Studies: Regional Sources of Telencephalic Afferents

1. Afferents via the Medial Forebrain Bundle

Anatomical studies using techniques which stain degenerating axoplasm have shown that the medial telencephalic wall, including the septum, medial pallium, and pars medialis of the amygdala, receives afferents via the medial forebrain bundle (mfb). These afferents arise from portions of the brainstem caudal to the isthmus and likely from the mesencephalon and diencephalon as well (Fig. 15). On entering the telencephalon the mfb partially decussates and so supplies afferents to the medial wall structures on both sides of the brain.

The first modern experimental study of ascending telencephalic afferents in amphibians was that of Vesselkin *et al.* (1971). After lesions of the posterior thalamus of *Rana temporaria,* these workers noted degeneration in the lateral septal nucleus and in the medial pallium. The interpretation given these results was that the posterior thalamus projected to the medial telencephalic wall. However, Northcutt (1972) reported essentially the same results from transections of the brainstem of *Rana catesbeiana* in the isthmal region. It is thus evident that thalamic lesions alone do not prove a thalamic projection to the medial telencephalic wall, as such lesions may destroy fibers ascending to the telencephalon from postthalamic levels of the brainstem. The amount of degenerative debris in the septum and medial pallium of *Rana pipiens* and *Rana catesbeiana* is substantially greater after thalamic lesions than after hemisections of the brainstem at the caudal border of the thalamus (Kicliter and Northcutt, 1975), but the point remains that thalamic lesions may interrupt fiber systems passing through the thalamus and thus do not provide

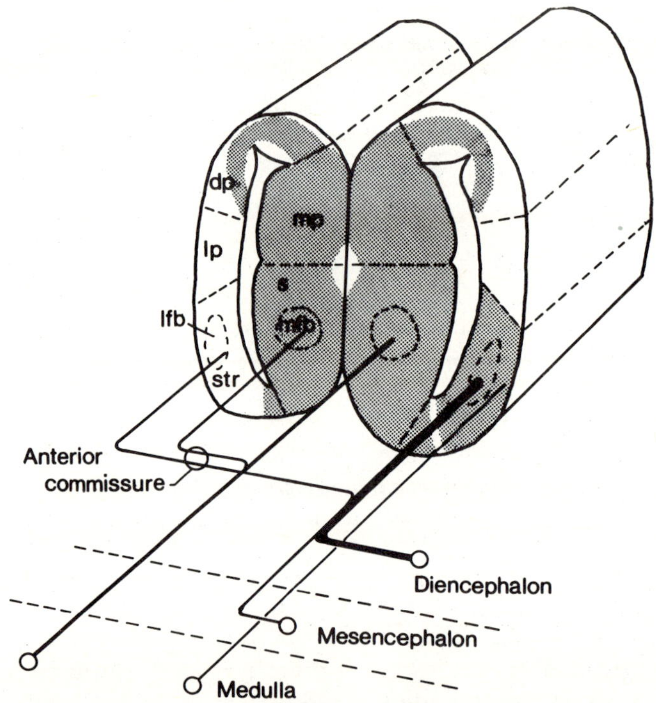

Figure 15. Diagram of sources and distribution of telencephalic afferents in *Rana* as revealed by anterograde degeneration studies. Sources are indicated by circles, pathways by lines, and distributions of lateral and medial forebrain bundles by shading. For clarity, distributions of mfb and lfb are not illustrated as overlapping, whereas they, in fact, do overlap as described in text. dp, Dorsal pallium; lfb, lateral forebrain bundle; lp, lateral pallium; mfb, medial forebrain bundle; mp, medial pallium; s, septum; str, striatum. Figure after Kicliter and Northcutt (1975).

conclusive evidence for a thalamo-telencephalic projection to the medial telencephalic wall. Within-subject control procedures are not feasible as the mfb distributes to both hemispheres. A final point regarding the mfb afferents is that when thalamectomies were performed in both *Rana pipiens* and *Rana catesbeiana,* the mfb could be shown to distribute not only to the septum and medial pallium but also to the dorsal pallium (Fig. 15). Figure 15 illustrates the large portion of the telencephalon supplied by ascending mfb afferents.

2. Afferents via the Lateral Forebrain Bundle

The lateral forebrain bundle (lfb) of the telencephalon distributes almost exclusively to the striatum, and this projection appears to be almost entirely ipsilateral (Northcutt, 1972; Kicliter, 1973; Gruberg and Ambros, 1974; Kicliter and Northcutt, 1975; Scalia, 1976*b*). Hemisections of the brainstem at the isthmus of *Rana pipiens* and *Rana catesbeiana* produce only sparse degeneration conveyed by the lfb to the dorsal border of the striatum, around the cells of the lateral pallial prominence (Kicliter and Northcutt, 1975). Brainstem hemisections at the caudal border of the thalamus produce sparse degeneration throughout the ipsilateral striatal neuropil and may produce a very small amount of debris in the contralateral striatal neuropil (Kicliter and Northcutt, 1975). Lesions of the lateral mesencephalic tegmentum of *Rana pipiens* produce a band of degeneration in the ipsilateral striatum on the periphery of the lateral forebrain bundle (Rubinson and Colman, 1972). Large lesions of the thalamus produce heavy degeneration in the ipsilateral striatum (Northcutt, 1972; Kicliter, 1973; Gruberg and Ambros, 1974; Kicliter and Northcutt, 1975). Since the lfb projection to the striatum is almost exclusively ipsilateral, a within-subject control experiment could be performed. Frogs sustaining hemisection of the brain at the caudal border of the thalamus, and a large thalamic lesion contralaterally, show far greater amounts of degenerative debris in the striatum ipsilateral to the thalamic lesion (Fig. 16). With smaller lesions of the dorsal thalamus it is possible to roughly localize the source of the thalamo-striatal afferents as cells of the posterocentral/posterolateral nuclear complex (Kicliter and Northcutt, 1975). This projection corresponds to Herrick's (1925, 1948) thalamofrontal tract, which he described in *Ambystoma* and *Rana*; Herrick believed the source of this projection was a diffusely constituted lateral geniculate body.

B. Cellular Sources of Telencephalic Afferents: The Horseradish Peroxidase Method

Anterograde degeneration studies reveal the terminal fields of ascending telencephalic afferents, but they yield only a gross indication of their sources. For precise identification of the sources of an afferent projection, no other neuroanatomical technique has enjoyed the success of the horseradish peroxidase (HRP) method (LaVail and LaVail, 1972; Lynch *et al.,* 1974). Scalia and Colman (1975) and Kicliter (1979) have employed this technique to examine the cellular sources of telencephalic afferents in *Rana pipiens.* The ascending afferents are illustrated schematically in Fig. 17.

1. Lateral Forebrain Bundle Afferents

Injections of concentrated HRP solution into the lateral forebrain bundle in the striatum reveal both afferent and efferent connections (Fig. 18). Prominent afferent cell groups are located in the ipsilateral posterocentral and posterolateral

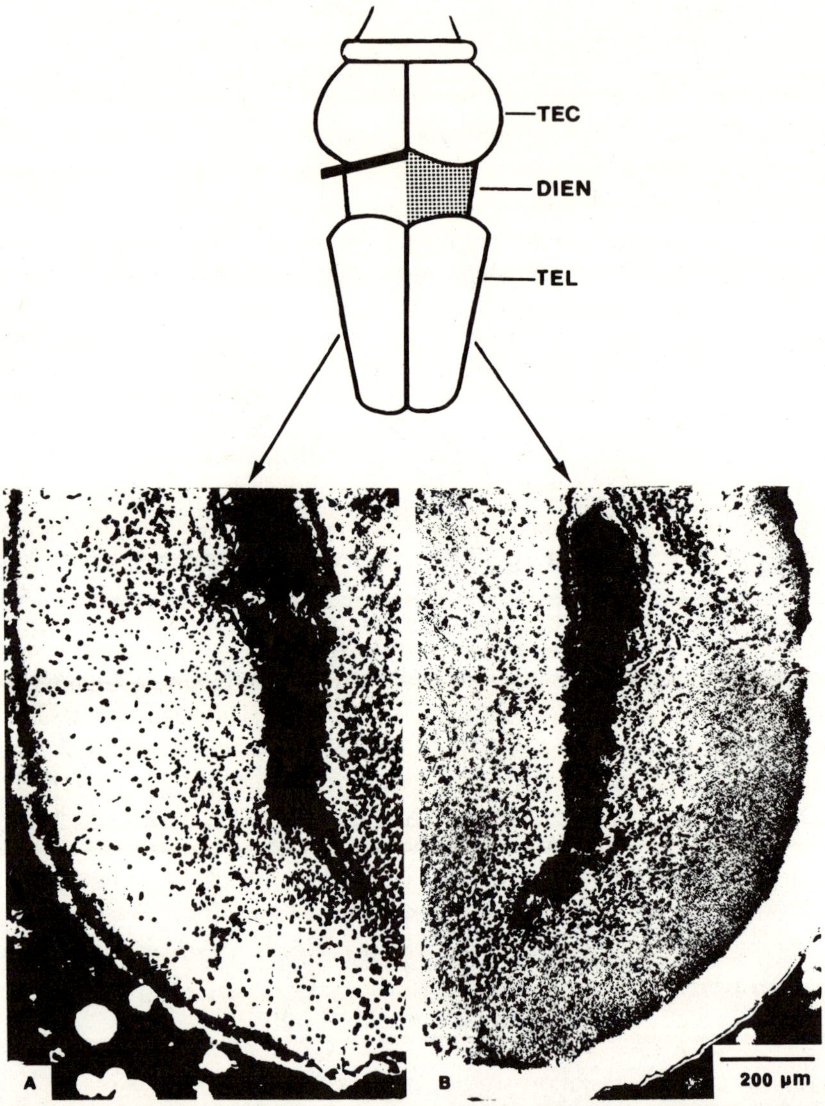

Figure 16. Results of a double-lesion experiment showing that dorsal thalamus projects to the striatum. The schematic dorsal view of the brain shows the lesion sites: hemisection at the caudal border of the thalamus on the left side of the brain; a large lesion of the dorsal thalamus on the right side of the brain. Photomicrographs A and B show the degeneration in the striata after these procedures. The striatum on the left (A) is almost free of degenerative debris while that on the right (B) is packed with degenerating terminal and preterminal elements (fine dots). DIEN, diencephalon; TEC, optic tectum; TEL, telencephalic hemisphere. Figure after Kicliter and Northcutt (1975).

nuclei of the dorsal thalamus (Figs. 18P,Q and 19). Figure 19 shows some of the cells of the posterolateral nucleus and the fibers ascending to them from the lfb, both filled with precipitate.

Lfb injections in the region of pars lateralis of the amygdala reveal—in addition to the posterocentral and posterolateral cells—a group of labeled cells in the ipsilateral rostral medulla (Figs. 20G,H and 21). This cell group does not fall within defined boundaries in any nomenclatural scheme. The most rostral of the labeled cells are located in what has been termed the cerebellar nucleus (e.g., Nieuwenhuys and Opdam, 1976). A column of labeled cells extends caudally from the cerebellar nucleus and may include some cells of the trigeminal principal sensory nucleus (Fuller and Ebbesson, 1973) or cells which receive primary statoacoustic projections (Campbell and Boord, 1974). Thalamic cells were filled after rostral injections of lfb, but the medullar cells were labeled only after injections of the caudal lfb in the

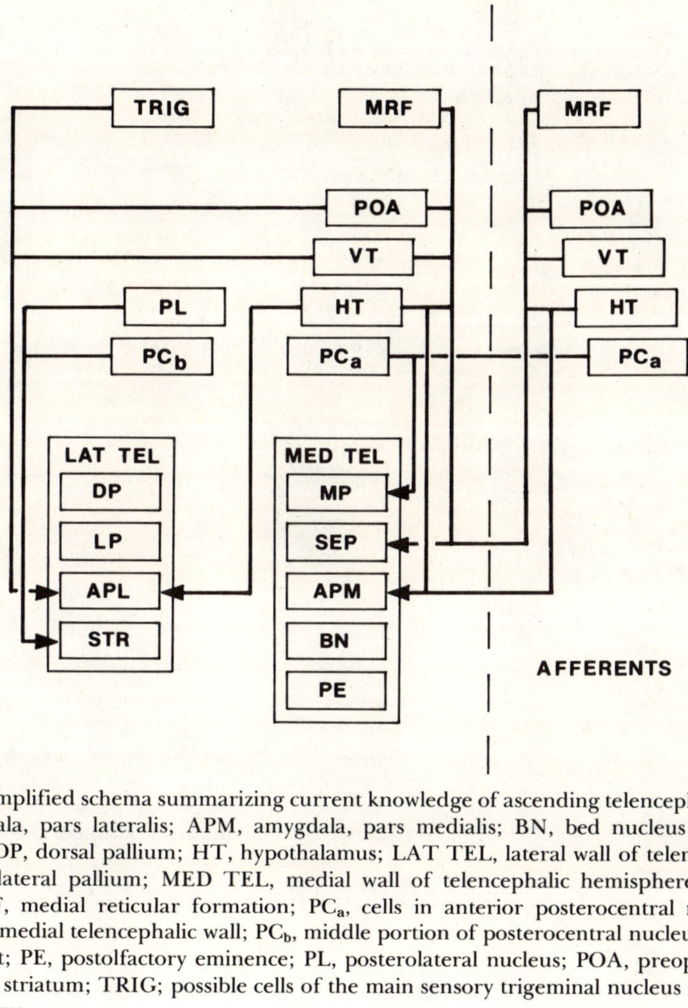

Figure 17. Simplified schema summarizing current knowledge of ascending telencephalic afferents. APL, Amygdala, pars lateralis; APM, amygdala, pars medialis; BN, bed nucleus of the pallial commissure; DP, dorsal pallium; HT, hypothalamus; LAT TEL, lateral wall of telencephalic hemisphere; LP, lateral pallium; MED TEL, medial wall of telencephalic hemisphere; MP, medial pallium; MRF, medial reticular formation; PC_a, cells in anterior posterocentral nucleus which project to the medial telencephalic wall; PC_b, middle portion of posterocentral nucleus that receives auditory input; PE, postolfactory eminence; PL, posterolateral nucleus; POA, preoptic area; SEP, septum; STR, striatum; TRIG; possible cells of the main sensory trigeminal nucleus (see text); VT, ventral thalamus.

region of pars lateralis of the amygdala. Thus it appears that the thalamic groups project to the striatum (although caudal telencephalic targets cannot be excluded), while the medullar group projects to the region of the neuropil of pars lateralis of the amygdala and, perhaps, to the caudal striatum.

Caudal lfb injections also labeled cells in the ventral thalamus and preoptic

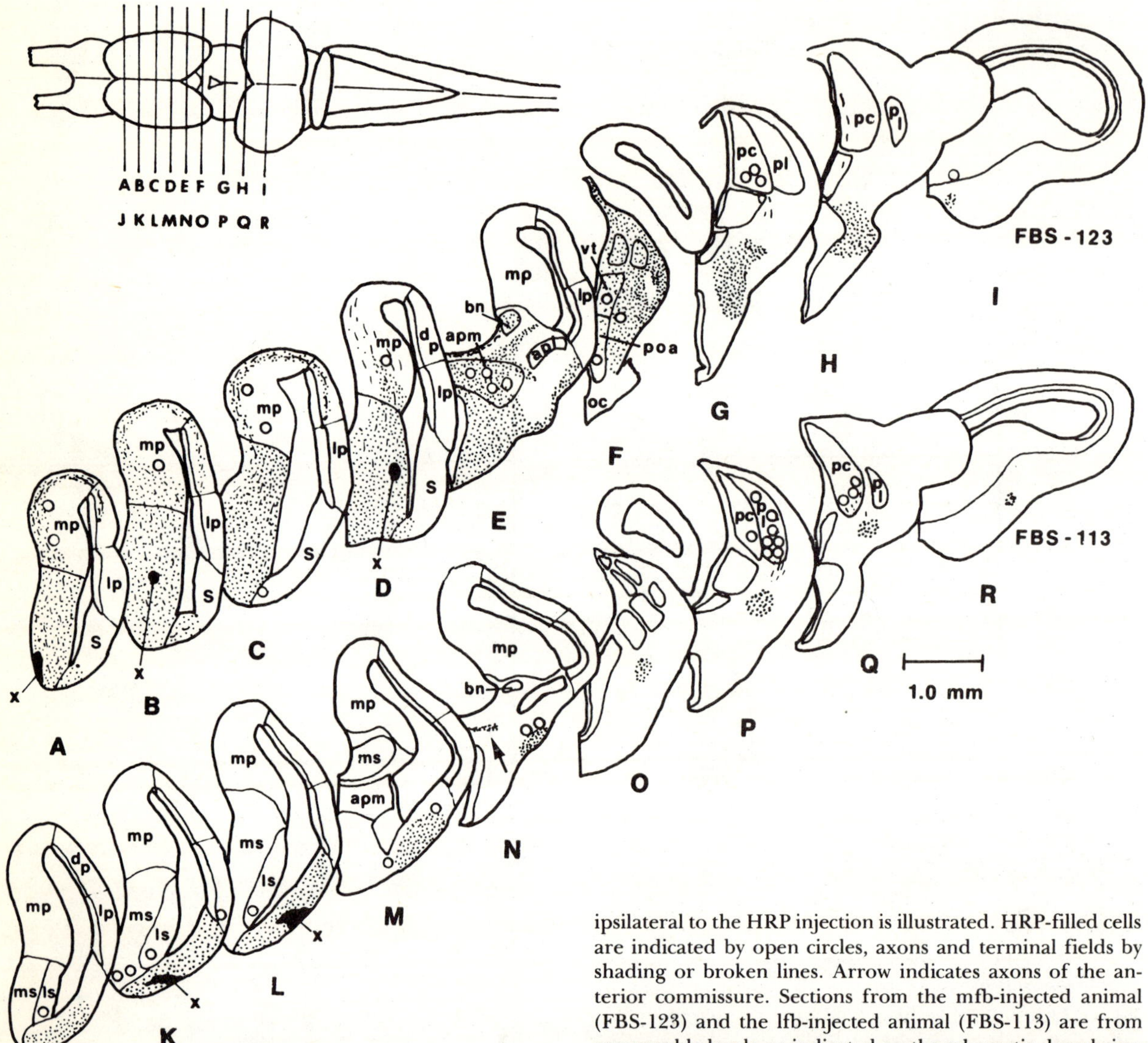

Figure 18. Outline drawings illustrating connections of the medial and lateral forebrain bundles revealed by the HRP technique. Whereas connections of the LFB are predominantly ipsilateral, many connections of the MFB are bilateral. For ease of comparison, only the side of the brain ipsilateral to the HRP injection is illustrated. HRP-filled cells are indicated by open circles, axons and terminal fields by shading or broken lines. Arrow indicates axons of the anterior commissure. Sections from the mfb-injected animal (FBS-123) and the lfb-injected animal (FBS-113) are from comparable levels, as indicated on the schematic dorsal view of the brain. Damage from needle tip, indicating injection sites, is labeled X. apl, Amygdala, pars lateralis; apm, amygdala, pars medialis; bn, bed nucleus of the pallial commissure; dp, dorsal pallium; lp, lateral pallium; ls, lateral septum; mp, medial pallium; ms, medial septum; oc, optic chiasm; pc, posterocentral nucleus; pl, posterolateral nucleus; S, striatum. Figure after Kicliter (1979).

area (Fig. 20B,C,D). It thus appears that both of these groups project to the region of pars lateralis of the amygdala.

2. Medial Forebrain Bundle Afferents

Injections of HRP into the medial forebrain bundle reveal both telencephalic afferents and efferents, as do injections into the lfb. In contrast to lfb connections, the mfb connections revealed are bilateral. Figure 18 shows outline drawings of a series of transverse hemisections through the brain of a *Rana pipiens* which sustained a double injection of the mfb. Only the side of the brain ipsilateral to the injection is illustrated, but all of the afferents revealed were labeled bilaterally. The label was more dense ipsilaterally, however. In the thalamus a group of labeled cells was located at the anterior extent of the posterocentral nucleus (Figs. 18G and 22). Locations of labeled cells within the posterocentral nucleus are, for the most part, different from the locations of cells in the posterocentral nucleus labeled after lfb injections. HRP studies also indicate that diencephalic afferents to the mfb are provided by the ventral thalamus and the preoptic area. Neary and Wilczynski (1977*a*) reported projections of the hypothalamus to the septum and pars medialis of the amygdala.

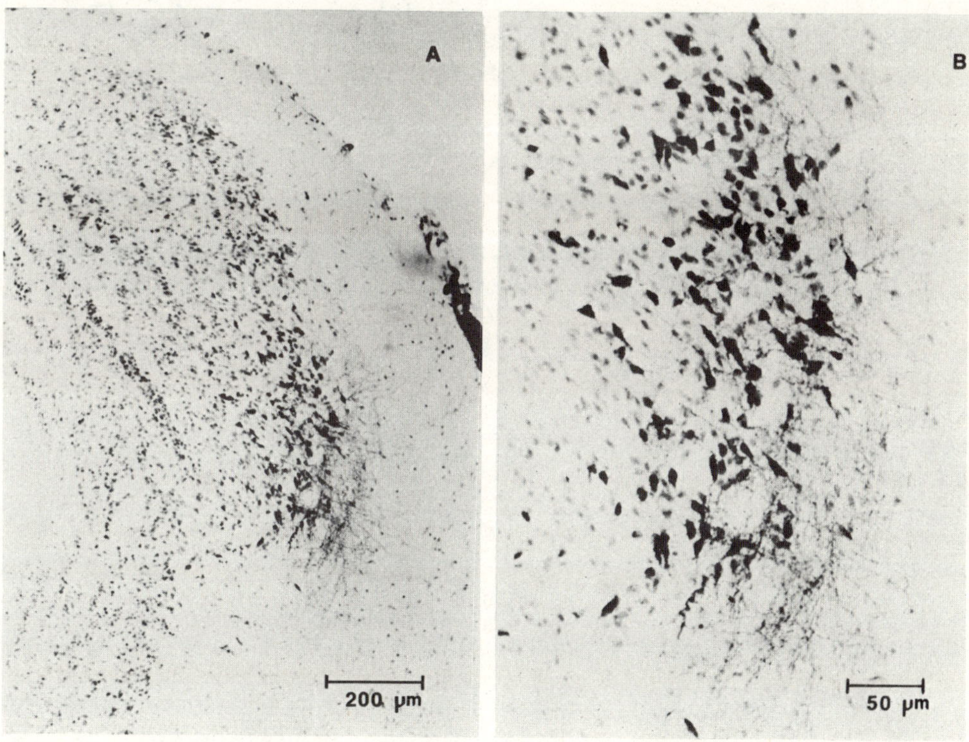

Figure 19. A: Photomicrographs of cells in the posterolateral nucleus filled with precipitate after HRP injection of the lateral forebrain bundle (FBS-113). Level of section is just anterior to section g in Fig. 18. B: Posterolateral cells at higher magnification showing their dendritic arborizations and their axons passing toward the lateral forebrain bundle. Figure after Kicliter (1979).

Medial forebrain bundle injections reveal a bilateral projection from a group of cells near the midline of the rostral medulla and mesencephalon (Fig. 181). Axons of these cells, as well as those of diencephalic afferents, appear to decussate in the anterior commissure; crossing axons were not observed at more caudal levels of the brain.

C. Ultrastructure of the Ascending Afferents

To date, only the lfb afferents have been investigated with ultrastructural methods (Kicliter and Kosaras, 1977). The lfb is composed of axons ranging in size from less than 1 μm to more than 6 μm. The larger fibers are usually myelinated. Both myelinated and unmyelinated fibers degenerate after dorsal thalamic lesions. Degenerating fibers are present throughout the lfb—both at the dien-telencephalic junction and further rostrally in the striatum—and do not appear to be concentrated in a specific portion of the bundle. Where synapses are observed with a

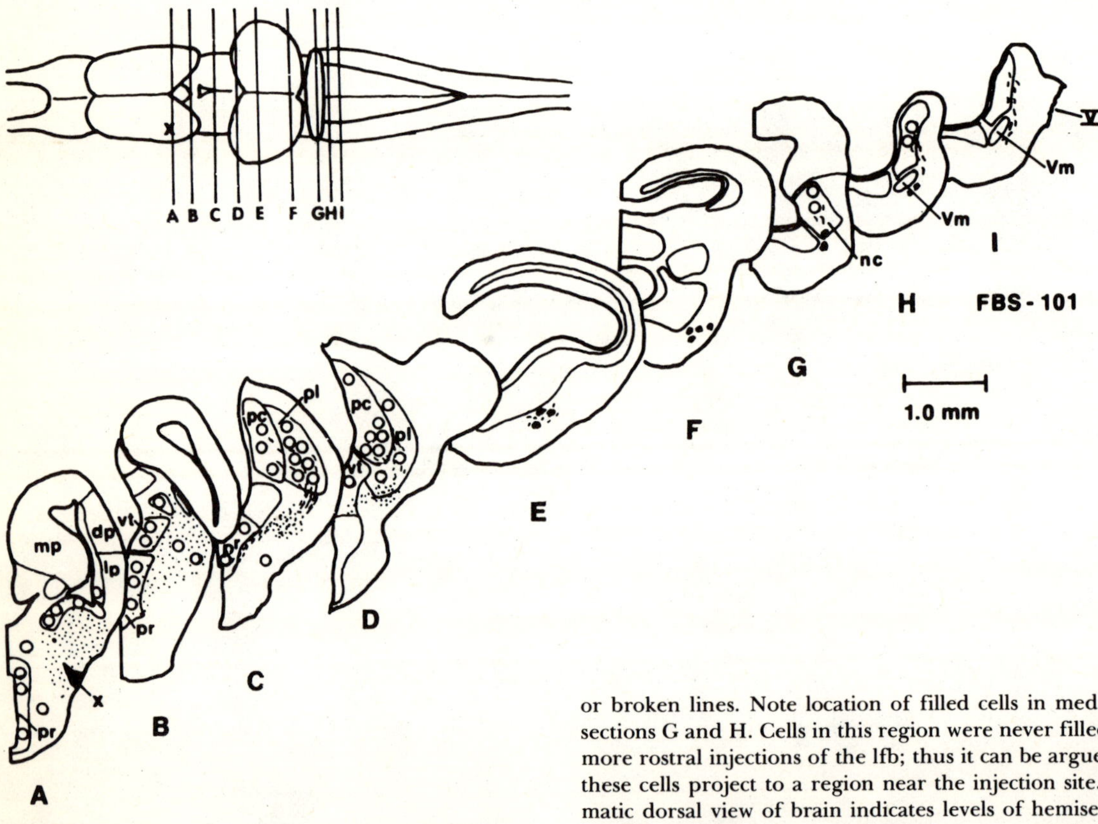

Figure 20. A: Series of hemisections illustrating connections of the lateral forebrain bundle after HRP injection into the region of pars lateralis of the amygdala. X marks needle damage made during injection indicated in section A. Labeled cells are indicated by circles, fibers by shading or broken lines. Note location of filled cells in medulla in sections G and H. Cells in this region were never filled after more rostral injections of the lfb; thus it can be argued that these cells project to a region near the injection site. Schematic dorsal view of brain indicates levels of hemisections. dp, Dorsal pallium; lp, lateral pallium; mp, medial pallium; nc, nucleus cerebelli; pc, posterocentral nucleus; pl, posterolateral nucleus; pr, preoptic area; V, trigeminal nerve; Vm, motor nucleus of the trigeminal; vt, ventral thalamus. Figure after Kicliter (1979).

degenerating presynaptic element, the predominant synaptic specialization is axodendritic (AD). A few axosomatic synapses with a degenerating presynaptic element are observed in the rostral striatum. The AD synapses are observed on both dendritic spines and dendritic shafts. These data correlate well with predictions made from light microscopic observations. The lfb afferents terminate in a region containing the radiating dendrites of striatal cells (Hoffman, 1963; Clairambault and Derer, 1968; Kicliter and Ebbesson, 1976); thus a predominance of AD synaptic specializations would be expected.

D. Other Ascending Afferents: A Quintofrontal Tract in Amphibians?

In addition to ascending thalamic afferents, the caudal lateral wall of the telencephalon, that region near the pars lateralis of the amygdala, receives ascending afferents from the ventral thalamus and preoptic area and from a cell group in the medulla. The latter projection may be homologous to the quintofrontal tract of birds (Cohen and Karten, 1974), which arises from cells of the principal sensory trigeminal nucleus and projects without synapse to the nucleus basalis in the telencephalon. Cohen and Karten (1974) proposed that this cell group in birds is homologous to the ventroposteromedial nucleus of mammals. As the amphibian

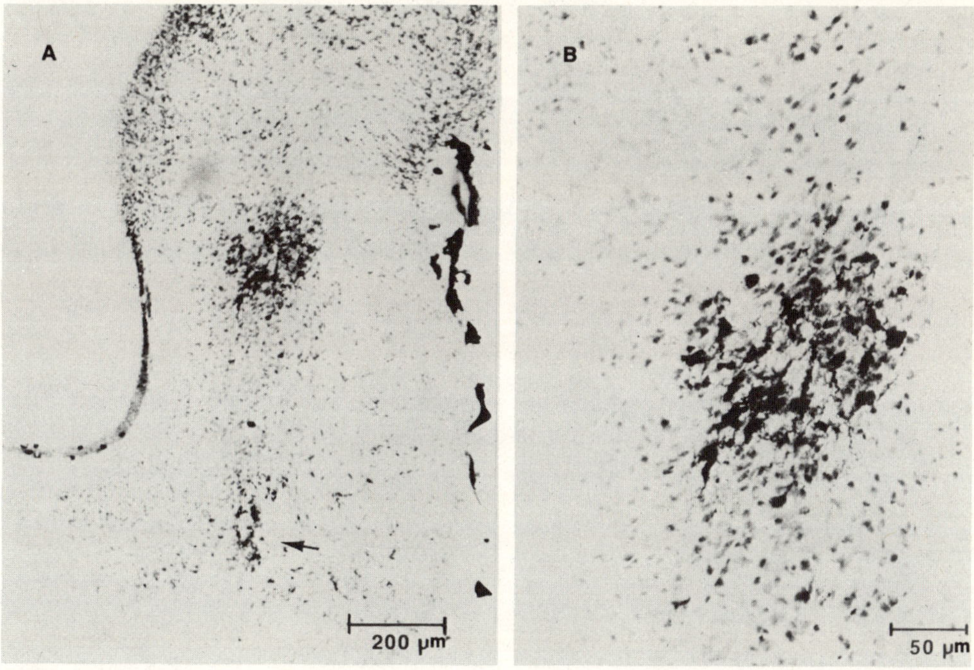

Figure 21. A: Photomicrograph of cells in medulla filled with precipitate after HRP injection into the lateral forebrain bundle in the region of pars lateralis of the amygdala. This is the same subject whose brain is illustrated in Fig. 20, and the level corresponds to section H, Fig. 20. Note lfb fibers (arrow) below labeled cells. B: Photomicrograph of these cells at higher magnification. Figure after Kicliter (1979).

medullary cells are located in a position to receive trigeminal afferents, their projection to the telencephalon may represent an amphibian quintofrontal tract.

E. Functional Significance of Telencephalic Afferents

The results of stimulation, ablation, and recording experiments in the telencephalon of amphibians have been recently reviewed (Kicliter and Ebbesson, 1976). Ascending afferents related to vision, audition, and somatic sensation have been localized in the telencephalon. Visually evoked potentials and visually driven units have been found in the medial telencephalic wall (Karamian *et al.*, 1966; Vesselkin *et al.*, 1971; Liege and Galand, 1972). Evoked potential latencies for electrical stimulation of the optic nerve are around 60 msec and thus are rather long to be consistent with a retino-thalamo-telencephalic pathway. However, nothing is known regarding the conduction time of thalamo-telencephalic axons or of the time required to generate an action potential in the thalamic cells after stimulation of retinal afferents.

The medial telencephalic wall also receives auditory and somatosensory affer-

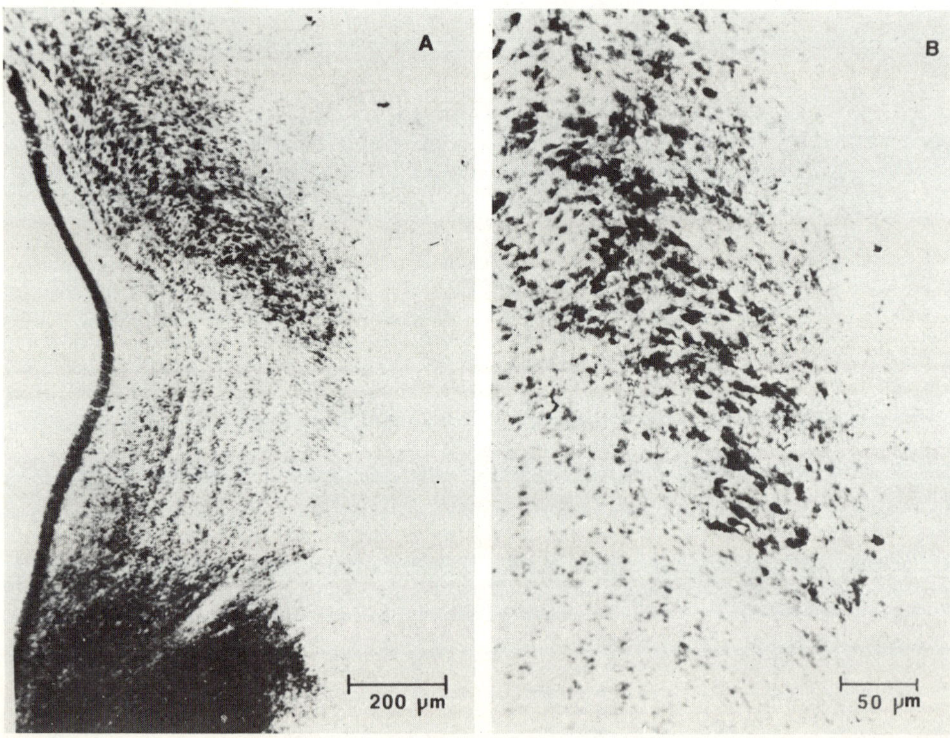

Figure 22. A: Cells in the anterior portion of the posterocentral nucleus filled with precipitate after HRP injections of the medial forebrain bundle. This subject (FBS-123) is illustrated in Fig. 18, and the level is just anterior to section G, Fig. 18. Heavy precipitate in mfb fibers is visible at the bottom of the figure. B: Photomicrograph, at higher magnification, of cells shown in A. Figure after Kicliter (1979).

ents (Karamian *et al.*, 1966; Northcutt, 1970). The middle portion of the thalamic nucleus posterocentralis is known to receive a projection from the torus semicircularis (Neary, 1974) and projects to the ipsilateral striatum. Thus the cells of the striatum may receive auditory as well as visual input. However, a thalamic cell group relaying auditory input to the medial telencephalic wall has not been identified anatomically.

The anterior portion of the thalamic nucleus posterocentralis receives an ascending projection from the obex region of the medulla (Neary and Wilczynski, 1977*b*). This projection is likely somatosensory in nature, and the anterior posterocentral nucleus is known to project to the medial pallium—thus possibly accounting for the somatosensory afferents recorded in this region.

The lateral forebrain bundle also carries visual afferents to the striatum and, perhaps, to pars lateralis of the amygdala (Gruberg and Ambros, 1974). The response characteristics of these afferents have not been delineated, and they are so complex (Gruberg and Ambros, 1974) that characterization will be difficult. Further comparative neurophysiological studies are needed to complement recent anatomical data.

VI. Some Intratelencephalic Connections in Amphibians

Intratelencephalic connections, excluding olfactory connections, have been studied with anterograde degeneration and horseradish peroxidase (HRP) techniques (Halpern *et al.*, 1968; Halpern, 1972; Kokoros, 1973; Kokoros and Northcutt, 1977; Kicliter, 1979). Both associative and commissural connections have been reported. The following discussion will be divided between pallial and subpallial projections. Intratelencephalic connections are presented schematically in Fig. 23.

A. Projections of the Pallium

Associative interpallial connections have been reported from dorsal pallium (as defined here) to ipsilateral medial pallium (Halpern, 1972; Kokoros, 1973; Kokoros and Northcutt, 1977; Kicliter, 1979). Lesions of the dorsal pallium produce degeneration in the medial pallium, and HRP injections of the medial pallium label most of the cells in the dorsal pallium. The dorsal pallium also projects to the dorsal portion of the septum (Halpern, 1972; Kokoros, 1973), and this projection appears to be topographically organized (Halpern, 1972).

The medial pallium has the most extensive intrinsic projections of any portion of the pallium. It projects massively throughout the ipsilateral septum, less densely to the contralateral septum, and to the ipsilateral postolfactory eminence (Halpern, 1972; Kokoros, 1973). The medial pallium also projects bilaterally to the bed nucleus of the pallial commissure (Kicliter, 1979).

Whether the medial pallium possesses commissural projections has been a subject of debate (Halpern *et al.*, 1968; Halpern, 1972; Kokoros, 1973; Kokoros and Northcutt, 1977; Scalia, 1976*a*). Such projections have been demonstrated in *Ambystoma, Rana,* and *Bufo* and thus would appear to be a general feature of amphibian telencephalic organization. Early failures to demonstrate the commissural projection are difficult to explain but may have resulted from the histochemical characteristics of these axons or their small size (Scalia, 1976*a*). The medial pallium itself also has intrinsic connections with other regions of the medial pallium (Halpern, 1972; Kokoros, 1973).

B. Projections of the Subpallium

Of the various subpallial nuclei, the striatal complex appears to have no projections to other telencephalic structures, whereas the nuclei of the medial wall have extensive intratelencephalic connections. Halpern (1972) reported a commissural projection of the striatum to the striatum of the opposite hemisphere—apparently connecting homologous regions of the striata. Injections of the lateral forebrain bundle with HRP did not reveal such a projection, though labeled axons were traced into the anterior commissure (Kicliter, 1979). Injections of HRP into the septum label most cells in pars medialis of the amygdala, and an extensive terminal field there is apparent. The septum also projects to the contralateral septum (Halpern, 1972; Kokoros, 1973; Kokoros and Northcutt, 1977; Kicliter, 1979). Injections of the medial pallium reveal labeled cells in the septum, thus

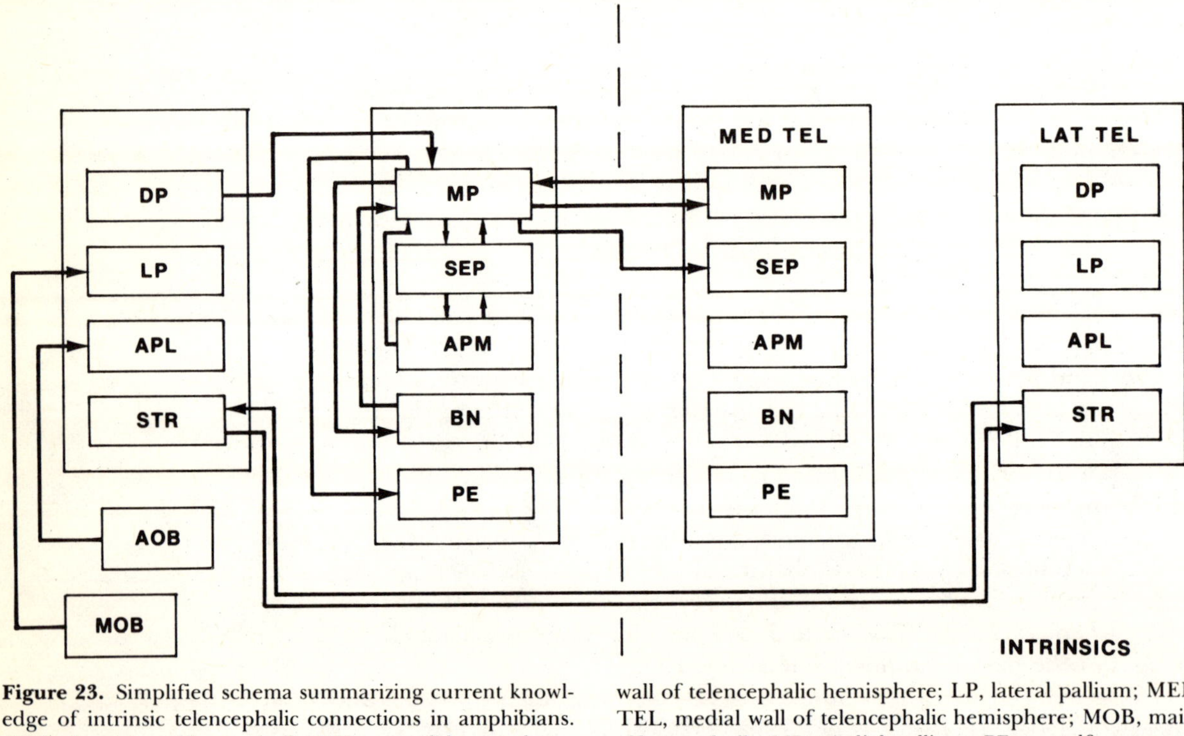

Figure 23. Simplified schema summarizing current knowledge of intrinsic telencephalic connections in amphibians. AOB, Accessory olfactory bulb; APL, amygdala, pars lateralis; APM, amygdala, pars medialis; BN, bed nucleus of the pallial commissure; DP, dorsal pallium; LAT TEL, lateral wall of telencephalic hemisphere; LP, lateral pallium; MED TEL, medial wall of telencephalic hemisphere; MOB, main olfactory bulb; MP, medial pallium; PE, postolfactory eminence; SEP, septum; STR, striatum.

indicating a septo-medial pallial projection. Finally, the bed nucleus of the pallial commissure has a reciprocal connection with the medial pallium, although it has not been determined if the bed nucleus connects with all portions of medial pallium or only with the caudal portion (Kicliter, 1979).

Intrinsic connections of the telencephalon clarify some features of telencephalic organization in amphibians. First, the telencephalon (at least in *Rana*) lacks the extensive secondary and tertiary olfactory association tracts once believed to exist. Second, the medial pallium resembles the hippocampus in its intrinsic telencephalic connections. A commissural connection, as well as a precommissural projection to septum and postolfactory eminence, has been demonstrated. The data on intrinsic connections complement earlier observations on the topography of this region, as well as the cytology and histochemistry. Third, data on the septum and amygdala, pars medialis, indicate that these two regions are reciprocally connected.

VII. Telencephalic Efferents

Data on telencephalic efferents are far scantier than on ascending afferents (see Fig. 24). The regional sources of telencephalic efferents in amphibians can be reviewed, but cellular sources have not been firmly established. The next few years should see more precise localization of the origins of telencephalic efferents as new experimental neuroanatomical techniques are applied to this problem.

Three major telencephalic efferent systems are characteristic of amphibians: the stria medullaris, the medial forebrain bundle, and the lateral forebrain bundle. The stria medullaris will not be discussed, as it appears to convey olfactory afferents destined for the habenula or crossing in the habenular commissure. These connections have been discussed above (see Section IV.B). The forebrain bundles carry descending as well as ascending fibers. As with the ascending afferents, the descending connections of the medial telencephalic wall are conveyed by the medial forebrain bundle, while the descending connections of the striatum and amygdala, pars lateralis, are carried in the lateral forebrain bundle.

There is some question whether telencephalic efferents arise from the medial pallium in all anurans. Halpern (1972) reported that the medial pallium in *Rana* does not project outside the telencephalon. However, Kokoros (1973) reported that the medial pallium in *Bufo* projects to the anterior dorsal thalamus, the ventral thalamus and the hypothalamus.

Lateral forebrain bundle efferents distribute ipsilaterally to dorsal and ventral thalamic nuclei and to the hypothalamus. Passing caudally, the lfb may project to cell groups in the mesencephalic tegmentum and medulla before terminating in the cervical segments of the spinal cord. Halpern (1972) reported that lesions confined to the striatum produced degeneration in the lateral forebrain bundle as far caudally as the mesencephalic tegmentum. This projection appears similar to pallidotegmental projections in mammals and birds (Nauta and Mehler, 1966; Karten and Dubbeldam, 1973). No distribution to thalamic groups was evident when the lesion was confined to the striatum. In contrast, when the lesion included the amygdala, pars lateralis, in the caudal telencephalon, projections to the posterocentral and posterolateral nuclei in the dorsal thalamus, and to the ventral thalamus, were observed (Halpern, 1972). The latter projections also resemble portions of pallidofugal projections in mammals. Kokoros (1973) confirmed these observations in *Bufo* and also reported a projection from the caudal telencephalon to the hypothalamus. This projection may correspond to the amygdalo-hypothalamic projection of the pars lateralis of the amygdala, which was also reported by Scalia (1976*a*).

A projection of the lateral forebrain bundle to upper cervical levels of the spinal cord has been reported in *Bufo* (Kokoros, 1973) and in *Ambystoma* (Kokoros and Northcutt, 1977). This projection was demonstrated only after hemispherectomies and is believed to arise from the caudal ventrolateral telencephalic wall. The projection travels ipsilaterally to the cord, and reportedly resembles corticobulbar and corticospinal tracts in mammals. Again, the application of retrograde techniques should provide more precise information on the origin(s) of this projection.

A projection from the telencephalon to the optic tectum appears to be lacking in anurans (Halpern, 1972; Kokoros, 1973), although such a projection does exist in urodeles (Kokoros and Northcutt, 1977).

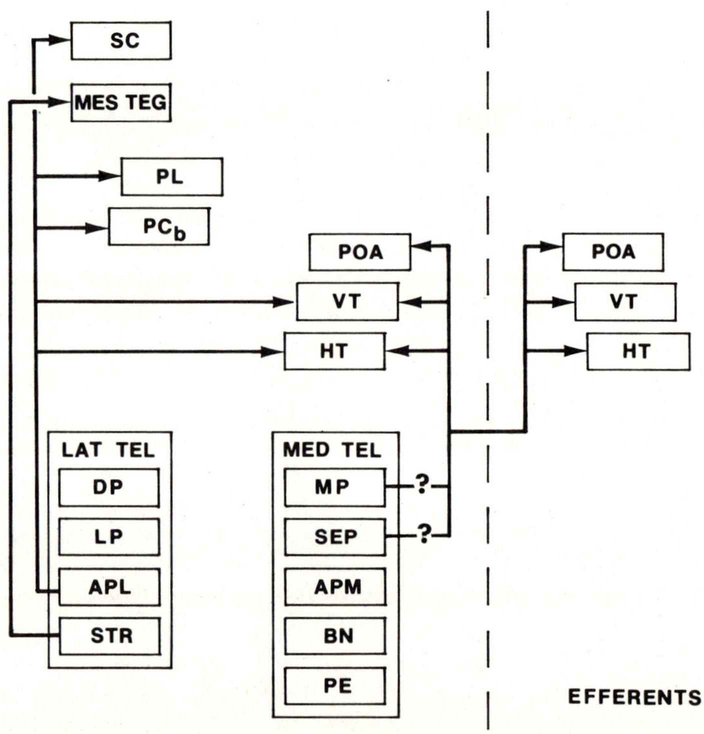

Figure 24. Simplified schema summarizing current knowledge of amphibian telencephalic efferents. APL, Amygdala, pars lateralis; APM, amygdala, pars medialis; BN, bed nucleus of the pallial commissure; DP, dorsal pallium; HT, hypothalamus; LAT TEL, lateral wall of the telencephalic hemisphere; LP, lateral pallium; MED TEL, medial wall of telencephalic hemisphere; MES TEG, mesencephalic tegmentum; MP, medial pallium; PC$_b$, that portion of PC which provides afferents to the lateral telencephalic wall; PE, postolfactory eminence; PL, posterolateral nucleus; POA, preoptic area; SC, spinal cord; SEP, septum; STR, striatum; VT, ventral thalamus.

VIII. Amphibian Telencephalic Organization

A. Telencephalic Organizational Pattern

In 1948, Herrick characterized the telencephalon of amphibians as a simple, unspecialized web of tissue that progressively elaborated in more advanced tetrapods. He believed that essentially the entire telencephalon received secondary or tertiary olfactory connections and that nonolfactory impulses reached striatal levels only after synapse in the dorsal thalamus. He further envisioned telencephalic efferents carrying primarily olfactory information to only hypothalamic or midbrain levels, to be integrated there with ascending gustatory information.

Thirty years later, after intensive testing of these hypotheses with increasingly sensitive experimental methods, a very different picture of amphibian telencephalic organization is emerging. Experimental studies have revealed the secondary olfactory projections to be far more limited than Herrick supposed, and, more importantly, we have begun to realize that two separate chemoreceptor systems—olfactory and vomeronasal—exist with separate pathways within the telencephalon. We have also discovered that the main telencephalic target of olfactory input—the lateral pallium—apparently does not possess direct connections with the hypothalamus and tegmentum but rather projects within the telencephalon to the medial pallium. Again we have been surprised, for the medial pallium is not a simple olfactory precursor of the mammalian hippocampus; instead, in amphibians it receives direct thalamic projections carrying visual and somatic information after relay in the dorsal thalamus. A picture seems to be emerging in which the amphibian medial pallium is a major multimodal target of ascending information, as well as being the sole output of the pallium, with the exception of the pars lateralis of the amygdala.

Herrick's hypothesis that dorsal thalamic pathways exist to the striatum has been experimentally confirmed; we now possess evidence that both visual and auditory information reaches the striatum from dorsal thalamic centers. However, the kind of visual and auditory information reaching the striatum and the utilization of this information remain mysteries. Experimental data on the primary striatal efferents do not particularly clarify the matter. We now know that these efferents are similar to the strio-nigral and pallidotegmental projections in other tetrapods, but the first pathway appears to be part of a feedback loop, and nothing is known about further connections of the second system. However, recent mammalian studies on connections of the substantia nigra with the superior colliculus raise the interesting possibility that the amphibian striatum may be linked with the tectum—a brain region mediating many orientation and recognition behaviors in amphibians.

There are still large gaps in our understanding of amphibian telencephalic organization. We know that the pars lateralis of the amygdala is the major, if not sole, target of information from the vomeronasal organ, but we still know virtually nothing regarding the sensory parameters of this organ.

Projections of the pars lateralis to the hypothalamus and caudal dorsal thalamus have been reported. Both of these areas project to different parts of the optic tectum. Again, this suggests the possibility that information from the vomeronasal organ may strongly affect tectal functions related to prey approach or avoidance behaviors. There are other amphibian telencephalic regions about which we are woefully ignorant. What is the nature of the ascending thalamic projections to the dorsal pallium? Does the lateral pallium receive other afferent sources? While these are anatomical questions, they raise a plethora of functional and behavioral questions which have yet to be answered.

B. Comparisons with Other Vertebrates

1. Anamniotic Comparisons

Amphibians possess small brains whose telencephalons can be characterized by a roof in which the medial pallium is hypertrophied and frequently marked by pronounced cellular migrations. The remaining portions of the pallium are characterized by periventricular cellular plates with little or no cellular migration. The striatum is well developed and receives ascending thalamic inputs as do the dorsal and medial pallial formations. When the telencephalon of amphibians is compared to the telencephalon of other tetrapods (Fig. 25), we are struck by the increased size and extensive cellular migrations that characterize amniotic telencephalons. However, we frequently forget that amphibians are the only anamniotes that have invaded a terrestrial ecosystem with even moderate success.

How does the telencephalon of amphibians compare to the telencephalon of other anamniotes? Recent data on brain–body ratios of amphibians and the sole living crossopterygian fish, *Latimeria,* reveal that both the brain–body ratio and the telencephalon–body ratio of amphibians and *Latimeria* are almost identical (Northcutt *et al.,* 1978). Further comparisons with *Ectosteorhachis,* a fossil rhipidistian and member of the group that gave rise to amphibians, reveal brain–body ratios (Jerison, 1973) similar to those of living amphibians and *Latimeria.* Thus the brains of modern amphibians are small, but they fall within the range of other closely related anamniotes and fossil crossopterygians.

Two additional groups of anamniotes possess similar telencephalic patterns—the polypteriform fishes and the most primitive living sharks (hexanchiforms and

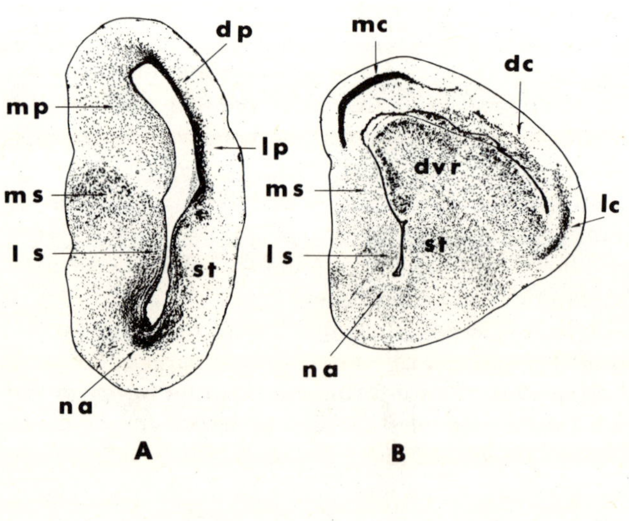

Figure 25. Representative transverse sections through the left telencephalic hemisphere of an amphibian, *Rana* (A), and a reptile, *Gekko* (B), illustrating differences in the development of the lateral hemispheric wall and the migration of neuronal populations from a periventricular position. dc, Dorsal cortex, dp, dorsal pallium; dvr, dorsal ventricular ridge; lc, lateral cortex; lp, lateral pallium; ls, lateral septum; mc, medial cortex; mp, medial pallium; ms, medial septum; na, nucleus accumbens; st, striatum. Figure after Northcutt and Royce (1975).

squaliforms). The polypteriform fishes are represented by two genera (*Polypterus* and *Erpetoichthys*) and are generally considered to be the most primitive living bony fishes. The telencephalon of *Polypterus,* although formed by an eversion process rather than by evagination as in amphibians, is remarkably similar to that of amphibians (see Chapter 3 of this volume). The pallium of *Polypterus* consists of a thin wall whose neurons do not migrate and thus form thick periventricular plates or sheets as in amphibians. The pallium of *Polypterus* is also divided into three components; the lateral component receives olfactory projections, whereas the dorsal and medial components receive nonolfactory ascending projections.

Finally, the pattern of telencephalic development in hexanchiform and squaliform sharks is remarkably similar to that of amphibians, as first noted by Johnston (1911). These sharks possess thin telencephalic walls with well-developed lateral ventricles. The pallial wall is characterized by a densely packed periventricular cellular plate and a more superficial zone with more scattered cells. The medial pallium is hypertrophied and is 3–4 times as thick as the remaining pallial formations (Northcutt, 1977, 1978).

Experimental neuroanatomical studies on the telencephalon of these sharks do not yet exist, but we do know that the advanced sharks are also characterized by restricted olfactory projections to the telencephalon, and that they possess ascending thalamo-telencephalic projections (Ebbesson, 1972).

All these data strongly suggest that the telencephalon of amphibians is not degenerate (i.e., secondarily simple) but that the amphibian pattern of telencephalic organization is characteristic of a primitive anamniotic level of telencephalic organization that repeatedly produced advanced forms in which the telencephalon underwent pallial hypertrophy and differentiation. This trend can now be documented for elasmobranchs (Northcutt, 1977, 1978), and bony fishes (see Chapter 3 of this volume), as well as the classic cases of birds and mammals.

2. Comparisons with Other Tetrapods

The amphibian–reptilian transition marks the beginning of a major adaptive radiation in vertebrate phylogeny. The emergence of reptiles correlates with striking morphological changes in the telencephalon (Fig. 25). The most striking difference among the telencephalons of amphibians, reptiles, and birds is the elaborate dorsal ventricular ridge. The ridge forms embryonically by a proliferation of the lateral pallial wall (Johnston, 1916; Källén, 1962). This proliferation almost obliterates the lateral ventricle and results in a mass of neural tissue with a variable number of distinct cytological fields. Despite this variability, all amniotic taxa examined experimentally possess a dorsal ventricular ridge whose rostral portion receives auditory and visual projections via the dorsal thalamus. In lizards and snakes a caudal portion of the dorsal ventricular ridge—nucleus sphericus—is the primary target of the accessory bulb. Does the telencephalon of amphibians possess a nueronal field homologous to the sauropsid dorsal ventricular ridge? If so, what is its topographical position and what are its connections?

If the telencephalon of modern amphibians is comparable to that of ancestral amphibians that gave rise to reptiles, two possibilities should be considered: (1) the dorsal ventricular ridge arose by migration of cells from the striatum; (2) the ridge arose by migration of cells from the lateral pallium.

At present, three lines of evidence suggest that the reptilian dorsal ventricular ridge is homologous to a field of cells in the amphibian lateral pallium: (1) similarities in the histochemistry of the anuran lateral pallium and the reptilian dorsal ventricular ridge, (2) cellular continuity of the anuran pars lateralis of the amygdala with the lateral pallium and the probable homology of the anuran pars lateralis with the reptilian nucleus sphericus, and (3) embryological evidence in reptiles that the lateral pallium and dorsal ventricular ridge represent subsequent migrations of the same matrix zone.

In both amphibians and reptiles the areas labeled as striatum in Fig. 25 contain high concentrations of acetylcholinesterase and biogenic monoamines, whereas neither the anuran lateral pallium nor reptilian dorsal ventricular ridge demonstrates such concentrations (Shen *et al.,* 1955; Braak, 1970; Parent and Olivier, 1970; Kusunoki, 1971; Parent, 1971, 1973; Northcutt, 1974).

In amphibians the accessory olfactory bulb projects to the pars lateralis of the amygdala and in reptiles to nucleus sphericus. It seems probable that these two nuclei are homologous as they both possess similar topographical positions within the telencephalon and both are the primary, if not sole, targets of the accessory olfactory bulb.

Recent studies on the embryogenesis of the reptilian telencephalon suggest that the lateral pallium forms by a migration of neuroblasts from a periventricular position in the dorsolateral hemispheric wall and that the remaining neuroblasts differentiate *in situ* to form the dorsal ventricular ridge (Källén, 1951*c*; Kirsche, 1972).

The most parsimonious interpretation is that the anuran lateral pallium and pars lateralis of the amygdala are field homologues of the reptilian dorsal ventricular ridge and lateral cortex. If this interpretation is correct, the amphibian–reptilian transition was marked by a shift of the ascending thalamic projections from a primary subpallial to a primary pallial target (the dorsal ventricular ridge) with retention of the subpallial (striatal) projection. We know that the sauropsid dorsal ventricular ridge input is segregated so that different regions of the ridge receive a single sensory modality. We know that several different modalities converge on the amphibian striatum, but we do not know if the striatal cells are multimodal. If these striatal cells are revealed to be multimodal, the amphibian–reptilian transition may also have been characterized by the evolution of new telencephalic cells.

A third possibility is that ancestral amphibians possessed a distinct dorsal ventricular ridge that was lost in modern amphibians. This interpretation will be indicated only if evidence emerges that the telencephalon of modern amphibians exhibits regressive tendencies, rather than retaining a large number of primitive tetrapod characters. Comparisons with bony fishes and sharks that retain the largest numbers of primitive telencephalic characters do not support an hypothesis of regressive telencephalic organization in modern amphibians (see Section VIII.B.1).

Demonstration of two telencephalic visual projections in amphibians allows us to compare amphibian telencephalic visual organization with that of birds and reptiles (sauropsids). Two telencephalic visual systems have also been identified in sauropsids (Fig. 26). The first, a retino-thalamo-telencephalic system, involves the lateral geniculate nucleus (reptiles, Hall and Ebner, 1970) or the lateral part of nucleus dorsolateralis anterior (birds, Karten and Nauta, 1968). This nucleus projects via the lateral forebrain bundle in the lateral wall of the hemisphere to the dorsal pallium (Hall and Ebner, 1970; Revzin, 1969; Karten *et al.,* 1973). The second, a retino-tecto-thalamo-telencephalic system, involves projection of the retina onto the optic tectum, which projects to nucleus rotundus in the thalamus (Karten and Revzin, 1966; Hall and Ebner, 1970). Nucleus rotundus, in turn, projects to ectostriatum in birds (Karten and Hodos, 1970) or dorsal ventricular ridge in reptiles (Hall and Ebner, 1970; Pritz, 1975). This second system also traverses the lateral forebrain bundle and the lateral telencephalic wall to reach its target and—in addition—provides collaterals to the striatum (Hall and Ebner, 1970).

Characteristics of sauropsid telencephalic visual systems provide criteria for proposing homologous systems in amphibians. The first system (retino-thalamo-telencephalic) should have the following characteristics:

1. The projection must be composed of the axons of thalamic cells which receive a direct projection from the retina.
2. The system must traverse the lateral forebrain bundle and the lateral wall of the telencephalon.
3. The system must terminate on a group of cells homologous to those of the sauropsid dorsal pallium.

The second system (retino-tecto-thalamo-telencephalic) must have the following

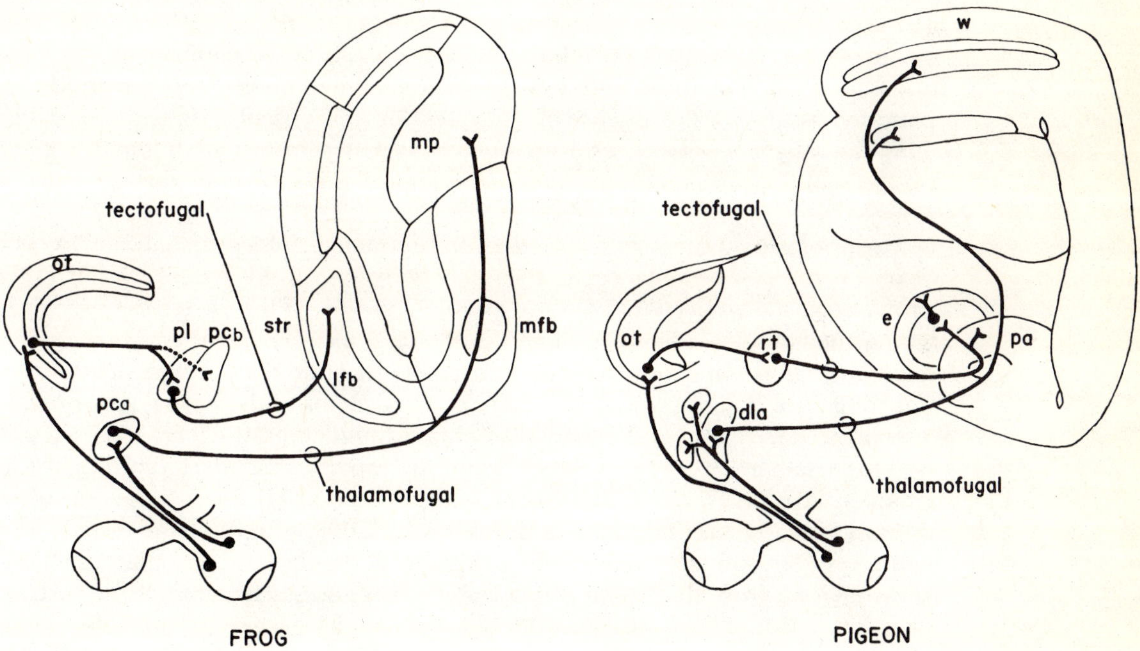

Figure 26. Comparison of thalamofugal and tectofugal visual systems in a frog (*Rana*) and a bird (*Columba livia*). Similarities and differences between the projections in the two species are described in text. dla, Anterior dorsolateral nucleus; e, ectostriatum; lfb, lateral forebrain bundle; mfb, medial forebrain bundle; mp, medial pallium; ot, optic tectum; pa, paleostriatum; pc_a, anterior posterocentral nucleus; pc_b, middle posterocentral nucleus; pl, posterolateral nucleus; rt, nucleus rotundus; str, striatum; w, wulst.

characteristics:

1. The projection must be composed of the axons of thalamic cells which receive a direct projection from the optic tectum, but not a direct retinal projection.
2. The system must traverse the lateral forebrain bundle and the lateral wall of the telencephalon.
3. The system must terminate on a group of cells homologous to those of sauropsid ectostriatum or dorsal ventricular ridge, and must provide collateral afferents to the striatum.
4. The striatum and DVR must be contiguous topologically.

If these criteria are rigidly applied, one must conclude that neither of the sauropsid systems is represented in amphibians. However, the amphibian retino-tecto-thalamo-telencephalic system comes closest to meeting the criteria. The optic tectum in *Rana* projects to a region of lateral thalamic neuropil which does not receive direct retinal projections (Rubinson, 1968; Lázár, 1969). The cells post-synaptic to this neuropil are located in the posterolateral nucleus and in portions of the posterocentral nucleus (Scalia and Gregory, 1970). These posterocentral/posterolateral cells project to the striatum via the lateral forebrain bundle. Thus these projections meet the criteria for the second system in terms of synaptic relays in tectum and thalamus. The projection travels to the telencephalon via the lateral forebrain bundle and terminates exclusively in a portion of the telencephalon which histochemically and topologically resembles the sauropsid striatum (Northcutt, 1974).

However, the retino-tecto-thalamo-telencephalic visual pathway in amphibians does not meet the third and fourth criteria of a homologous sauropsid visual pathway, because of the absence of a distinct dorsal ventricular ridge in amphibians. This discrepancy will be resolved only by further information on the general problem of a possible amphibian homologue of the sauropsid dorsal ventricular ridge.

Amphibians also possess a retino-thalamo-telencephalic visual system, but it bears even less resemblance to the analogous sauropsid system. Scalia (1976*b*) proposed that a projection from the anterior portion of the posterocentral nucleus to the medial telencephalic wall represents a geniculo-cortical pathway in *Rana*. This projection appears to represent a retino-thalamo-telencephalic pathway terminating in a pallial region, but there are problems with Scalia's interpretation. The projection traverses the medial forebrain bundle and the medial telencephalic wall to terminate in a region which, in most respects, resembles the hippocampal complex of reptiles, birds, and mammals (see Section III.B). Another problem is that whereas some cells in the anterior portion of the posterocentral nucleus supply dendrites to the anterior thalamic neuropil, most dendrites in the anterior thalamic neuropil arise from the lateral geniculate nucleus and nucleus rotundus (Scalia and Gregory, 1970). The projections of these latter nuclei have not been determined. At present it seems premature to claim that the posterocentral-medial pallial system is homologous to the geniculo-cortical pathway of amniotes.

Acknowledgments. Preparation of the manuscript and unpublished research cited here were supported, in part, by NIH Grants R01-NS11006 to R. G. N. and

R01-EY02500 to E. K. and by NSF Grant GB-40134 to R. G. N. We thank Linda Hanna, Nancy Mathews, and Mary Sue Northcutt for technical assistance, Donald Luce for preparation of some of the illustrations, and Neima Lacomba for secretarial assistance. We appreciate the helpful comments of Dr. Boyd Campbell on an earlier version of the manuscript. The Wistar Press kindly gave permission for reproduction of Figs. 2–7, 13, 15, 16, 18–22, and 25.

IX. References

Ariëns Kappers, C. U., Huber, G. C., and Crosby, E. C., 1936, *The Comparative Anatomy of the Nervous System of Vertebrates, Including Man,* reprinted 1960, Hafner, New York.

Baroz, C., Bauchot, R., and Clairambault, P., 1969, Étude architecturale du prosencéphale de *Nectophrynoides occidentalis* Angel, *J. Hirnforsch.* **11:**227.

Braak, H., 1970, Biogene Amine im Gehirn vom Frosch (*Rana esculenta*), *Z. Zellforsch.* **106:**269.

Broadwell, R. D., 1975, Olfactory relationships of the telencephalon and diencephalon in the rabbit. I. An autoradiographic study of the efferent connections of the main and accessory olfactory bulbs, *J. Comp. Neurol.* **163:**329.

Campbell, C. B. G., and Boord, R. L., 1974, Central auditory pathways of nonmammalian vertebrates, in: *Handbook of Sensory Physiology, V/1,* pp. 337–362, Springer-Verlag, Berlin.

Clairambault, P., 1967, Le complexe strio-amygdalaire des anoures, in: *Problèmes Actuels de Paléontologie* (*Évolution des Vertébrés*), pp. 281–294, Éditions du Centre National de la Recherche Scientifique, Paris.

Clairambault, P., 1968, Morphogenèse du télencéphale. Morphogenèse expérimentale du télencéphale des Ranidés, *Arch. Biol.* (*Liège*) **79:**537.

Clairambault, P., 1969, Étude architectonique du télencéphale de Rana pipiens en début de métamorphose, *J. Hirnforsch.* **11:**203.

Clairambault, P., 1976, Development of the prosencephalon, in: *Frog Neurobiology* (R. Llinás and W. Precht, eds.), pp. 924–945, Springer-Verlag, New York.

Clairambault, P., and Capanna, E., 1970, Aspetti della neuroistogenesi del Pallio telencefalico in dueRànidi, *R. C. Accad. Naz. Lincei* **48:**727.

Clairambault, P., and Derer, P., 1968, Contributions à l'étude architectonique du télencéphale des Ranidés, *J. Hirnforsch.* **10:**123.

Cohen, D. H., and Karten, H. J., 1974, The structural organization of avian brain: An overview, in *Birds, Brain and Behavior* (I. J. Goodman and M. W. Schein, eds.), pp. 29–73, Academic Press, New York.

Daval, G., Leveteau, J., and MacLeod, P., 1970, Electro-olfacto-gramme local et discrimination olfactive chez la Grenouille, *J. Physiol.* (*Paris*) **62:**477.

De Beer, G., 1958, *Embryos and Ancestors,* 3rd ed., Oxford University Press, London.

Ebbesson, S. O. E., 1972, New insights into the organization of the shark brain, *Comp. Biochem. Physiol.* **42A:**121.

Estes, R., and Reig, O. A., 1973, The early fossil record of frogs: A review of the evidence, in: *Evolutionary Biology of the Anurans* (J. L. Vial, ed.), pp. 11–63, University of Missouri Press, Columbia, Mo.

Ewert, J.-P., 1970, Neural mechanisms of prey-catching and avoidance behavior in the toad (*Bufo bufo* L.), *Brain Behav. Evol.* **3:**36.

Fish, P. A., 1895, The central nervous system of *Desmognathus fusca, J. Morphol.* **10:**231.

Fuller, P. M., and Ebbesson, S. O. E., 1973, Central projections of the trigeminal nerve in the bullfrog (*Rana catesbeiana*), *J. Comp. Neurol.* **152:**193.

Gans, C., 1970, Strategy and sequence in the evolution of the external gas exchangers of ectothermal vertebrates, *Forma Functio* **3:**61.

Gesteland, R. C., 1976, Physiology of olfactory reception, in: *Frog Neurobiology* (R. Llinás and W. Precht, eds.), pp. 234–250, Springer-Verlag, New York.

Graziadei, P., 1971, The olfactory mucosa of vertebrates, in: *Handbook of Sensory Physiology,* Vol. IV: *Chemical Senses,* Part 1: *Olfaction* (L. M. Beidler, ed.), pp. 27–58, Springer-Verlag, New York.

Graziadei, P., and DeHan, R., 1973, Neuronal regeneration in frog olfactory system, *J. Cell Biol.* **59:**525.

Graziadei, P., and Metcalf, J., 1971, Autoradiographic and ultrastructural observations on the frogs olfactory mucosa, *Z. Zellforsch.* **116:**305.

Grubb, J. C., 1973*a*, Olfactory orientation in breeding Mexican toads, *Bufo valliceps, Copeia,* **1973:**490.

Grubb, J. C., 1973*b*, Olfactory orientation in *Bufo woodhousei fowleri, Pseudacris clarki* and *Pseudacris streckeri, Anim. Behav.* **21:**726.

Gruberg, E. R., and Ambros, V. R., 1974, A forebrain visual projection in the frog (*Rana pipiens*), *Exp. Neurol.* **44:**187.

Hall, E., 1972, Some aspects of the structural organization of the amygdala, in: *The Neurobiology of the Amygdala* (B. E. Eleftheriou, ed.), pp. 95–121, Plenum Press, New York.

Hall, W. C., and Ebner, F. F., 1970, Thalamotelencephalic projections in the turtle (*Pseudemys scripta*), *J. Comp. Neurol.* **140:**101.

Halpern, M., 1972, Some connections of the telencephalon of the frog, *Rana pipiens, Brain Behav. Evol.* **6:**42.

Halpern, M., Scalia, F., and Riss, W., 1968, On the nature of the hippocampal commissure in the frog, *Brain Behav. Evol.* **1:**155.

Haslam, G., 1889, Eckers *Anatomy of the Frog* (translation, with additions), Oxford University Press, London.

Hecht, M. K., 1969, The living lower tetrapods: Their interrelationships and phylogenetic position, *Ann. N.Y. Acad. Sci.* **167:**74.

Herrick, C. J., 1910, The morphology of the forebrain in Amphibia and Reptilia, *J. Comp. Neurol.* **20:**413.

Herrick, C. J., 1921, The connections of the vomeronasal nerve, accessory olfactory bulb and amygdala in Amphibia, *J. Comp. Neurol.* **33:**213.

Herrick, C. J., 1925, The amphibian forebrain. III. The optic tracts and centers of *Amblystoma* and the frog, *J. Comp. Neurol.* **39:**433.

Herrick, C. J., 1933, The amphibian forebrain. VI. *Necturus, J. Comp. Neurol.* **58:**1.

Herrick, C. J., 1948, *The Brain of the Tiger Salamander,* University of Chicago Press, Chicago.

Hoffman, H. H., 1963, The olfactory bulb, accessory olfactory bulb, and hemisphere of some anurans, *J. Comp. Neurol.* **120:**317.

Hoffman, H. H., 1966, The structure of the forebrain of *Bufo marinus, Ala. J. Med. Sci.* **3:**286.

Hoffman, A., 1973, Stereotaxic atlas of the toad's brain, *Acta Anat.* **84:**416.

Howell, E. M., and Hoffman, H. H., 1966, The forebrain of *Hyla cinerea, Ala. J. Med. Sci.* **3:**270.

Ingle, D., 1973, Disinhibition of tectal neurons by pretectal lesions in the frog, *Science* **180:**422.

Jarvik, E., 1960, *Théories de l'Évolution des Vertébrés, Réconsidérées à la Lumière des Récentes Découvertes sur les Vertébrés Inférieurs,* Masson, Paris.

Jerison, H. J., 1973, *Evolution of the Brain and Intelligence,* Academic Press, New York.

Johnston, J. B., 1911, The telencephalon of selachians, *J. Comp. Neurol.* **21:**1.

Johnston, J. B., 1916, The development of the dorsal ventricular ridge in turtles, *J. Comp. Neurol.* **26:**481.

Källén, B., 1951*a*, The nuclear development in the mammalian forebrain with special regard to the subpallium, *K. Fysiogr. Saellsk. Foerh.* **61:**1.

Källén, B., 1951*b*, Embryological studies on the nuclei and their homologization in the vertebrate forebrain, *K. Fysiogr. Saellsk. Foerh.* **62:**1.

Källén, B., 1951*c*, On the ontogeny of the reptilian forebrain. Nuclear structures and ventricular sulci, *J. Comp. Neurol.* **95:**307.

Källén, B., 1962, Embryogensis of brain nuclei in the chick telencephalon, *Ergeb. Anat. Entwicklungsgesch.* **36:**62.

Karamian, A. I., Vesselkin, N. P., Belekhova, M. G., and Zagorulko, T. M., 1966, Electrophysiological characteristics of tectal and thalamo-cortical divisions of the visual system in lower vertebrates, *J. Comp. Neurol.* **127:**559.

Karten, H. J., and Dubbeldam, J. L., 1973, The organization and projections of the paleostriatal complex in the pigeon (*Columba livia*), *J. Comp. Neurol.* **148:**61.

Karten, H. J., and Hodos, W., 1970, Telencephalic projections of the nucleus rotundus in the pigeon (*Columba livia*), *J. Comp. Neurol.* **140:**35.

Karten, H. J., and Nauta, W. J. H., 1968, Organization of the retinothalamic projections in the pigeon and owl, *Anat. Rec.* **160:**373.

Karten, H. J., and Revzin, A. M., 1966, The afferent connections of the nucleus rotundus in the pigeon, *Brain Res.* **2:**368.

Karten, H. J., Hodos, W., Nauta, W. J. H., and Revzin, A. M., 1973, Neural connections of the "visual wulst" of the avian telencephalon. Experimental studies in the pigeon (*Columba livia*) and owl (*Speotyto cunicularia*), *J. Comp. Neurol.* **150:**253.

Kicliter, E., 1973, An anatomical connection between the anterior thalamus and the telencephalon in the frog, *Soc. Neurosci. Prog. Abstr. 3rd Meet.*, p. 410.

Kicliter, E., 1979, Some telencephalic connections in the frog, *Rana pipiens: J. Comp. Neurol.* **185:**75.

Kicliter, E., and Ebbesson, S. O. E., 1976, Organization of the "non-olfactory" telencephalon, in: *Frog Neurobiology* (R. Llinás and W. Precht, eds.), pp. 946–972, Springer-Verlag, New York.

Kicliter, E., and Kosaras, B., 1977, Ultrastructural features of the striatum and the thalamostriatal projection of ranid frogs, *Anat. Rec.* **187:**769.

Kicliter, E., and Northcutt, R. G., 1975, Ascending afferents to the telencephalon of ranid frogs: An anterograde degeneration study, *J. Comp. Neurol.* **161:**239.

Kirsche, W., 1972, Die Entwicklung des Telencephalons der Reptilien und deren Beziehung zur Hirn-Bauplanlehre, *Nova Acta Leopold.* **37:**9.

Kokoros, J. J., 1973, Efferent projections of the telencephalon in the toad (*Bufo marinus*) and tiger salamander (*Ambystoma tigrinum*), Ph.D. dissertation, Department of Anatomy, Case Western Reserve University.

Kokoros, J. J., and Northcutt, R. G., 1977, Telencephalic efferents of the tiger salamander *Ambystoma tigrinum tigrinum* (Green), *J. Comp. Neurol.* **173:**613.

Kreht, H., 1931, Über die Faserzüge im Zentralnervensystem von *Proteus anguineus* Laur, *Z. Mikrosk. Anat. Forsch.* **25:**375.

Kuhlenbeck, H., 1922, Zur Morphologie des Gymnophionengehirns, *Jen. Z. Naturwiss., Neue Folge* **51:**453.

Kuhlenbeck, H., 1953, The telencephalic zonal system of the gymnophione *Siphonops annulatus, Anat. Rec.* **115:**399.

Kuhlenbeck, H., Malewitz, T. D., and Beasley, A. B., 1967, Further observations on the morphology of the forebrain in Gymnophiona, with reference to the topologic vertebrate forebrain pattern, in: *Evolution of the Forebrain* (R. Hassler and H. Stephan, eds.), pp. 9–19, Plenum Press, New York.

Kusunoki, T., 1971, The chemoarchitectonics of the turtle brain, *Yokohama Med. Bull.* **22:**1.

Lascano, E., Segura, E. T., and Ferrario, J. A., 1971, Organización anatómica del encéfalo del *Bufo arenarum* Hensel, *Rev. Soc. Argent. Biol.* **47:**70.

LaVail, J. H., and LaVail, M. M., 1972, Retrograde axonal transport in the central nervous system, *Science* **176:**1416.

Lázár, G., 1969, Efferent pathways of the optic tectum in the frog, *Acta Biol. Acad. Sci. Hung.* **20:**171.

Liege, B., and Galand, G., 1972, Single-unit visual responses in the frog's brain, *Vision Res.* **12:**609.

Lynch, G., Gall, C., Mensah, P., and Cotman, C. N., 1974, Horseradish peroxidase histochemistry: A new method for tracing efferent projections in the central nervous system, *Brain Res.* **65:**373.

McCotter, R. E., 1917, The vomero-nasal apparatus in *Chrysemys punctata* and *Rana catesbeiana, Anat. Rec.* **13:**51.

Medvedeva, I. M., 1968, Die Homologie des Jacobsonschen Organs bei Anura und Urodela, in: *Current Problems of Lower Vertebrate Phylogeny* (T. Ørvig, ed.), pp. 331–340, Interscience, New York.

Mustaparta, H., 1971, Spatial distribution of receptor-responses to stimulation with different odours, *Acta Physiol. Scand.* **82:**154.

Nauta, W. J. H., and Mehler, W. R., 1966, Projections of the lentiform nucleus in the monkey, *Brain Res.* **1:**3.

Neary, T. J., 1974, Diencephalic efferents of the torus semicircularis in the bullfrog, *Rana catesbeiana, Anat. Rec.* **178:**425.

Neary, T. J., and Wilczynski, W., 1977*a*, Autoradiographic demonstration of hypothalamic efferents in the bullfrog, *Rana catesbeiana, Anat. Rec.* **187:**665.

Neary, T. J., and Wilczynski, W., 1977*b*, Ascending thalamic projections from the obex region in ranid frogs, *Brain Res.* **138:**529.

Nieuwenhuys, R., 1967, Comparative anatomy of olfactory centres and tracts, in: *Sensory Mechanisms* (Y. Zotterman, ed.), Vol. 23 of *Progress in Brain Research,* pp. 1–64, Elsevier, New York.

Nieuwenhuys, R., and Opdam, P., 1976, Structure of the brain stem, in: *Frog Neurobiology* (R. Llinás and W. Precht, eds.), pp. 811–855, Springer-Verlag, New York.

Northcutt, R. G., 1970, Pallial projections of the sciatic, ulnar and mandibular branch of the trigeminal afferents in the frog (*Rana catesbeiana*), *Anat. Rec.* **166:**356.

Northcutt, R. G., 1972, Afferent projections of the telencephalon of the bullfrog, *Rana catesbeiana, Anat. Rec.* **172:**374.

Northcutt, R. G., 1974, Some histochemical observations on the telencephalon of the bullfrog, *Rana catesbeiana* Shaw, *J. Comp. Neurol.* **157:**379.

Northcutt, R. G., 1977, Elasmobranch central nervous system organization and its possible evolutionary significance, *Am. Zool.* **17:**411.

Northcutt, R. G., 1978, Brain organization in the cartilaginous fishes, in: *Sensory Biology of Sharks, Skates, and Rays* (E. S. Hodgson and R. F. Mathewson, eds.), pp. 117–193, Office of Naval Research, Department of the Navy, Arlington, Va.

Northcutt, R. G., and Royce, G. J., 1975, Olfactory bulb projections in the bullfrog *Rana catesbeiana, J. Morphol.* **145:**251.

Northcutt, R. G., Neary, T. J., and Senn, D. G., 1978, Observations on the brain of the coelacanth, *Latimeria chalumnae:* External anatomy and quantitative analysis, *J. Morphol.* **155:**181.

Oldham, R. S., 1967, Orienting mechanisms in the green frog, *Rana clamitans, Ecology* **48:**477.

Olivecrona, H., 1964, Notes on forebrain morphology in the gymnophion (*Ichthyophis glutinosus*), *Acta Morphol. Neerl. Scand.* **6:**45.

Ørvig, T. (ed.), 1968, *Current Problems of Lower Vertebrate Phylogeny,* Nobel Symposium 4, Interscience, New York.

Ottoson, D., 1956, Analysis of the electrical activity of the olfactory epithelium, *Acta Physiol. Scand.* **35:**1 (Suppl. 122).

Parent, A., 1971, Comparative histochemical study of the amygdaloid complex, *J. Hirnforsch.* **13:**89.

Parent, A., 1973, Distribution of monoamine-containing neurons in the brain stem of the frog, *Rana temporaria, J. Morphol.* **139:**67.

Parent, A., 1975, The monoaminergic innervation of the telencephalon of the frog, *Rana pipiens, Brain Res.* **99:**35.

Parent, A., and Olivier, A., 1970, Comparative histochemical study of the corpus striatum, *J. Hirnforsch.* **12:**73.

Parsons, T. S., 1970, The nose and Jacobson's organ, in: *Biology of the Reptilia, Morphology B,* Vol. 2 (C. Gans and T. S. Parsons, eds.), pp. 99–191, Academic Press, New York.

Parsons, T. S., and Williams, E. E., 1963, The relationships of the modern amphibia, *Q. Rev. Biol.* **38:**26.

Pritz, M. B., 1975, Anatomical identification of a telencephalic visual area in crocodiles: Ascending connections of nucleus rotundus in *Caiman crocodilus, J. Comp. Neurol.* **164:**323.

Ramón Y Cajal, P., 1922, *El Cerebro de los Batracios, Libro en Honor de D. S. Ramón y Cajal,* Tomo 1, pp. 13–59, Madrid.

Revzin, A. M., 1969, A specific visual projection area in the hyperstriatum of the pigeon (*Columba livia*), *Brain Res.* **15:**246.

Risser, J., 1914, Olfactory reactions in amphibians, *J. Exp. Zool.* **16:**617.

Romer, A. S., 1966, *Vertebrate Paleontology,* 3rd ed., University of Chicago Press, Chicago.

Röthig, P., 1912, Beiträge zur Studium des Zentralnervensystems der Wirbelthiere. 5. Die Zellanordnungen im Vorderhirn der Amphibien, mit besonderer Berücksichtigung der Septumkerne und ihr Vergleich mit den Verhältnissen bei *Testudo* und *Lacerta, Verh. K. Akad. Wet. Amsterdam* (*Ser. 2*) **17:**3.

Röthig, P., 1926, Beiträge zum Studium des Zentralnervensystems der Wirbeltiere. 10. Über die Faserzüge im Vorder-und Zwischenhirn der Anuren. *Jahrb. Morphol. Mikr. Anat. Abt. 2 Z. Mikrosk. Anat. Forsch.* **5:**23.

Royce, G. J., and Northcutt, R. G., 1969, Olfactory bulb projections in the tiger salamander (*Ambystoma tigrinum*) and the bullfrog (*Rana catesbeiana*), *Anat. Rec.* **163:**254.

Rubaschkin, W., 1903, Zur Morphologie des Gehirns der Amphibien, *Arch. Mikrosk. Anat.* **62:**207.

Rubinson, K., 1968, Projections of the tectum opticum of the frog, *Brain Behav. Evol.* **1:**529.

Rubinson, K., and Colman, D. R., 1972, Designated discussion: A preliminary report on ascending thalamic afferents in *Rana pipiens, Brain Behav. Evol.* **6:**69.

Scalia, F., 1972, The projection of the accessory olfactory bulb in the frog, *Brain Res.* **36:**409.

Scalia, F., 1976*a*, Structure of the olfactory and accessory olfactory systems, in: *Frog Neurobiology* (R. Llinás and W. Precht, eds.), pp. 213–233, Springer-Verlag, New York.

Scalia, F., 1976*b*, The optic pathway of the frog: Nuclear organization and connections, in: *Frog Neurobiology* (R. Llinás and W. Precht, eds.), pp. 386–406, Springer-Verlag, New York.

Scalia, F., and Colman, D. R., 1975, Identification of telencephalic-afferent thalamic nuclei associated with the visual system of the frog, *Neurosci. Abstr.* **1:**46.

Scalia, F., and Gregory, K., 1970, Retinofugal projections in the frog: Location of the postsynaptic neurons, *Brain Behav. Evol.* **3:**16.

Scalia, F., Halpern, M., Knapp, H., and Riss, W., 1968, The efferent connexions of the olfactory bulb in the frog: A study of degenerating unmyelinated fibers, *J. Anat.* **103:**245.

Schnitzlein, H. N., Hamel, E. G., Jr., Carey, J. H., Brown, J. W., Hoffman, H. H., Faucette, J. R., and Showers, M. J. C., 1973, The interrelations of the striatum with subcortical areas through the lateral forebrain bundle, *J. Hirnforsch.* **13:**409.

Shen, S. C., Greenfield, P., and Boell, E. J., 1955, The distribution of cholinesterase in the frog brain, *J. Comp. Neurol.* **102:**717.

Skeen, L. C., and Hall, W. C., 1977, Efferent projections of the main and the accessory olfactory bulb in the tree shrew (*Tupaia glis*), *J. Comp. Neurol.* **172:**1.

Söderberg, G., 1922, Contributions to the forebrain morphology in amphibians, *Acta Zool. Stockholm* **3:**65.

Sternthal, D. E., 1974, Olfactory and visual cues in the feeding behavior of the leopard frog (*Rana pipiens*), *Z. Tierpsychol.* **34:**239.

Thireau, M., 1976, L'encéphalisation chez les Urodèles. I. Analyse volumétrique de l'encéphale et de ses étages: Recherche d'un lot d'espèces de "base," *Bull. Mus. Hist. Nat. Paris Zool.* **266:**527.

Thireau, M., Bauchot, R., Platel, R., and Ridet, J.-M., 1973, L'encéphale de *Salamandra salamandra fastuosa* Schreiber, 1912 (Amphibia, Caudata, Salamandridae): Étude préalable à des recherches quantitatives, *Bull. Mus. Hist. Nat. Paris Zool.* **80:**49.

Thomson, K. S., 1968, A critical review of the diphyletic theory of rhipidistian–amphibian relationships, in: *Current Problems of Lower Vertebrate Phylogeny* (T. Ørvig, ed.), pp. 285–306, Interscience, New York.

Tracy, C. R., and Dole, J. W., 1969, Orientation of displaced California toads, *Bufo boreas,* to their breeding sites, *Copeia* **1969:**693.

Vesselkin, N. P., Agayan, A. L., and Nomokonova, L. M., 1971, A study of thalamo-telencephalic afferent systems in the frogs, *Brain Behav. Evol.* **4:**295.

Wake, D., 1966, Comparative osteology and evolution of the lungless salamanders, family Plethodontidae, *Mem. South. Calif. Acad. Sci.* **4:**1.

Wilczynski, W., and Northcutt, R. G., 1977, Afferents to the optic tectum of the leopard frog: An HRP study, *J. Comp. Neurol.* **173:**219.

Winans, S., and Scalia, F., 1970, Amygdaloid nucleus: New afferent input from the vomeronasal organ, *Science* **170:**330.

9

The Telencephalon of Snakes

MIMI HALPERN

I. Introduction

Reptiles, as a group, are most interesting subjects for the study of telencephalic development, because it is in reptiles that the differentiation of cortical regions first becomes obvious. The relative simplicity of the reptilian telencephalon and its position intermediate between amphibian and mammalian telencephalic development offer further inducements to its study. Of particular interest to students of development of the central nervous system and those attempting to define homologous structures is the observation that the development of the reptilian brain parallels the development of mammalian brains (Warner, 1946) and that many similarities exist between the final adult reptilian telencephalon and intermediate stages of mammalian telencephalic ontogenetic development (Humphrey, 1967). Interestingly, reptiles differ among themselves considerably and must be considered an exceptionally heterogeneous group. It is therefore somewhat surprising that with the exception of a few scattered reports (Meyer, 1892, 1895; Rabl-Ruckhard, 1894; Edinger, 1896; Ariëns Kappers and Theunissen, 1908; DeLange, 1911; Rose, 1923; Ariëns Kappers *et al.*, 1960), one serious series of investigations (Warner, 1931, 1946, 1947), and a short paper by Carey (1967) little attention has been paid in the past to the study of the ophidian telencephalon. It has only been within the past 3–4 years that experimental work has been reported on the telencephalon of snakes. It will become clear as this chapter progresses that the major current work on the ophidian telencephalon is occurring in Dr. Philip Ulinski's laboratory and my own.

The present chapter will survey the ophidian telencephalon in terms of its normal anatomy and its fiber connections, to the extent that these are known. The

MIMI HALPERN • Department of Anatomy and Program in Biological Psychology, Downstate Medical Center, Brooklyn, New York 11203.

purpose of this chapter is to serve as a guide to the reader in exploring the snake brain. Wherever possible, I have cited the details of studies of the snake brain, but, as all who work in this area realize, enormous gaps remain. Thus this survey through the ophidian telencephalon cannot be and is not intended to be exhaustive.

As each region of the telencephalon is surveyed, I will summarize findings of previous investigators and discuss my own observations as well. The normal material from which my own observations are made has been stained with cresyl violet, and by the methods of Weil, Klüver-Barrera, and Ramón y Cajal. Whenever possible, horizontal and sagittal sections were made in addition to coronal sections. I have examined Golgi-impregnated material but not sufficiently to add significantly to the literature at this time. I have therefore relied entirely on the studies emanating from Dr. Ulinski's laboratory for description of neuronal morphology of those telencephalic regions for which studies have been reported. Similarly, I have not examined electron micrographs of snake telencephalon and have relied again on Dr. Ulinski's published work on this subject.

The vast majority of the material gathered in my laboratory is from snakes of the genus *Thamnophis,* with the following species represented: *Thamnophis radix, Thamnophis sirtalis sirtalis, Thamnophis parietalis, Thamnophis elegans.* I have in addition obtained a few specimens of *Typhlops punctata, Natrix sipedon, Boa constrictor constrictor, Elaphe obsoleta rosalleni, Coluber constrictor,* and *Pituophis catonifer catonifer.* Examination of the brains of these other snakes has permitted me a somewhat broader view of ophidians than would be obtained from a study restricted to one genus. The reader will note that the vast majority of photomicrographs of the normal brain are coronal sections through the telencephalon of the rat snake (*Elaphe obsoleta rosalleni*) (Fig. 1; see Table I for list of abbreviations used in figures). Although my greatest familiarity is with the brain of *Thamnophis* and the bulk of my material is also from snakes of the genus *Thamnophis,* the brain of the rat snake offered several advantages that I could not overlook. To my knowledge, no detailed description of this brain has ever been published. The brain and animal itself are larger than in the species of the genus *Thamnophis.* The advantage of large brain size is obvious: discrete lesions, discrete injections, and discrete stimulation are facilitated. On a more subjective and qualitative level, the nuclear regions of the telencephalon and diencephalon appear to be better differentiated from each other. Although this is an advantage in terms of labeling discrete areas, it may prove to be a disadvantage if what superficially appear to be separable regions turn out to be a single region. Compare, for example, Figs. 2 and 3. Figure 3 is a series of sections through the brain of *Natrix sipidon* and shows many fewer distinct subdivisions than the telencephalon of *Elaphe.* Several specific areas of the rat snake brain appear to be particularly well developed compared to that of other species. These include the lateral pallium, which can easily be subdivided into five parts—the ventral amygdaloid nucleus, and the posterior colliculus, to mention a few.

The experimental material from which statements based on my own studies of fiber connections are made has been obtained solely from snakes of the genus *Thamnophis* and should not be generalized for snakes as a group until supportive evidence is obtained from other species. All of the fiber connection studies reported in this chapter from my own laboratory or from that of Dr. Ulinski utilize the same general approach. Lesions are placed in the structure whose efferent connections are under study. The lesion is made either by heat coagulation or by passing a current through the exposed tip of a metal electrode. The animal survives under constant environmental conditions for a number of days. The optimal survival interval for demonstrating the degenerating efferent fibers is determined experimentally by sampling over a broad range of survival times. Each area of the brain, each system within an area, may have a different survival interval at which the degenerating fibers and terminals are maximally demonstrable. Animals are killed by perfusion with saline followed by formol-saline, stored in fixative, embed-

Table I. List of Abbreviations

A	Nucleus accumbens (of Warner, 1946, 1947)	MS	Medial superposition
AC	Anterior commissure	nAOT	Nucleus of the accessory olfactory tract
aDVR	Anterior dorsal ventricular ridge	nDB	Nucleus of the diagonal band of Broca?
aDVRl	Anterior dorsal ventricular ridge, lateral portion	nHC	Nucleus of the hippocampal commissure
		nLOT	Nucleus of the lateral olfactory tract
		NS (NSp)	Nucleus sphericus
aDVRm	Anterior dorsal ventricular ridge, medial portion	NSh	Nucleus sphericus, hilar layer
		NSm	Nucleus sphericus, mural layer
AM	Angulostriatal mass	NSma	Nucleus sphericus, marginal layer
AOB	Accessory olfactory bulb	OG	Olfactory gray
AOT	Accessory olfactory tract	OpCh (opc)	Optic chiasm
bAC	Bed nucleus of the anterior commissure	OpN	Optic nerve
D	Dorsal cortex	OpTr	Optic tract
Dc	Dorsal cortex, cortical layer	OS	Olfactostriatum
DM	Dorsomedial nucleus of thalamus	OT	Olfactory tubercle
Dp	Dorsal cortex, polymorphic layer	OV	Olfactory ventricle
DVR	Dorsal ventricular ridge	pDVR	Posterior dorsal ventricular ridge
eg	External granular layer	PED	Peduncle of the lateral forebrain bundle
En	External nucleus of optic tract	Pn	Paraterminal nucleus
ep	External plexiform layer	po	Preoptic area
gl	Glomerular layer	PS	Paleostriatum
H (Hy,hy)	Hypothalamus	PSb	Paleostriatum, bed nucleus of stria terminalis?
ig	Internal granular layer		
ip	Internal plexiform layer	PSd	Paleostriatum, dorsal portion
IVF	Interventricular foramen	PSv	Paleostriatum, ventral portion
L (lp)	Lateral pallium	RA	Rostral amygdaloid nucleus
Ld	Lateral pallium, dorsal portion	Rdi	Retrobulbar region pars dorsalis internus
Le	Lateral pallium, external portion	Rdm	Retrobulbar region pars dorsomedialis
LFB	Lateral forebrain bundle	S	Septum
Li	Lateral pallium, internal portion	SCn	Suprachiasmatic nucleus
Ll	Lateral pallium, lateral portion	Sd	Dorsal septal nucleus
LM	Lateral mammillary nucleus	Sf	Medial septal nucleus pars fimbriae
LPO	Lateral preoptic area	Sl	Lateral septal nucleus
LS	Lateral superposition	Sm	Medial septal nucleus
LV	Lateral ventricle	SOn	Supraoptic nucleus
Lv	Lateral pallium, ventral portion	Sr	Rostral septal nucleus
m	Mitral cell layer	Th	Thalamus
M	Medial cortex	V	Ventral cortex
MFB	Medial forebrain bundle	VA	Ventral amygdaloid nucleus
Ml	Medial cortex, lateral portion	VAl	Ventral amygdaloid nucleus, lateral portion
Mm	Medial cortex, medial portion	VAm	Ventral amygdaloid nucleus, medial portion
MM	Medial mammillary nucleus	VM	Ventromedial nucleus of the hypothalamus
MOB	Main olfactory bulb	VNn (vn)	Vomeronasal nerve
MOT	Main olfactory tract	ZLi	Zona limitans interstriata
MPO	Medial preoptic area	III	Third ventricle

ded in a gelatin and/or egg yolk matrix, cut frozen, and stained. Normally a closely spaced series of sections is stained by one of the modifications of the Fink–Heimer (1967) procedure for demonstrating degenerating axons and terminals. Adjacent sections are stained for Nissl substance with cresyl violet.

II. Normal Anatomy

A. Gross Appearance

The telencephalon of all snakes examined conforms to a general pattern as follows: An olfactory bulb is situated at the rostral end of an elongated but relatively broad olfactory peduncle. The accessory olfactory bulb occupies the medial aspect of the entire length of the olfactory peduncle. As the peduncle attaches to the

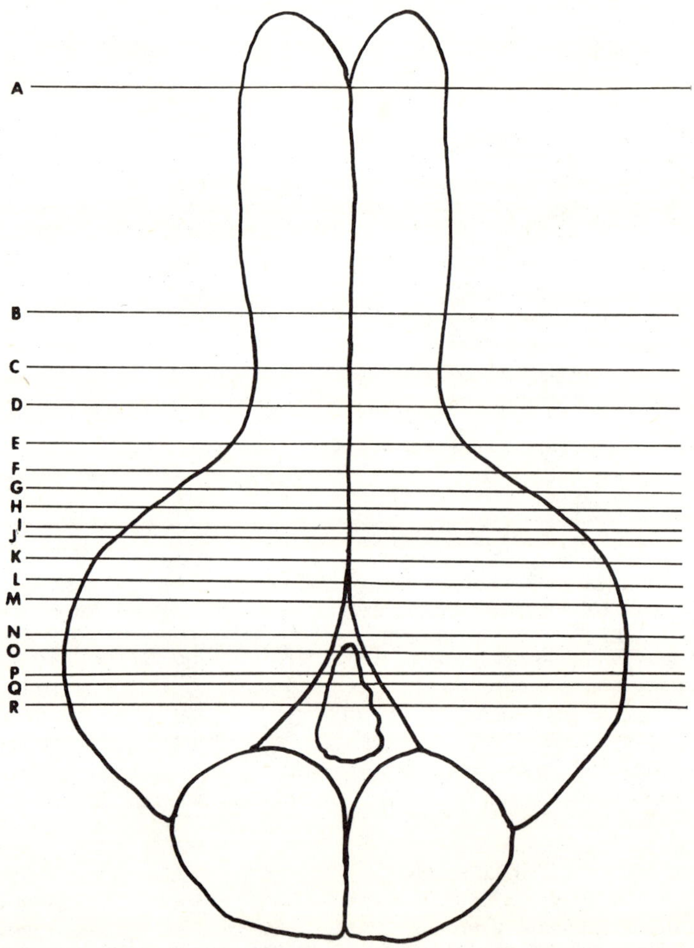

Figure 1. Dorsal reconstruction of the telencephalon of the rat snake (*Elaphe obsoleta rosalleni*). Lines transverse to the longitudinal axis indicate levels from which photomicrographs in Fig. 2A–G are taken.

retrobulbar telencephalon, there is an expansion of the brain tissue in a lateral direction as well as in a ventral direction. This expansion continues to approximately the level of the anterior commissure, at which point there is a slight and gradual reduction of the lateral expansion of the telencephalic hemisphere.

At caudal diencephalic levels the cerebral hemispheres diminish markedly along their medial wall, making room for the developing optic tectum medially. The caudal telencephalic pole persists for a considerable distance alongside the optic tectum.

In general terms the telencephalon can be partitioned into the following regions: main olfactory bulb, accessory olfactory bulb, retrobulbar region (anterior olfactory nucleus of most authors), cortical mantle, septum, dorsal ventricular ridge (neostriatum), amygdala (archistriatum), basal lateral telencephalic structures (paleostriatum), and preoptic area.

B. Lateral Ventricle

The lateral ventricle occupies the entire extent of the telencephalic hemisphere. In the main olfactory bulb the ventricle occupies a central position and is oval in cross section. The ventricle expands dorsoventrally in its course through the olfactory peduncle, separating the accessory olfactory bulb formation medially from the olfactory tract fibers which occupy the lateral wall of the olfactory peduncle. As seen in cross section, the ventricle rapidly changes shape in the retrobulbar region, becoming slit shaped, angled mediodorsal to ventrolateral in the rostral retrobulbar region, and assuming a C shape more caudally with the arms of the C pointing laterally and ventrolaterally. As midtelencephalic levels are approached, the cross-sectional appearance of the ventricle becomes "wishbone shaped," with the handle representing the medial expansion of the ventricle. The lateral extension of the ventricle separates the cortical mantle dorsally from the ventricular ridge ventrally, and the ventral extension of the ventricle separates the septum medially from the ventricular ridge dorsolaterally. The ventral extension of the ventricle develops a medial pocket at the level of the anterior commissure, which expands behind the commissure to become the interventricular foramen, connecting the two lateral ventricles with the medianly situated third ventricle. The development of the interventricular foramen separates the postcommissural septum dorsally from the rostral, dorsal diencephalon ventrally. Caudal to the interventricular foramen, the postcommissural septum gradually disappears and with it the medial wing of the lateral ventricle. The lateral aspect of the ventricle continues to expand laterally and ventrolaterally until it reaches the ventral border of the hemisphere, where its wall becomes thinned to a tela choroidea. At the caudal pole of the telencephalon the lateral ventricle totally separates the nucleus sphericus from the remaining cortical mantle.

C. Main Olfactory Bulb

The olfactory nerves are formed by the axons of bipolar neurons situated in the posterior part of the nasal chamber. The nerves travel a relatively short distance to terminate along the periphery of the main olfactory bulb.

Crosby and Humphrey (1939) described the olfactory bulbs of the copperhead (*Agkistrodon mokasen*), the water moccasin (*Natrix*), and the garter snake (*Thamnophis sirtalis*). In each snake six layers were identified from the periphery to the ventricular surface: (1) a nerve fiber layer, (2) a glomerular layer containing periglomerular cells, (3) an external molecular (plexiform) layer with few neuronal perikarya but occasional "displaced mitral cells," (4) a mitral cell layer, whose cell bodies are widely scattered, (5) an internal molecular (plexiform) layer with few cell bodies, and (6) a densely packed periventricular internal granular layer. An external granular layer, sandwiched between the glomerular layer and the external molec-

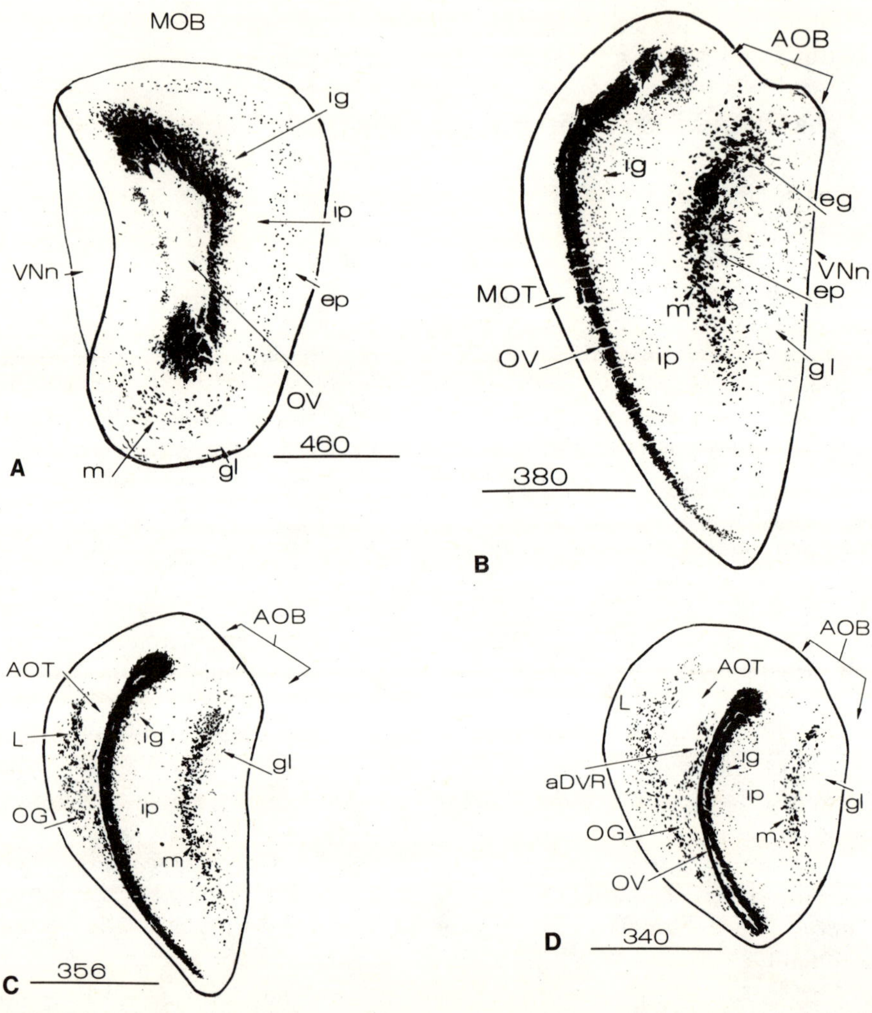

Figure 2. Series of photomicrographs of cresyl violet-stained sections through the telencephalon of the rat snake (*Elaphe obsoleta rosalleni*). With the exception of A, all sections represent the left side of the brain. The bars at the lower portion of the figures represent 500 μm, and the numbers represent the position of the section in the original sequence of sections cut from the brain. A few photomicrographs have been "touched up" because handling of the tissue damaged them.

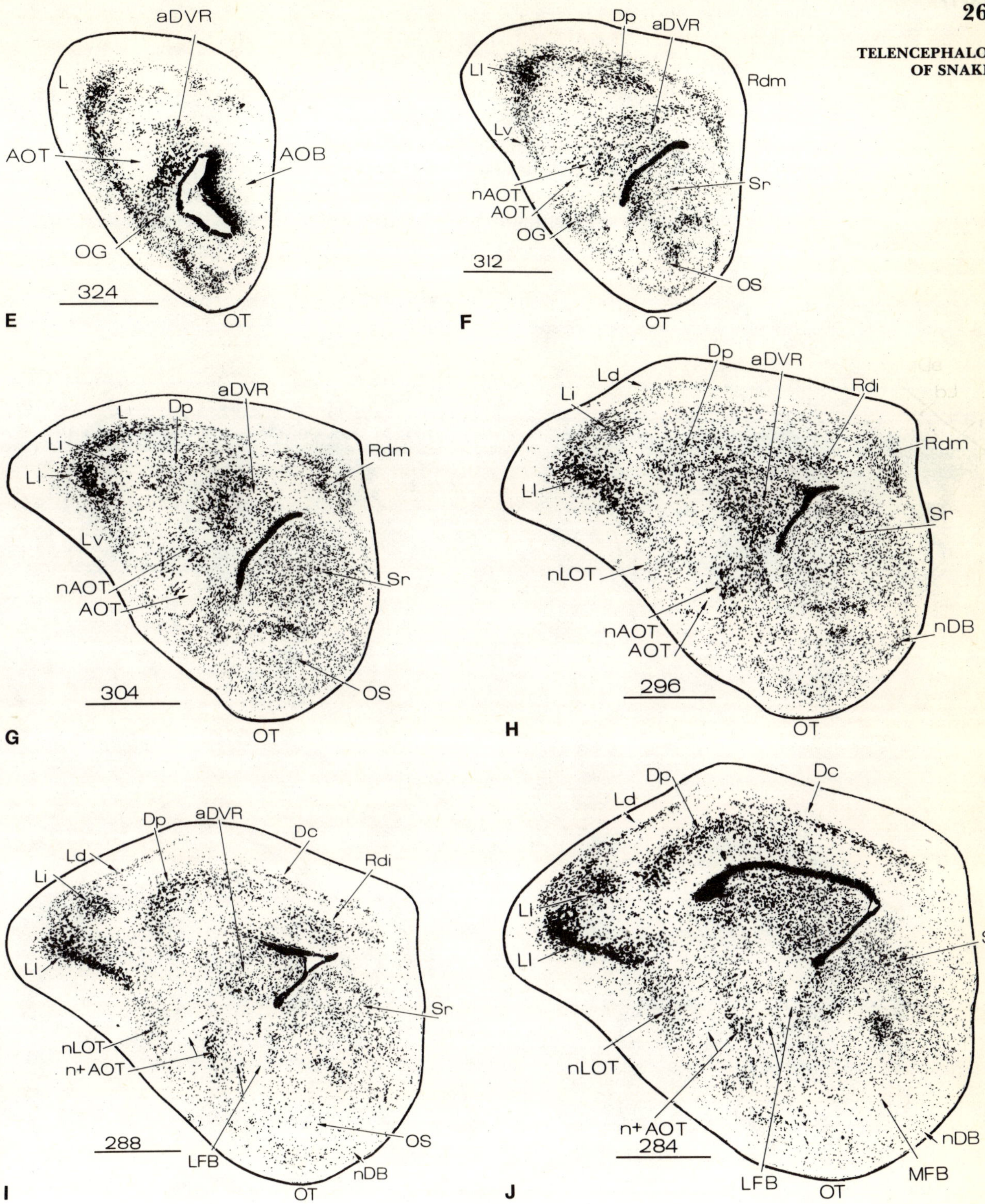

Figure 2. (*cont.*)

ular layer, is illustrated by Crosby and Humphrey (their Fig. 2A) but not described in the text. Rudin (1974) similarly describes six layers of the olfactory bulb in a large variety of ophidian species.

The rostral portions of the main olfactory bulb of the rat snake (Fig. 2B) are surrounded on all sides by olfactory nerve fibers. These olfactory nerve fibers terminate in well-formed glomeruli situated along the periphery of the main olfactory bulb. A single layer of small periglomerular cells surrounds each glomerulus. Internal to the glomerular layer of the main olfactory bulb, small- to medium-sized cells form an outer granular layer. A narrow outer plexiform layer containing few cell bodies separates the outer granular layer from the mitral cell layer. The

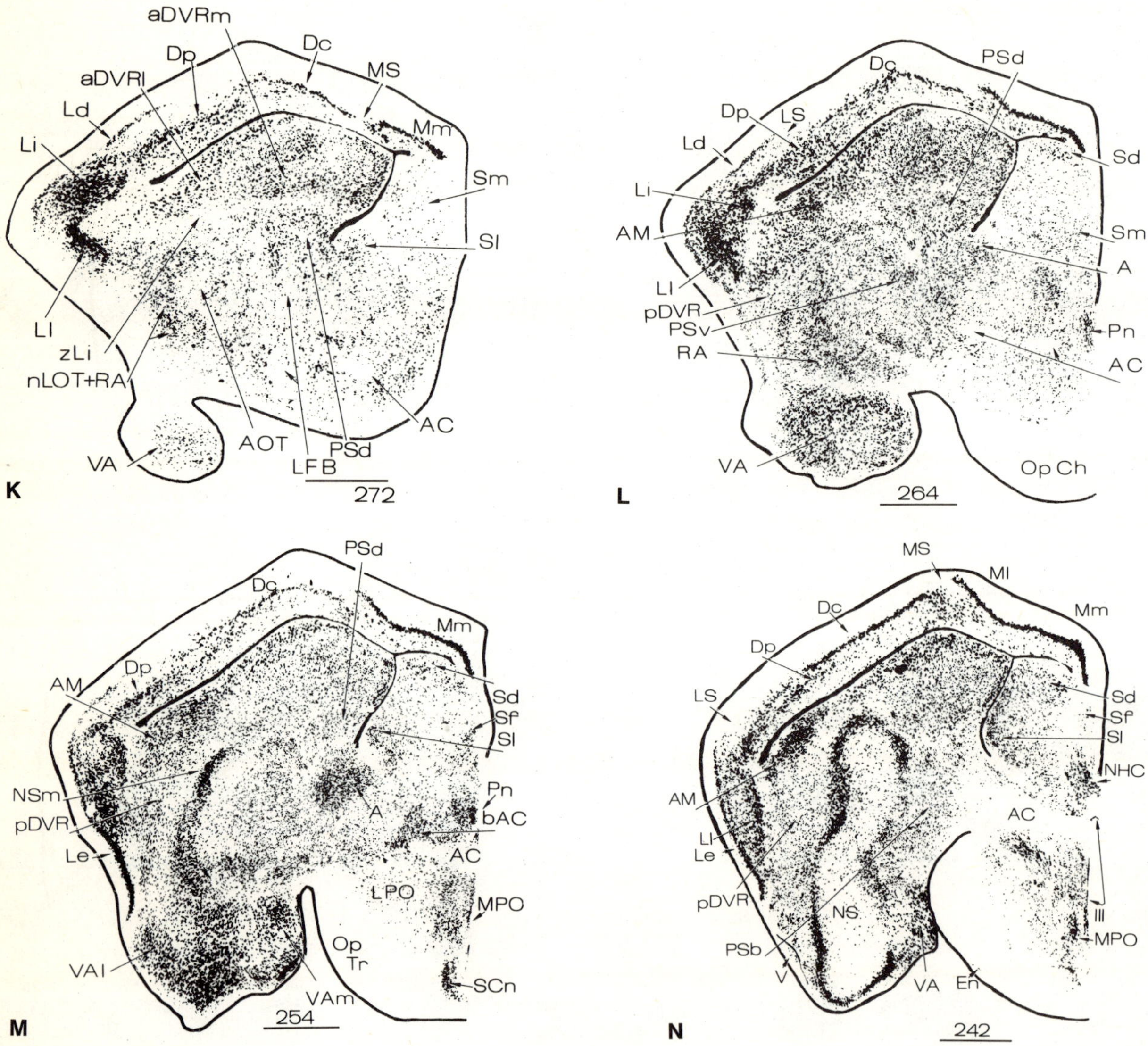

Figure 2. (*cont.*)

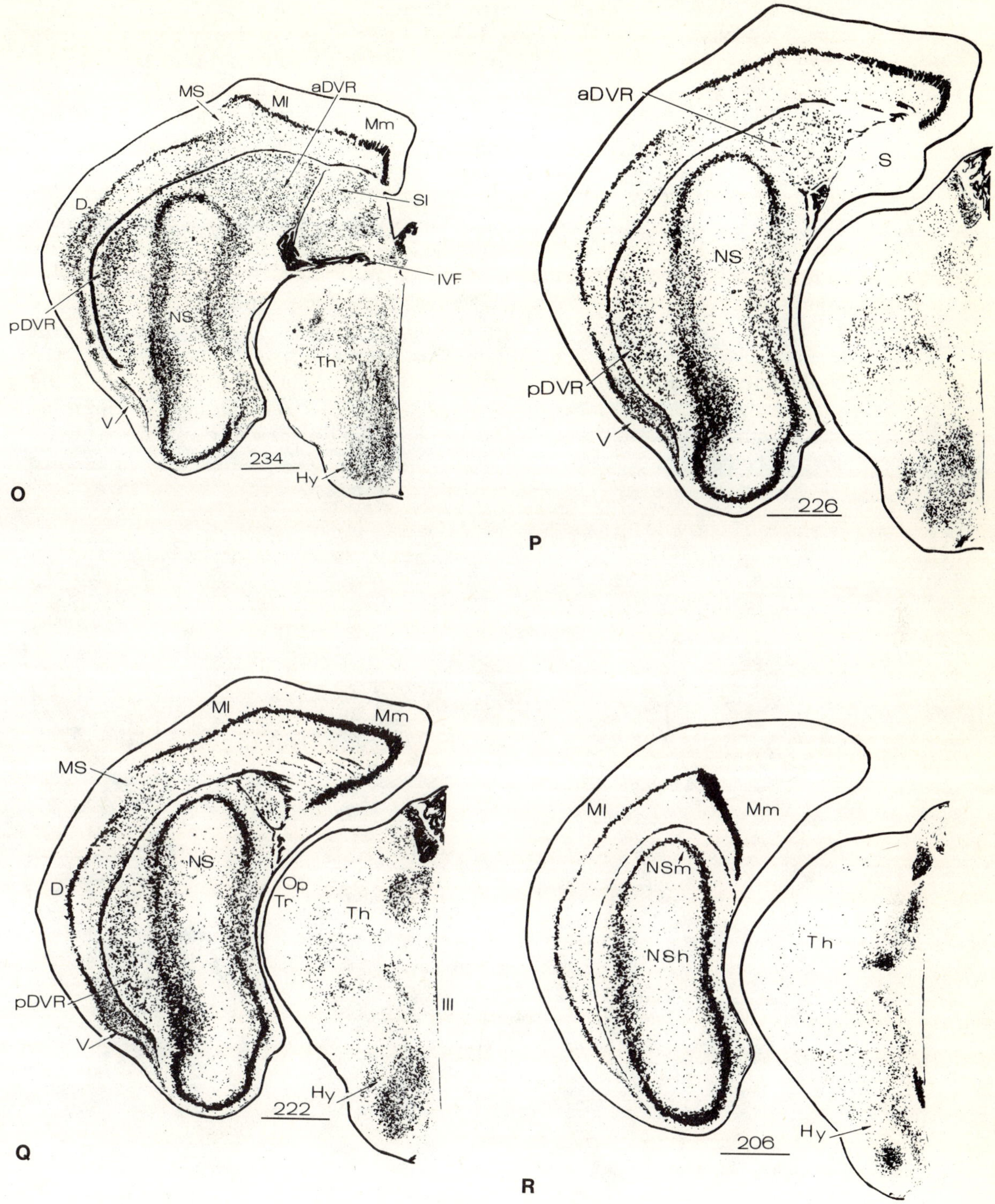

Figure 2. *(cont.)*

mitral cell layer is approximately eight cells deep. The cell bodies (15–20 μm along their long axis and 8–12 μm along their short axis) are not tightly packed, and an extensive neuropil containing axons forming a loose feltwork exists between the cell bodies. The internal plexiform layer, which lies just internal to the mitral cell layer, is broader than the outer plexiform layer but narrower than the mitral cell layer. The internal plexiform layer contains many small, pale-staining cells, very loosely packed with an occasional "displaced mitral cell" present. The neuropil of the internal plexiform layer is occupied by a dense fiber bundle which, when traced caudally, appears continuous with the olfactory tract. The internal granular layer, situated between the internal plexiform layer and the lumen of the olfactory ventricle, is composed of small cells whose nuclei are usually the only visible components. The nucleolus is barely visible. When the perinuclear Nissl substance does stain, it forms a very thin cuff around the nucleus. The outer two-thirds of the granular layer shows a gradation of packing density from moderate adjacent to the internal plexiform layer to very dense closer to the ependymal lining of the olfactory ventricle. The inner one-third of the internal granular layer is uniformly dense with virtually no discernible neuropil, in light microscopic sections, between the cell bodies.

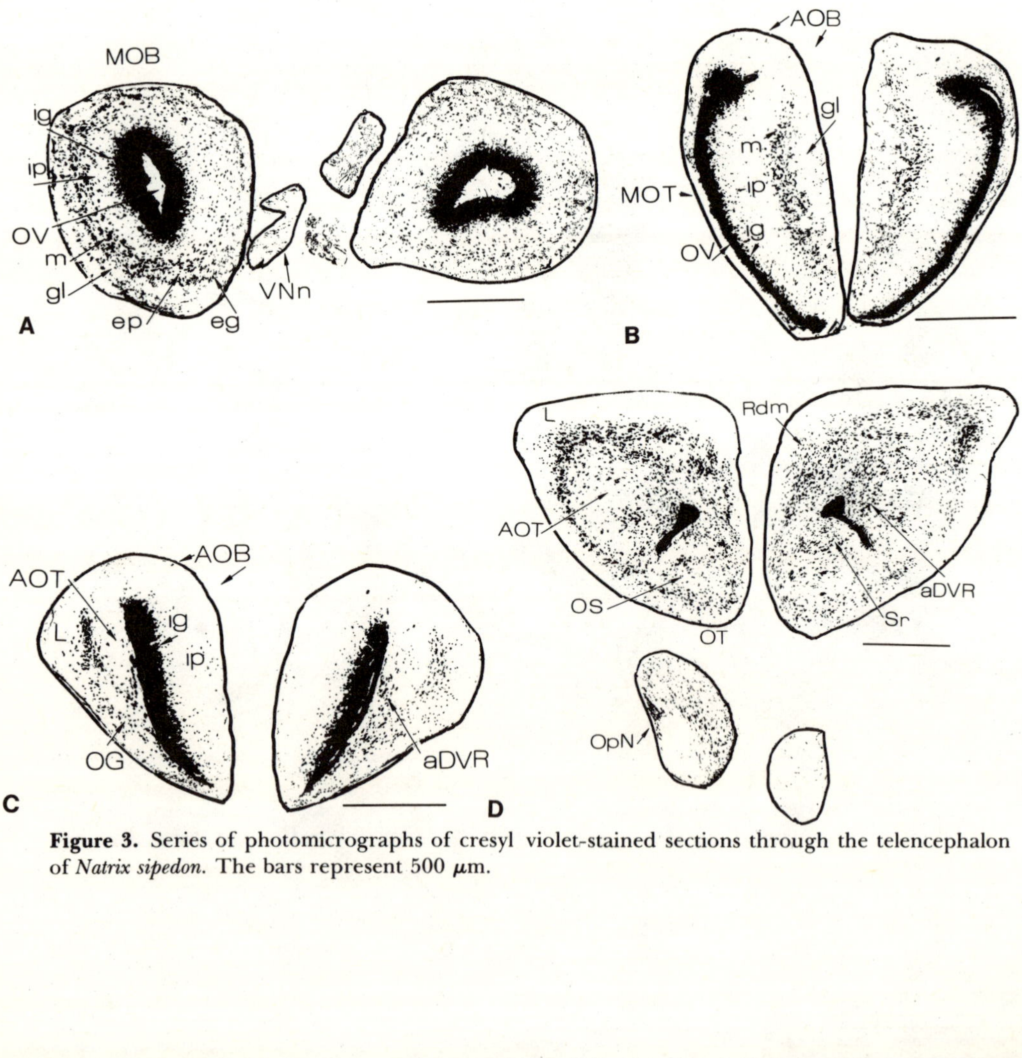

Figure 3. Series of photomicrographs of cresyl violet-stained sections through the telencephalon of *Natrix sipedon*. The bars represent 500 μm.

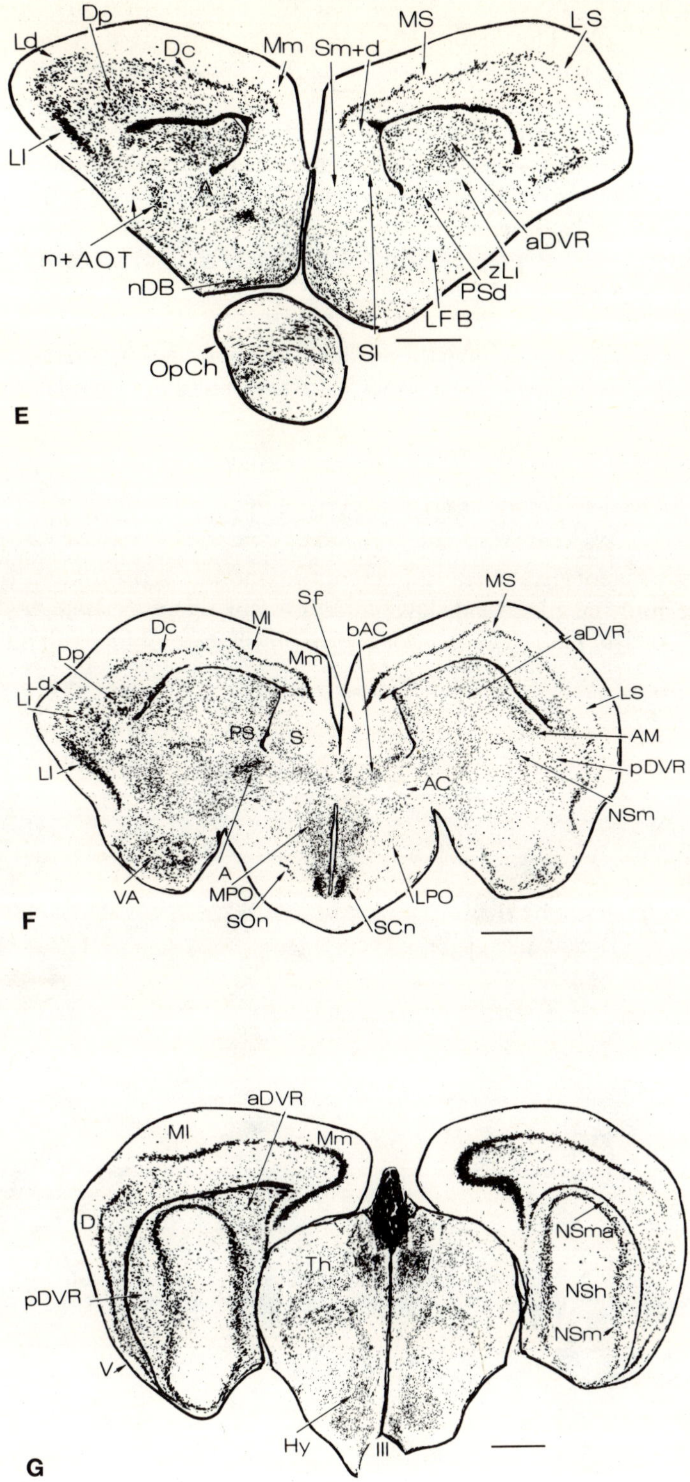

Figure 3. (*cont.*)

The vomeronasal nerve courses medial to the main olfactory bulb at all but the most rostral levels. The medial surface of the main olfactory bulb adjacent to the vomeronasal nerve is devoid of glomeruli. At caudal levels of the main olfactory bulb the external granular layer and mitral cell layer disappear medially, leaving only internal plexiform and granular layers. Laterally, dorsally and ventrally all layers remain. As the accessory olfactory bulb develops medially, the main olfactory bulb tissue disappears, first dorsally, then laterally, and finally ventrally.

The olfactory bulbs of *Natrix sipedon* (Fig. 3A) and *Typhlops punctata* (Fig. 4A) are illustrated for the purpose of comparison with the rat snake (Fig. 2A). The olfactory bulbs of *Natrix* and *Elaphe* are very similar in both differentiation and size of cellular components. The layers of the olfactory bulb of *Typhlops,* however, are more difficult to distinguish, the cellular elements being smaller overall and having few distinguishable characteristics. The internal plexiform layer in *Typhlops* is almost entirely absent.

D. Main Olfactory Tract

The main olfactory tract is a caudal continuation of a prominent fiber bundle located in the internal plexiform layer of the main olfactory bulb. Following the disappearance of the lateral portion of the main olfactory bulb, the olfactory tract

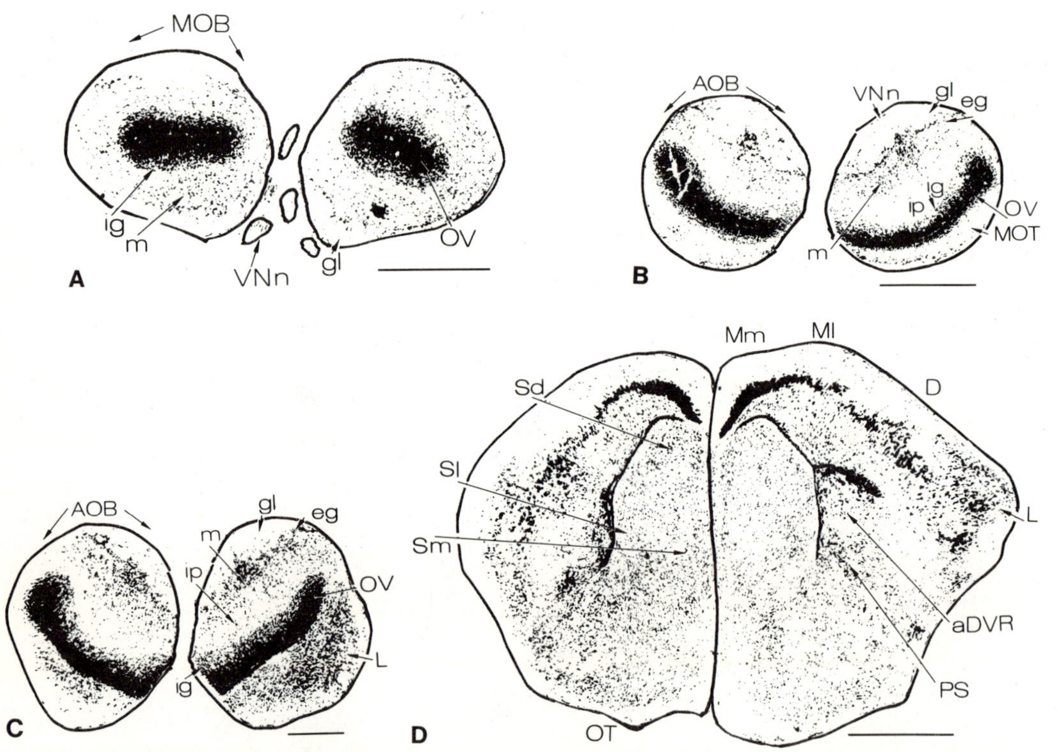

Figure 4. Series of photomicrographs of cresyl violet-stained sections through the telencephalon of *Typhlops punctata.* The bars represent 500 μm.

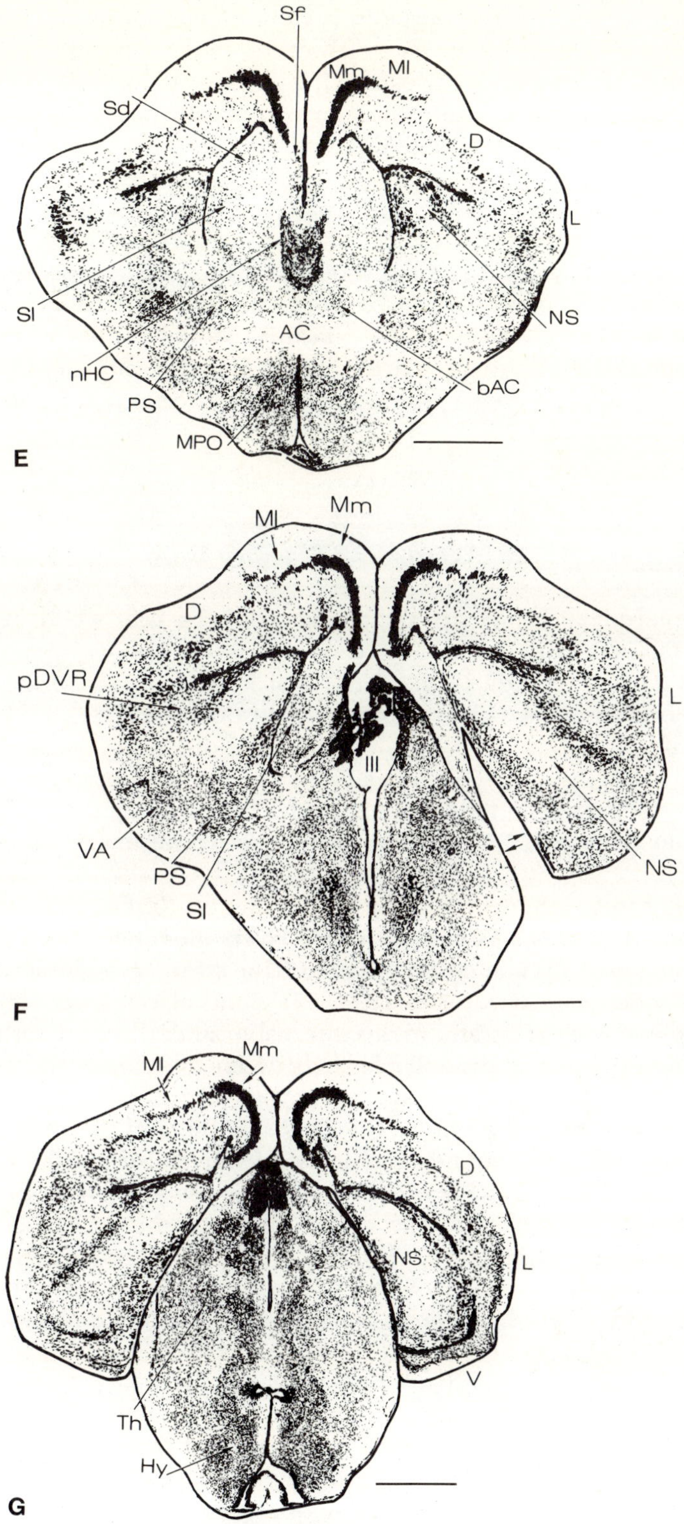

Figure 4. (*cont.*)

occupies a thin portion of the olfactory peduncle between the olfactory ventricle and pial surface. Many of the fibers which make up the olfactory tract at the level of the olfactory peduncle are myelinated, as observed in Weil-stained material. Most of the fibers, however, lose their myelin sheaths as retrobulbar levels are approached and travel considerable distances to their target neurons as unmyelinated fibers.

Immediately posterior to the main olfactory bulb, the main olfactory tract occupies the entire lateral wall of the olfactory peduncle (Figs. 2B and 3B). In *Typhlops* the main olfactory tract runs ventrally in the olfactory peduncle (Fig. 4B). As the accessory bulb develops, its accessory olfactory tract begins to occupy the dorsal and dorsolateral aspects of the olfactory peduncle. It is at this point and only at this point that the two tracts are adjacent. With the subsequent development of the lateral pallium (see below) the two tracts are effectively separated by the cell bodies of the lateral pallium.

E. Accessory Olfactory Bulb

The vomeronasal nerves are the axons of bipolar cells whose cell bodies are found in the sensory epithelium of the vomeronasal (Jacobson's) organ. This organ, in snakes, is located on either side of the septal bone just above the hard palate. The nerves exit from the organ's dome-shaped dorsal surface and course dorsocaudally along the septal bone for a considerable distance. The nerves enter the cranial cavity alongside the most medial fibers of the olfactory nerve. Their intracranial course is parallel to the horizontal axis of the brain just medial to the main olfactory bulb (Figs. 2A, 3A, and 4A) within a groove in the bony intracranial septum.

According to Crosby and Humphrey (1939) and Rudin (1974), the accessory olfactory bulb of snakes is composed of six layers identified, from the medial to ventricular surface, as (1) an entering nerve fiber layer, (2) a glomerular layer, (3) an external molecular (plexiform) layer, (4) a mitral cell layer, (5) an internal molecular (plexiform) layer, and (6) an internal granular layer. Crosby and Humphrey include an external granular layer between the glomerular layer and the external molecular layer in their illustration (their Fig. 2B).

The accessory olfactory bulb of the rat snake replaces the medial part of the main olfactory bulb and extends for a considerable rostrocaudal distance. The accessory olfactory bulb in total rostrocaudal extent is more than $2\frac{1}{2}$ times longer than the main olfactory bulb. The major layers of the two bulbs are similar, although their extent differs.

The layers of the accessory olfactory bulb differ somewhat when rostral and caudal sections are compared. The rostral accessory olfactory bulb lacks an external plexiform layer and has a very poorly developed external granular layer. Thus the mitral cell layer is found closely apposed to the glomerular cell layer. The mitral cells (20–25 μm along their long axis and 7–12 μm along their short axis) stain darkly with cresyl violet and are more tightly packed than the mitral cells of the main olfactory bulb. The internal plexiform layer, which is broader than the equivalent main olfactory bulb layer, contains a dorsoventrally oriented prominent fiber bundle. A narrow internal granular layer intervenes between the internal plexiform layer and ependymal lining of the olfactory ventricle.

In more caudal sections through the accessory olfactory bulb a prominent vomeronasal nerve layer is present medial to a glomerular layer which is two to four glomeruli broad in mediolateral extent. Small cells are present between and around the glomeruli. An external granular layer and very narrow external plexiform layer intervene between the glomerular and mitral cell layers. The internal plexiform layer is divisible into a medial portion and lateral portion by the fibers of the accessory olfactory tract which travel dorsoventrally through the middle of the internal plexiform layer. The medial portion of the internal plexiform layer is relatively cell free and contains a fine neuropil as seen in Ramón y Cajal-stained sections. The lateral portion of this layer contains more perikarya, which are scattered in the neuropil. The internal granular layer is thinner (five to eight cells thick) than the comparable layer of the main olfactory bulb, and contains small, tightly packed cell bodies.

The structure of the accessory olfactory bulb changes gradually in appearance. A progression of changes, beginning with a thinning of the vomeronasal nerve layer, followed by a diminution of the glomerular layer and then the disappearance of the mitral cell layer, ensues as the retrobulbar region is approached. The internal plexiform layer and granular layers extend well into retrobulbar levels.

F. Accessory Olfactory Tract

The accessory olfactory tract (lateral olfactory tract of Warner, 1947) takes origin from the mitral cells of the accessory olfactory bulb. The tract forms as a distinctive structure lateral to the olfactory ventricle shortly after the accessory olfactory bulb has developed its full complement of layers (Fig. 2C). The fibers which travel in the accessory olfactory tract course first in the internal plexiform layer of the accessory olfactory bulb, travel dorsocaudally over the dorsal edge of the olfactory ventricle, and enter the caudally directed accessory olfactory tract. This tract is heavily myelinated at the level of the accessory olfactory bulb and continues to be myelinated until rostral levels of the nucleus sphericus are reached. The tract lacks myelin throughout its long course within the hilar layer of the nucleus sphericus. In its rostral trajectory through the retrobulbar region the accessory olfactory tract is sandwiched between the cells of the anterior dorsal ventricular ridge and the innermost cells of the lateral pallium (Fig. 2D,E). At caudal levels of the retrobulbar region the tract lies ventral to the cells of the anterior dorsal ventricular ridge and medial to the most ventral cells of the lateral pallium (Fig. 2F–H). At midtelencephalic levels the accessory olfactory tract occupies a ventrolateral position bordered medially by the lateral cells of the olfactory tubercle and laterally by cells associated with the "nucleus of the lateral olfactory tract" (Fig. 2I,J). As the rostral and ventral amygdaloid nuclei develop caudally (Fig. 2K), the tract loses its relatively superficial position, expands dorsally, and, once the nucleus sphericus is fully developed, occupies virtually the entire depth of the ventricular ridge (Fig. 2N–R).

The accessory olfactory tract contains a prominent interstitial nucleus along most of its course (Fig. 2F–J). It is first observed at retrobulbar levels and extends to midtelencephalic levels. The nucleus is quite distinctive, being composed of dark-staining medium-sized scattered cells. It is almost always found in the dorsomedial portion of the accessory olfactory tract. The nucleus is most easily identified in Ramón y Cajal-stained sections or sections from brains in which the accessory olfactory bulb has been damaged and the tissue stained by the Fink–Heimer method.

G. Retrobulbar Region

The region behind the olfactory bulb and accessory olfactory bulb is probably best termed the retrobulbar region, although it has typically been called the anterior olfactory nucleus. This region contains so many diverse parts, some of which may have no relation to the main olfactory bulb, that it is important to carefully scrutinize the nomenclature being used at this time. Certainly my own studies on the efferent connection of the olfactory bulb in *Thamnophis sirtalis* and *Thamnophis radix* indicate that just caudal to the termination of the accessory olfactory bulb a ringlike cortical mantle appears which receives on its subpial surface efferent fibers from the olfactory bulb. This region, however, is continuous and indistinguishable from some telencephalic areas which develop caudal to the retrobulbar region. In an earlier paper (Halpern, 1976*b*) I have taken the liberty of not using the term "anterior olfactory nucleus" to describe this retrobulbar region. It is clear from my own observations in *Thamnophis sirtalis* and *Thamnophis radix* that the lateral pallium actually forms rostrally in the retrobulbar region, extending medially to form a semicircle on the dorsal surface of the anterior telencephalon. This appearance is not the same in all snakes; i.e., in the rat snake, for which I have no experimental data, the region just behind the accessory bulb is exceedingly complex, and it is not clear at this point that in fact thet lateral pallium extends as far medially along the dorsal convexity of the retrobulbar region as this structure does in *Thamnophis.*

Crosby and Humphrey (1939) describe the region just posterior to the olfactory formation in garter snake (*Thamnophis sirtalis*), python (*Python molurus*), copperhead (*Agkistrodon mokasen*), and water moccasin (*Natrix*). In *Thamnophis* they describe an anterior olfactory nucleus divided into a pars medialis, a pars dorsalis, a pars lateralis, and a pars ventralis. The pars lateralis appears most rostrally in the lateral wall of the telencephalic vesicle and is continuous caudally with the pyriform cortex. The pars dorsalis can be traced caudally into the general cortex. The pars ventralis lies just ventral to the ventricle and is continuous caudally with the tuberculum olfactorium. The pars medialis is represented by periventricular gray matter. The anterior olfactory nucleus of the python and copperhead appears to be similar in general outline to that of garter snakes. In the water moccasin the nucleus appears to be somewhat less well developed than in the garter snake. Warner in his 1931 article does not deal with the details of the structure of the anterior olfactory nucleus.

Following a series of coronal sections of the rat snake caudally through posterior accessory olfactory bulb levels, the first structure encountered is a cellular aggregation which accompanies a gradual thickening of the tissue lateral to the olfactory ventricle. The cell bodies first appear adjacent to the ventricle approximately midway between the dorsal and ventral surfaces of the olfactory peduncle

(Fig. 2C). In more caudal sections the number of cell bodies increases dorsally, and these cells take a more lateral position, although they never reach the pial surface (Fig. 2D). The fibers of the olfactory tract are always found external to these cell bodies, and at rostral levels the accessory olfactory tract lies medial to these cells. The mass is composed of cells with ovoid nuclei and a cap of Nissl substance at each pole. The orientation of the long axis of these cells is parallel to the pial surface. This cell group develops into a massive structure caudally and is continuous, without interruption, with the cells forming the lateral pallium (Fig. 2E). At most rostral retrobulbar levels these cells could easily be labeled anterior olfactory nucleus pars lateralis; however, it is impossible to determine where the anterior olfactory nucleus ends and the lateral pallium begins. As stated previously, I have used the term "lateral pallium" throughout. The accessory olfactory tract lies between the cells of the rostral lateral pallium and the olfactory ventricle (Fig. 2C).

Shortly after the lateral pallial cells appear, a second group of cell bodies develops between the fibers of the accessory olfactory tract and the olfactory ventricle. This group of cells may be traced into caudal continuity with the cells of the anterior dorsal ventricular ridge (Fig. 2D). It will be described in detail below in the section on the anterior dorsal ventricular ridge.

As the lateral pallium enlarges caudally it develops a heterogeneity of appearance and expands medially to cover most of the dorsal aspect of the retrobulbar telencephalon (Fig. 2F,G). It is composed at this level of several distinct subdivisions, all of which contain a broad molecular layer. The lateral pallium in the rostral retrobulbar region contains a dorsal portion (Ld) composed of small light-staining scattered cells forming a thin sheet along the dorsal aspect of the telencephalon (Fig. 2H), a lateral portion (Ll) composed of a thick sheet of dark-staining tightly clumped cells (Fig. 2F–I), and a ventral portion (Lv) of light-staining moderate-sized cells with a moderate packing density (Fig. 2F,G). At caudal levels through the retrobulbar region a dense clump of perikarya appear dorsomedial to the lateral portion of the lateral pallium. This clump is identified here as the internal portion (Li) of the lateral pallium (Fig. 2G–J).

The ventral portion of the retrobulbar portion of the lateral pallium is continuous with a distinctive cell cluster of medium- and small-sized cells packed moderately in the shape of an elongated triangle, the olfactory gray (Fig. 2D–F). The long axis of the triangle follows the contour of the lateral pial surface and contains a cell-free molecular layer between the pia and its cellular mass. Rostrally this nucleus originates at the junctional region between the developing anterior dorsal ventricular ridge and lateral pallium (Fig. 2D). A similar region in *Thamnophis* was identified by me in an earlier paper (Halpern, 1976*b*) as olfactory gray (see also Fig. 3C for this structure in *Natrix*). This nuclear region disappears as the accessory olfactory tract approaches the pial surface caudally.

The ventral portion of the retrobulbar region was designated anterior olfactory nucleus pars ventralis by Crosby and Humphrey (1939) and noted by them to be in continuity caudally with the olfactory tubercle. Here again, I have omitted the anterior olfactory nucleus designation and utilized the term "olfactory tubercle" throughout. In rat snake, more than in *Thamnophis,* the olfactory tubercle is very well developed and composed of several subdivisions. The structure as a whole (Fig. 2E–G) has at least three layers: an outer (subpial) molecular layer, which may vary in thickness; a cortical layer, which not only varies in thickness but also may, at some levels, be readily divided into medial and lateral portions; and an inner plexiform layer, which contains cell-free regions, scattered cell bodies, and occasionally dense aggregations of neuronal perikarya. Caudally in the retrobulbar region the olfactory tubercle's cortical layer becomes less distinct and its molecular layer narrower (Fig. 2H). The olfactory tubercle continues caudally, losing its laminated appearance until rostral levels of the preoptic area, where it disappears.

Internal to the olfactory tubercle is a complex region which contains the bulk of the rostral portion of the medial forebrain bundle. Following Durward (1930) this region is labeled olfacto-striatum (Fig. 2F,G,I). Durward includes in his olfacto-striatum the nucleus accumbens septi. This nucleus is represented by Durward in a more rostral position than the nucleus accumbnes of Warner (1947) and this chapter, and these probably are not homologous structures. On the other hand, the olfacto-striatum of Durward appears similar to that observed here in snakes and probably contains similar structures.

The dorsomedial portion of the retrobulbar region presents a more complex problem of nomenclature because several cell groups appear in this area which do not have a clear continuity with named structures caudally. Thus, just as the accessory olfactory bulb disappears, a dorsomedially placed cell mass appears, composed of perikarya which stain deeply with cresyl violet and are relatively tightly clustered. The overall shape of this cell mass (labeled here retrobulbar region pars dorsomedialis, Fig. 2G,H) is triangular in cross section, with its long axis parallel to the medial wall. It is tempting to consider this cell group the rostral continuation of the medial or dorsomedial cortex; however, it disappears prior to the emergence of those cortices in more caudal sections. One could identify this cell group as the pars medialis of the anterior olfactory nucleus, but this would lead to a conflict with the previous description of the pars medialis as represented by periventricular gray matter (Crosby and Humphrey, 1939). As a result, I have introduced the term "retrobulbar region pars dorsomedialis" to distinguish it from the previous designations of other authors.

Along the dorsal surface of middle to caudal levels of the retrobulbar region a thin layer of pale-staining medium-sized cells appears (see Fig. 2F,H, unlabeled dorsalmost cells). External to this cell layer is a molecular layer and internal to it is a variably constituted plexiform layer (Fig. 2I). Progressing caudally in the telencephalon, this region contains more dark-staining neurons until it clearly forms the cortical layer of the dorsal cortex (DC, Fig. 2I). The anterior portion of this cell plate was identified by Crosby and Humphrey (1939) as anterior olfactory nucleus pars dorsalis. As explained previously, I prefer to consider this region as part of the dorsal cortex because its caudal boundary is inseparable from the dorsal cortex as usually defined.

Ventral to the dorsal cell plate of the retrobulbar region and just dorsal to the lateral ventricle, a thick, dark-staining band of cells is present for a short rostrocaudal distance. This cell mass, labeled here "retrobulbar region pars dorsalis internus" (Fig. 2H,I), does not appear to have a caudal continuity with any named structure, although it has a superficial resemblance, in light microscopic sections stained for Nissl substance, with the mass of cells just lateral to it which forms more caudally the polymorphic layer of the dorsal cortex. This suggests that the retrobulbar region pars dorsalis internus may merge into the polymorphic layer of the dorsal cortex. Rostrally these two structures, the polymorphic layer of the dorsal cortex and the retrobulbar regions pars dorsalis internus, are in fact adjacent to each other.

The polymorphic layer of the dorsal cortex is a prominent structure in the retrobulbar region and appears rostral to the level where a cortical layer of the dorsal cortex can be clearly distinguished (Fig. 2F). It is first observed in coronal sections as an oval cluster of dark-staining perikarya just ventral to the dorsal cortical portion of the rostral lateral pallium and dorsal to the lateral margin of the rostral anterior dorsal ventricular ridge. In Ramón y Cajal-stained sections one gains the distinct impression that fibers of the LFB travel through the anterior dorsal ventricular ridge to gain access to this region. The polymorphic layer of the dorsal cortex at rostral levels resembles the pallial thickening of other reptiles (Riss *et al.*, 1969) and may be considered homologous to it, although one should exercise caution here as in other places prior to suggesting a functional homology on the basis of superficial resemblance. The polymorphic layer of the dorsal cortex will be dealt with in more detail in Section II.I.

H. Septum

The septal region is defined here as that portion of the telencephalon which lies medial to the lateral ventricle, ventral to the cortical mantle, and dorsal to the olfactostriatum and olfactory tubercle in the rostral telencephalon and dorsal to the anterior commissure and interventricular foramen in the caudal telencephalon.

Carey (1967) identified eight distinct septal nuclei in the brain of the black snake (*Coluber constrictor constrictor*). Lateral and medial nuclei were described as extending through the septum, with the medial nucleus larger than the lateral nucleus. A dorsal septal nucleus was identified and illustrated at a level which corresponds to the dorsal part of rat snake section 272 (Fig. 2K). The nucleus is illustrated as medially placed in the dorsal septum adjacent to the most ventral cells of the cornu ammonis (medial cortex of the present chapter). Since there is no verbal description of the dorsal septal nucleus in the Carey chapter and there are no further illustrations, its rostral–caudal extent and morphological characteristics are not ascertainable. A well-developed nucleus accumbens septi was identified and described as extending from the rostral septum to the level of the anterior commissure, where it becomes indistinct and merges with the bed nucleus of the anterior commissure. The latter nucleus and the nucleus of the hippocampal commissure are both identified by Carey in the blacksnake septum. The nucleus of the diagonal band of Broca "extends over the caudal border of the tuberculum olfactorium" from the ventral margin of the medial septal nucleus to the ventral border of the pyriform area (lateral cortex of the present chapter) and neostriatum. This latter relationship is not clear from Carey's illustrations as the nucleus of the diagonal band of Broca is not labeled in his illustrations. The nucleus hippocamposeptalis, "actually intermediate between the septum and the hippocampus," lies, according to Carey, at levels through the posterior portion of the olfactory tubercle just ventral to the dorsomedial tip of the hippocampal formation (my retrobulbar region pars dorsomedialis). The section in which Carey labels the nucleus hippocamposeptalis is, as close as I can determine, comparable in level to the rat snake section 312 (Fig. 2F), which, in fact, is not a level through the caudal olfactory tubercle. In the blacksnake this nucleus is better developed caudally. In the rat snake I have been unable to identify this nucleus caudal to section 316 (just rostral to Fig. 2F).

Crosby *et al.* (1967) identify nine septal nuclei in *Boa constrictor,* adding to Carey's list a nucleus triangularis, which lies just dorsomedial to the bed nucleus of the anterior commissure. Warner (1947) describes, in the septum, four major nuclei: medial and lateral septal nuclei, the nucleus accumbens septi, and a paraterminal nucleus. The last nucleus is described as being oval in shape, lying dorsal to the anterior commissure close to the midline. The nucleus accumbens of Warner does not coincide with other descriptions but is described as "a small oval cell mass situated at the ventral extremity of the lateral ventricle, at the precommissural level of the telencephalon. . . . It lies just medial to the paleostriatum, and just ventral to the lateral septal nucleus."

In examining the septal region of the rat snake the following clear subdivisions can be made: (1) a rostral nucleus, (2) a dorsal nucleus, (3) a lateral nucleus, (4) a medial nucleus, (5) a nucleus accumbens septi, (6) a nucleus of the hippocampal commissure or nucleus of the posterior pallial commissure, (7) a nucleus of the anterior commissure, (8) a nucleus of the diagonal band, and (9) a paraterminal nucleus.

The rostral septal nucleus (Figs. 2F–J and 3D) is found just caudal to the accessory olfactory bulb and appears basically homogeneous in cresyl violet-stained sections. In a few rostral sections (Fig. 2F) a densely staining small lateral subdivision can be distinguished (rostral septal nucleus pars lateralis, but not labeled). This subdivision is *not* continuous caudally with the lateral septal nucleus and therefore does not bear that name. Just ventral to the rostral nucleus a densely stained band of small cells is invariably present as well (Fig. 2F–J, but not labeled). I have been unable to find this nucleus described previously, and since it does not appear to be associated consistently with a fiber bundle I have simply considered it a ventral subdivision of the rostral septal nucleus. The bulk of the rostral septal nucleus is semicircular to circular in shape, consisting of moderately packed nondescript cells. Its neuropil, in Ramón y Cajal-stained sections, is intensely stained, setting it apart from adjoining regions. It appears from the normal material as if the fibers of the medial forebrain bundle which course through the telencephalon just ventral to the rostral nucleus are terminating densely in the neuropil between the cell bodies and thus contribute to the dark background.

Ventromedial to the rostral septal nucleus a cluster of cells can be observed which follows the ventromedial curve of the medial wall of the rostral telencephalon. This nucleus appears in Ramón y Cajal-stained sections to be associated with a fiber bundle running in a similar pattern, i.e., from a dorsal medial position to a ventral position along the ventromedial curvature of the telencephalon and then laterally along the olfactory tubercle. On the basis of this observation I have labeled this the "nucleus of the diagonal band of Broca" (Fig. 2H–J), although without any assurance that this fiber bundle is the diagonal band.

The rostral septal nucleus is replaced caudally, at a level coincident with the appearance of a definitive medial cortex, by the medial, lateral, and dorsal septal nuclei (Figs. 2K and 3E). These three nuclei represent cellular aggregations within the septal mass in medial, lateral, and dorsal positions. Use of these terms here is consistent with use by the previous authors already discussed; however, I intend no homology with similarly named septal nuclei of other vertebrates. The terms are utilized here purely to communicate to the reader their location within the septum.

The lateral septal nucleus extends from just caudal to the rostral septal nucleus to almost the caudal pole of the postcommissural septum. It is characterized rostrally by dark-staining, closely packed cells lying along the ventral margin of the ventral wing of the lateral ventricle. In the postcommissural region the lateral nucleus occupies the entire lateral wall of the septum, its cells are less darkly stained with cresyl violet, and the cells are less tightly packed. The pre- and postcommissural portions of the lateral septal nucleus blend gradually into each other; however, they do have differing gross morphological appearances and should probably be considered as distinctive subdivisions of a single larger structure.

The dorsal septal nucleus (Fig. 2L,M) is a moderate aggregation of cells in the dorsal aspect of the septum just ventral to the medial wing of the lateral ventricle. It extends from just caudal to the rostral septal nucleus to the level of the hippocampal (or posterior pallial) commissure and is not found in the postcommissural septum.

The medial septal nucleus is a heterogeneous structure occupying rostrally a large portion of the septum as an amorphous mass (Fig. 2K). Rapidly, however, dense aggregations develop in the medial region, forming subdivisions of the medial nucleus (Fig. 2D,N). In the commissural region a distinctive subnucleus of the medial septal nucleus is seen dorsally in a paramedian position and appears to correspond to the nucleus fimbriae of Frederikse (1931) (Figs. 2M,N, 3F, and 4E).

The paraterminal nucleus (Fig. 2L,M) appears just rostral to the closure of the interhemispheric fissure precommissurally and extends into the commissural ridge as a distinctive medially placed, darkly staining nucleus.

The nucleus of the hippocampal (Figs. 2N and 4E) or pallial commissure replaces the paraterminal nucleus caudally. Warner (1931) does not distinguish between the paraterminal nucleus and the nucleus of the hippocampal commissure, but they appear so distinctive from each other in the rat snake as to be easily differentiated. The nucleus of the hippocampal commissure is distinctively H shaped, and in Ramón y Cajal-stained sections can be seen to be pervaded by crossing fibers originating in septal and cortical regions.

The bed nucleus of the anterior commissure (Figs. 2M, 3F, and 4E) lies just dorsal and just ventral to the anterior commissure on either side of the paraterminal nucleus and nucleus of the hippocampal commissure.

The nucleus accumbens (Figs. 2L,M and 3F) is a dark-staining aggregate of neuronal perikarya which bridges between the septum and paleostriatum. In fact, the structure may be more appropriately designated a part of the paleostriatum. The nucleus originates at midtelencephalic levels and extends to the level of the anterior commissure. In identifying this structure as nucleus accumbens, I arbitrarily followed the labeling of Warner (1947, his Fig. 6). This label should be considered very tentative and awaits comparative studies of histochemical identification and experimental studies of interconnections with other telencephalic studies.

I. Cortical Mantle

Warner (1931) following Meyer (1892) separated the cortical mantle into three distinct parts. The medial part was separated from the dorsal portion by the superposito-medialis. The dorsal cortex was separated from the lateral cortex by the superposito-lateralis. The medial cortex was described by Warner as containing two parts, a medial portion in which the cells were small and tightly packed and a more dorsal portion in which the cells were larger and less crowded. Warner divides the lateral cortex into an area praepiriformis and a ventrally placed dark-staining region with crowded cells, the ventrolateral cortex.

Ulinski (1974) has described the cytoarchitecture of the cerebral cortex of snakes of the families Boidae and Colubridae using electron microscopy and Golgi-impregnated material in addition to cresyl violet- and Klüver-Barrera-stained material. The four cortices described are a medial, a dorsal medial, a dorsal, and a lateral cortex. Each cortex contains three neuronal layers: an outer layer (layer 1), containing primarily axons and dendrites from lower layers and other CNS structures; a middle layer (layer 2), characterized by the presence of many densely packed somata; and an inner layer (layer 3), frequently containing many loosely packed somata. The somata of cells in medial cortex appear confined almost exclusively to layer 2. These cells have a candelabra appearance when their dendritic organization is viewed. Most of the dendrites reach toward the pial surface of layer 1. A few dendrites descend toward the ventricular surface. The cells of layer 2 of the dorsal medial cortex are characterized by a double pyramidal dendritic field. The upper dendritic arbors extend into the subpial layer while the lower arbors extend into the periventricular region. The dorsal medial cortex also contains stellate-type cells in layer 3 adjacent to the ventricle. The dorsal cortex, which lies lateral to the dorsal medial cortex, is characterized by the presence in the subpial layer of a myelinated fibrous system. This subpial layer contains relatively few neuronal cell bodies. On the other hand, layer 2 is quite broad, about four cells thick. The shape of the cells varies from fusiform to circular. The fusiform somata have dendrites which go to layer 1 or layer 2, while the more rounded somata have dendrites forming a stellate pattern. The innermost layer of dorsal cortex contains a relatively large number of neurons which vary in shape and size and dendritic field. The lateral cortex lies just lateral to the dorsal cortex and is separated from it by the lateral superposition. Ulinski subdivides the lateral cortex into a dorsal portion, which is relatively thin with small densely packed cells, an intermediate portion, which is very wide and contains loosely packed cells, and a thinner ventral portion. The outer layer of lateral cortex is approximately 200 μm thick and contains few somata, if any at all. It is mainly composed of fiber bundles. The neuronal somata of layer 2 are predominantly circular, but double pyramidal cells are also present. Layer 3 of lateral cortex contains large numbers of scattered circular somata.

The first cortical area to appear as one views the rat snake brain in coronal section, progressing from rostral to caudal, is the lateral cortex or pallium (Fig. 2C). As noted above, the lateral pallium is first observed lateral to the olfactory ventricle at levels through the caudal accessory olfactory bulb. The lateral pallium of the retrobulbar region was described previously as heterogeneous. This heterogeneity continues into more caudal portions of the telencephalon, with some subdivisions disappearing and others appearing for the first time caudal to the retrobulbar region. The ventral portion of the lateral pallium does not extend caudally to midtelencephalic levels. Otherwise, all portions of the lateral pallium described in the retrobulbar region extend caudally to midtelencephalic levels. The dorsal portion is the first to disappear, being last seen at the level of crossing of the anterior commissure. Just before the dorsal portion disappears, however, a new portion appears which is characterized by exceptionally dark-staining, very tightly packed perikarya forming a dorsoventrally oriented band approximately six cells thick. This external portion of the lateral pallium (first illustrated but not labeled in Fig. 2L, labeled in Fig. 2M,N as Le) forms a lateral margin to the cellular layers of the lateral pallium. Very soon after the disappearance of the dorsal portion of the lateral pallium, the internal portion disappears as a separate entity. These changes leave the lateral pallium with a subpial molecular layer, a cortexlike external portion, and a nuclearlike lateral portion. Prior to the disappearance of the lateral portion of the lateral pallium, a transition region (intermediate portion) develops between the external and lateral regions (Fig. 2N). This portion and the external layer cannot be clearly distinguished in the most caudal levels of the telencephalon but do not end abruptly.

In Ramón y Cajal- and Weil-stained sections the entire length of lateral pallium is notable for its relative paucity of well-stained axons. The molecular layer contains a very fine, loosely woven neuropil while the internal and lateral portions have a somewhat closer-knit but still exceedingly fine neuropil. The appearance of the neuropil is quite striking and characteristic of the lateral pallium as contrasted to the other portions of the cortical mantle.

The lateral pallium of *Natrix* and *Typhlops,* as illustrated in Figs. 3E,F and 4C–F, suggests some of the variability this structure may evince. The lateral pallium of *Natrix* has all the sublayers described for *Elaphe* except that the external and lateral portions are less differentiated. *Typhlops,* on the other hand, has a poorly differentiated but nonetheless extensive lateral pallium. The poor differentiation of the lateral pallium of *Typhlops* with its narrow molecular layer reminds one of the poorly differentiated main olfactory bulb and narrow internal plexiform layer.

The development of the dorsal cortex of the rat snake has been described in Section II.G. At midtelencephalic levels the dorsal cortex is characterized by a subpial molecular layer, a cortical layer containing medium-sized, moderately dark-staining cells arranged in a sheet parallel to the pial surface. A polymorphic layer lies between the cortical layer and the ependymal lining of the dorsal wing of the lateral ventricle. This polymorphic layer is populated with numerous dark-staining, closely packed perikarya laterally, but is sparsely populated medially. At the medial superposition (Fig. 2N) the medial edge of the cortical layer of the dorsal cortex underlies the lateral border of the cortical layer of the medial cortex. At the lateral superposition (not labeled in Fig. 2 but labeled in Fig. 3E,F) the medial edge of the lateral pallium overlies the polymorphic layer of the dorsal cortex. At the medial superposition a loose cluster of cells can be observed just medial to the medial edge of the cortical layer of the dorsal cortex and just ventral to the lateralmost portion of the medial cortex. In Ramón y Cajal-stained sections the dorsal cortex is characterized by an intensely stained, very intricate fiber plexus in its supraventricular layer. Since the polymorphic layer laterally lies along the dorsal bank of the lateral ventricle, this region does not contain a well-developed fiber plexus. The middle portion of the molecular layer of the dorsal cortex also contains a well-developed fiber plexus, although it does not stain with the intensity of the supraventricular plexus.

The dorsal cortex extends a considerable distance in the caudal telencephalon, following the curvature of the lateral ventricle as this latter structure encircles the ventricular ridge. The cortical layer, which is abbreviated in medio-lateral extent rostrally, expands considerably caudally. The polymorphic layer, at postcommissural levels, moves away from the ventricular layer and occupies a position adjacent to the lateral limit of the cortical layer. Thus, at caudal levels, the polymorphic layer does not represent the supraventricular layer of the dorsal cortex but rather a lateral extension of the cortical layer. Eventually, the dorsal cortex is replaced entirely by the medial cortex, which expands laterally at caudal levels of the telencephalon and almost completely encircles the nucleus sphericus.

The dorsal cortex of *Natrix,* as illustrated in Fig. 3E–G, is in all ways comparable to the dorsal cortex of *Elaphe. Typhlops,* on the other hand, has a less extensive dorsal cortex, although further analysis is needed before stating that it is in fact more poorly developed or differentiated. The dorsal cortical structure most obvious by its reduction or absence in *Typhlops* is the polymorphic layer, which in other snakes is so well developed.

The medial cortex is customarily subdivided into a medial (small-celled) portion and a lateral (large-celled) portion. Ulinski (1974) refers to the medial portion as the medial cortex and the lateral portion as the dorsomedial cortex. As previously stated by others, the medial part of the medial cortex is distinguished from the lateral portion by the relatively small size and greater packing density of the neurons of the medial portion. The cortical layer of the medial portion of the medial cortex is frequently eight cells thick (10–12 caudally) while the lateral portion of the medial cortex is more frequently two or three cells thick. In Ramón y Cajal-stained sections a well-formed fiber bundle running parallel to the dorsal pial surface can be seen below the cortical cell layer of the medial portion of the medial cortex. This fiber bundle (the alveus of Warner, 1946) extends medially to the pial surface of the midline and bends ventrally in the septum. The molecular layer of the rostral medial cortex contains a moderately well-developed fiber plexus in its inner half: the subpial portion is sparsely populated with axons as seen in Ramón y Cajal-stained coronal sections. In caudal sections through the medial cortex the supraventricular fiber bundle (alveus?) becomes very well developed and is clearly related (originating from and/or terminating in) the internal portion of the medial cortex. A similar relationship exists between this fiber bundle and the dorsal cortex. The molecular layer of the lateral portion of the medial cortex develops a unique appearance in caudal sections. A fiber bundle with axons running in not perfect parallel array is seen medially adjacent to the cell layer, and progressing closer and closer to the pial surface as one follows the lateral portion of the medial cortex laterally. The cortical layer of the lateral portion of the medial cortex also approaches the pial surface, but no so rapidly as this fiber bundle. This bundle is at least partially composed of commissural fibers from the contralateral medial cortex (Ulinski, 1976*b*; Halpern, 1974).

At postcommissural levels the medial cortex extends laterally along the dorsal surface of the telencephalon. Just caudal to the disappearance of the septum the medial portion of the medial cortex bends in on itself, forming a J-shaped hook (Figs. 2Q and 3G). Its polymorphic layer, which is relatively narrow rostrally and sparsely populated with perikarya, contains a massive fiber bundle running mediolaterally, forming what is commonly called the postcommissural fornix. The fibers of this bundle are clearly related to the lateral portion of the medial cortex. Whereas rostrally the polymorphic layer of the medial part of the medial cortex is virtually nonexistent, caudally it is broad and well populated with cells. The lateral portion also expands its polymorphic layers caudally. The cortical layer (layer 2) of the lateral portion does not appear, in Nissl-stained coronal sections, to be composed of a homogeneous population of cells. The more medially placed cells are more darkly stained and larger than the more tightly stained, smaller, laterally placed cells.

In the most caudal sections of the telencephalon the medial cortex swings around laterally, replacing both dorsal and lateral cortices, to encircle the dorsal and lateral aspects of the nucleus sphericus.

A small ventral region of the cortical mantle is seen only at midcaudal levels of the telencephalon (Fig. 2N–P). This ventral cortex is associated in coronal section with the appearance of the ventral aspect of the lateral ventricle. It is distinguished from the adjacent lateral cortex by its exceptionally well-populated polymorphic layer. Caudally it joins the more dorsally situated cortex but continues to be identifiable by its well populated polymorphic layer. In Ramón y Cajal-stained sections this ventral cortex is also distinguished by having a very dense plexus of fibers within its polymorphic layer and another dense plexus associated with its dorsal aspect in the molecular layer.

J. Dorsal Ventricular Ridge

The dorsal ventricular ridge is composed of three distinct structures, the anterior dorsal ventricular ridge (neostriatum of Warner, 1931, 1947), the posterior dorsal ventricular ridge,* and the angulostriatal mass (the latter two composing the angulostriatal cells of Warner). Warner describes in the neostriatum a dorsal lateral cell group which is larger than the smaller central cells. These dorsal lateral cells form a cap over the smaller central cells. Warner also describes a cell group in the dorsal lateral aspect of the ventricular ridge which he labels the "angulostriatal cells." In his (1931) illustration No. 8 he indicates that these cells are continuous with the cells that we currently call the posterior dorsal ventricular ridge. Ulinski (1976*a*) has described in detail the structure of the anterior dorsal ventricular ridge (aDVR) in snakes. Ulinski finds in his studies of both light microscopic sections and electron microscopic sections that the neuronal somata of the anterior dorsal ventricular ridge show the same cytological characteristics in all regions of the aDVR. However, the distribution of these neurons within the aDVR is not homogeneous. There is a great deal of clustering of cells, two to five in each cluster throughout the aDVR. This clustering is particularly apparent at the periphery of the aDVR along the ventricular surface. Ulinski describes two fiber bundles afferent to the aDVR. One comes from the lateral forebrain bundle and enters the aDVR rostrally, curving backward to reach caudal portions of aDVR. The second system of afferents to the aDVR comes from the anterior commissure and enters aDVR caudally.

The aDVR of the rat snake, as described in the section on the retrobulbar region, first develops lateral to the olfactory ventricle at caudal accessory olfactory

* The posterior dorsal ventricular ridge is commonly considered a part of the amgydala (Senn and Northcutt, 1973).

bulb levels (Fig. 2D). In the retrobulbar region, the aDVR is found dorsolateral to the slit-shaped lateral ventricle (Fig. 2E–H). When the lateral ventricle develops its lateral extension, the aDVR is situated ventral to the lateral extension and lateral to the ventromedial arm of the ventricle (Fig. 2I–O). The aDVR is separated from the telencephalic structures lying ventral to it by a cell-free zone (zona limitans interstriata of Ariëns Kappers *et al.*, 1960) (Fig. 2K). In the rat snake the zona limitans becomes obscured caudally (Fig. 2L,M) at approximately the level that the mural layer of the nucleus sphericus first becomes distinctive. When the dorsal aspect of the mural layer of the nucleus sphericus reaches the lateral ventricle (Fig. 2N), the aDVR is found medial to the nucleus sphericus. The aDVR becomes smaller (Fig. 2P,Q) and gradually disappears (Fig. 2R) caudal to the interventricular foramen.

The cells of the rostral part of the aDVR are medium sized (about 10 μm in their long axis) with round nuclei and relatively abundant perinuclear Nissl substance. They are moderately well packed and do not give the corticoid appearance which becomes characteristic more caudally of the subventricular layer. Ramón y Cajal-stained sections of this rostral portion of the aDVR reveal a rich fiber plexus in its neuropil with many of these fibers traceable to the lateral forebrain bundle situated in the ventral portion of the rostral telencephalon.

At a level approximately coincident with the definitive development of a medial cortex (Fig. 2K) the aDVR reaches its broadest, medial to lateral, development. At this level it is clear that the aDVR is a heterogeneous structure composed of a medial portion containing smaller (about 10 μm in their long axis) and more light-staining cells than the lateral portion, in which not only are the cells larger (14–20 μm in their long axis), more darkly stained, with a more distinctive perinuclear cytoplasm, but also the perikarya are more irregularly packed, giving the general appearance of greater scatter with occasional clumps. At telencephalic levels through the anterior commissure the lateral portion of the aDVR assumes a dorsolateral position subjacent to the lateral ventricle and is flanked laterally by the angulostriatal mass (Fig. 2L–N). As the mural layer of the nucleus sphericus develops, the lateral part of the aDVR diminishes in size until it is represented by a few darkly stained cells interposed between the rest of the aDVR and the angulostriatal mass. At these midtelencephalic levels the dorsal and medial aspect of the aDVR takes on a corticoid appearance, with many clumps of cells appearing in the subventricular zone. The core of the aDVR remains relatively homogeneous in appearance.

The aDVR of *Natrix* is very similar in appearance to that of *Elaphe* (Fig. 3E,F). On the other hand, in *Typhlops*, as noted previously by Senn and Northcutt (1973), the aDVR is markedly reduced (Fig. 4D).

The angulostriatal mass is situated just below the lateral ventricle lateral to the aDVR at midtelencephalic levels (Fig. 2L) and is composed of medium-sized, very dark-staining, tightly clumped cells. It extends caudally to a level when the mural layer of the nucleus sphericus reaches the ventricular surface (Fig. 2O), where it blends indistinguishably into the dorsal part of the posterior dorsal ventricular ridge.

The posterior dorsal ventricular ridge is composed of a loose aggregation of moderately to lightly stained cells (Fig. 2L–Q). It is sandwiched between the lateral wall of the mural layer of the nucleus sphericus and the lateral portion of the lateral pallium (rostrally) or the lateral extension of the lateral ventricle caudally. In its rostral portion the cells of pDVR are similar in size and staining properties to the cells of the core of aDVR, while the caudal portions of pDVR contain larger, more darkly stained cells which tend to be found in small aggregations.

K. Paleostriatum

The basal lateral telencephalon contains a variety of structures which together could be considered part of the paleostriatum. Warner (1947) describes a triangular area of densely packed cells located medial and ventral to the anterior dorsal ventricular ridge (his neostriatum). This area is illustrated by him in two figures (his Figs. 6 and 7, which correspond approximately to the dorsal portions of Fig. 2L and Fig. 2N of the present chapter). In the more rostral illustration he identifies the paleostriatum as an area dorsolateral to nucleus accumbens septi and ventral to neostriatum. In the more caudal section the paleostriatum is figured ventral to the neostriatum, medial to nucleus sphericus, and bridging the region between the ventricular ridge and the preoptic area.

That region of the ventral telencephalon not belonging to the amygdaloid complex (see below) or septum is designated here as paleostriatum. Although clear subdivisions can be identified, their relationship (homologous or analogous) to similarly situated structures in the telencephalon of other vertebrates cannot be determined in the present study. Connectivity studies and histochemical analysis of this region will help immeasurably in understanding the significance of the various subdivisions. In general, the paleostriatum is situated ventral to the aDVR, lateral to the septum, and medial to the accessory olfactory tract. A large portion of the paleostriatum is found interstitial to the fibers of the lateral forebrain bundle as that fiber tract travels dorsally to reach the aDVR. Another large part of the paleostriatum (as defined by Warner) is a nucleus medial to the midportion of the nucleus sphericus. This triangular-shaped nucleus (in cross section) extends from the medial wall of the nucleus sphericus to the lateral preoptic region. The efferent fibers of the nucleus sphericus form a fiber bundle similar to the stria terminalis (Halpern and Silfen, 1974) of other vertebrates. This fiber bundle courses through the triangular-shaped nucleus, and therefore this portion of the paleostriatum may be considered comparable to the bed nucleus of the stria terminalis* of other vertebrates. It has been so labeled here (PSb) tentatively.

At levels rostral to the bed nucleus of the stria terminalis the paleostriatum is composed of two portions. The dorsal part (Fig. 2K–M) is found adjacent to the ventral arm of the lateral ventricle just ventral to the zona limitans intrastriata. The ventral portion is found ventral to the dorsal part of the paleostriatum and medial to the accessory olfactory tract (Fig. 2L). It is composed of very darkly staining cells which are frequently clumped. Both dorsal and ventral portions of the paleostriatum are interstitial to the LFB as seen in Ramón y Cajal-stained material.

* The bed nucleus of the stria terminalis is generally considered a part of the preoptic area (Crosby *et al.*, 1962).

L. Archistriatum or Amygdala

Warner (1947) includes the nucleus sphericus and the nucleus ventromedialis (ventral amygdaloid nucleus of present chapter) in the archistriatum. Following Curwen (1939) one would also include the posterior dorsal ventricular ridge in the archistriatum or amygdala. I have chosen to discuss the posterior DVR above and to include the nucleus of the lateral olfactory tract* in the amygdaloid region.

The nucleus of the lateral olfactory tract (of Warner) is situated along the ventral border of the telencephalon from rostral (precommissural) levels (Fig. 2H) to a level coincident with the appearance of the ventral amygdaloid nucleus (Fig. 2K). Since no lateral olfactory tract exists at these levels, the nucleus is misnamed. Its position lateral to the accessory olfactory tract would make a name such as "lateral nucleus of the accessory olfactory tract" more appropriate. It remains to be demonstrated, however, that this nucleus has any relationships other than proximity to the accessory olfactory tract.

Just caudal to the nucleus of the lateral olfactory tract (Fig. 2H) a second nucleus appears which occupies a position lateral and ventral to the accessory olfactory tract and dorsal to the ventral amygdaloid nucleus. I have labeled this nucleus the "rostral amygdaloid nucleus" (Fig. 2L) to indicate its position. Its cells are of moderate to small size and are moderately clumped.

The ventral amygdaloid nucleus first appears at levels through the most rostral anterior commissure (Fig. 2K). In coronal sections its most rostral aspect appears to hang off the ventrolateral border of the telencephalon. The nucleus is separated dorsally from the rest of the telencephalon by a relatively cell-free zone through which fibers travel to and from the lateral pallium (Halpern, 1976*b*). The ventral amygdaloid nucleus is not a homogeneous structure. The cells in its ventral portion are more rounded and somewhat larger than the cells in its dorsal portion. The perikarya in the dorsomedial portion are elongated, with their long axis parallel to the cell-free zone dorsal to them. The cells in the dorsolateral region are more tightly packed, and the neuropil in this region is marked by a very dense and intricate fiber plexus. In caudal sections through the ventral amygdaloid nucleus the middle portion of the nucleus is replaced by the ventral portion of the mural layer of the nucleus sphericus. The nucleus sphericus thus splits the ventral amygdaloid nucleus into medial and lateral caudal segments (Fig. 2M) prior to the disappearance of the nucleus entirely (Fig. 2O).

The nucleus sphericus is probably the most prominent and most constant feature of the snake telencephalon. It occupies virtually the entire ventricular ridge of the caudal telencephalon. The nucleus is clearly laminated, consisting of an outer marginal layer, an inner hilar layer, and a dense cellular mural layer (Ulinski and Kanarek, 1973). Ulinski and Kanarek describe the nucleus sphericus of the common boa (*Constrictor constrictor*) as a cup-shaped aggregation of cells found posterior to the anterior commissure. The cells of the marginal layer are fusiform in shape, with their long axes oriented tangential to the mural layer. These cells have three to five primary dendrites with secondary and tertiary dendrites. The dendritic field is oriented tangential to the mural layer. The mural layer contains the vast majority

* The nucleus of the lateral olfactory tract is commonly considered a subdivision of the amgydala (Crosby *et al.*, 1962.)

of the cells of the nucleus sphericus. These cells have three sets of dendrites: one set which extends into the marginal layer, a second set of dendrites which run horizontally within the mural layer, and a third set of dendrites which enter the hilar layer. There are relatively few cells in the hilar layer. As seen in our own material, the hilar layer is occupied almost entirely by the unmyelinated portions of the axons of the accessory olfactory tract (lateral olfactory tract of Warner and others). The accessory olfactory tract enters the nucleus sphericus rostrally, where the nucleus is incomplete in its circumference. The mural layer cells are first clearly distinguishable at a level corresponding to the most rostral crossing fibers of the anterior commissure (Fig. 2M). At this level only the dorsolateral mural cells are clearly distinguishable. Subsequently the ventral portion of the nucleus sphericus becomes formed both in its medial and in its lateral aspect, and finally at the level of the hippocampal commissure the entire nucleus is seen in cross section. Examination of Nissl-stained sections makes it quite clear that the mural layer is not homogeneous in packing density or thickness. Dorsal and ventral portions appear more uniformly densely packed while the medial and lateral walls vary considerably in both packing density and thickness. At rostral levels through the anterior commissure the medial wall appears continuous with the cells of the bed nucleus of the stria terminalis.

M. Preoptic Area

Surrounding the preoptic recess of the third ventricle is a dense core of periventricular gray matter, the medial preoptic nucleus. Along the ventral aspect of the medial preoptic nucleus the densely stained suprachiasmatic nucleus is located. Lateral to the medial preoptic nucleus the forebrain bundles and stria terminalis course through the cell-poor lateral preoptic area. The supraoptic nucleus, a flat oval-shaped nucleus lying along the optic tracts as they course toward the diencephalon, separates the lateral preoptic area from the underlying optic tracts. The preoptic area blends imperceptibly into the anterior hypothalamus.

III. Fiber Connections

A. Main Olfactory Bulb

The efferent connections of the main olfactory bulb of snakes have recently been studied (Kowell, 1974; Halpern, 1973, 1976*b*). Following lesions restricted to the main olfactory bulb, degeneration (Fig. 5) is observed in the main olfactory tract, which lies lateral to the olfactory ventricle in the olfactory peduncle. As the retrobulbar region is approached and the lateral pallium develops, the degeneration is restricted to the peripheral portions of the retrobulbar region and almost completely encircles this area (anterior olfactory nucleus of most authors). In the region of the olfactory gray and olfactory tubercle, degenerating terminals invade the cellular areas. Otherwise, the degeneration is restricted to the molecular layer of the pallium. More caudally in the retrobulbar region the lateral pallium occupies a more restricted lateral position, and the degeneration of main olfactory bulb origin is associated with the lateral pallium and olfactory tubercle exclusively. The lateral pallium extends posteriorly to a level caudal to the hippocampal commissure, and degeneration of olfactory bulb origin is always associated with it. The olfactory tubercle extends to the level of the optic chiasma and has associated with it degeneration of main olfactory bulb origin. This degeneration continues caudally in the stria medullaris thalami, which is situated dorsal to the dorsal aspect of the optic tract. The degenerating fibers travel in the stria medullaris to the level of the habenular commissure, where they cross the midline and enter the contralateral stria medullaris. The stria medullaris thalami contralateral to the main olfactory bulb lesion contains degenerating fibers which traverse the base of the telencephalon dorsal to the ventral amygdaloid nucleus to gain access to the lateral pallium where they terminate.

B. Accessory Olfactory Bulb

The efferent fibers from the accessory olfactory bulb (Kowell, 1974; Halpern, 1973, 1976*b*) travel exclusively in the accessory olfactory tract (Fig. 6). The nucleus interstitial to the accessory olfactory tract is, in all probability, a major recipient of accessory olfactory bulb efferents. The remaining fibers continue caudally in the accessory olfactory tract and terminate within the hilar layer of the nucleus sphericus. A degeneration-free zone surrounds the core degeneration in the hilar layer.

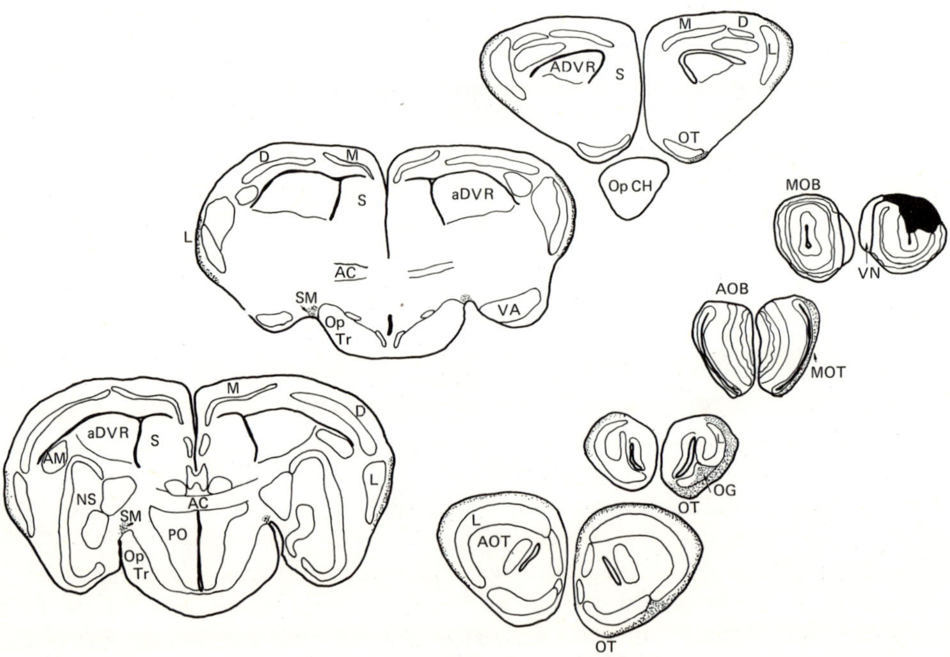

Figure 5. Series of projection drawings through the telencephalon of a garter snake (*Thamnophis sirtalis sirtalis*) that survived 7 days following main olfactory bulb ablation. The lesion area is indicated in black. The location of the resulting degeneration is marked by black dots.

No degeneration is seen in the contralateral telencephalon following accessory olfactory bulb lesions. Although the nucleus of the lateral olfactory tract is adjacent to the accessory olfactory tract for a considerable rostro-caudal distance, there appear to be no terminations of accessory olfactory bulb efferents in its immediate vicinity.

C. Nucleus Sphericus

The nucleus sphericus is the major recipient of efferent fibers from the accessory olfactory bulb (Halpern, 1973, 1976*b*; Kowell, 1974). In order to trace the further connections of the vomeronasal–accessory olfactory bulb system, electrolytic lesions were placed in the nucleus sphericus of 17 garter snakes (*Thamnophis sirtalis sirtalis* and *Thamnophis radix*) (Halpern and Silfen, 1974). Since considerable damage to the overlying cortices accompanies such ablation, lesions were placed in the dorsal and medial cortices of additional subjects, avoiding involvement of the nucleus sphericus. The results of these ablations are reported in the sections devoted to the connections of those cortices. Although the anterior dorsal ventricular ridge sustained damage in some of the animals with nucleus sphericus lesions, a sufficient number of brains containing nucleus sphericus lesions without anterior dorsal ventricular ridge damage were available for identification of the pathways. Animals in this study survived 7 and 9 days.

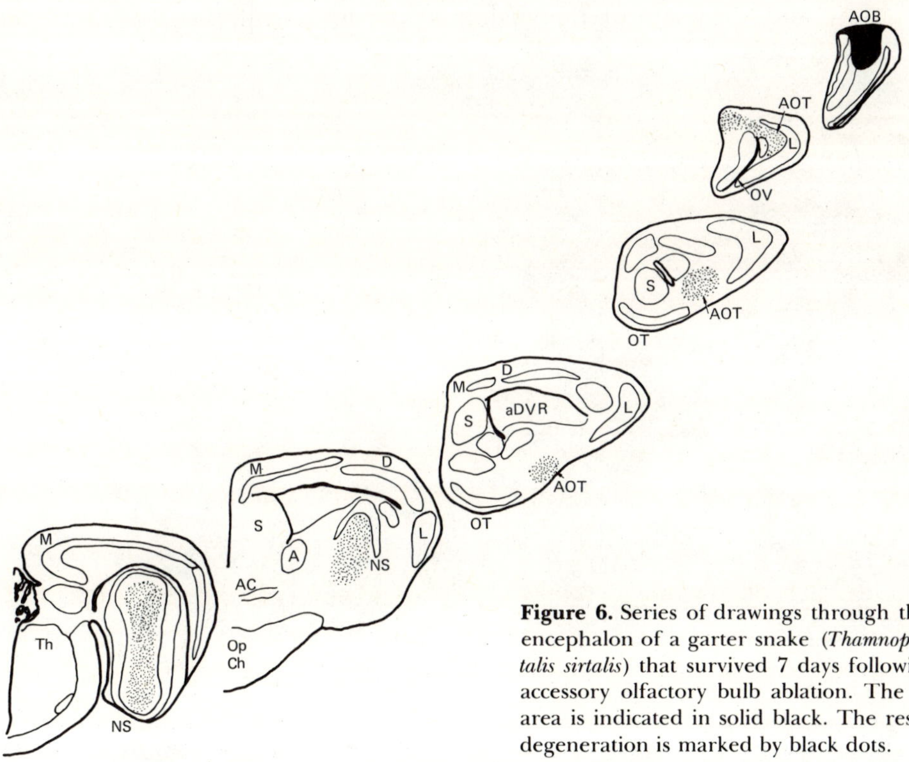

Figure 6. Series of drawings through the telencephalon of a garter snake (*Thamnophis sirtalis sirtalis*) that survived 7 days following an accessory olfactory bulb ablation. The lesion area is indicated in solid black. The resulting degeneration is marked by black dots.

Figure 7 is a series of projection drawings through the forebrain of a snake with a lesion (indicated in solid black) of the nucleus sphericus. Ipsilaterally, degeneration can be traced within the nucleus sphericus rostral and caudal to the lesion. The central core of degeneration is identical in location to that observed after accessory olfactory bulb lesions. However, additional degeneration not seen after accessory olfactory bulb lesions is observed in the more superficial portions of the hilar layer, the mural layer, and the marginal layer of the nucleus.

Degenerating fibers leaving the nucleus sphericus pass through the nucleus we have tentatively identified as the bed nucleus of the stria terminalis, which lies just medial to the nucleus sphericus at preoptic levels. These fibers pass medially into the preoptic area and hypothalamus, terminating in a ventromedially placed hypothalamic nucleus located midway through the rostral–caudal extent of the hypothalamus. This nucleus will be referred to as the ventromedial hypothalamic nucleus. No degeneration is observed in the contralateral hypothalamus, thalamus, or preoptic area.

Degeneration ipsilateral to the nucleus sphericus can also be followed rostrally to terminate in the ipsilateral accessory olfactory bulb. These degenerating axons surround the core of the accessory olfactory tract, and a few degenerating fibers are found within the tract. This rostrally traveling degeneration terminates in the internal granular layer and the adjacent portion of the internal plexiform layer of the accessory olfactory bulb. No degeneration is observed in the contralateral accessory olfactory bulb or either main olfactory bulb following nucleus sphericus lesions.

Efferent fibers from the nucleus sphericus cross the midline in the anterior commissure and terminate predominantly in the more superficial layers of the

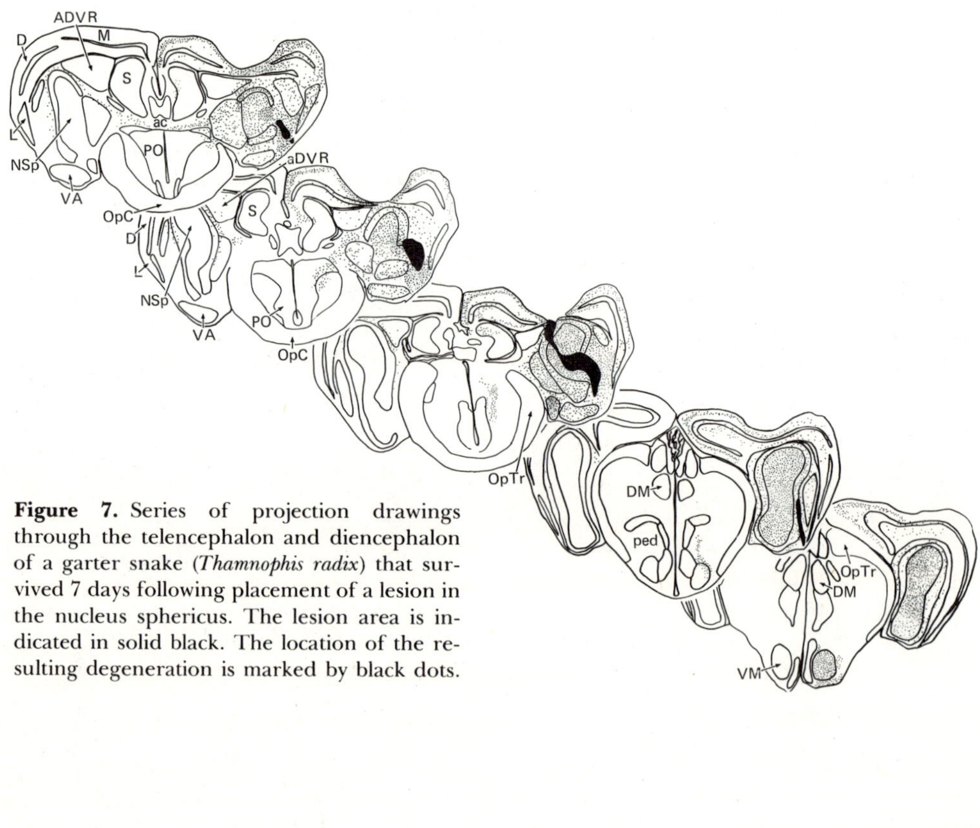

Figure 7. Series of projection drawings through the telencephalon and diencephalon of a garter snake (*Thamnophis radix*) that survived 7 days following placement of a lesion in the nucleus sphericus. The lesion area is indicated in solid black. The location of the resulting degeneration is marked by black dots.

contralateral nucleus sphericus. The hilar layer is relatively clear of degeneration; the few particles present in this layer appear to be axons crossing to the lateral aspect of the nucleus. Contralateral degeneration predominates in the marginal and mural layers. Degeneration on the side contralateral to the lesion is not widespread throughout the nucleus sphericus, but is located at those levels corresponding to the lesion levels.

D. Medial Cortex

The medial cortex is a major recipient of efferent fibers from the dorsal and lateral cortices (Ulinski, 1976*b*). The terminations of ipsilateral cortico-cortical and commissural fibers on the dendrites of these cells occur in a highly organized manner, suggesting that the cells of the medial cortex are capable of integrating information derived from diverse sources and modulating their own output in response to differing patterns of stimulation. Nothing is known at present, however, of additional noncortical sources of input to the medial cortex. Ulinski (1976*b*) reports as well that medial cortex projects to the ipsilateral, dorsal, and lateral cortices.

Laminar heat lesions were placed in the medial cortex of 16 garter snakes. The animals survived 2–21 days at 22–24°C. Large lesions of the medial cortex produce the pattern of degeneration shown in Fig. 8. Ipsilaterally the degeneration extends the entire length of the medial cortex rostral to and caudal to the lesion. Degeneration is also seen at the level of the lesion in the ipsilateral dorsal cortex in its molecular layer. The appearance of degeneration in the lateral cortex is variable and appears to be related to the size and lateral placement of the lesion.

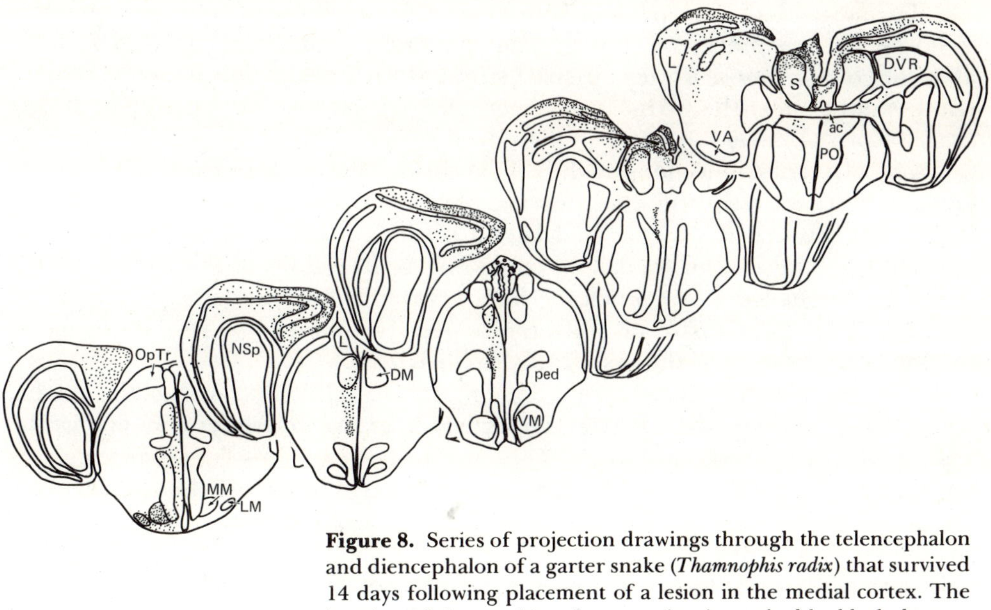

Figure 8. Series of projection drawings through the telencephalon and diencephalon of a garter snake (*Thamnophis radix*) that survived 14 days following placement of a lesion in the medial cortex. The location of the resulting degeneration is marked by black dots.

Degenerating efferent fibers leave the medial cortex and terminate in the dorsal and intermediate regions of the septum ipsilaterally. In Fig. 8 the degeneration in the postcommissural septum is in all likelihood due to the interruption by the lesion of fibers originating in the dorsal cortex and traversing the supraventricular layer of the medial cortex. Axons are seen crossing the midline in the nucleus of the hippocampal commissure, a cellular commissural area dorsal to the anterior commissure. These crossing fibers distribute to the contralateral septum and medial cortex. Within the medial cortex the axons of contralateral origin terminate in a lamina adjacent to the cell bodies of the medial cortex.

Fibers destined for the hypothalamus travel medial to the septal nuclei, above the anterior commissure, and pass ventrally behind the commissure to enter the anterior thalamus. Degeneration is observed in this anterior thalamic area following dorsal cortex lesions as well as following medial cortex lesions and may therefore be the result of interruption of fibers from the dorsal cortex. The degenerating fiber bundle descends medially in the thalamus and periventricular region of the hypothalamus, continuing in a ventrocaudal direction until it passes caudal to the ventromedial nucleus of the hypothalamus. Caudal to the ventromedial nucleus, the fiber bundle flares out laterally prior to terminating in two nuclei identified by Crosby and Woodburne (1940) as the medial and lateral mammillary nuclei. The medial cortex to hypothalamus connection is entirely ipsilateral.

The small amount of degeneration illustrated in the ventricular ridge in Fig. 8 is the result of heat damage to the aDVR and should not be considered part of the efferent connections of the medial cortex.

E. Dorsal Cortex

To date, with the exception of Ulinski's (1976*b*) demonstration of medial cortex to dorsal cortex connections, no experimental evidence has been presented of the afferents of the dorsal cortex in snakes. Based on information in other reptiles (Butler and Ebner, 1972; Hall and Ebner, 1970), however, one would expect that thalamocortical fibers terminate in the dorsal cortex.

The efferent connections of the dorsal cortex (Fig. 9) were studied by placing laminar heat lesions in the dorsal cortex. Since this region is relatively small and interposed between the medial and lateral cortices, many of the lesions included either the medial part of the lateral cortex or the lateral tip of the medial cortex. A few fortuitous lesions in which the dorsal cortex alone was damaged combined with the ability to compare two different types of contaminated lesions permitted the following analysis of the results (Halpern, 1976*a*).

The major intracortical connection of the dorsal cortex is with the medial cortex. Degeneration arising from a dorsal cortex lesion occupies a lamina in the middle part of the molecular layer of the medial cortex. Thus dorsal cortex axons terminate between the subpial lamina formed by terminals from the lateral cortex and the deep lamina formed by terminals from the contralateral medial cortex and the lateral part of the ipsilateral medial cortex. The dorsal cortex itself contains degeneration both rostral to and caudal to the lesion in all of its layers.

Dorsal cortex lesions result in an abundance of degeneration in the medial and ventrolateral portions of the precommissural septum, the rostral septal nucleus, and the dorsal intermediate postcommissural septum.

The posterior dorsal ventricular ridge contains a considerable amount of degeneration following dorsal cortex lesions while the anterior dorsal ventricular ridge and angulostriatal mass rarely contain degeneration following such lesions. These structures did not contain degeneration in the case illustrated in Fig. 9.

A small but consistent amount of degeneration can be traced out of the septum running in the lateral portion of the nucleus of the hippocampal commissure, above the anterior commissure and just rostral to the interventricular foramen. This degeneration appears to terminate at the most rostral dorsal limit of the diencephalon in a small, poorly defined nucleus which probably corresponds to a rostral extension of Warner's nucleus anterior of the thalamus (Warner, 1931).

F. Lateral Cortex

The major known sources of afferents to the lateral cortex are the ipsilateral and contralateral main olfactory bulbs (Halpern, 1973, 1976*b*; Kowell, 1974). The axons from the main olfactory bulb terminate in the outermost portion of the

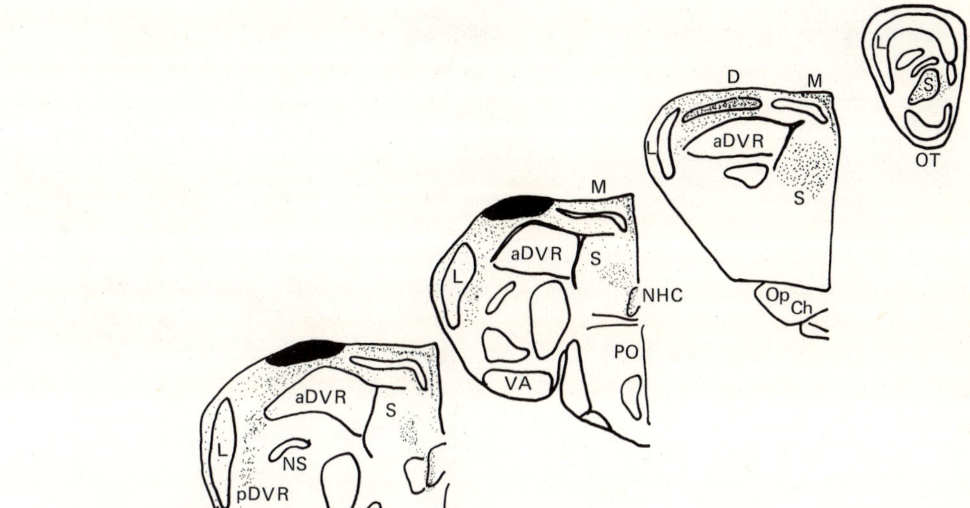

Figure 9. Series of projection drawings through the telencephalon and diencephalon of a garter snake (*Thamnophis radix*) that survived 7 days following placement of a lesion in the dorsal cortex. The lesion area is indicated in solid black. The location of the resulting degeneration is marked by black dots.

molecular layer. Ulinski (1976*b*) reports a source of afferents to the lateral pallium from the ipsilateral medial cortex. Following lesions of the rostral lateral pallium (Fig. 10), the pattern of degeneration indicates that the lateral pallium is heavily interconnected. The degeneration fills the molecular layer between the outer third, which contains degeneration of main olfactory bulb origin, and the outer cellular layer along its entire rostrocaudal extent.

The other cortical recipient of lateral cortex efferents is the medial portion of the medial cortex. The subpial portion of its molecular layer contains a dense accumulation of degenerating terminals for its entire rostrocaudal extent following lateral pallial lesions.

In the retrobulbar region relatively dense degeneration encircles all but the most ventral portion and invades most of the peripherally-lying cell groups. The olfactory tubercle is devoid of degeneration except for some scattered particles most rostrally. Degeneration following lateral cortex lesions can be followed rostrally in the main olfactory tract to the main olfactory bulb, where it is found in the internal granular layer and adjacent portions of the internal plexiform layer.

No contralateral degeneration is seen following lateral pallial lesions, nor is there any evidence of a diencephalic projection.

G. Septum

Ulinski (1975) reports a topographic heterogeneity in cortico-septal projections. The dorsal and medial cortices appear to be the major sources of cortico-septal fibers. The medial cortex projects bilaterally to the dorsal precommissural septum,

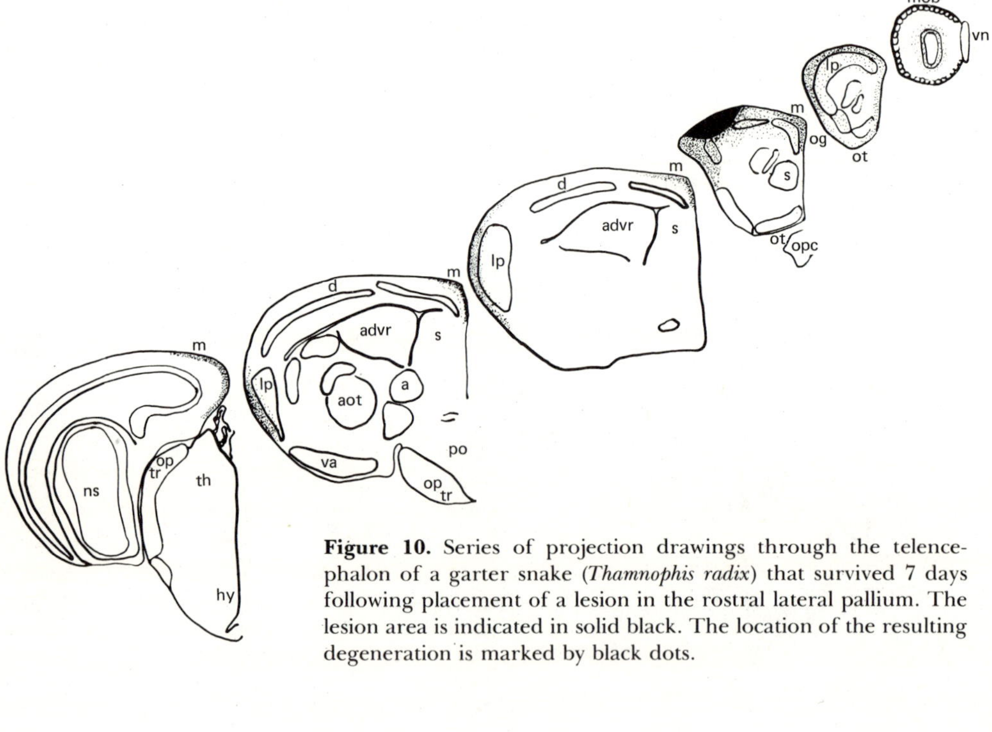

Figure 10. Series of projection drawings through the telencephalon of a garter snake (*Thamnophis radix*) that survived 7 days following placement of a lesion in the rostral lateral pallium. The lesion area is indicated in solid black. The location of the resulting degeneration is marked by black dots.

and the dorsal cortex projects to the ipsilateral dorsal postcommissural septum and a strip of septum which becomes more ventral at more rostral levels.

Although no restricted lesions of DM cortex were made, Ulinski (1975) argues from Golgi material and combined dorsal cortex–dorsomedial cortex lesions in which all septal degeneration terminates in dorsal cortex termination sites that dorsomedial cortex does not send axons to the septum. He remains equivocal on whether lateral cortex sends axons to the septum. Our own data suggest that this is not the case.

To date, no experimental study of the efferent connections of the septum has been reported.

IV. Concluding Remarks

The telencephalon of snakes shares much in common with the telencephalon of other reptiles but is distinctly different as well. A considerable amount of work is needed before we can feel entirely comfortable with the use of a universal nomenclature for all reptiles. Comparative histochemical studies of the telencephalon will aid in identifying structures of similar chemical constitution. Connectivity studies such as those described in Section III of this chapter will also facilitate comparisons between reptile groups and the development of a single system of nomenclature. Several structures within the telencephalon of snakes have remained relatively unstudied because of technical difficulties involved in placing restricted lesions within their borders. The application to snakes of the newer histochemical and autoradiographic techniques for describing axonal connections within the central nervous system will permit easier access to those structures which have, up to now, been relatively inaccessible. For example, in my laboratory we have been injecting horseradish peroxidase (HRP) into the dorsolateral thalamus. The HRP is transported in both an orthograde (Colman *et al.,* 1976) and a retrograde (Kristensson and Olsson, 1971) direction. The HRP transported in an orthograde manner can be traced from the thalamus through the lateral forebrain bundle to the anterior dorsal ventricular ridge, where the fibers terminate in a fine plexus. HRP transported in a retrograde manner can be traced to the cells of the paleostriatum surrounding the lateral forebrain bundle (Wang and Halpern, unpublished observations).

Acknowledgments. The work described in this chapter was supported by NINDS Grant NS1215201 and a SUNY Grain-in-Aid. Dr. Walter Riss generously gave of his time to read and criticize the manuscript. I am deeply appreciative of the histological assistance of Natalie Frumin, the photographic work of Jack Illari, and the secretarial assistance of Ida Muntner and Rose Kraus.

V. References

Ariëns Kappers, C. U., and Theunissen, W. F., 1908, Die Phylogenese des Rhombencephalons, des Corpus striatum und der Vorderhirn Kommissuren, *Folia Neurobiol.* **1:**173.

Ariëns Kappers, C. U., Huber, G. C., and Crosby, E. C., 1960, *The Comparative Anatomy of the Nervous System of Vertebrates, Including Man,* Hafner, New York.

Butler, A. B., and Ebner, F. F., 1972, Thalamotelencephalic projections in the lizard *Iguana iguana. Anat. Rec.* **172:**282.

Carey, J. H., 1967, The nuclear pattern of the telencephalon of the Blacksnake, *Coluber constrictor constrictor,* in: *Evolution of the Forebrain* (R. Hassler and H. Stephan, eds.), pp. 73–80, Plenum Press, New York.

Colman, D. R., Scalia, F., and Cabrales, E., 1976, Light and electron microscopic observations on the anterograde transport of horseradish peroxidase in the optic pathway in the mouse and rat, *Brain Res.* **102:**156.

Crosby, E. C., 1917, The forebrain of *Alligator mississippiensis, J. Comp. Neurol.* **27:**325.

Crosby, E. C., and Humphrey, T., 1939, Studies of the vertebrate telencephalon. I. The nuclear configuration of the olfactory and accessory olfactory formations and of the nucleus olfactorius anterior of certain reptiles, birds, and mammals, *J. Comp. Neurol.* **71:**121.

Crosby, E. C., Humphrey, T., and Lauer, E. U., *Correlative Anatomy of the Nervous System,* Macmillan, New York.

Crosby, E. C., and Woodburne, R. T., 1940, The comparative anatomy of the preoptic area and the hypothalamus, in: The Hypothalamus and Central Levels of Autonomic Function, *Res. Publ. Assoc. Res. Nerv. Ment. Dis.* **20:**52.

Crosby, E. C., DeJonge, B. R., and Schneider, R. C., 1967, Evidence for some of the trends in the phylogenetic development of the vertebrate telencephalon, in: *Evolution of the Forebrain* (R. Hassler and H. Stephan, eds.), pp. 117–135, Plenum Press, New York.

Curwen, A. O., 1939, The telencephalon of *Tupinambis nigropunctatus.* III. Amygdala, *J. Comp. Neurol.* **71:**613.

DeLange, S. J., 1911, Das Vorderhirn der Reptilien, *Folia Neurobiol.* **5:**548.

Durward, A., 1930, The cell masses in the forebrain of *Sphenodon punctatum, J. Anat.* **65:**8.

Edinger, L., 1896, Untersuchungen über die vergleichende Anatomie des Gehirns. III. Neue Studien über das Vorderhirn der Reptilien, *Abh. Senckenb. Naturforsch. Ges.* **19:**313.

Fink, R. P., and Heimer, L., 1967, Two methods for selective silver impregnation of degenerating axons and their synaptic endings in the central nervous system, *Brain Res.* **4:**369.

Frederikse, A., 1931, *The Lizard's Brain: An Investigation of the Histological Structure of the Brain of Lacerta vivipara,* C. C. Callenback, Nijerk.

Hall, W. C., and Ebner, F. F., 1970, Thalamotelencephalic projections in the turtle (*Pseudemys scripta*), *J. Comp. Neurol.* **140:**101.

Halpern, M., 1973, Olfactory bulb and accessory olfactory bulb projections in the snake, *Thamnophis sirtalis, Anat. Rec.* **175:**337.

Halpern, M., 1974, An experimental demonstration of the fornix system in a snake, *Soc. Neurosci. 4th Annu. Meet.*

Halpern, M., 1976*a*, Efferent connections of the lateral and dorsal cortices of snakes of the genus *Thamnophis, Anat. Rec.* **184:**421.

Halpern, M., 1976*b*, The efferent connections of the olfactory bulb and accessory olfactory bulb in the snakes, *Thamnophis sirtalis* and *Thamnophis radix, J. Morphol.* **150:**553.

Halpern, M., and Silfen, R., 1974, The efferent connections of the nucleus sphericus in the garter snake, *Thamnophis sirtalis, Anat. Rec.* **178:**368.

Humphrey, T., 1967, The development of the human hippocampal formation correlated with some aspects of its phylogenetic history, in: *Evolution of the Forebrain* (R. Hassler and H. Stephan, eds.), pp. 104–116, Plenum Press, New York.

Kowell, A. P., 1974, The olfactory and accessory olfactory bulbs in constricting snakes: Neuroanatomic and behavioral observations, *Diss. Abstr.* **35(4):**1490B.

Kristensson, K., and Olsson, J. 1971, Retrograde axonal transport of protein, *Brain Res.* **29:**363.

Meyer, A., 1892, Über das Vorderhirn einiger Reptilien, *Z. Wiss. Zool.* **55:**63.

Meyer, A., 1895, Zur Homologie der Fornixcommissur und des Septum lucidum bei den Reptilien und Säugern, *Anat. Anz.* **10:**474.

Pritz, M. D., 1973, Connections of the alligator visual system: Telencephalic projections of nucleus rotundus, *Anat. Rec.* **175:**416.

Rabl-Ruckhard, H., 1894, Einiges über das Gehirn der Riesenschlange, *Z. Wiss. Zool.* **58:**694.

Riss, W., Halpern, M., and Scalia, F., 1969, The quest for clues to forebrain evolution—The study of reptiles, *Brain Behav. Evol.* **2:**1.

Rose, M., 1923, Histologische Lokalisation des Vorderhirns der Reptilien, *J. Psychol. Neurol. Lpz.* **29:**219.

Rudin, W., 1974, Untersuchungen am olfaktorischen System der Reptilien. III. Differenzierungsformen einiger olfaktorischer Zentren bei Reptilien, *Acta. Anat.* **89:**481.

Senn, D. G., and Northcutt, R. G., 1973, The forebrain and midbrain of some squamates and their bearing on the origin of snakes, *J. Morphol.* **140:**135.

Ulinski, P. S., 1974, Cytoarchitecture of cerebral cortex in snakes, *J. Comp. Neurol.* **158:**243.

Ulinski, P. S., 1975, Corticoseptal projections in the snakes *Natrix sipedon* and *Thamnophis sirtalis, J. Comp. Neurol.* **164:**375.

Ulinski, P. S., 1976*a*, Structure of the anterior dorsal ventricular ridge in snakes, *J. Morphol.* **148:**1.

Ulinski, P. S., 1976*b*, Intracortical connections in the snakes *Natrix sipedon* and *Thamnophis sirtalis, J. Morphol.* **150:**463.

Ulinski, P. S., and Kanarek, D. A., 1973, Cytoarchitecture of nucleus sphericus in the common boa, *Constrictor constrictor, J. Comp. Neurol.* **151:**159.

Warner, F. J., 1931, The cell masses of the telencephalon and diencephalon of the rattlesnake, *Crotalus atrox, Proc. Acad. Sci. Amsterdam* **34:**1156.

Warner, F. J., 1946, The development of the forebrain of the American diamond-back rattlesnake, *Proc. Zool. Soc. London* **116:**22.

Warner, F. J., 1947, The fiber tracts of the forebrain of the American diamond-back rattlesnake (*Crotalus adamanteus*), *Proc. Zool. Soc. London* **116:**22.

10

Cytoarchitectonic and Connectional Organization of the Lacertilian Telencephalon with Comments on Vertebrate Forebrain Evolution

ANN B. BUTLER

I. Introduction

Two assumptions regarding nonmammalian vertebrates have long been held to be true. The first of these is that nonmammals, as opposed to mammals, behave in stereotyped ways and have little capacity to modify their behavior through learning. The second assumption is that nonmammals are "lower" vertebrates, representing evolutionary stages that gave rise to the "higher" vertebrates, i.e., mammals. Both of these assumptions suggest that the brains of nonmammalian vertebrates (1) are much more simply organized than the brains of mammals and (2) lack any structures which would be comparable to the "higher" (different usage than above but not easily definable) centers of mammalian brains, such as the cerebral neocortex. Thus there would seem to be little reason to study the organization of nonmammalian brains other than out of historical, evolutionary interest.

Were either of the above assumptions true, one might indeed make a good case for such a line of reasoning. However, behavioral and anatomical studies, most of which have been carried out within the last 10 years, in addition to the basic flaw of reasoning above in terms of evolutionary mechanisms, have cast grave doubt on these assumptions. There are now sufficient data to warrant a revision of a number of previously held concepts regarding the organization and evolution of vertebrate brains.

ANN B. BUTLER • Department of Anatomy, Georgetown University, Washington, D.C. 20007.

Most of the experimentally determined data on the connectional organization of reptilian telencephalons deal with ascending sensory system projections; while some data have been obtained in lizards, several of the major projection systems have been more thouroughly worked out in other reptiles and in birds. Thus these data will be reviewed here and compared to the data on forebrain connections in lizards.

II. Anatomy of the Lacertilian Forebrain

Before discussion of the presently known telencephalic connections in reptiles and other vertebrates, the normal anatomical structure of the forebrain should be considered. A number of excellent descriptive papers on reptilian telencephalons are available in the literature (e.g., Unger, 1906; Johnston, 1915; Crosby, 1916; Cairney, 1926; Warner, 1931; Curwen, 1937; Armstrong *et al.*, 1953; Goldby and Gamble, 1957; Northcutt, 1967, 1970; Ebbesson and Voneida, 1969; Platel, 1969; Riss *et al.*, 1969; Beckers *et al.*, 1971; Platel *et al.*, 1973; Ulinski, 1974, 1976*b*; Ulinski and Kanarek, 1973), so, for the present purpose, I will emphasize only the major pallial areas in two representative types of lizards.

Figure 1 shows photomicrographs of transverse Nissl-stained sections through midtelencephalic levels of the lizards *Gekko gecko* (on the left) and *Iguana iguana*. In these and other species of lizards, the pallium is composed of three cortical regions and a relatively massive protrusion into the lateral ventricle, the dorsal ventricular ridge (DVR). The pallial cortical areas of the medial, dorsal, and lateral

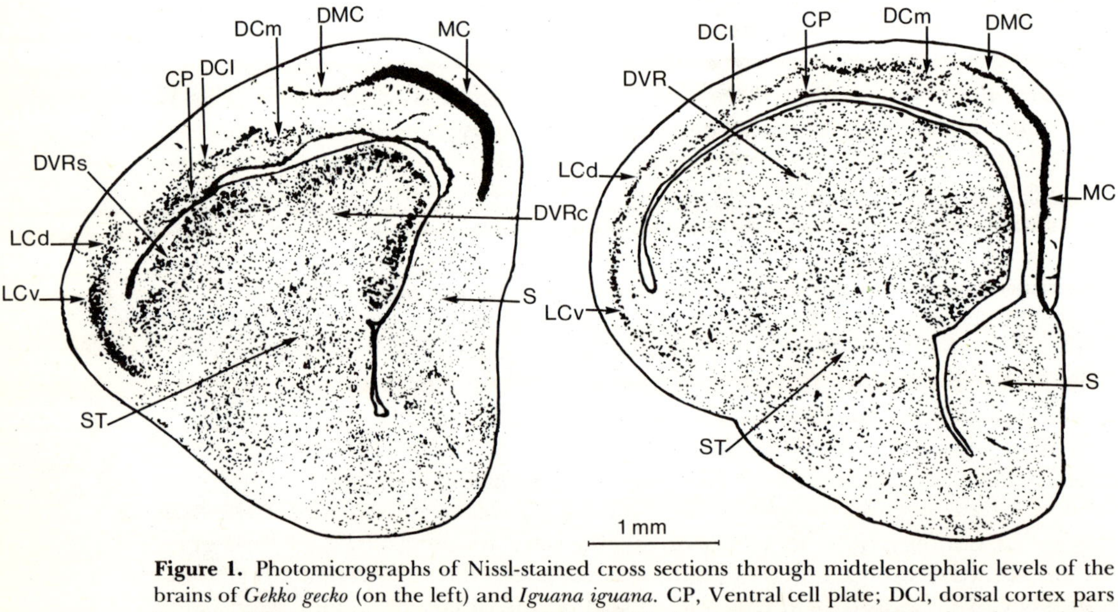

Figure 1. Photomicrographs of Nissl-stained cross sections through midtelencephalic levels of the brains of *Gekko gecko* (on the left) and *Iguana iguana*. CP, Ventral cell plate; DCl, dorsal cortex pars lateralis; DCm, dorsal cortex pars medialis; DMC, dorsomedial cortex; DVR, dorsal ventricular ridge; DVRc, core nucleus of dorsal ventricular ridge; DVRs, surrounding corticoid band of dorsal ventricular ridge; LCd, lateral cortex pars dorsalis; LCv, lateral cortex pars ventralis; MC, medial cortex; S, septum; ST, striatum.

walls can each be subdivided on the basis of cytoarchitectonics. The medial wall is composed of medial cortex (MC, Fig. 1) and dorsomedial cortex (DMC). Dorsal cortex has three subdivisions: dorsal cortex pars medialis (DCm), dorsal cortex pars lateralis (DCl), and the ventral cell plate (CP), which was described by Unger (1906). Lateral cortex can be divided into a pars dorsalis (LCd) and a pars ventralis (LCv), on the basis of cell-packing density. LCd overlies part of the dorsal cortex pars lateralis, and DMC overlies part of dorsal cortex pars medialis, complicating the analysis of efferent connections of these subdivisions. These cortical regions have been given a variety of names in the literature, and some of these are summarized in Table I.

The dorsal ventricular ridge is generally divided into three major regions—pars anterior, pars posterior, and nucleus sphericus. (The pallial origin of pars posterior and nucleus sphericus has not been established: Northcutt, 1978.) Nucleus sphericus, which has been shown to be the target of accessory olfactory bulb projections in lizards and snakes (Gamble, 1952; Heimer, 1969; Halpern, 1973), occupies the caudal, ventral portion of the ridge, and the pars posterior is defined as that part of the dorsal ventricular ridge dorsal to nucleus sphericus. In comparing *Gekko* and *Iguana* (Fig. 1) differences in the cytoarchitectonic organization of the dorsal ventricular ridge pars anterior can be seen. In *Gekko* the ridge is composed of a core neuropil (DVRc), which is surrounded by a band of clumped and relatively unmigrated cells (DVRs). In *Iguana* the cells are relatively more migrated from the ventricular surface and form nuclear areas. Only traces of a corticoid band structure are present in the DVR in *Iguana,* such as that seen along the medioventral portion of its surface. Variation in terminology applied to the dorsal ventricular ridge is summarized in Table II.

Gekko and *Iguana* are representative of two types of lizards, each recognizable by a number of features, including the differences in the cytoarchitecture of the dorsal ventricular ridge, the relative development of the medial cortex and septum, and differences in tectal lamination (Senn and Northcutt, 1973; Northcutt, 1978). The core neuropil–corticoid band arrangement of the DVR is the type I, or lacertid, pattern and is found in the Anguidae, Cordylidae, Dibamidae, Gekkonidae, Helodermatidae, Lacertidae, Lanthanotidae, Pygopodidae, Scincidae, Xantusidae, and Xenosauridae. The more migrated, nuclear arrangement of the DVR is the type II, or iguanid, pattern and characterizes the Agamidae, Chameleonidae, Iguanidae, Teiidae, and Varanidae (Northcutt, 1977). As the type I, lacertid pattern is also found in turtles and in the rhynchocephalian *Sphenodon,* it is considered to be the more generalized (ancestral) pattern. The significance of this variation in morphology will be considered below.

The subpallium of the telencephalon is composed mainly by the septum (S) and striatal regions (ST, Fig. 1). While the septum will be considered here in relation to the medial cortex, few studies have yet been carried out on the connections of other regions of the lacertilian subpallium (e.g., Parent, 1976). Histochemical studies have demonstrated that the striatum has a high content of both succinate dehydrogenase and acetylcholinesterase (Northcutt, 1978); it is therefore thought to be homologous to the paleostriatal complex of birds (Karten, 1969; Karten and Dubbeldam, 1973) and the basal ganglia of mammals.

Diencephalic and pretectal nuclei have been described in a variety of species of lizards (*Chameleon vulgaris*: Shanklin, 1930; *Lacerta sicula*: Senn, 1968; *Iguana*

Table I. Nomenclature of the Pallial Cortical Areas in Reptiles

Current usage in *Iguana iguana* and *Gekko gecko*	Medial Cortex	Dorsomedial cortex	Dorsal cortex pars medialis	Ventral cell plate	Dorsal cortex pars lateralis	Lateral cortex pars dorsalis	Lateral cortex pars ventralis
Unger (1906): *Gekko gecko*	Mediodorsal cell plate, small cells	Mediodorsal cell plate, large cells	Dorsal cell plate	Ventral cell plate	Dorsal cell plate	Lateral cell plate	
Johnston (1915): *Cistudo carolina*	Hippocampal formation	Subiculum cornu ammonis	General pallium			Lobus piriformis	
Crosby (1916): *Alligator mississippiensis*	Hippocampus pars dorsomedialis	Hippocampus pars dorsalis	General cortex			Pyriform lobe cortex	
Cairney (1926): *Sphenodon punctatus*	Hippocampus		General cortex			Pyriform cortex	
Northcutt (1967): *Iguana iguana*	Hippocampus pars dorsomedialis	Hippocampus pars dorsalis	Dorsomedial cortex		Dorso-lateral cortex	Pyriform cortex	
Ebbesson and Voneida (1969): *Tupinambis nigropunctatus*	Medial cortex	Dorsomedial cortex + ventral cortex	Dorsal cortex, layers 1 and 2	Dorsal cortex layer 3	Dorsolateral cortex + layer 3 of lateral cortex	Lateral cortex, layers 1 and 2	
Ulinski (1974): Families Boidae and Colubridae	Medial cortex	Dorsomedial cortex	Dorsal cortex	Ventral cell plate	Dorsal cortex	Lateral cortex	
Lohman and Van Woerden-Verkley (1976): *Tupinambis nigropunctatus*	Cortex mediodorsalis, small-celled part	Cortex mediodorsalis, large-celled part	Dorsal cortex			Lateral cortex	
Northcutt (1978): *Iguana iguana* and *Gekko gecko*	Medial cortex, ventral small-celled component (C2)	Medial cortex, dorsal large-celled component (Cl)	Dorsal cortex, subdivision C3		Dorsal cortex, subdivisions C2 and C1	Lateral cortex	

iguana: Butler and Northcutt, 1973; *Tupinambis nigropunctatus*: Cruce, 1974; *Gekko gecko*: Northcutt and Butler, 1974*a*). Some of the nuclei described in *Iguana* (Butler and Northcutt, 1973) are shown in Fig. 2. A number of these nuclei have been found to be targets of visual, auditory, or somesthetic projections. Projections of some of the visual and auditory thalamic nuclei to parts of the telencephalic cortices and dorsal ventricular ridge have also been traced.

III. Connections of the Lacertilian Forebrain

Figure 3 presents a summary of some of the known ascending sensory, corticocortical, and descending projections in lizards. Pretectal nuclei have been omitted, but those which receive retinal projections may well be part of an additional visual pathway to the telencephalon.

A. Ascending Sensory Projections

Retinal projections have been studied in a variety of lizard species (Armstrong, 1950; Ebbesson, 1970; Butler and Northcutt, 1971*a*; Butler, 1974; Northcutt and Butler, 1974*a*; Cruce and Cruce, 1975). In the thalamus, the retina (RET, Fig. 3) has been found to project to the pars dorsalis and pars ventralis of the lateral geniculate nucleus (LGN, Fig. 3), and to the nucleus ventrolateralis pars ventralis. Nucleus geniculatus lateralis pars dorsalis receives a bilateral retinal input, via the optic chiasm (OC), and this nucleus has been thought to be a good candidate for a homologue of the dorsal lateral geniculate nucleus in mammals. However, retinal

Table II. Nomenclature of the Subcortical Pallium in Reptiles

Current usage in *Iguana iguana* and *Gekko gecko*	Dorsal ventricular ridge
Unger (1906): *Gekko gecko*	Epistriatum
Johnston (1915): *Cistudo carolina*	Dorsal ventricular ridge
Crosby (1916): *Alligator mississippiensis*	Dorsolateral area
Cairney (1926): *Sphenodon punctatus*	Hypopallium
Northcutt (1967): *Iguana iguana*	Hyperstriatum anterior
Ulinski (1976*b*): Families Boidae and Colubridae	Dorsal ventricular ridge
Lohman and Van Woerden-Verkley (1976): *Tupinambis nigropunctatus*	Dorsal striatum
Northcutt (1970, 1978): *Chrysemys picta, Iguana iguana,* and *Gekko gecko*	Dorsal ventricular ridge

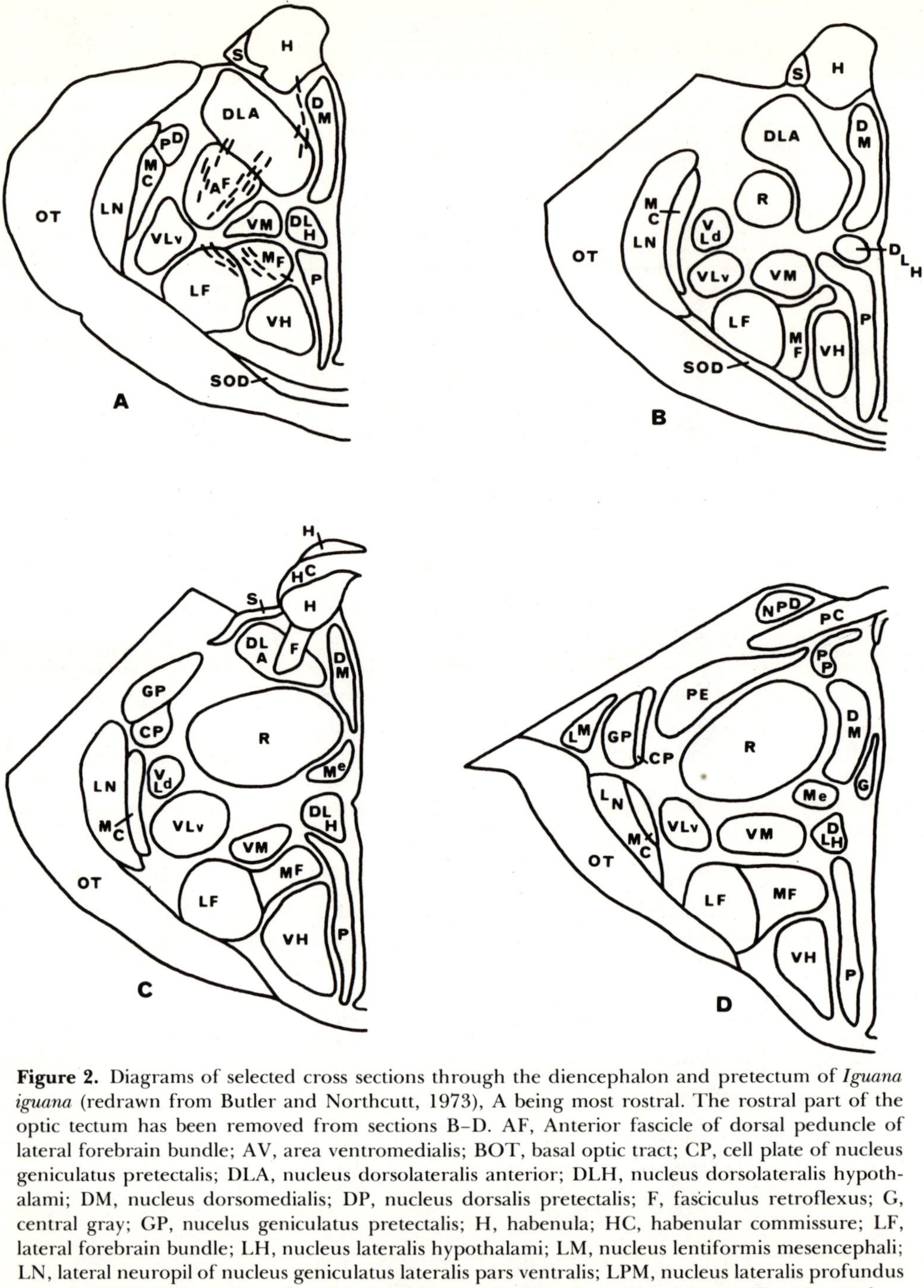

Figure 2. Diagrams of selected cross sections through the diencephalon and pretectum of *Iguana iguana* (redrawn from Butler and Northcutt, 1973), A being most rostral. The rostral part of the optic tectum has been removed from sections B–D. AF, Anterior fascicle of dorsal peduncle of lateral forebrain bundle; AV, area ventromedialis; BOT, basal optic tract; CP, cell plate of nucleus geniculatus pretectalis; DLA, nucleus dorsolateralis anterior; DLH, nucleus dorsolateralis hypothalami; DM, nucleus dorsomedialis; DP, nucleus dorsalis pretectalis; F, fasciculus retroflexus; G, central gray; GP, nucelus geniculatus pretectalis; H, habenula; HC, habenular commissure; LF, lateral forebrain bundle; LH, nucleus lateralis hypothalami; LM, nucleus lentiformis mesencephali; LN, lateral neuropil of nucleus geniculatus lateralis pars ventralis; LPM, nucleus lateralis profundus mesencephali; MC, medial cell plate of nucleus geniculatus lateralis pars ventralis; Me, nucleus medialis; MF, medial forebrain bundle; MP, nucleus medialis pretectalis; NPD, nucleus posterodorsalis; OT, optic tract; P, nucleus periventricularis; PC, posterior commissure; PD, nucleus geniculatus lateralis pars dorsalis; PE, nucleus lentiformis thalami pars extensa; PP, nucleus lentiformis thalami pars plicata; R, nucleus rotundus; S, stria medullaris; SOD, supraoptic decussation;

projections were also traced to an area dorsal to the dorsal geniculate nucleus in *Xantusia* (Butler, 1974) and *Gekko* (Northcutt and Butler, 1974*a*); subsequently, Northcutt (1978) has identified this and an additional region as two additional dorsal thalamic retinal targets in lizards and other reptiles—the dorsal optic nucleus, laterally adjacent to nucleus dorsolateralis anterior, and nucleus dorsocentralis, dorsal to nucleus rotundus. Thus there are now three possible candidates for a homologue of the mammalian dorsal lateral geniculate nucleus, and there is a question as to the nature of the other two nuclei. The efferent projections of these thalamic visual nuclei have not been determined in lizards.

The retina also projects to the superficial layers (8–13) of the optic tectum via the medial and lateral optic tracts (layer 14), and in some species this projection has been found to be bilateral (Butler, 1974; Northcutt and Butler, 1974*a*; Cruce and Cruce, 1975). Efferents from the tectum (TeO, Fig. 3) project bilaterally, via the supraoptic decussation (SOD), on nucleus rotundus (ROT) in the dorsal thalamus, as well as to some pretectal nuclei and other targets (Ebbesson, 1970; Butler and Northcutt, 1971*b*; Butler, 1976*a*). Nucleus rotundus then projects to a lateral region of the dorsal ventricular ridge (Distel and Ebbesson, 1975).

The auditory projection pathway to the thalamus has been traced in the lizard

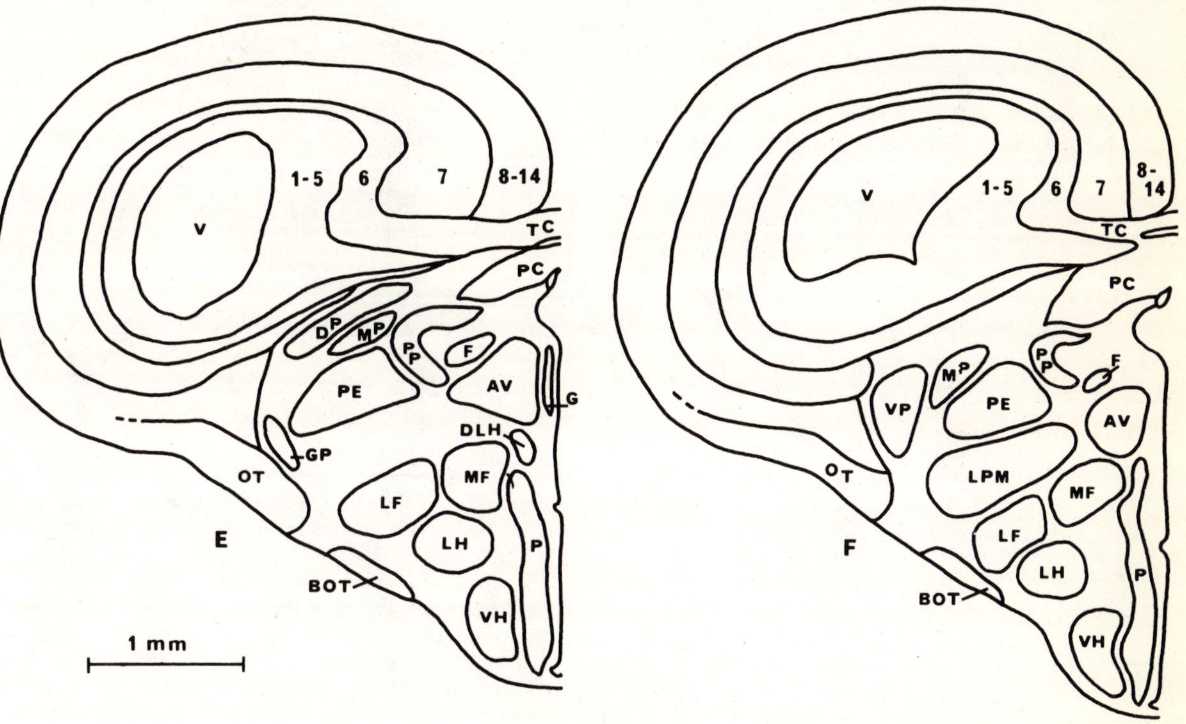

Figure 2. (*cont.*)

TC, tectal commissure; V, tectal ventricle; VH, nucleus ventralis hypothalami; VLd, nucleus ventrolateralis pars dorsalis; VLv, nucleus ventrolateralis pars ventralis; VM, nucleus ventromedialis; VP, nucleus ventralis pretectalis; 1–5, layers 1–5 of the optic tectum (periventricular gray and white); 6, layer 6 of the optic tectum (central white); 7, layer 7 of the optic tectum (central gray); 8–14, layers 8–14 of the optic tectum (superficial gray and white).

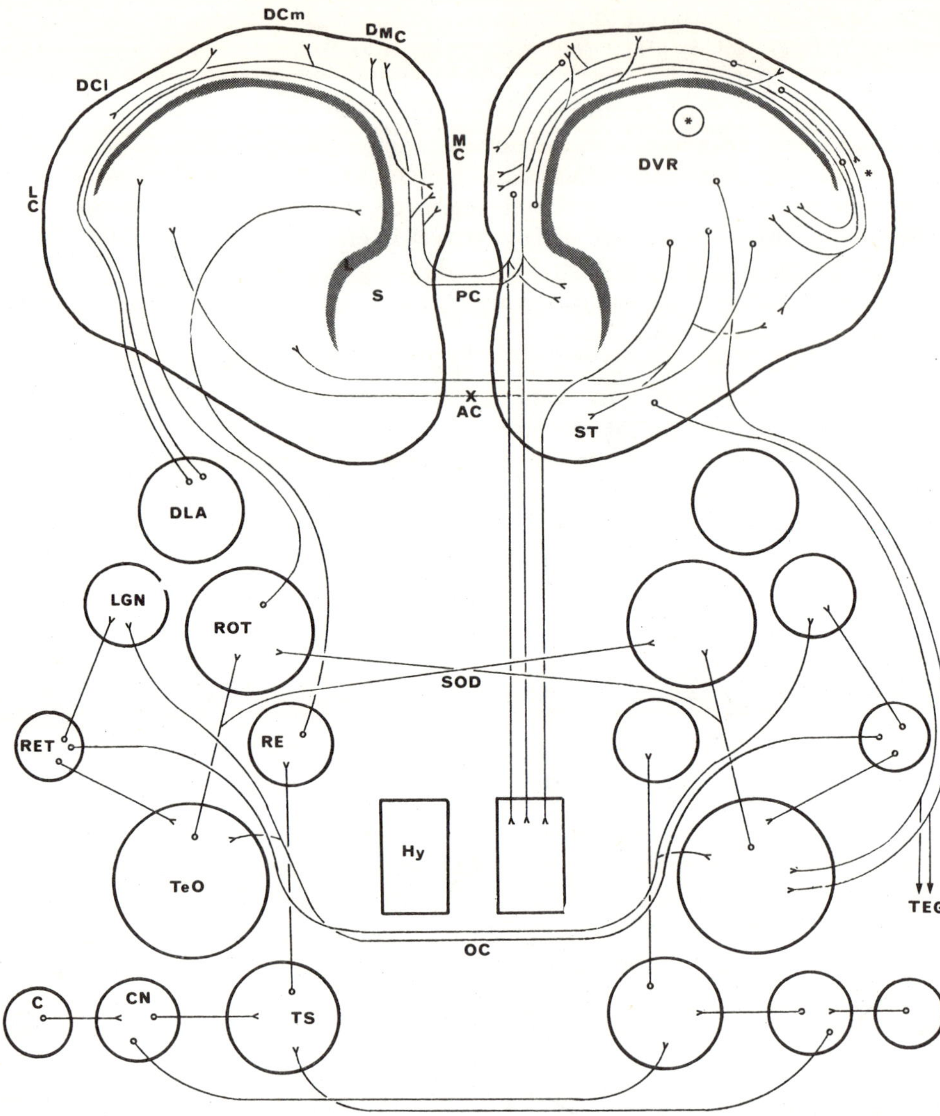

Figure 3. Schematic representation of organization of the telencephalon in lizards with ascending afferent pathways. Ascending systems include both ipsilateral and contralateral projections to the thalamic level. Efferent and commissural connections of the telencephalon are shown originating from the right hemisphere (diagrammed in transverse section), and afferent telencephalic connections are shown to the left hemisphere. Small circles denote cell bodies of origin and small v's at the end of lines denote termination. An X across a line (shown at AC) indicates that this connection has been found to be absent. AC, Anterior commissure; C, cochlea; CN, cochlear nuclei; DCl, dorsal cortex pars lateralis; DCm, dorsal cortex pars medialis; DLA, nucleus dorsolateralis anterior; DMC dorsomedial cortex; DVR, dorsal ventricular ridge; Hy, hypothalamus; L, lateral ventricle; LGN, lateral geniculate nucleus; LC, lateral cortex; MC, medial cortex; OC, optic chiasm; PC, anterior pallial commissure; RE, nucleus reuniens; RET, retina; ROT, nucleus rotundus; S, septum; SOD, supraoptic decussation; ST, striatum; TEG, mesencephalic tegmentum; TeO, optic tectum; TS, central nucleus of torus semicircularis; * encircled, site of recording of visual evoked potentials (Peterson and Rowe, 1976); * in lateral cortex on right, site of projection from DMC. Data on connections are from the following. Retinal projections: Ebbesson (1970); Butler and Northcutt

Iguana (Foster, 1974). Cochlear receptors (C) project on the cochlear nuclei (CN), which in turn project bilaterally to the central nucleus of the torus semicircularis (TS) in the midbrain, the homologue of the mammalian inferior colliculus. Efferents of the torus semicircularis then project to nucleus reuniens (RE), alternately termed "nucleus medialis," in the dorsal thalamus. In both *Iguana* (Foster and Peele, 1975) and *Varanus* (Distel and Ebbesson, 1975) projections from nucleus reuniens have been traced to a medioventral portion of the dorsal ventricular ridge.

Somesthetic efferents from the spinal cord and dorsal column nuclei (not shown in Fig. 3) have also been traced to lateral regions of the thalamus in *Tupinambis* (Ebbesson, 1967, 1976); however, the projections to the telencephalon have not yet been determined.

Nuclei dorsolateralis anterior (DLA, Fig. 3) and dorsomedialis occupy a large volume of the dorsal thalamus, and have long been considered possible homologues of the anterior thalamic group in mammals. While the afferent connections are unknown, efferent projections of nucleus dorsolateralis anterior have been traced with the anterograde degeneration method to a portion of dorsal cortex in *Varanus* (Distel and Ebbesson, 1975). However, different results have been obtained in *Tupinambis;* using both anterograde degeneration and retrograde horseradish peroxidase methods, nucleus dorsolateralis anterior was found to project to the outer, molecular layer of medial cortex (MC), the fibers having passed ventral to both the lateral and dorsal cortices (Lohman, personal communication).

B. Intrahemispheric Corticocortical Projections

The efferent projections of the medial wall cortices—medial cortex and dorsomedial cortex—have been described in the tegu lizard, *Tupinambis* (Lohman and Mentink, 1972; Lohman and Van Woerden-Verkley, 1976). The small-celled, medial cortex (MC, Fig. 3) projects dorsally and laterally to the dorsomedial and dorsal cortices (DMC, DCm, DCl). The large-celled, dorsomedial cortex projects reciprocally to medial cortex and laterally to the dorsal part of lateral cortex (asterisk in LC, Fig. 3), but not to the dorsal cortices.

Efferents of dorsal and lateral cortices have been studied in *Tupinambis* (Lohman and Mentink, 1972; Lohman and Van Woerden-Verkley, 1976) and *Gekko* (Butler, 1975, 1976*b*). Lesions involving dorsal cortex pars medialis and pars lateralis result in terminal degeneration in dorsomedial and medial cortices in *Gekko,* as

(1971*a*); Butler (1974); Northcutt and Butler (1974*a*); Cruce and Cruce (1975). Tectal projections: Ebbesson (1970); Butler and Northcutt (1971*b*); Foster and Hall (1975); Butler (1976*a*). Auditory projection pathway to the thalamus: Foster (1974). Projections of nuclei reuniens (medialis) and rotundus to the DVR and of nucleus dorsolateralis anterior to dorsal cortex: Distel and Ebbesson (1975); Foster and Peele (1975). Projection of nucleus dorsolateralis anterior to medial cortex: Lohman (personal communication). Commissural and intrahemispheric connections of cortices: Voneida and Ebbesson (1969); Lohman and Mentink (1972); Butler (1976*b*); Lohman and Van Woerden-Verkley (1976). Descending efferent projections of cortices: Lohman and Mentink (1972); Lohman and Van Woerden-Verkley (1976). Efferent projections of the dorsal ventricular ridge: Hoogland (1975); Butler (1976*a*); Lohman and Van Woerden-Verkley (1976); Sligar and Voneida (1976). Efferent projections of striatum: Hoogland (1975). Olfactory input to lateral cortex is not shown here but has been reported by Heimer (1969). Lizard species studied include *Anolis carolinensis, Gekko gecko, Iguana iguana, Tupinambis nigropunctatus, Varanus benegalensis,* and *Xantusia vigilis.*

will be discussed further below, but not in *Tupinambis.* In *Gekko* the dorsal cortex was also found to project to the dorsal part of lateral cortex.

More laterally placed lesions in *Gekko* involved both dorsal cortex pars lateralis (DCl) and lateral cortex pars dorsalis. This region was found to project medially to dorsal cortex pars medialis (DCm), dorsomedial cortex (DMC), and medial cortex (MC). However, lesions confined to lateral cortex in *Tupinambis* produced terminal degeneration only in the medial cortex.

Thus, at present, it is probable that in lizards there are (1) reciprocal connections between the medial and dorsomedial cortices, (2) reciprocal connections between the medial and lateral parts of dorsal cortex, and (3) a circuit of projections from medial cortex to dorsomedial cortex to lateral cortex and back to medial cortex. Reciprocal connections between the dorsal and medial cortices are also a possibility.

C. Interhemispheric Corticocortical Connections

In *Tupinambis* commissural connections, from either hemispherectomy or medial wall lesions, have been found to be restricted to the medial and dorsomedial cortices (Voneida and Ebbesson, 1969; Lohman and Mentink, 1972; Lohman and Van Woerden-Verkley, 1976). In *Gekko,* however, the entire dorsal cortex is also in receipt of commissural projections which arise, at least in part, from the contralateral dorsal cortex (Butler, 1975, 1976*b*).

D. Descending Telencephalic Projections

The medial, dorsal, and lateral cortices project into the dorsal ventricular ridge, and dorsal cortical fibers have additionally been traced into the striatum (ST). The dorsal and medial cortices also project to the septum (Butler, 1976*b*; Lohman and Van Woerden-Verkley, 1976).

The hypothalamus (Hy) is one of the major extratelencephalic targets of the cortices, as well as of the dorsal ventricular ridge (Northcutt, 1968; Lohman and Mentink, 1972; Lohman and Van Woerden-Verkley, 1976; Sligar and Voneida, 1976). The DVR also projects to the striatum bilaterally, and both the DVR and striatum have long descending projections which have been traced as far as the tegmentum (TEG) in the mesencephalon (Hoogland, 1975; Sligar and Voneida, 1976).

It is possible that parts of the cortex and the DVR project reciprocally to dorsal thalamic nuclei, such as nucleus dorsolateralis anterior and rotundus, but such connections have not yet been reported in a lizard.

IV. Forebrain Organization in Other Reptiles and Birds

The pathways of ascending sensory systems to the telencephalon have also been traced in crocodiles, turtles, and birds. Visual system projections from the contralateral retina have been traced to a number of targets in the diencephalon and mesencephalon, including the pars dorsalis of the lateral geniculate nucleus and the optic tectum (Kosareva, 1967; Karten and Nauta, 1968; Knapp and Kang, 1968*a,b*; Hall and Ebner, 1970*a;* Braford, 1973). Similar retinal projections, bilateral to some sites, have also been traced in snakes (Repérant, 1972; Halpern and Frumin, 1973; Northcutt and Butler, 1974b; Repérant and Rio, 1976).

In the turtle *Pseudemys* (Hall and Ebner, 1970*a*; Foster *et al.,* 1976) and in birds (Karten *et al.,* 1973) the pars dorsalis of the lateral geniculate nucleus has been found to project to part of the cortical pallium—general (dorsal) cortex in turtles and the visual wulst in birds. This pathway would appear to correspond to the retino-geniculostriate pathway in mammals; however, in *Pseudemys* horseradish peroxidase placed in general cortex resulted in reaction product in nucleus dorsolateralis anterior as well as in the dorsal geniculate nucleus (Foster *et al.,* 1976). In birds nucleus dorsolateralis anterior projects to a portion of the wulst, just medial to but discrete from the geniculate target (Karten *et al.,* 1973), and it is thus possible that similar discrete portions of general cortex in turtles receive nonoverlapping inputs from these two nuclei. As will be discussed further below, overlapping inputs to general cortex could suggest that this region is actually a limbic visual area, rather than a discrete homologue of the striate cortex in mammals. Additional data are needed to resolve this problem.

A second visual pathway to the telencephalon, via a tectal projection to nucleus rotundus, has also been traced in turtles (Hall and Ebner, 1970*b*), crocodiles (Braford, 1972; Pritz, 1973, 1975), and birds (Karten and Revzin, 1966; Karten and Hodos, 1970; Karten *et al.,* 1973; Benowitz and Karten, 1976). Nucleus rotundus projects to the core of the dorsal ventricular ridge in turtles and to a lateral portion of the ridge in crocodiles and in birds (termed ectostriatum).

Ascending auditory projections from the torus semicircularis (inferior colliculus) have been traced to the thalamic nucleus reuniens in crocodiles (Pritz, 1974*a*) and nucleus ovoidalis in birds (Karten, 1967). From these nuclei, fibers project to a medioventral portion of the dorsal ventricular ridge (Pritz, 1974*b*; Karten, 1968), termed "field L of Rose" in birds. Auditory evoked potentials have been recorded from this area in crocodiles (Weisbach and Schwartzkopff, 1967).

Ascending projections of the dorsal column nuclei to the telencephalon have not yet been studied in reptiles, but in birds an ascending trigeminal pathway, via nucleus basalis (Zeigler and Karten, 1973), to a laterodorsal portion of the ridge (Zeier and Karten, 1971) and ascending somesthetic projections to the ridge (Delius and Bennetto, 1972) have been found.

Review of a number of other studies on descending and commissural connections of the telencephalon of reptiles and birds (e.g., Zeier and Karten, 1971, 1973) is beyond the scope of this chapter. The morphological organization of the ascending sensory recipient targets, particularly the medial and dorsal cortical zones and the dorsal ventricular ridge, will be focused on here.

A. Cortex

In all reptiles medial, dorsal, and lateral cortical zones are present, but are less easily divisible morphologically in some orders than they are in lizards. In crocodiles (Crosby, 1916) and in turtles such as *Chrysemys* (Northcutt, 1970), for example, the cortical plate is periventricular in position, and divisions between medial, dorsomedial, and dorsal cortex are not readily apparent. In birds parts of the medial and dorsal pallial zones are hypertrophied into an enlarged, laminated structure, the wulst. The precise correspondence of pallial regions among orders of reptiles and birds awaits elucidation from further connectional studies.

There have been several studies of the intrahemispheric corticocortical connections in turtles and snakes which allow preliminary comparisons with the corticocortical organization in lizards. In snakes (Ulinski, 1976*a*) medial cortex has been found to project to the dorsomedial and dorsal cortices and the dorsomedial cortex to medial cortex, as in the tegu lizard (Lohman and Van Woerden-Verkley, 1976). In snakes, however, medial cortex, rather than dorsomedial cortex, was found to project to lateral cortex. Additionally, septal and medial cortical projections to dorsal cortex have been found in snakes by Repérant (1976).

Lesions involving dorsal cortex (pars medialis and pars lateralis) in the turtle *Chrysemys* (Northcutt, 1970) result in terminal degeneration in medial, dorsomedial, and lateral (pars dorsalis) cortices, as is the case in *Gekko* (Butler, 1975, 1976*b*), but only in medial cortex in snakes (Ulinski, 1976*a*). More laterally placed lesions in turtles (Northcutt, 1970), involving dorsal cortex pars lateralis and lateral cortex pars dorsalis, result in projections to dorsal cortex pars medialis and medial cortex, as in *Gekko,* and additionally to dorsomedial cortex. Finally, lesions confined to lateral cortex pars dorsalis in snakes (Ulinski, 1976*a*) result in degeneration only in medial cortex, as is the case in the tegu lizard (Lohman and Van Woerden-Verkley, 1976).

Thus an overview of all species of reptiles studied to date allows only tentative conclusions regarding intracortical connections. Medial cortex projects to the dorsomedial and dorsal cortices, and perhaps to the dorsal part of lateral cortex; it in turn may receive projections from the dorsomedial, dorsal, and/or lateral cortices, but the problem of interruption of fibers of passage passing medially, even of possible thalamic origin, has not yet been dealt with. Similarly, lesions of dorsal cortex generally result in terminal degeneration in medial, dorsomedial, and lateral cortices but could simply be interrupting both medially and laterally passing fiber systems. Finally, commissural and ascending projection systems are likewise interrupted with lesions of the medial and dorsomedial cortices. Until anterograde and retrograde intraneuronal transport methods are applied to a number of species of reptiles, corticocortical circuitry will remain unclear.

B. Dorsal Ventricular Ridge

The morphological organization of the dorsal ventricular ridge within lizards is, as discussed above, of either a corticoid band–core (lacertid) or a nuclear (iguanid) arrangement (Northcutt, 1978). In comparing the morphology of the dorsal ventricular ridge in other reptiles and birds, one finds that the corticoid band–core arrangement also generally occurs in turtles, *Sphenodon,* and snakes, whereas the nuclear arrangement occurs in the thecodonts—crocodiles and birds.

As shown in Fig. 4, thecodonts diverged from the line of cotylosaur stem reptiles well before the time of the radiation of the presently known forms of lizards during the Cretaceous (Romer, 1966). As *Sphenodon,* snakes, and the majority of lizards have the corticoid band–core (type I) dorsal ventricular ridge, it is probable that the lepidosauria did also. Turtles diverged from the stem reptiles very early, and since they also have the type I DVR, it is more probable that the type I vs. the nuclear (type II) DVR was the ancestral, cotylosaur condition. Thus the type II DVR configuration has probably been independently achieved by the thecodonts and the type II lizards as the result of parallel evolution.

The type II, nuclear arrangement of the ridge involves not only a migration of cells away from the ventricular surface but also a quantitative increase in the size of the ridge (Platel, personal communication). Since it is likely that the ridge is the target of ascending visual, auditory, trigeminal, and probably somatosensory projections, as are some of the cell populations in mammalian neocortex, the adaptive pressures influencing its cytoarchitectonic organization are in all probability related to the use of these sensory systems.

At first glance, birds and crocodiles do not have strikingly similar adaptive zones. However, crocodiles and birds are all either active predators or foragers which must avoid other predators. Also, crocodiles and birds may both have been derived from a single arboreal ancestral stock. *Sphenosuchus* and other Upper Triassic crocodilomorphs have a high degree of pneumatization of the skull, as well as slender, hollow limb and girdle bones, suggesting an arboreal adaption (Walker, 1972).

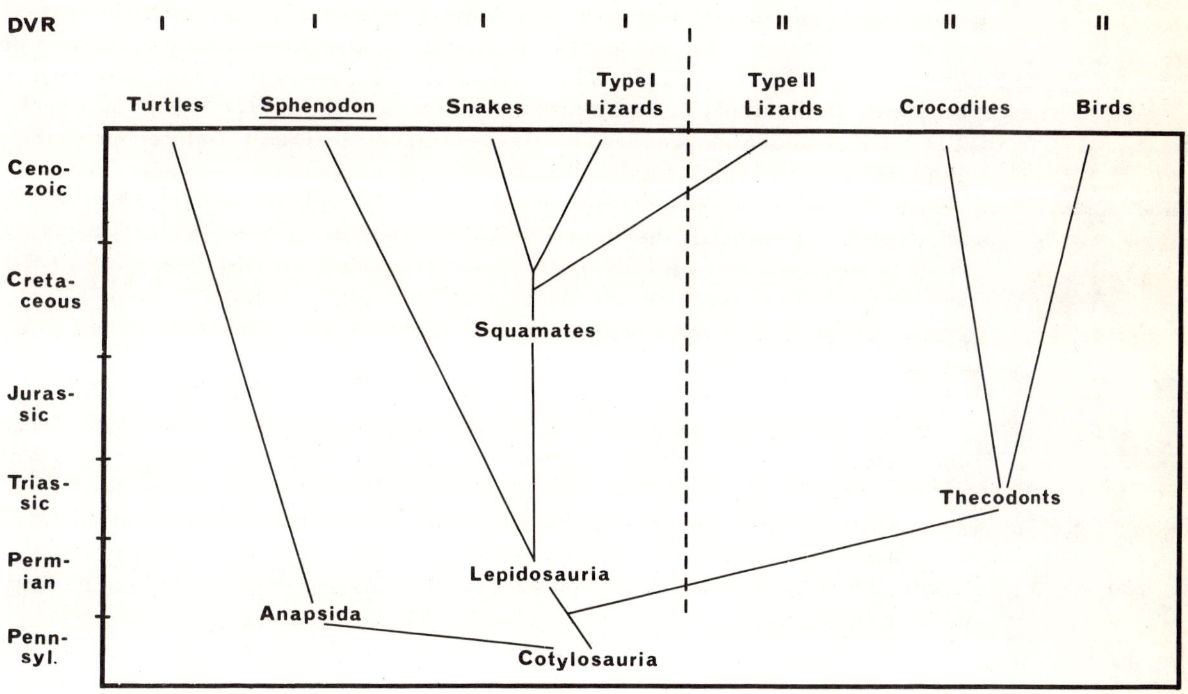

Figure 4. Dendrogram of reptilian radiations. The Cenozoic era and periods of the Mesozoic era are shown on the left. The vertical dashed line shows the division between the occurrence of type I (core nucleus–corticoid band) dorsal ventricular ridges and type II(nuclear) dorsal ventricular ridges.

The type II lizards—Iguanidae, Chameleonidae, Teiidae, Varanidae, and Agamidae—have some members which are arboreal, active foragers and/or predators. *Tupinambis,* a teiid, while being mostly terrestrial, is a powerful and swift lizard which preys on a variety of smaller vertebrates and insects, as well as on chickens and their eggs (Schmidt and Inger, 1966), using highly developed senses of vision and audition along with olfaction. It has the quantitatively largest dorsal ventricular ridge of all lizards (Platel, personal communication). Also, of type I lizards, geckos are among the most similar to iguanas in their arboreal, actively foraging behavior; they also use vocalization for communication. Among type I lizards, they have the quantitatively largest ridge, overlapping the range of the lower ridge sizes in type II lizards (Platel, personal communication).

Snakes are a somewhat special case as regards the morphology of the DVR. They originated in the Cretaceous (Romer, 1966), most probably from fossorial lizards (Bellairs and Underwood, 1951). Analysis of a number of brain characters in the forebrain and midbrain in a representative variety of snakes and lizards (Senn and Northcutt, 1973) indicates that snakes most probably arose from the same ancestral stock as the lizard *Dibamus.* The period of burrowing existence in primitive snakes resulted in marked reduction of a number of sensory systems, particularly vision, followed by selective redevelopment of these systems with subsequent reinvasion of terrestrial and arboreal habitats (Walls, 1942; Senn, 1966). In the water snake *Natrix,* for example, the pars dorsalis of the lateral geniculate nucleus is relatively very large, while the optic tectum is reduced and nucleus rotundus is extremely small (Northcutt and Butler, 1974*b*). Additionally, the torus semicircularis (inferior colliculus) is very reduced in snakes, and a paratorus, formed by the caudal continuation of different tectal laminae than the torus, is present (Senn and Northcutt, 1973). Thus, although the function of the paratorus is unknown, the auditory pathway present in lizards (Foster, 1974; Foster and Peele, 1975; Distel and Ebbesson, 1975) is also probably markedly reduced in snakes. Both the tecto-rotundal visual system and the auditory system project to the dorsal ventricular ridge. In extant burrowing snakes the ridge remains reduced, but although the volume of the ridge is relatively expanded in the more specialized snakes, elaphids and colubrids, this expansion is not necessarily the result of the same selective pressures as resulted in the type II ridge morphology in some lizards, crocodiles, and birds (Northcutt, personal communication). In most snakes some migration of neurons away from the ventricular surface occurs, resulting in a less clearly discernable corticoid band–core arrangement (Ulinski, 1976*b*). While the DVR of these snakes could thus be argued to have developed a type II, nuclear morphology, we cannot presently determine whether this is the result of parallelism or convergence. It can still be noted, as regards selective pressures, that volumetric increase and a trend toward a nuclear configuration of the dorsal ventricular ridge are correlated in snakes, as in lizards, crocodiles, and birds, with terrestrial and/or arboreal habits combined with active predation and/or the exposure to and necessity to avoid predators.

The rhynchocephalian *Sphenodon,* on the other hand, leads a terrestrial and partly burrowing existence. This species is now confined to a few islands off the coast of New Zealand; it was pitifully unable to avoid mammalian predators introduced to New Zealand by European settlers, to the point of its extinction on the main islands. The DVR in *Sphenodon* has an extremely prominent corticoid band–

core, or type I, arrangement (Cairney, 1926; Durward, 1930). Turtles, which also have a type I DVR, evolved their protective carapace in the early Permian (Romer, 1966) and are able to forage for food without great threat from predators, and they have never invaded an arboreal habitat.

In summary, the volumetric increase and cellular migration in the type II dorsal ventricular ridge of some lizards, crocodiles, and birds and the similar morphological trends in the ridge of some snakes appear to be generally correlated with behaviors and habitat requiring relatively more complex sensory processing. Detection and capture of prey and the detection of predators, reproductive and social behavior, and individual recognition, for example, require the abilities to detect, shift, and/or fix attention to novel stimuli, while filtering out nonrelevant, potentially distracting stimuli.

Similar morphological trends, due to similar adaptive pressures, may well have occured in the ancestral stock which gave rise to mammals. The mammallike reptiles—synapsids—diverged from the reptilian cotylosaur stock in the Pennsylvanian, and mammals arose from them much later in the Triassic. Mesozoic mammals were small in size, fed on insects, small birds, fruit, and eggs, and are presumed to have been nocturnal and somewhat arboreal; they were continually threatened by carnivorous reptiles and therapsids (Romer, 1966). The early placental mammals, which probably arose in the Cretaceous and became well established in the Tertiary, had similar habits (Romer, 1966). The early divergence of the synapsids was probably accomplished before the dorsal ventricular ridge was well developed, but the trends discussed above of (1) migration away from the ventricular matrix of sensory-recipient cells in the telencephalon, to form laminae here instead of nuclei (Karten, 1969), and (2) an increase in volume of the telencephalic pallium were both followed.

V. Telencephalic Connections in *Iguana* and *Gekko*

The pattern of ascending projections seen following transections of the thalamus or midbrain and some of the inter- and intrahemispheric connections have been studied in the lizards *Iguana* (Butler and Ebner, 1972) and *Gekko* (Butler, 1975, 1976*b*), and these data will now be reviewed here. In both lizards retinal projections have been traced to sites in the dorsal thalamus and optic tectum (Butler and Northcutt, 1971*a*; Northcutt and Butler, 1974*a*), and the optic tectum has been found to project bilaterally to nucleus rotundus (Butler and Northcutt, 1971*b*; Foster and Hall, 1975; Butler, 1976*a*). Auditory projections from the cochlear nuclei, via the nucleus of the torus semicircularis and nucleus medialis (reuniens), to the medial part of the dorsal ventricular ridge have also been reported in *Iguana* (Foster, 1974; Foster and Peele, 1975).

A. Ascending Projections

Thalamic transections carried out in *Iguana* (Butler and Ebner, 1972), an example of which is shown in Fig. 5, result in a complex pattern of degeneration in the cortex, dorsal ventricular ridge, and subpallium of the ipsilateral telencephalon (Figs. 6 and 7). Ascending fibers reach their targets by two courses. Projections to the subpallium and the dorsal ventricular ridge remain within the lateral forebrain bundle until turning dorsalward to their point of termination (Fig. 6C–E). Fibers projecting to the pallial cortices, however, leave the lateral forebrain bundle to enter the hemisphere via the posterior pallial commissure (arrow in Fig. 6G). They turn caudally and then dorsally over the caudal pole of the telencephalon (Fig. 6K). The fibers then traverse both the medial and lateral walls of the telencephalon (Fig. 6H–J) to form a dorsal bundle, over the dorsomedial cortical cell plate (Fig. 6E), which runs rostrally, terminating in the cortical zones along its course. The fibers are of both large and small caliber, and terminal degeneration is present to some degree in all cortical zones. The medial cortex (MC, Fig. 6E) receives a relatively sparse projection, mostly confined to its ventral and rostral portion (Fig. 6D–F), from fibers passing dorsally through it in the alveus. The majority of terminal degeneration in cortex is confined, however, to the dorsomedial (DMC, Figs. 6E and 8) and dorsal (DC, Fig. 6E; DCm, CP, DCl, Fig. 8) cortices. The dorsalmost part of the cell plate of medial cortex (MC, Fig. 8) also contains degeneration. Terminal debris is distributed throughout the depths of the cortices and extends from their caudal (Fig. 6G–K) to their rostral (Fig. 6A,B) extents.

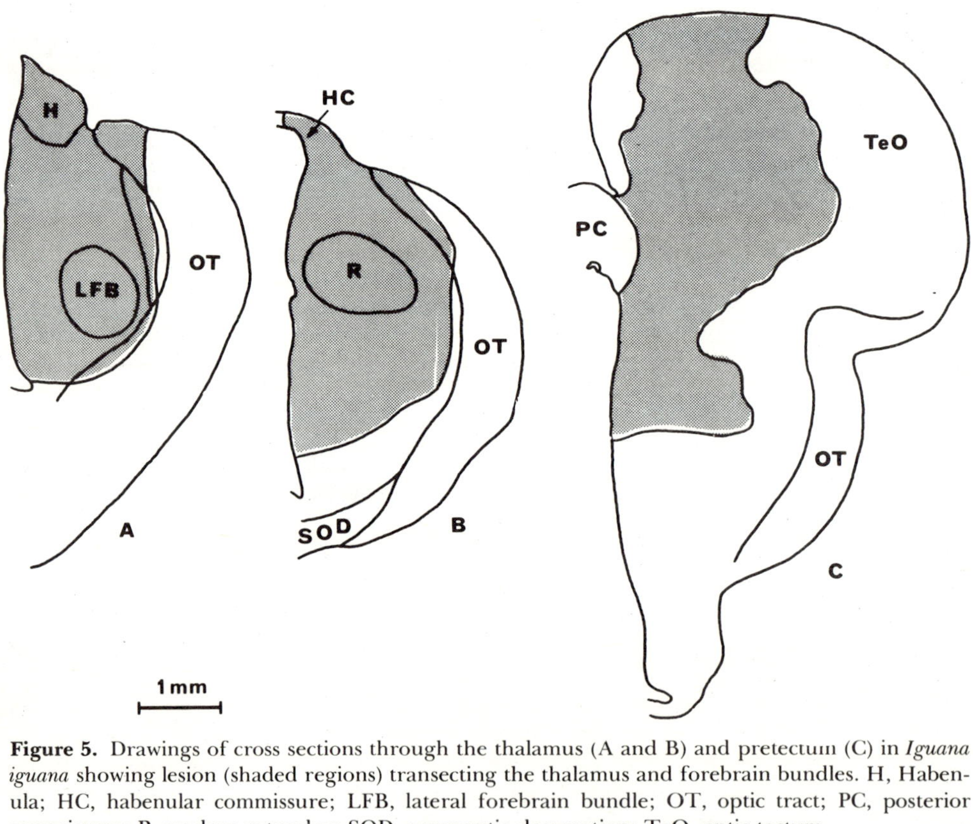

Figure 5. Drawings of cross sections through the thalamus (A and B) and pretectum (C) in *Iguana iguana* showing lesion (shaded regions) transecting the thalamus and forebrain bundles. H, Habenula; HC, habenular commissure; LFB, lateral forebrain bundle; OT, optic tract; PC, posterior commissure; R, nucleus rotundus; SOD, supraoptic decussation; TeO, optic tectum.

Within the dorsal ventricular ridge (DVR, Figs. 6E and 8), two very dense fields of degeneration are present, one along the medioventral wall of the ridge (Figs. 6D,E and 8) and one in the central portion of the ridge (Figs. 6C,D and 8). A third, but less dense terminal field is present in the lateral part of the ridge (Figs. 6B–D and 8). The medioventral field corresponds in position to the target of the auditory projection from nucleus medialis (reuniens) found in *Caiman* (Pritz, 1974*b*) and lizards (Distel and Ebbesson, 1975; Foster and Peele, 1975). The central field is somewhat more medial in position than the visual target of nucleus rotundus in *Caiman* (Pritz, 1973, 1975) and *Varanus* (Distel and Ebbesson, 1975); however, visual evoked potentials have been recorded from this central area (encircled asterisk in Fig. 3) in the desert iguana *Dipsosaurus* (Peterson and Rowe, 1976).

Ascending fibers also terminate in a number of regions in the subpallium, including the septum, nucleus accumbens, and lateral striatal areas (S, A, and ST in Figs. 6E and 8).

Midbrain transections, such as that shown in Fig. 9, result in a somewhat similar pattern of degeneration in the telencephalon, but with several important differences. In contrast to degeneration seen following thalamic transection, this projection is (1) bilateral, (2) composed of only large-caliber fibers, (3) sparse within the cortical cell plates, and (4) diffuse rather than to specific targets in the DVR. Fibers decussate through a ventral midbrain commissure. They travel rostrally and enter the subpallium and dorsal ventricular ridge from the lateral forebrain bundle (Fig. 10B), terminating diffusely in these areas.

Those fibers projecting to cortex enter the hemispheres via the posterior pallial commissure (PPC, Figs. 10D and 11A). Fibers then turn caudally and dorsally over the caudal pole (Figs. 10E–G and 11B) and run rostrally in a dorsal bundle (Fig. 10A–E) over the cell plate of the dorsomedial cortex (DMC, Fig. 10D). Caudally, terminal degeneration is primarily confined to the dorsomedial (DMC) and dorsal (DC) cortices but is also present in the cell-free region deep to the cell plate of medial cortex (MC, Fig. 10E,F). [The dorsomedial cortex fuses caudally with a ventral plate of similar, large neurons (Fig. 10E,F), which Ebbesson and Voneida (1969) termed "ventral cortex." As there is no discernable morphological variation within the fused cell plate (Fig. 10F), and as both populations of neurons are contiguous medially with medial cortex and laterally with dorsal cortex (Fig. 10E), both are regarded here as parts of dorsomedial cortex.] More rostrally, terminal fields of degeneration in the cortex are mostly confined to the dorsomedial and dorsal cortices, becoming quite sparse in the lateral part of dorsal cortex, and also present in the rostral, ventral portion of medial cortex (Fig. 10A–D).

Midbrain transections in *Gekko* (Butler, 1975), such as that shown in Fig. 12, also result in bilateral, large-caliber fiber projections to the telencephalon. Fibers decussate in a ventral midbrain commissure and reach the telencephalic cortical pallium via the posterior pallial commissure (PPC, Fig. 13B); the fibers traverse the caudal pole of the hemispheres (Fig. 14A) and run dorsally in the medial and lateral walls to terminate primarily in the dorsomedial and dorsal cortices (DMC, DC, Figs. 13 and 14B) and sparsely in medial cortex (MC). Diffuse terminal degeneration is also present in subpallial regions of the telencephalon and in the dorsal ventricular ridge, more densely in the core neuropil (DVRc, Fig. 13A) than in the corticoid band (DVRs). While ascending projections to the DVR from mid-

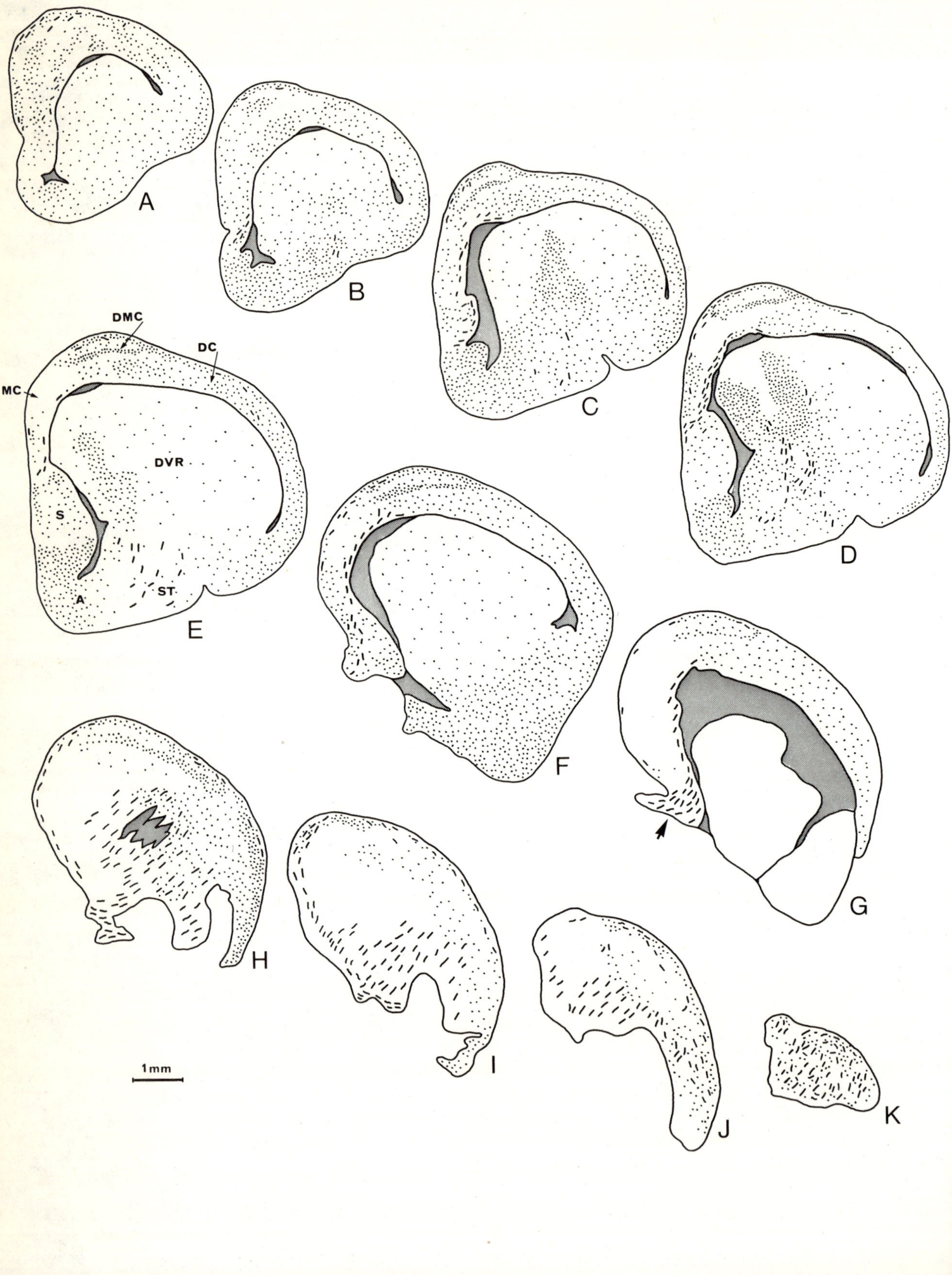
A
B
C
D
DMC
DC
MC
DVR
S
A
ST
E
F
G
H
I
J
K
1mm

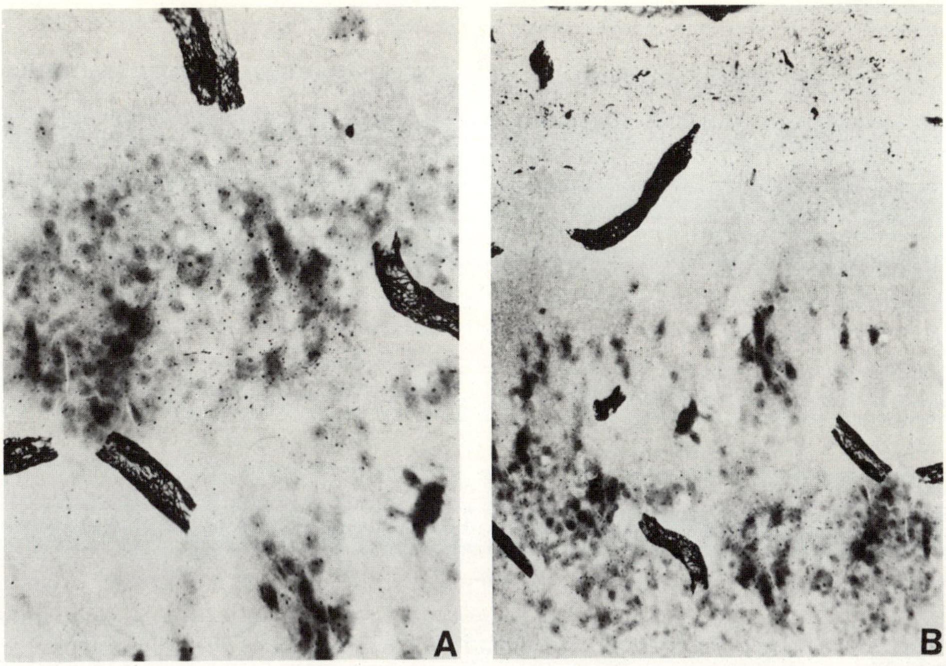

Figure 7. Photomicrographs of degeneration in the dorsalmost part of medial cortex (A) and in the outer layer of the cortex over the medial and dorsomedial cortical cell plates (B), at a level similar to that shown in Fig. 6D,E, following thalamic transection in *Iguana,* ipsilateral to the lesion.

brain lesions have thus been found in both *Iguana* and *Gekko,* such a projection system seems to be absent in turtles (Hall and Ebner, 1970*b*; Parent, 1976).

B. Cortical Efferent Projections

Lesions which involve the dorsal cortex in *Gekko* (Fig. 15) result in ipsilateral projections to the more lateral and medial cortical areas as well as less dense projections to the septum and dorsal ventricular ridge. The pattern of contralateral projections arising from such a lesion is comparable to that seen following much larger lesions of the cortices and dorsal ventricular ridge (Butler, 1975, 1976*b*). Fibers enter the contralateral alveus (A, Fig. 15B) via the hippocampal commissure (HC) and terminate primarily in the medial, dorsomedial, and dorsal cortices. Sparse terminal degeneration is also present in the lateralmost portion of the dorsal ventricular ridge (DVRc, DVRs).

More laterally placed lesions do not result in contralateral projections to the

Figure 6. Chartings of degeneration seen in *Iguana* in the ipsilateral telencephalon in cross sections following the lesion shown in Fig. 5. Section A is most rostral and section K most caudal. The lateral ventricle is indicated by shading. A, Nucleus accumbens; DC, dorsal cortex; DMC, dorsomedial cortex; DVR, dorsal ventricular ridge; MC, medial cortex; S, septum; ST, striatum; arrow in section G, posterior pallial commissure. In this and following figures, terminal degeneration is represented by stippling and degenerated fibers of passage by dashes.

medial, dorsomedial, or dorsal cortices, and it can thus be concluded that in *Gekko* the dorsal cortex does have interhemispheric commissural connections.

The pattern of terminal degeneration in medial cortex is variable, depending on the site of the lesion, and complex. A summary diagram interpreting the results in *Gekko* is shown in Fig. 16.

VI. Discussion

A. Dorsal Ventricular Ridge

A number of recent anatomical and electrophysiological studies have demonstrated that the dorsal ventricular ridge in reptiles is in receipt of ascending sensory projections relayed from dorsal thalamic nuclei (e.g., Hall and Ebner, 1970*b*; Pritz, 1974*b*, 1975; Foster and Peele, 1975; Distel and Ebbesson, 1975; Peterson and Rowe, 1976), as discussed above. The view that the reptilian dorsal ventricular ridge is homologous to mammalian basal ganglia has long been held. However, the evidence from connectional and histochemical studies is now compelling enough to render this concept untenable. The current view—that the dorsal ventricular ridge is homologous to parts of mammalian neocortex—is gaining wider acceptance. This view does not encompass the ideas, however, that all cell populations present in neocortex are present in the ridge or that neocortex evolved from the ridge. The latter statement is obviously as meaningless as it would be to say that modern

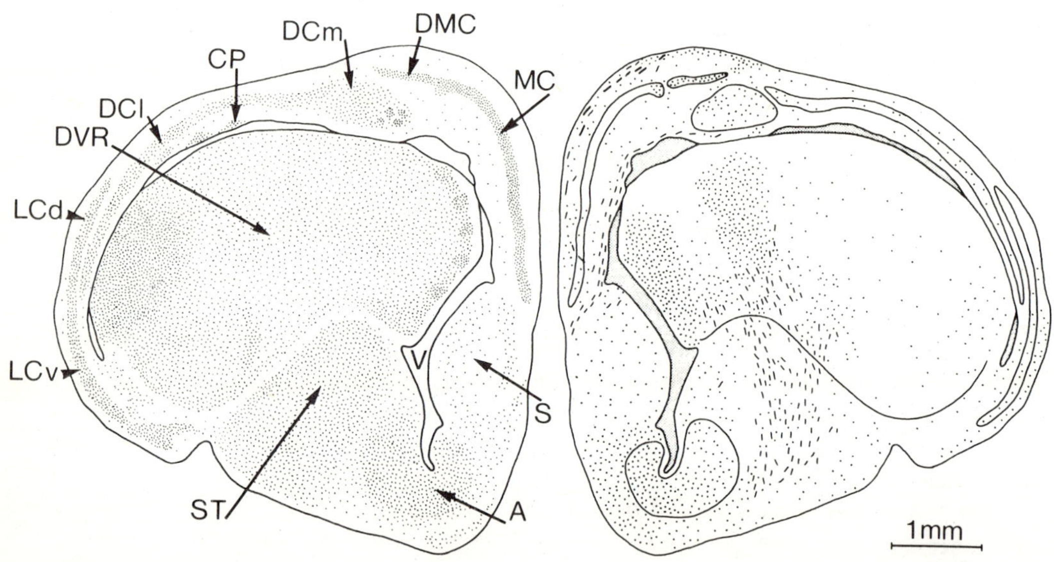

Figure 8. Enlargement of charting shown in Fig. 6D (on right) and camera lucida drawing of adjacent Nissl-stained section. On the right the lateral ventricle is indicated by shading. A, Nucleus accumbens; CP, ventral cell plate; DCl, dorsal cortex pars lateralis; DCm, dorsal cortex pars medialis; DMC, dorsomedial cortex; DVR, dorsal ventricular ridge; LCd, lateral cortex pars dorsalis; LCv, lateral cortex pars ventralis; MC, medial cortex; S. septum: ST, striatum; V, lateral ventricle.

mammals evolved from modern reptiles. Rather, it is thought possible that the cell populations in the DVR which receive ascending sensory projections in reptiles and birds and the primary sensory-recipient cells in the neocortex in mammals both evolved from a cell population present in the common ancestor of these two vertebrate radiations. Other cell populations, such as commissural projection cells and interneuron associational cells, may also be present in the dorsal ventricular ridge and may either have been present in the ancestral stock common to mammals or have evolved independently. Identification of and study of the distribution of these cell populations in reptiles can help to answer this question.

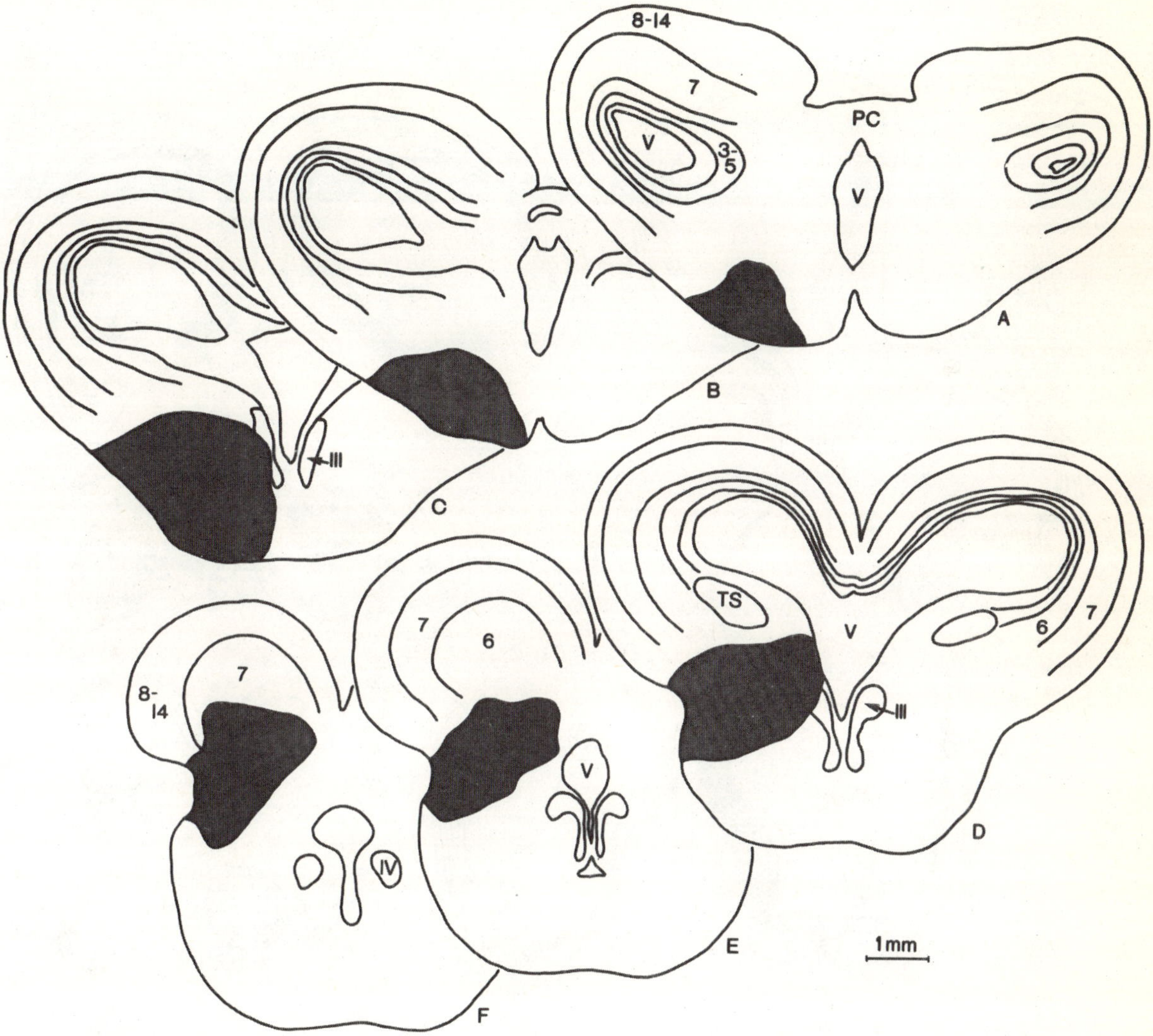

Figure 9. Drawings of cross sections through the midbrain in *Iguana,* A being most rostral and F most caudal, showing lesion (shaded region) transecting the midbrain. Surgical approach was made dorsally, caudal to the level of section F. PC, Posterior commissure; TS, central nucleus of torus semicircularis; V, ventricle; III, oculomotor nucleus, IV, trochlear nucleus; 3–5, 6, 7, and 8–14, layers of optic tectum.

Few studies of the efferent projections of the ridge have yet been done; however, in addition to descending projections, commissural projections of the DVR have been found only in turtles (Northcutt, 1970; Ware, 1974). The dorsal ventricular ridge has been found to project to the contralateral striatum but not to the contralateral ridge in lizards (Butler, 1975, 1976*b*; Sligar and Voneida, 1976). Further, in birds, transection of the anterior commissure does not result in degeneration in any of the sensory-recipient regions of the dorsal ventricular ridge (Zeier and Karten, 1973).

It is interesting to note, in this regard, that in those mammals considered to be most primitivelike, major portions of the primary sensory cortices are in receipt of commissural connections, whereas in other mammals, such as primates, com-

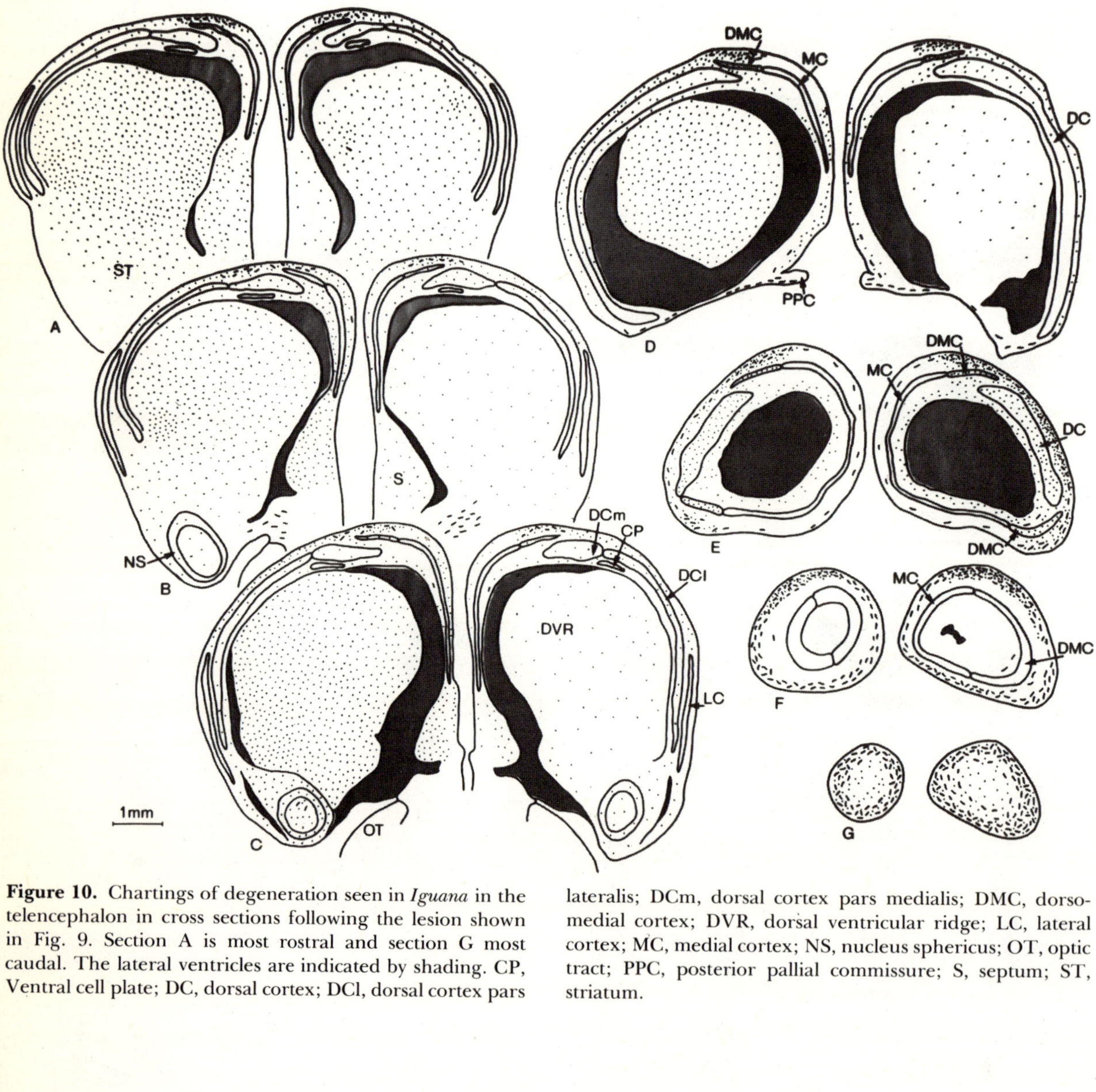

Figure 10. Chartings of degeneration seen in *Iguana* in the telencephalon in cross sections following the lesion shown in Fig. 9. Section A is most rostral and section G most caudal. The lateral ventricles are indicated by shading. CP, Ventral cell plate; DC, dorsal cortex; DCl, dorsal cortex pars lateralis; DCm, dorsal cortex pars medialis; DMC, dorsomedial cortex; DVR, dorsal ventricular ridge; LC, lateral cortex; MC, medial cortex; NS, nucleus sphericus; OT, optic tract; PPC, posterior pallial commissure; S, septum; ST, striatum.

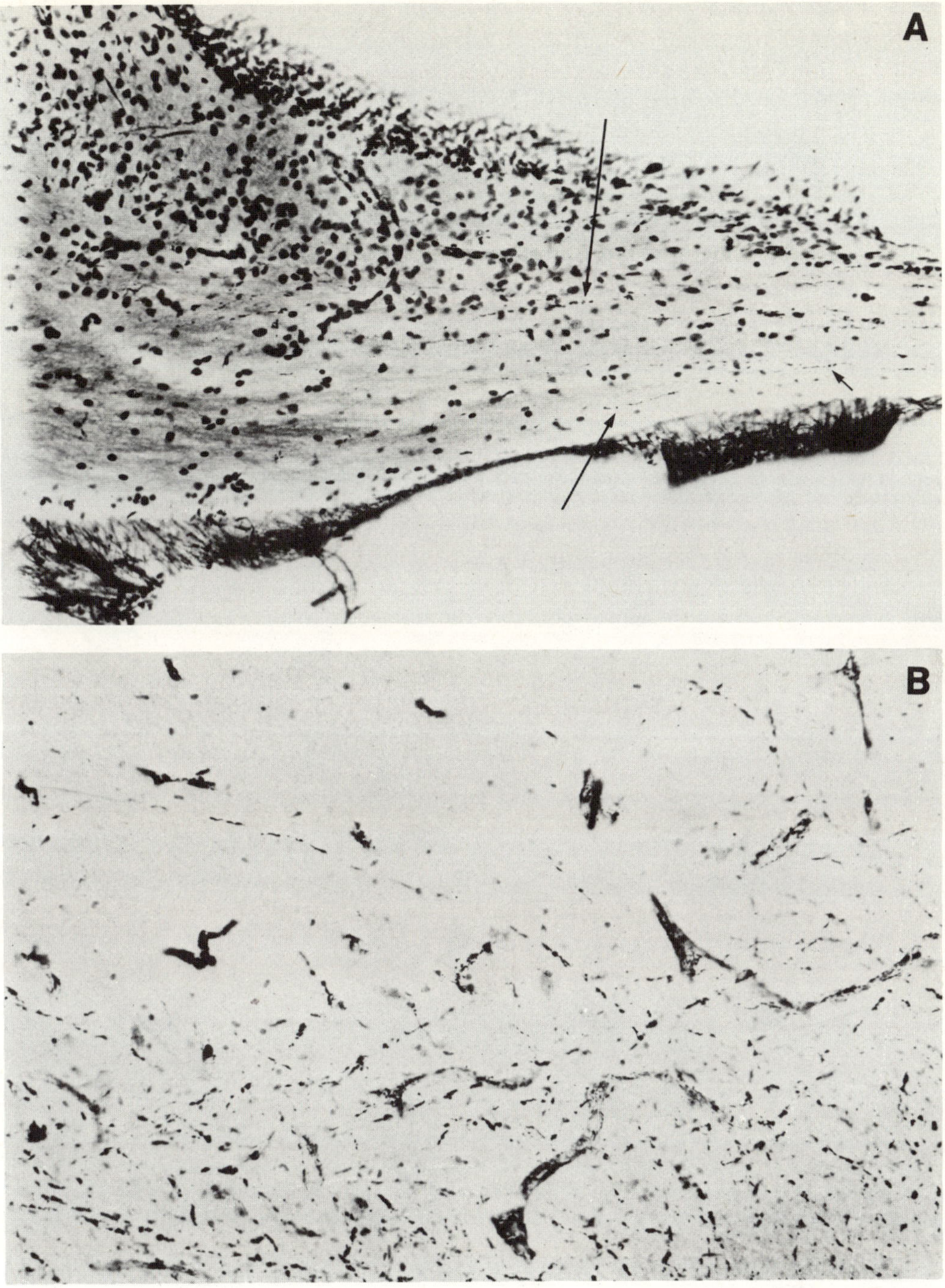

Figure 11. Photomicrographs of degeneration entering the telencephalon via the posterior pallial commissure (A), indicated by arrows, and passing over the caudal pole of the telencephalon (B), at levels similar to those shown in Fig. 10D,G, respectively, following midbrain transection in *Iguana*, ipsilateral to the lesion.

missural connections tend to be limited to association cortices (Myers, 1965, 1972; Ebner, 1969). It is thus possible that a similar trend has occurred in the connectional organization of the reptilian and avian telencephalon. Turtles are generally regarded as more similar to the ancestral reptilian stock than other reptilian orders and birds. As was discussed above, the trends of (1) cellular migration away from the ventricular matrix to form nuclei and/or laminae and (2) volumetric increase (type I vs. type II DVR, Fig. 4) have occurred in the telencephalon in the mammalian, lacertilian, and thecodont radiations. A third trend—that of (3) progressive decrease of commissural connections of primary sensory-receptive telencephalic regions—may also have occurred in these radiations independently, as the result of parallel evolution. More species will need to be studied in order to test this hypothesis. This interpretation would suggest that interhemispheric commissural connections between sensory-receptive regions may have been established very early in ancestral reptiles, and their presence may well be a primitive character.

B. Dorsal Cortex

The dorsal cortex of lizards is a complex region cytoarchitectonically, including the pars medialis, pars lateralis, ventral cell plate of Unger (1906), and the pallial thickening rostrally (Northcutt, 1967). It was classically considered to be the only part of the reptilian brain which could be homologous to mammalian neocortex

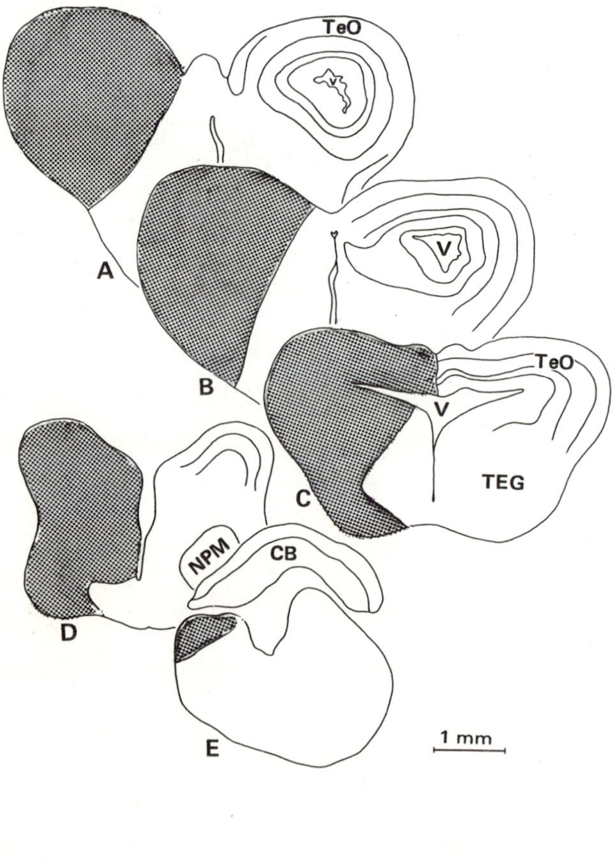

Figure 12. Drawings of cross sections through the midbrain in *Gekko gecko,* A being most rostral and E most caudal, showing lesion (shaded regions) transecting the midbrain. CB, Cerebellum; NPM, nucleus profundus mesencephali; TEG, tegmentum; TeO, optic tectum, V, ventricle.

(Elliot Smith, 1910; Ariëns Kappers *et al.,* 1936). Some recent evidence supports the idea that part or all of dorsal cortex in turtles is homologous to mammalian visual cortex, because of its reciprocal connections with the dorsal lateral geniculate nucleus (Hall and Ebner, 1970*b*, 1974; Northcutt, 1970; Ware, 1974; Foster *et al.,* 1976). Other evidence suggests, however, that dorsal cortex in snakes, lizards, and turtles may have reciprocal connections with part of the anterior nuclear group in the thalamus, particularly nucleus dorsolateralis anterior (Distel and Ebbesson, 1975; Foster *et al.,* 1976; Halpern, 1976), and that dorsal cortex projects to the medial cortex, septum, and hypothalamus (Northcutt, 1970; Lohman and Mentink, 1972; Butler, 1975, 1976*b*; Halpern, 1976; Lohman and Van Woerden-Verkley, 1976; Ulinski, 1976*a*). This latter set of projections is consistent with the idea that dorsal cortex is associated with the medial telencephalic wall and homologous to part(s) of the mammalian limbic system rather than to neocortex.

There are several possible interpretations of the present data. Firstly, the lateral part of dorsal cortex may be homologous to part of mammalian visual cortex and the medial part of dorsal cortex to part of the hippocampal formation. In birds the medial and lateral parts of the wulst (a dorsal telencephalic region) receive separate, nonoverlapping inputs from anterior and visual thalamic nuclei, respectively (Karten *et al.,* 1973). Additional studies in lizards and turtles, using smaller, more discrete injections of horseradish peroxidase and/or tritiated amino acids, may reveal similar segregation of inputs to the dorsal cortex.

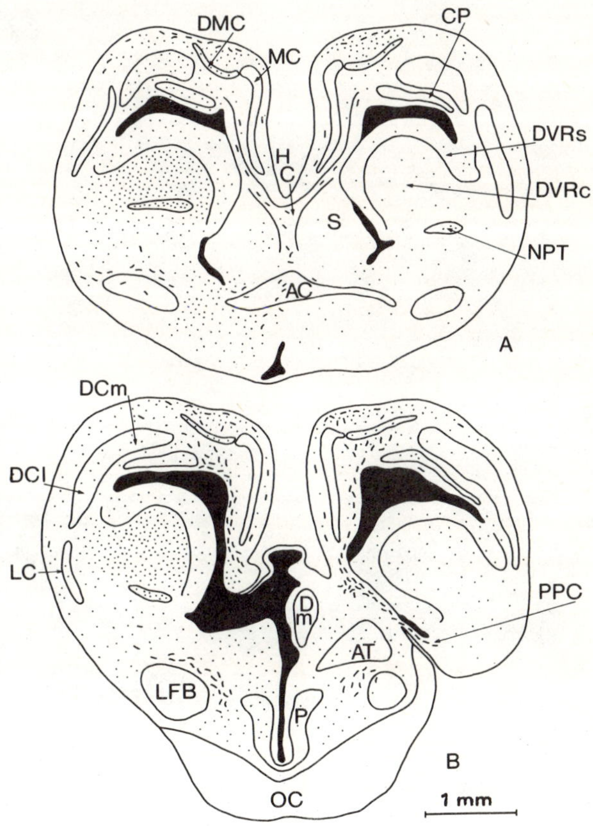

Figure 13. Chartings of degeneration seen in *Gekko* in the telencephalon in cross sections, A being more rostral, following the lesion shown in Fig. 11. The lateral and third ventricles are indicated by shading. AC, Anterior commissure; AT, area triangularis; CP, ventral cell plate; DCl, dorsal cortex pars lateralis; DCm, dorsal cortex pars medialis; Dm, nucleus dorsomedialis; DMC, dorsomedial cortex; DVRc, core nucleus of dorsal ventricular ridge; DVRs, surrounding corticoid band of dorsal ventricular ridge; HC, hippocampal commissure; LC, lateral cortex; LFB, lateral forebrain bundle; MC, medial cortex; NPT, nucleus parvocellularis telencephali; OC, optic chiasm; P, nucleus periventricularis; PPC, posterior pallial commissure; S, septum.

A second possibility is that reptilian dorsal cortex is homologous as a field of cells to parts of both mammalian striate cortex and the hippocampal formation. The demonstration that the same population of cells in dorsal cortex of lizards or turtles which receives visual input also receives anterior thalamic input and/or projects to the hypothalamus would support this hypothesis. If this were the case, the lateral part of the wulst in birds, which receives a discrete visual input from the thalamus (Karten *et al.*, 1973) might well not be a homologue of mammalian striate cortex but rather have been acquired as the result of parallel evolution.

Finally, a corollary to the latter possibility is that all of the dorsal cortex in reptiles may be homologous to mammalian limbic structures and that the so-called dorsal geniculate nucleus in the thalamus may be part of a limbic visual pathway not found in mammals. Clearly, additional data are needed before any coherent picture regarding the nature and organization of reptilian dorsal cortex can be formulated.

C. Trends in Forebrain Evolution

Among all vertebrates there appear to be several common features of forebrain organization. One of these features is that ascending sensory information (visual, auditory, somesthetic) is relayed through dorsal thalamic nuclei to parts of both

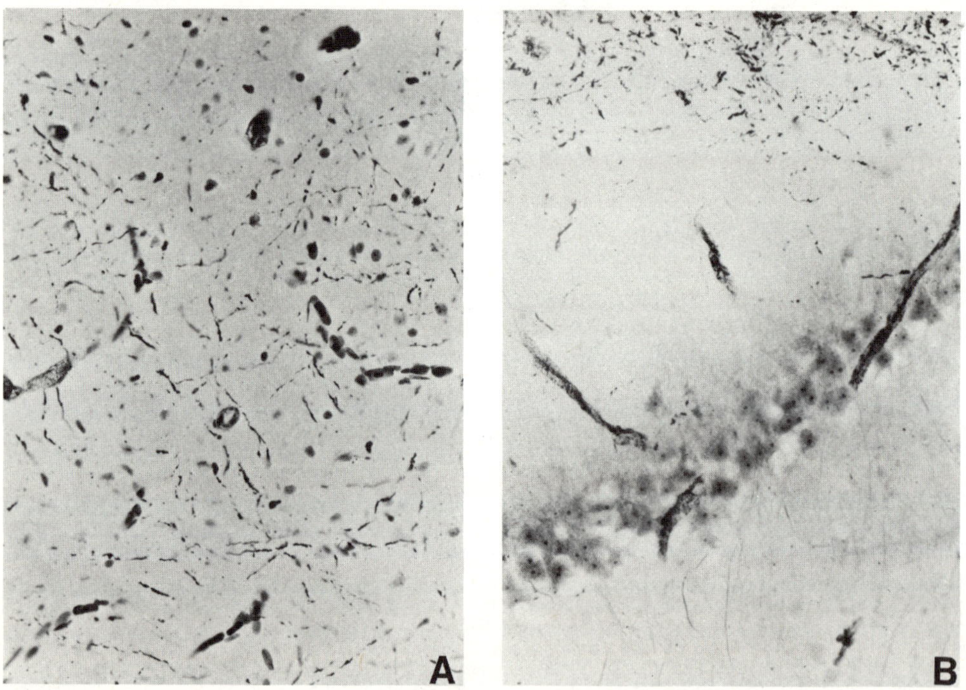

Figure 14. Photomicrographs of degeneration passing over the caudal pole of the telencephalon (A) and in the outer layer of the cortex over the dorsomedial cortical cell plate (B), at levels similar to those in Fig. 13, following midbrain transection in *Gekko*. The degeneration in A is on the side contralateral to the lesion and that in B is on the side ipsilateral to the lesion.

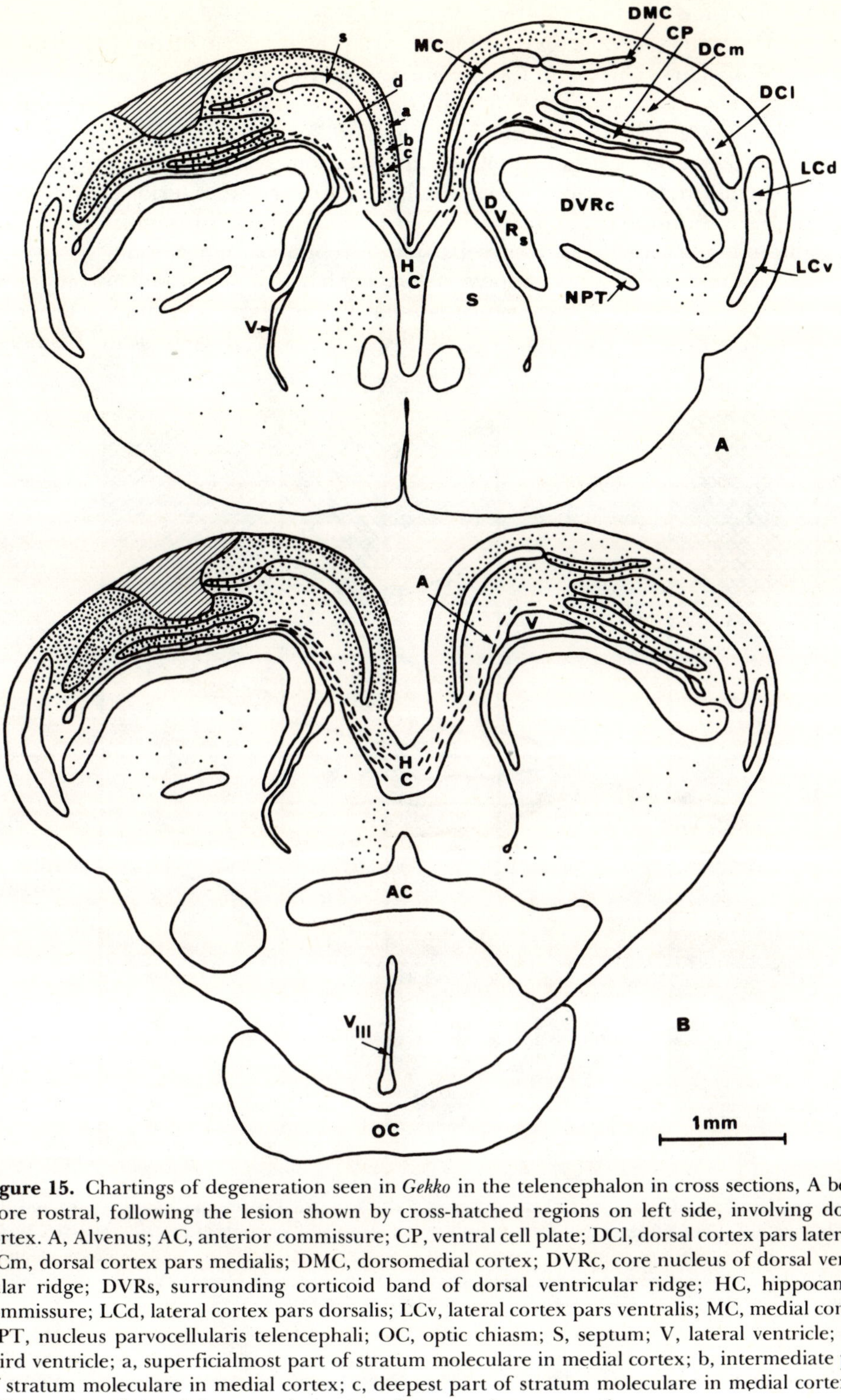

Figure 15. Chartings of degeneration seen in *Gekko* in the telencephalon in cross sections, A being more rostral, following the lesion shown by cross-hatched regions on left side, involving dorsal cortex. A, Alvenus; AC, anterior commissure; CP, ventral cell plate; DCl, dorsal cortex pars lateralis; DCm, dorsal cortex pars medialis; DMC, dorsomedial cortex; DVRc, core nucleus of dorsal ventricular ridge; DVRs, surrounding corticoid band of dorsal ventricular ridge; HC, hippocampal commissure; LCd, lateral cortex pars dorsalis; LCv, lateral cortex pars ventralis; MC, medial cortex; NPT, nucleus parvocellularis telencephali; OC, optic chiasm; S, septum; V, lateral ventricle; V_{III}, third ventricle; a, superficialmost part of stratum moleculare in medial cortex; b, intermediate part of stratum moleculare in medial cortex; c, deepest part of stratum moleculare in medial cortex; s, cell soma layer in medial cortex; d, stratum album et griseum centrale.

the subpallium and pallium, and that the pallial targets of these systems are discrete and separate from the olfactory-recipient area. This pattern of organization has been found in sharks (Heimer, 1969; Ebbesson and Heimer, 1970; Ebbesson and Schroeder, 1971; Cohen *et al.*, 1973; Schroeder and Ebbesson, 1974) and amphibians (Scalia *et al.*, 1968; Kicliter and Northcutt, 1975; Northcutt and Royce, 1975; Kicliter and Ebbesson, 1976), as well as in reptiles, birds, and mammals. Commissural interhemispheric connections via the hippocampal and anterior commissures have also been found in amphibians (Halpern, 1972), and if present in sharks and teleosts would be a basic feature of vertebrate forebrain organization.

Among amniotes, several trends in telencephalic organization are apparent within the lacertilian, thecodont, and mammalian radiations. As discussed above, two of these trends are an increase of the migration of cells away from the

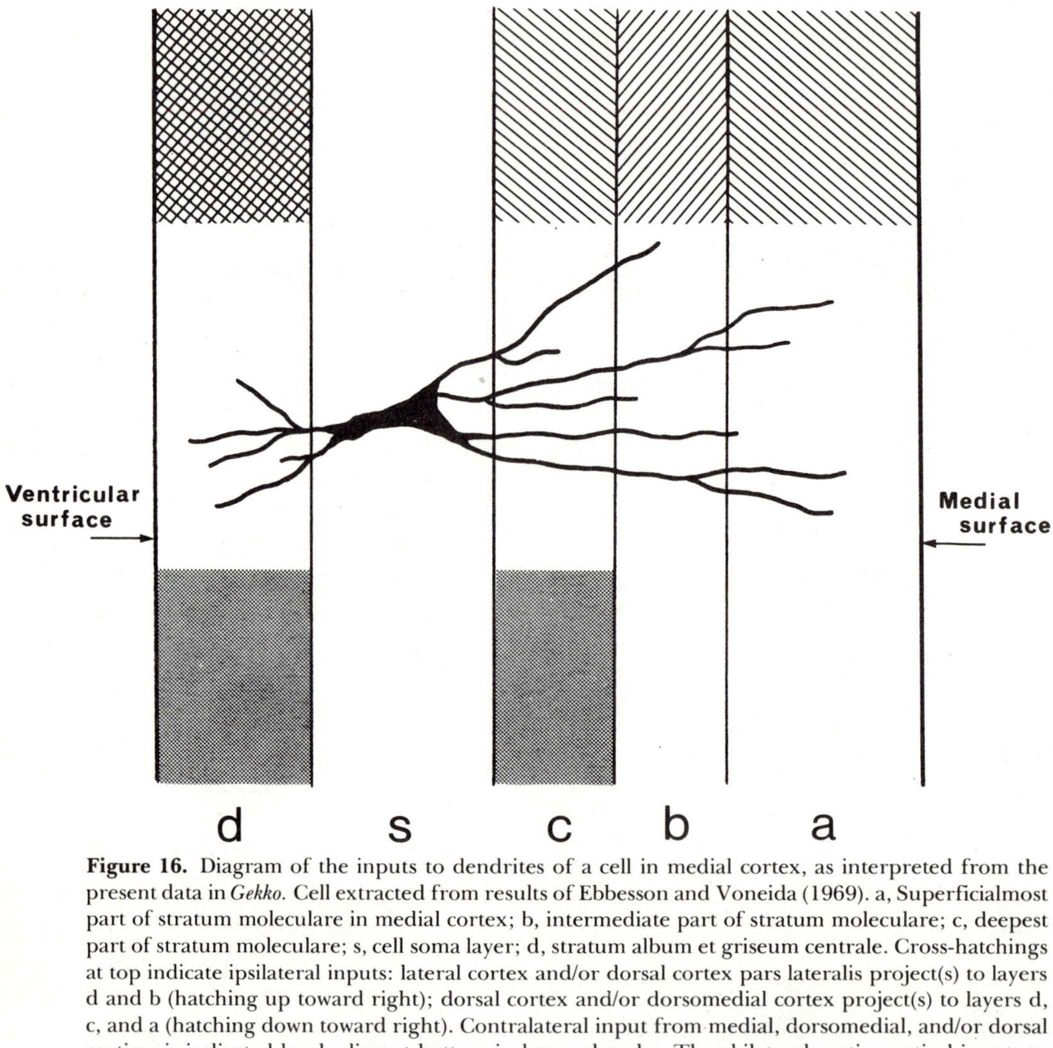

Figure 16. Diagram of the inputs to dendrites of a cell in medial cortex, as interpreted from the present data in *Gekko.* Cell extracted from results of Ebbesson and Voneida (1969). a, Superficialmost part of stratum moleculare in medial cortex; b, intermediate part of stratum moleculare; c, deepest part of stratum moleculare; s, cell soma layer; d, stratum album et griseum centrale. Cross-hatchings at top indicate ipsilateral inputs: lateral cortex and/or dorsal cortex pars lateralis project(s) to layers d and b (hatching up toward right); dorsal cortex and/or dorsomedial cortex project(s) to layers d, c, and a (hatching down toward right). Contralateral input from medial, dorsomedial, and/or dorsal cortices is indicated by shading at bottom in layers d and c. Thus bilateral corticocortical inputs to medial cortical neurons appear to be restricted to the more proximal portions of the dendrites.

ventricular matrix and volumetric increase of the pallium. Cellular migration may be a mechanism to achieve dendritic polarity, even though this could be achieved in two of three planes (rostrocaudal and either medio-lateral or dorso-ventral) by periventricular cells, depending on established fiber system orientation. Migration would, however, give a neuron an additional hemisphere of volume through which dendrites could radiate. Volumetric increase would allow for an increased space for a given cell's dendrites to occupy, along with glial elements, and/or an increased number of neurons. Whether or not the development of new types of neurons, e.g., Golgi type II neurons, is correlated with volumetric increase remains to be determined. Finally, while the presence of interhemispheric commissural connections may be a generalized vertebrate character, the elimination of such connections between primary pallial sensory-recipient regions may have occurred independently in the lacertilian, thecodont, and mammalian radiations.

In conclusion, we now have identified the dorsal ventricular ridge as a major target of ascending sensory systems in reptiles and birds and can begin to relate the variation in its cytoarchitectonic organization to adaptive pressures and evolutionary trends among vertebrates. The dorsal cortex of reptiles, on the other hand, appears to be more complexly organized than previously realized, and interpreting present data in relation to mammalian brain evolution is difficult. Further studies of the connectional organization of the telencephalon in a wide variety of reptiles must be completed before an understanding of this dorsal pallial region can be achieved.

ACKNOWLEDGMENTS. This work was supported by NIH Grants Nos. 1 RO1 NS11686-01 and 7 RO1 NS12966-01, and by the author. The author wishes to thank Dr. R. Glenn Northcutt for helpful comments on the manuscript.

VII. References

Ariëns Kappers, C. U., Huber, G. C., and Crosby, E. C., 1936, *The Comparative Anatomy of the Nervous System of Vertebrates, Including Man,* Hafner, New York.

Armstrong, J. A., 1950, An experimental study of the visual pathways in a reptile (*Lacerta vivipara*), *J. Anat.* **84:**146.

Armstrong, J. A., Gamble, H. J., and Goldby, F., 1953, Observations on the olfactory apparatus and the telencephalon of *Anolis,* a microsmatic lizard, *J. Anat.* **87:**288.

Beckers, H. J. A., Platel, R., and Nieuwenhuys, R., 1971, Les aires corticales de quelques reptiles squamates (*Lacerta viridis, Chamaeleo lateralis, Monopeltis guentheri*), *Acta Morphol. Neerl. Scand.* **9:**337.

Bellairs, A. d'A., and Underwood, G. L., 1951, The origin of snakes, *Biol. Rev.* **26:**193.

Benowitz, L. I., and Karten, H. J., 1976, Organization of the tectofugal visual pathway in the pigeon: A retrograde transport study, *J. Comp. Neurol.* **167:**503.

Braford, M. R., Jr., 1972, Ascending efferent tectal projections in the South American spectacled caiman, *Anat. Rec.* **172:**275.

Braford, M. R., Jr., 1973, Retinal projections in *Caiman crocodilus, Am. Zool.* **13:**1345.

Butler, A. B., 1974, Retinal projections in the night lizard, *Xantusia vigilis* Baird, *Brain Res.* **80:**116.

Butler, A. B., 1975, Telencephalic afferents in *Gekko gecko, Anat. Rec.* **181:**323.

Butler, A. B., 1976*a*, Ascending efferent tectal projections in the lizard *Gekko gecko* (L.), *Neurosci. Abstr.* **2:**171.

Butler, A. B., 1976*b*, Telencephalon of the lizard *Gekko gecko* (Linnaeus): Some connections of the cortex and dorsal ventricular ridge, *Brain Behav. Evol.* **13:**396.

Butler, A. B., and Ebner, F. F., 1972, Thalamotelencephalic projections in the lizard *Iguana iguana, Anat. Rec.* **172:**282.

Butler, A. B., and Northcutt, R. G., 1971*a*, Retinal projections in *Iguana iguana* and *Anolis carolinensis, Brain Res.* **26:**1.

Butler, A. B., and Northcutt, R. G., 1971*b*, Ascending tectal efferent projections in the lizard *Iguana iguana, Brain Res.* **35:**597.

Butler, A. B., and Northcutt, R. G., 1973, Architectonic studies of the diencephalon of *Iguana iguana* Linnaeus, *J. Comp. Neurol.* **149:**439.

Cairney, J., 1926, A general survey of the forebrain of *Sphenodon punctatum, J. Comp. Neurol.* **42:**255.

Cohen, D. H., Duff, T. A., and Ebbesson, S. O. E., 1973, Electrophysiological identification of a visual area in shark telencephalon, *Science* **182:**492.

Crosby, E. C., 1916, The forebrain of *Alligator mississippiensis, J. Comp. Neurol. 27:*325.

Cruce, J. A. F., 1974, A cytoarchitectonic study of the diencephalon of the tegu lizard, *Tupinambis nigropunctatus, J. Comp. Neurol.* **153:**215.

Cruce, W. L. R., and Cruce, J. A. F., 1975, Projections from the retina to the lateral geniculate nucleus and mesencephalic tectum in a reptile (*Tupinambis nigropunctatus*): A comparison of anterograde transport and anterograde degeneration, *Brain Res.* **85:**221.

Curwen, A. O., 1937, The telencephalon of *Tupinambis nigropunctatus.* I. Medial and cortical areas, *J. Comp. Neurol.* **66:**375.

Delius, J. D., and Bennetto, K., 1972, Cutaneous sensory projections to the avian forebrain, *Brain Res.* **37:**205.

Distel, H., and Ebbesson, S. O. E., 1975, Connections of the thalamus in the monitor lizard, *Neurosci. Abstr.* **1:**559.

Durward, A., 1930, The cell masses in the forebrain of *Sphenodon punctatum, Engl. J. Anat.* **65:**8.

Ebbesson, S. O. E., 1967, Ascending axon degeneration following hemisection of the spinal cord in the tegu lizard (*Tupinambis nigropunctatus*), *Brain Res.* **5:**178.

Ebbesson, S. O. E., 1970, On the organization of central visual pathways in vertebrates, *Brain Behav. Evol.* **3:**178.

Ebbesson, S. O. E., 1976, The somatosensory thalamus in reptiles, *Anat. Rec.* **184:**395.

Ebbesson, S. O. E., and Heimer, L., 1970, Projections of the olfactory tract fibers in the nurse shark (*Ginglymostoma cirratum*), *Brain Res.* **17:**47.

Ebbesson, S. O. E., and Schroeder, D. M., 1971, Connections of the nurse shark's telencephalon, *Science* **173:**254.

Ebbesson, S. O. E., and Voneida, T. J., 1969, The cytoarchitecture of the pallium in the tegu lizard (*Tupinambis nigropunctatus*), *Brain Behav. Evol.* **2:**431.

Ebner, F. F., 1969, A comparison of primitive forebrain organization in metatherian and eutherian mammals, *Ann. N.Y. Acad. Sci.* **167:**241.

Elliot Smith, G., 1910, Some problems relating to the evolution of the brain, *Lancet* **1.**

Foster, R. E., 1974, The ascending brainstem auditory pathways in a reptile, *Iguana iguana, Anat. Rec.* **178:**357.

Foster, R. E., and Hall, W. C., 1975, The connections and laminar organization of the optic tectum in a reptile (*Iguana iguana*), *J. Comp. Neurol.* **163:**397.

Foster, R. E., and Peele, T. L., 1975, Thalamotelencephalic auditory pathways in the lizard (*Iguana iguana*), *Anat. Rec.* **181:**531.

Foster, R. E., Hall, J. A., and Ebner, F. F., 1976, Visual cortex in the turtle (*Pseudemys scripta* and *Chrysemys picta*), *Anat. Rec.* **184:**405.

Gamble, H. J., 1952, An experimental study of the secondary olfactory connexions in *Lacerta viridis, J. Anat.* **86:**180.

Golby, F., and Gamble, H. J., 1957, The reptilian cerebral hemispheres, *Biol. Rev.* **32:**383.

Hall, W. C., and Ebner, F. F., 1970*a*, Parallels in the visual afferent projections of the thalamus in the hedgehog (*Paraechinus hypomelas*) and the turtle (*Pseudemys scripta*), *Brain Behav. Evol.* **3:**135.

Hall, W. C. and Ebner, F. F., 1970*b*, Thalamotelencephalic projections in the turtle (*Pseudemys scripta*), *J. Comp. Neurol.* **140:**101.

Hall, J. A., and Ebner, F. F., 1974, The efferent projections of general cortex to the brainstem in the turtle, *Pseudemys scripta, Anat. Rec.* **178:**513.

Halpern, M., 1972, Some connections of the telencephalon of the frog, *Rana pipiens, Brain Behav. Evol.* **6:**42.

Halpern, M., 1973, Olfactory bulb and accessory olfactory bulb projections in the snake, *Thamnophis sirtalis, Anat. Rec.* **175:**337.

Halpern, M., 1976, Efferent connections of the lateral and dorsal cortices of snakes of the genus *Thamnophis, Anat. Rec.* **184:**421.

Halpern, M., and Frumin, N., 1973, Retinal projections in a snake, *Thamnophis sirtalis, J. Morphol.* **141:**359.

Heimer, L., 1969, The secondary olfactory connections in mammals, reptiles and shark, *Ann. N.Y. Acad. Sci.* **167:**129.

Hoogland, P. V. J. M., 1975, Efferent connections of the striatum in *Tupinambis nigropunctatus,* dissertation, Nijmegen (published by G. Peeters en S. v. Kaauwen).

Johnston, J. B., 1915, The cell masses in the forebrain of the turtle, *Cistudo carolina, J. Comp. Neurol.* **25:**393.

Karten, H. J., 1967, The organization of the ascending auditory pathway in the pigeon (*Columba livia*). I. Diencephalic projections of the inferior colliculus (nucleus mesencephali lateralis pars dorsalis), *Brain Res.* **6:**409.

Karten, H. J., 1968, The ascending auditory pathway in the pigeon (*Columba livia*). II. Telencephalic projections of the nucleus ovoidalis thalami, *Brain Res.* **11:**134.

Karten, H. J., 1969, The organization of the avian telencephalon and some speculations on the phylogeny of the amniote telencephalon, *Ann. N.Y. Acad. Sci.* **167:**164.

Karten, H. J., and Dubbeldam, J. L., 1973, The organization and projections of the paleostriatal complex in the pigeon (*Columba livia*), *J. Comp. Neurol.* **148:**61.

Karten, H. J., and Hodos, W., 1970, Telencephalic projections of the nucleus rotundus in the pigeon (*Columba livia*), *J. Comp. Neurol.* **140:**35.

Karten, H. J., and Nauta, W. J. H., 1968, Organization of retinothalamic projections in the pigeon and owl, *Anat. Rec.* **160:**373.

Karten, H. J., and Revzin, A. M., 1966, The afferent connections of the nucleus rotundus in the pigeon, *Brain Res.* **2:**368.

Karten, H. J., Hodos, W., Nauta, W. J. H., and Revzin, A. M., 1973, Neural connections of the "visual Wulst" of the avian telencephalon: Experimental studies in the pigeon (*Columba livia*) and owl (*Speotyto cunicularia*), *J. Comp. Neurol.* **150:**253.

Kicliter, E., and Ebbesson, S. O. E., 1976, Organization of the "nonolfactory" telencephalon of "the frog," in: *Handbook of Frog Neurobiology* (R. Llinas and W. Precht, eds.), pp. 946–972, Springer-Verlag, New York.

Kicliter, E., and Northcutt, R. G., 1975, Ascending afferents to the telencephalon of ranid frogs: An anterograde degeneration study, *J. Comp. Neurol.* **161:**239.

Knapp, H., and Kang, D. S., 1968*a*, The retinal projections of the side-necked turtle (*Podocnemis unifilis*) with some notes on the possible origin of the pars dorsalis of the lateral geniculate body, *Brain Behav. Evol.* **1:**369.

Knapp, H., and Kang, D. S., 1968*b*, The visual pathways of the snapping turtle (*Chelydra serpentina*), *Brain Behav. Evol.* **1:**19.

Kosareva, A. A., 1967, Projections of optic fibers to visual centers in a turtle (*Emys orbicularis*), *J. Comp. Neurol.* **130:**263.

Lohman, A. H. M., and Mentink, G. M., 1972, Some cortical connections of the tegu lizard (*Tupinambis teguixin*), *Brain Res.* **45:**325.

Lohman, A. H. M., and Van Woerden-Verkley, I., 1976, Further studies on the cortical connections of the tegu lizard, *Brain Res.* **103:**9.

Myers, R. E., 1965, Phylogenetic studies of commissural connections, in: *CIBA Foundation Study Group No. 20: Functions of the Corpus Callosum* (G. Ettlinger, ed.), pp. 138–143, Churchill, London.

Myers, R. E., 1972, The forebrain commissures and their functions, in: *Cerebral Interhemispheric Relations,* pp. 15–20, Publishing House of the Slovak Academy of Sciences, Bratislava.

Northcutt, R. G., 1967, Architectonic studies of the telencephalon of *Iguana iguana, J. Comp. Neurol.* **130:**109.

Northcutt, R. G., 1968, Descending axon degeneration following ablation of the telencephalic cortex in the horned lizard (*Phrynosoma cornutum*), *Anat. Rec.* **160:**400.

Northcutt, R. G., 1970, The telencephalon of the Western painted turtle (*Chrysemys picta belli*), *Ill. Biol. Monogr.,* No. 43.

Northcutt, R. G., 1978, Forebrain and midbrain organization in lizards and its possible evolutionary significance, in: *The Behavior and Neurology of Lizards* (N. Greenberg and P. D. MacLean, eds.), pp. 11–64, U.S. Dept. H.E.W., Washington, D.C.

Northcutt, R. G., and Butler, A. B., 1974*a*, Evolution of reptilian visual systems: Retinal projections in a nocturnal lizard, *Gekko gecko* (Linnaeus), *J. Comp. Neurol.* **157:**453.

Northcutt, R. G., and Butler, A. B., 1974*b*, Retinal projections in the Northern water snake, *Natrix sipedon sipedon* (L.), *J. Morphol.* **142:**117.

Northcutt, R. G., and Royce, G. J., 1975, Olfactory bulb projections in the bullfrog *Rana catesbeiana* Shaw, *J. Morphol.* **145:**251.

Parent, A., 1976, Striatal afferent connections in the turtle (*Chrysemys picta*) as revealed by retrograde axonal transport of horseradish peroxidase, *Brain Res.* **108:**25.

Peterson, E., and Rowe, M., 1976, Electrophysiological evidence for a visual projection to the dorsal ventricular ridge in a lizard, *Dipsosaurus dorsalis, Anat. Rec.* **184:**500.

Platel, R., 1969, Étude cytoarchitectonique qualitative et quantitative des aires corticales d'un Saurien: *Scincus scincus* (L.) Scincides, *J. Hirnforsch.* **11:**31.

Platel, R., Beckers, H. J. A., and Nieuwenhuys, R., 1973, Les champs corticaux chez *Testudo hermanii* (Reptile Chélonien) et chez *Caiman crocodylus* (Reptile Crocodilien), *Acta Morphol. Neerl. Scand.* **11:**121.

Pritz, M. B., 1973, Connections of the alligator visual system: Telencephalic projections of nucleus rotundus, *Anat. Rec.* **150:**416.

Pritz, M. B., 1974*a*, Ascending connections of a midbrain auditory area in a crocodile, *Caiman crocodilus, J. Comp. Neurol.* **153:**179.

Pritz, M. B., 1974*b*, Ascending connections of a thalamic auditory area in a crocodile, *Caiman crocodilus, J. Comp. Neurol.* **153:**199.

Pritz, M. B., 1975, Anatomical identification of a telencephalic visual area in crocodiles: Ascending connections of nucleus rotundus in *Caiman crocodilus, J. Comp. Neurol.* **164:**323.

Repérant, J., 1972, Étude expérimentale des projections visuelles chez la vipère (*Vipera aspis*), *C. R. Acad. Sci.* **275:**695.

Repérant, J., 1976, Afférences et efférences télencéphaliques du cortex dorsal de la vipère (*Vipera aspis* L.), données préliminaires, *C. R. Acad. Sci.* **283:**809.

Repérant, J., and Rio, J.-P., 1976, Retinal projections in *Vipera aspis*: A reinvestigation using light radioautographic and electron microscopic degeneration techniques, *Brain Res.* **107:**603.

Riss, W., Halpern, M., and Scalia, F., 1969, The quest for clues to forebrain evolution—The study of reptiles, *Brain Behav. Evol.* **2:**1.

Romer, A. S., 1966, *Vertebrate Paleontology,* 3rd ed., University of Chicago Press, Chicago.

Scalia, F., Halpern, M., Knapp, H., and Riss, W., 1968, The efferent connections of the olfactory bulb in the frog: A study of degenerating unmyelinated fibers, *J. Anat.* **103:**245.

Schmidt, K. P., and Inger, R. F., 1966, *Living Reptiles of the World,* 3rd ed., Doubleday, New York.

Schroeder, D. M., and Ebbesson, S. O. E., 1974, Nonolfactory telencephalic afferents in the nurse shark (*Ginglymostoma cirratum*), *Brain Behav. Evol.* **9:**121.

Senn, D. G., 1966, Über das optische System im Gehirn squamater Reptilien, *Acta Anat.* **65:**1 (Suppl. 52).

Senn, D. G., 1968, Bau und Ontogenese von Zwischen- und Mittelhirn bei *Lacerta sicula* (Rafinesque), *Acta Anat. Suppl.* **55:**1.

Senn, D. G., and Northcutt, R. G., 1973, The forebrain and midbrain of some squamates and their bearing on the origin of snakes, *J. Morphol.* **140:**135.

Shanklin, W. M., 1930, The central nervous system of *Chameleon vulgaris, Acta Zool.* **11:**426.

Sligar, C. M., and Voneida, T. J., 1976, Efferent projections of the dorsal ventricular ridge in *Tupinambis nigropunctatus, Anat. Rec.* **184:**532.

Ulinski, P. S., 1974, Cytoarchitecture of cerebral cortex in snakes, *J. Comp. Neurol.* **158:**243.

Ulinski, P. S., 1976*a*, Intracortical connections in the snakes *Natrix sipedon* and *Thamnophis sirtalis, J. Morphol.* **150:**463.

Ulinski, P. S., 1976*b*, Structure of anterior dorsal ventricular ridge in snakes, *J. Morphol.* **148:**1.

Ulinski, P. S., and Kanarek, D. A., 1973, Cytoarchitecture of nucleus sphericus in the common boa, *Constrictor constrictor, J. Comp. Neurol.* **151:**159.

Unger, L., 1906, Untersuchungen über die Morphologie und Faserung des Reptiliengehirns. I. Das Vorderhirn des Gecko, *Anat. Hefte* **31:**271.

Voneida, T. J., and Ebbesson, S. O. E., 1969, On the origin and distribution of axons in the pallial commissures in the tegu lizard (*Tupinambis nigropunctatus*), *Brain Behav Evol.* **2:**467.

Walker, A. D., 1972, New light on the origin of birds and crocodiles, *Nature (London)* **237:**257.

Walls, G. L., 1942, *The Vertebrate Eye,* Cranbrook Institute of Science, Cranbrook, Mich.

Ware, C. B., 1974, Projections of dorsal cortex in the side necked turtle (*Podocenmis unifilis*), *Soc. Neurosci. 4th Annu. Meet.,* St. Louis, p. 466.

Warner, J. F., 1931, The cell masses in the telencephalon and diencephalon of the rattlesnake, *Crotalus atrox, Proc. Acad. Sci. Amsterdam* **34:**1156.

Weisbach, W., and Schwartzkopff, J., 1967, Nervose Antworten auf Schallreiz im Groshirn von Krokodilen, *Naturwissenschaften* **54:**650.

Zeier, H., and Karten, H. J., 1971, The archistriatum of the pigeon: Organization of afferent and efferent connections, *Brain Res.* **31:**313.

Zeier, H., and Karten, H. J., 1973, Connections of the anterior commissure in the pigeon (*Columba livia*), *J. Comp. Neurol.* **150:**201.

Zeigler, H. P., and Karten, H. J., 1973, Brain mechanisms and feeding behavior in the pigeon (*Columba livia*). I. Quintofrontal structures, *J. Comp. Neurol.* **152:**59.

11

Parallels in the Organization of Auditory and Visual Systems in Crocodiles

MICHAEL B. PRITZ

I. Introduction

Vertebrates are thought to have had a unimodal origin; that is, they are thought to have arisen only once in time (Romer, 1966). Therefore, all vertebrate nervous systems should exhibit certain features in common which reflect their common genetic inheritance. Indeed, at a certain level of examination this appears to be the case. Thus all vertebrate brains that have been examined reveal the same gross brain regions: prosencephalon, mesencephalon, and rhombencephalon. Furthermore, additional subdivisions such as the telencephalon and optic tectum can readily be identified in all vertebrates. Soon, however, a point is reached where clear-cut divisions are not obvious. For example, the dorsal division of the lateral geniculate nucleus, which is easily identified in many mammals because of its striking pattern of lamination, may or may not be present in other vertebrate classes. Therefore, one task for comparative vertebrate neuroanatomy is to identify and describe which neuronal aggregates and neural circuits are or are not present in various vertebrates. This approach, which will document similarities as well as differences, requires comparison of similar findings not only in other members of a particular class but also in species in other vertebrate classes. In this manner, similarities may reveal basic features of neural organization common to all vertebrate central nervous systems whereas differences may reveal important aspects or trends in the evolution of vertebrate nervous systems.

MICHAEL B. PRITZ • University Hospitals, University of Michigan Medical Center, Ann Arbor, Michigan 48109.

With this in mind, experiments were undertaken to determine the organization of two sensory systems, audition and vision, in a single group of reptiles, *Caiman crocodilus*. Initially, two questions were addressed: (1) Are these structures which subserve audition and vision anatomically separate in the thalamus and telencephalon? (2) Are there any similarities in the organization of these two sensory systems? The latter comparison would, it was hoped, reveal certain features in common between the two sensory systems which might be generalizable to the same sensory systems in other amniotes and to other sensory systems in crocodiles and other amniotes. While these questions could have been approached in several ways so as to reveal different aspects of neuronal organization, they were addressed in this case by making small stereotaxic lesions and using a modification of the Nauta method (Fink and Heimer, 1967) to determine the locus and trajectory of degenerated axons and axon terminals.

The subsequent sections summarize experiments that determined ascending connections of midbrain and thalamic auditory and visual areas in crocodiles (Pritz, 1974*a,b,* 1975). These studies demonstrate the following points: (1) Audition and vision do remain separate in the thalamus and telencephalon. (2) Parallels in ascending fiber connections do exist for these midbrain and thalamic auditory and visual areas. Additional comparisons demonstrate other similarities between auditory and visual systems in *Caiman*. A comparison with other nonmammalian amniotes points out that some of these findings are generalizable to other groups of reptiles and birds. A comparison with mammals demonstrates some similarities and differences in the organization of these two sensory systems and points out the possible evolutionary implications of these findings.

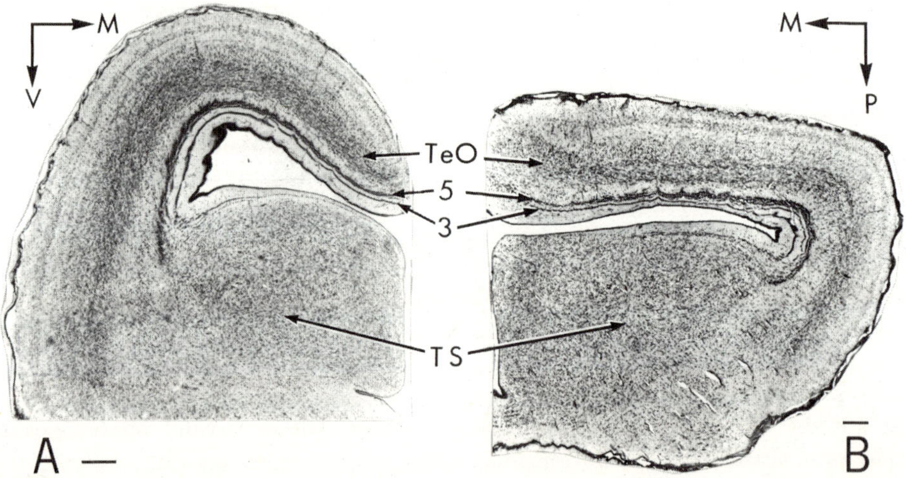

Figure 1. Cytoarchitecture of midbrain auditory and visual areas in *Caiman*. A: Transverse section stained with cresyl violet that corresponds to line drawing C4 in Fig. 4. B: Horizontal section stained with cresyl violet. Bar scale in A and B represents 300 μm. M, Medial; P, posterior; TeO, optic tectum; TS, central nucleus of the torus semicircularis; V, ventral; 3, lamina 3 of the optic tectum; 5, lamina 5 of the optic tectum.

II. Parallels in the Organization of Midbrain Auditory and Visual Areas in *Caiman*

Auditory and visual space are precisely organized in the midbrain of crocodiles. Audition is represented tonotopically in the torus semicircularis (Manley, 1971) while vision is organized retinotopically in the optic tectum (Heric and Kruger, 1965). Not only are the torus semicircularis and optic tectum similar in certain physiological properties and topographic location (see Fig. 1), but also they share similar ascending connections. Each midbrain sensory region projects bilaterally to a prominent neuronal aggregate in the caudal thalamus. In each case, contralateral connections occur via the supraoptic decussation. The central nucleus of the torus semicircularis, the midbrain auditory area, projects to nucleus reuniens pars centralis (Pritz, 1974*a*) whereas the optic tectum, the midbrain visual region, sends axons to terminate in nucleus rotundus (Braford, 1972). No overlap was found in the projections of the central nucleus of the torus semicircularis and optic tectum to the caudal thalamus or to any other region of the diencephalon of *Caiman*. Thus audition and vision remain segregated in the thalamus of *Caiman*.

III. Parallels in the Organization of Thalamic Auditory and Visual Regions in *Caiman*

Nucleus reuniens pars centralis, the thalamic auditory region, and nucleus rotundus, the thalamic visual area, which share similar inputs from the midbrain and similar topographic location in the caudal thalamus, exhibit similar outputs to the telencephalon. In each case ascending axons enter the dorsal peduncle of the lateral forebrain bundle, travel rostrally in the lateral forebrain bundle, swing dorsally through the ventrolateral area, and terminate in the ipsilateral dorsolateral area. Moreover, in each case the trajectory and locus of termination in the telencephalon of axons from these sensory nuclei reflect the topographical location in the diencephalon of each respective nucleus. Thus axons from nucleus reuniens pars centralis, which is located in a caudal and medial part of the diencephalon (see Fig. 2), remain restricted to a medial part of the lateral forebrain bundle and end in a caudal and medial part of the dorsolateral area (Pritz, 1974*b*). On the other hand, axons from nucleus rotundus, which is located anterior and lateral to nucleus reuniens pars centralis (see Fig. 2), remain restricted to a lateral part of the lateral forebrain bundle and terminate in an anterior and lateral part of the dorsolateral area (Pritz, 1975). No overlap in the telencephalic projections of nucleus reuniens pars centralis and nucleus rotundus could be demonstrated. Thus audition and vision, which are separate in the midbrain and thalamus, are also segregated in the telencephalon (see Fig. 3). These regions of the dorsolateral area in *Caiman* that receive auditory and visual input from the thalamus correspond to the dorsal ventricular ridge of other reptiles and birds. These ascending connections of auditory and visual systems that synapse in the midbrain of *Caiman* are summarized in Fig. 4.

The parcellation of sensory modalities in the midbrain, thalamus, and telencephalon was once felt to be a unique property of mammalian sensory systems.

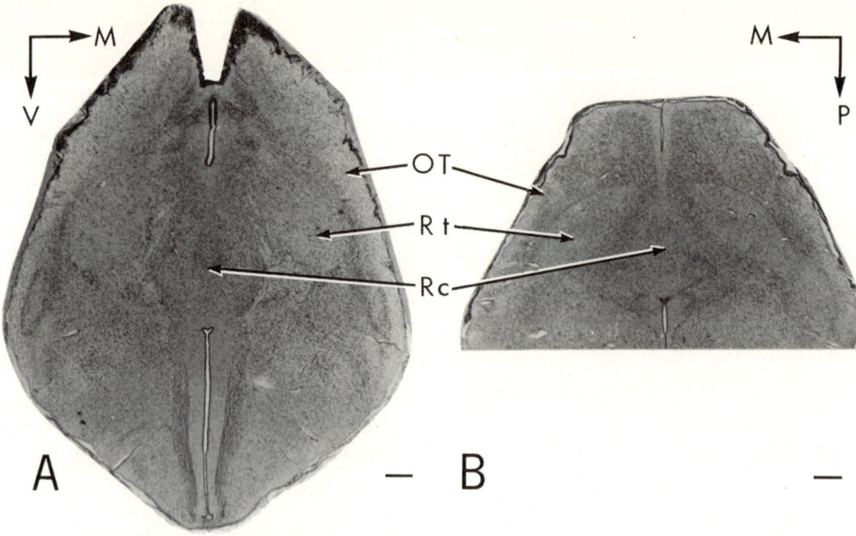

Figure 2. Cytoarchitecture of thalamic auditory and visual areas in *Caiman*. A: Transverse section stained with cresyl violet that corresponds to line drawing C3 in Fig. 4. B: Horizontal section stained with cresyl violet. Bar scale in A and B represents 300 μm. M, Medial; OT, optic tract; P, posterior; Rc, nucleus reuniens pars centralis; Rt, nucleus rotundus; V, ventral.

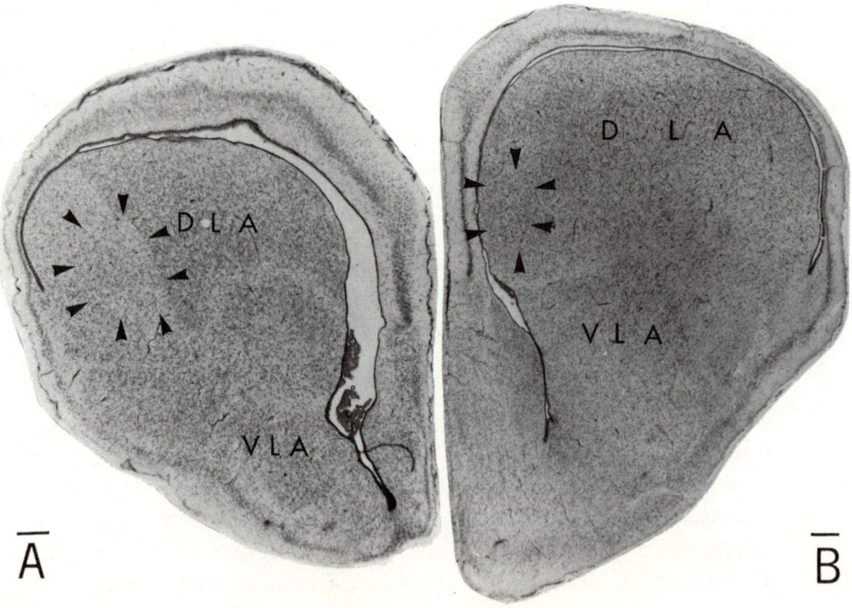

Figure 3. Cytoarchitecture of telencephalic auditory and visual areas in *Caiman*. A: Cresyl violet-stained section that corresponds to line drawing C1 in Fig. 4, illustrating the telencephalic visual area. B: Cresyl violet-stained section that corresponds to line drawing C2 in Fig. 4, illustrating the telencephalic auditory area. The boundaries of these sensory areas are marked by arrowheads. Bar scale in A and B represents 300 μm. DLA, Dorsolateral area; VLA, ventrolateral area.

However, experiments in pigeons demonstrated that audition and vision were segregated in these brain regions in this group of birds (Karten, 1967, 1968; Karten and Revzin, 1966; Karten and Hodos, 1970). The present series of experiments (Pritz, 1974*a,b,* 1975) is the first account to demonstrate that a similar organization applies to members of the class Reptilia. Whether other nonmammalian amniote sensory systems will prove to be as segregated and highly organized as those of crocodiles and pigeons remains to be seen. Nevertheless, the findings of a separation of audition and vision in the midbrain and forebrain of pigeons and crocodiles cast considerable doubt on a commonly held belief that the forebrain of nonmammalian amniotes is a diffusely organized sensory-motor amalgam.

IV. Other Parallels in the Organization of Auditory and Visual Systems That Synapse in the Midbrain of *Caiman*

The foregoing account, which has emphasized certain similarities in the organization of auditory and visual systems in *Caiman,* has focused on parallels in fiber connections from the midbrain centrally to the telencephalon. An examination of more peripheral synaptic elements demonstrates additional similarities between these two sensory systems. These similarities can be viewed in terms of a generalized pattern composed of six elements that extend from the periphery to the telencephalon: receptor cells, bipolar cells, long axon cells, and neuronal aggregates in the midbrain, thalamus, and telencephalon (see Tables I and II, column 1). These last three structures and their respective counterparts in auditory and visual systems of *Caiman* have already been discussed (see Tables I and II, column 4) while the three more peripheral synaptic elements have not. In auditory and visual systems of *Caiman* the respective counterparts for each of these synaptic elements in this generalized pattern are as follows: receptor cells—rods and cones and hair cells; bipolar cells—retinal bipolar cells and spiral ganglion cells; long axon cells—retinal ganglion cells and cochlear nuclei neurons (see Tables I and II, column 4).

Table I. Generalized Pattern of Synaptic Elements of Sensory Systems That Synapse in the Midbrain of Amniotes and the Specific Structures in Auditory Systems That Correspond to This Generalized Scheme

(1) Generalized pattern of synaptic elements	(2)	(3) Audition	(4)
	Mammals	Birds	Reptiles
Receptor cells	Hair cells	Hair cells	Hair cells
Bipolar cells	Spiral ganglion cells	Spiral ganglion cells	Spiral ganglion cells
Long axon cells	Cochlear nuclei cells	Cochlear nuclei cells	Cochlear nuclei cells
Midbrain	Inferior colliculus central nucleus	Nucleus lentiformis mesencephali pars dorsalis	Torus semicircularis central nucleus
Thalamus	Medial geniculate body ventral division	Nucleus ovoidalis	Nucleus reuniens pars centralis (posterior)
Telencephalon	Auditory cortex	Dorsal ventricular ridge	Dorsal ventricular ridge

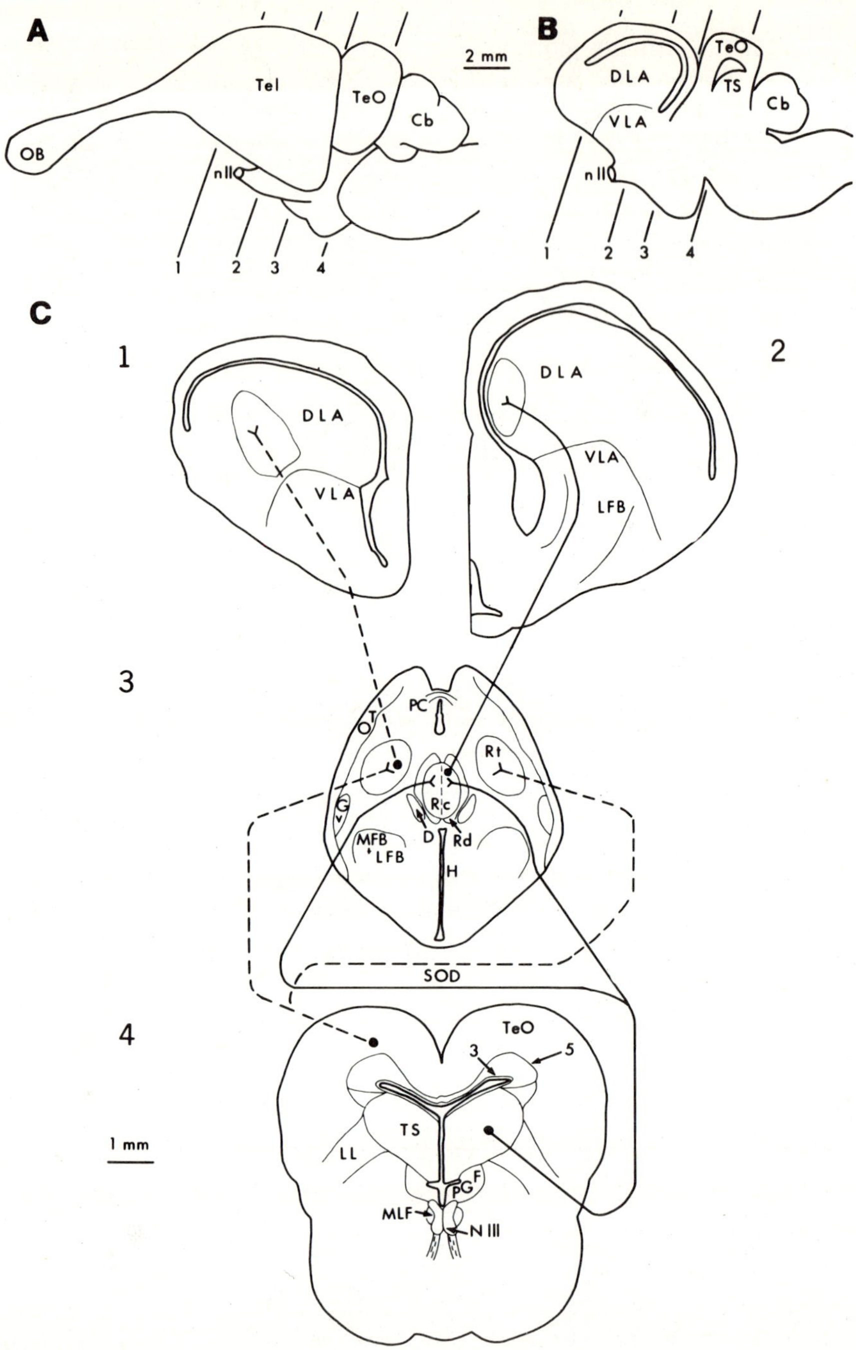

Figure 4. Summary of ascending connections of auditory and visual systems that synapse in the midbrain of *Caiman*. A,B: Outline drawings of *Caiman* brains drawn to scale that illustrate the plane of section and brain levels, 1–4, of similarly labeled transverse sections in C. Lateral (A) and parasagittal (B) views are figured. C: Diagram of composite transverse sections, 1–4, that show the auditory (solid lines) and visual (broken lines) pathways from the midbrain and their major connections. Cb, Cerebellum; D, nucleus diagonalis; DLA, dorsolateral area; Gv, ventral geniculate

Table II. Generalized Pattern of Synaptic Elements of Sensory Systems That Synapse in the Midbrain of Amniotes and the Specific Structures in Visual Systems That Correspond to this Generalized Scheme

(1) Generalized pattern of synaptic elements	(2) Vision: Mammals	(3) Vision: Birds	(4) Vision: Reptiles
Receptor cells	Rods and cones	Rods and cones	Rods and cones
Bipolar cells	Bipolar cells	Bipolar cells	Bipolar cells
Long axon cells	Ganglion cells	Ganglion cells	Ganglion cells
Midbrain	Superior colliculus	Optic tectum	Optic tectum
Thalamus	"Pulvinar"	Nucleus rotundus	Nucleus rotundus
Telencephalon	Nonstriate visual cortex	Dorsal ventricular ridge	Dorsal ventricular ridge

V. Comparison with Other Reptiles and Birds

These parallels in synaptic elements and ascending fiber connections described in previous sections are not unique to auditory and visual systems of *Caiman*. Similar patterns of organization have been described in other nonmammalian amniotes, although identical fiber connections are not present in all cases.

Ascending connections of midbrain and thalamic auditory areas have been investigated in lizards (*Iguana iguana*) and pigeons (*Columba livia*). In each case certain of the fiber connections parallel the trajectory and locus of termination described for *Caiman*. In both *Iguana* and *Columba* midbrain auditory areas project to a prominent nucleus in the caudal diencephalon which sends axons via the lateral forebrain bundle to terminate in a medial portion of the ipsilateral dorsal ventricular ridge. In *Iguana* preliminary evidence indicates that the central nucleus of the torus semicircularis terminates in nucleus reuniens posterior (Foster, 1974). No mention is made in this account (Foster, 1974) as to whether the projection to nucleus reuniens posterior is bilateral and, if so, whether contralateral connections are achieved by way of the supraoptic decussation. Ascending connections of this thalamic auditory area in *Iguana* end in a medial portion of the ipsilateral dorsal ventricular ridge. However, the terminal field observed after nucleus reuniens posterior lesions may not be restricted only to this area (Foster and Peele, 1975). In *Columba* the midbrain auditory area, nucleus mesencephali lateralis pars dorsalis, not only projects bilaterally to nucleus ovoidalis but also does so via the supraoptic decussation (Karten, 1967). Axons from nucleus ovoidalis terminate in field L, a caudal and medial region in the ipsilateral dorsal ventricular ridge (Karten, 1968).

In an analogous fashion, ascending connections of midbrain and thalamic visual areas in turtles (*Pseudemys scripta*) and pigeons (*Columba livia*) not only

nucleus; H, hypothalamus; LFB, lateral forebrain bundle; LL, lateral lemniscus; MFB, medial forebrain bundle; MLF, medial longitudinal fasciculus; N III, oculomotor nucleus; n II, optic nerve; OB, olfactory bulb; OT, optic tract; PC, posterior commissure; PGF, periventricular gray and fibers; Rc, nucleus reuniens pars centralis; Rd, nucleus reuniens pars diffusa; Rt, nucleus rotundus, SOD, supraoptic decussation; Tel, telencephalon; TeO, optic tectum; TS, torus semicircularis; VLA, ventrolateral area; 3, lamina 3 of the optic tectum; 5, lamina 5 of the optic tectum. This figure is reprinted from Pritz (1975, Fig. 9) with permission of the Wistar Institute Press.

parallel certain fiber connections described for *Caiman* but also parallel those of the auditory system. Axons from the midbrain visual area, the optic tectum, terminate in a prominent nucleus in the posterior thalamus which projects to the ipsilateral dorsal ventricular ridge by way of the lateral forebrain bundle. In *Pseudemys* the optic tectum projects bilaterally to nucleus rotundus, although the trajectory of this contralateral component could not be identified (Hall and Ebner, 1970*b*). Ascending fibers of nucleus rotundus in *Pseudemys* end in the core of the ipsilateral dorsal ventricular ridge (Hall and Ebner, 1970*a*). In *Columba* the optic tectum also establishes connections with nucleus rotundus, but these are made only ipsilaterally (Karten and Revzin, 1966). Nucleus rotundus projects onto the core of the ipsilateral ectostriatum (Karten and Hodos, 1970). These similarities in sensory system organization are summarized in Table I for audition (columns 3 and 4) and in Table II for vision (columns 3 and 4) in these nonmammalian amniotes.

The foregoing account emphasizes certain features of sensory system organization in *Caiman* and in other nonmammalian amniotes. In all these instances auditory and visual information terminates in the dorsal ventricular ridge. However, other experimental evidence (Hall and Ebner, 1970*a*; Hunt and Webster, 1972; Karten *et al.*, 1973; Meier *et al.*, 1974; Repérant *et al.*, 1974) indicates that sensory information also reaches the telencephalon by way of other thalamic nuclei that do not receive input from the midbrain. In these latter cases the locus of telencephalic termination is in cortex. These two regions of the telencephalon, cortex and the dorsal ventricular ridge, differ from each other in several ways in these reptiles and birds. First, cortex possesses distinct laminae that include a surface fiber layer and neurons with dendritic trees that are polarized toward the pial surface. On the other hand, the dorsal ventricular ridge, which lacks the lamination and orientation of dendrites characteristic of cortex, is organized as a nucleus (which in certain reptiles is ensheathed by a band of neurons). Second, cortex, which is located between the lateral ventricle and the meninges, is a surface structure, while the dorsal ventricular ridge, which is located near the lateral ventricle but never near the meninges, is a deep brain structure. Third, cortex receives input from sensory systems that bypass the midbrain and synapse directly in the thalamus (Hall and Ebner, 1970*a;* Hunt and Webster, 1972; Karten *et al.*, 1973; Meier *et al.*, 1974; Repérant *et al.*, 1974) while the dorsal ventricular ridge receives input from sensory systems that synapse in the midbrain (Hall and Ebner, 1970*a*; Pritz, 1974*b*, 1975; Foster and Peele, 1975; Karten, 1968; Karten and Hodos, 1970).

VI. Comparison with Mammals

A comparison of the organization of auditory and visual systems between *Caiman* and certain mammals demonstrates similarities as well as differences. Tables I and II indicate that the synaptic elements from the periphery to the midbrain are readily comparable. Comparisons of midbrain, thalamic, and telencephalic structures, however, pose more difficult problems, which are dealt with in depth in previous reports (Pritz, 1974*a,b*, 1975). These papers should be consulted for a more detailed discussion of this point.

In mammals each of these midbrain sensory regions projects to a prominent neuronal aggregate in the caudal thalamus. The midbrain auditory area, the central nucleus of the inferior colliculus, projects to the ventral (inferior) division of the medial geniculate body (Morest, 1964; Ramón y Cajal, 1966) while the midbrain visual area, the superifical layers of the superior colliculus, sends axons to terminate in the "pulvinar"* (Harting *et al.*, 1973*b*; Benevento and Fallon, 1975; Glendenning *et al.*, 1975). Midbrain auditory connections with the posterior thalamus are bilateral, but unlike in *Caiman* and *Columba* they are achieved not by way of the supraoptic decussation but rather via the commissure of the inferior colliculus (Moore and Goldberg, 1963, 1966; Tarlov and Moore, 1966; Powell and Hatton, 1969; van Noort, 1969; Carey and Webster, 1971). On the other hand, midbrain visual connections to the "pulvinar" are only ipsilateral (Harting *et al.*, 1973*b*; Benevento and Fallon, 1975; Glendenning *et al.*, 1975). Both auditory and visual thalamic nuclei project to ipsilateral regions of neocortex. The medial geniculate body sends axons to terminate in auditory cortex (Wilson and Cragg, 1969; Mesulam and Pandya, 1973; Niimi and Naito, 1974; Ryugo and Killackey, 1974) whereas the "pulvinar" projects to nonstriate visual cortex, a cortical region between striate cortex (area 17) and auditory cortex (Harting *et al.*, 1973*a*; Rezak and Benevento, 1975; Glendenning *et al.*, 1975).

This latter point, the locus of termination of these sensory thalamic efferents in the telencephalon, demonstrates the most striking difference between these sensory systems in *Caiman* and these mammals. Both auditory cortex and nonstriate visual cortex receive input from sensory systems that synapse in the midbrain. However, these cortical regions differ markedly from sensory areas in the dorsal ventricular ridge of *Caiman* in terms of cytoarchitecture and topographic location. These neocortical areas are multilaminated regions that include a surface fiber layer and neurons with dendritic trees that are oriented toward the pial surface, whereas the dorsal ventricular ridge, which lacks the lamination and orientation of dendrites characteristic of neocortex, is organized as a nucleus. Furthermore, these neocortical areas are surface structures that are located between the lateral ventricle and the meninges, whereas the dorsal ventricular ridge is a deep brain structure that is located near the lateral ventricle but not near the meninges.

These striking differences in morphology between telencephalic sensory areas in mammals and nonmammalian amniotes have not prevented comparisons between these regions, because criteria other than myelo- and cytoarchitecture are important in the assessment of homologies† between these areas in amniotes (see Campbell and Hodos, 1970). Should these telencephalic sensory areas in mammals and nonmammals indeed prove to be homologous, then the visual region in the dorsal ventricular ridge and the cortical visual area in *Pseudemys,* for example, would be homologous to nonstriate and striate visual cortices in rhesus monkey.

* "Pulvinar" used in this context is a generalized term that refers to a portion of the dorsal thalamus in tree shrew, rhesus monkey, and bushbaby that receives visual input from the superficial layers of the superior colliculus but not from the retina. This region is designated as the pulvinar in tree shrew (Harting *et al.*, 1973*b*) while in rhesus monkey and bushbaby this area refers to a portion of the inferior pulvinar (Benevento and Fallon, 1975; Glendenning *et al.*, 1975).

† "Homology" refers to structures or other entities in two or more organisms which can be traced back through a genealogical series to a stipulated common ancestral precursor or particular neuroanatomical entity irrespective of morphological similarity (Campbell and Hodos, 1970). While several types of homology have been noted, only a few are applicable to the nervous system. Discussions of these various types can be found in papers by Northcutt (1969) and Campbell and Hodos (1970).

This comparison would raise an interesting paradox because in *Pseudemys* the dorsal ventricular ridge is better developed than the cortical visual area. On the other hand, just the reverse is true of rhesus monkey. Although nonstriate visual cortex, a so-called association area, is well developed in monkeys, striate cortex, a so-called primary area, is the more specialized and more highly developed (Sanides, 1970). A continuation of this logic suggests that one feature in the evolution of the telencephalon of amniotes then is the development and expansion of certain of the so-called primary areas while the so-called association areas may have been present and fairly well developed for millions of years. Such a notion is quite the opposite of most popular views of cortical organization and evolution but is not unique. Similar conclusions were reached previously by different investigators, who used quite different approaches (Woolsey and Fairman, 1946; Bishop, 1959; Sanides, 1970).

VII. Summary

Ascending connections of midbrain and thalamic auditory and visual areas in crocodiles (*Caiman crocodilus*) were summarized. These studies demonstrate the following points: (1) Audition and vision remain anatomically separate in the midbrain, thalamus, and telencephalon. (2) Parallels exist in the ascending fiber connections of midbrain and thalamic auditory and visual nuclei. (3) Additional similarities are present in the organization of more peripheral synaptic elements of these two sensory systems.

A comparison of these results in *Caiman* with similar studies in other non-mammalian amniotes indicates that many of these findings are generalizable to other groups of reptiles and birds. A comparison of these findings in *Caiman* with similar data on mammals demonstrates not only similarities but also differences in the organization of audition and vision in these two classes of vertebrates. The evolutionary implications of these findings were discussed.

Note Added in Proof. Since this manuscript was submitted, several studies on amniote sensory systems have been published that relate directly to the topics discussed in this paper. Nevertheless, the hypotheses suggested and the conclusions reached in this summary remain the same.

ACKNOWLEDGMENTS. Much of the research described in this chapter was done in the Department of Anatomy, Case Western Reserve University. I am grateful to Professor M. Singer for the use of laboratory space and photographic facilities. I also thank T. J. Voneida, R. B. Freeman, and E. M. Pritz. I thank the Wistar Institute Press for permission to reproduce the illustration used as Fig. 4.

VIII. References

Benevento, L. A., and Fallon, J. H., 1975, The ascending projections of the superior colliculus in the Rhesus monkey (*Macaca mulatta*), *J. Comp. Neurol.* **160:**339.

Bishop, G. H., 1959, The relation between nerve fiber size and sensory modality: Phylogenetic implications of the afferent innervation of cortex, *J. Nerv. Ment. Dis.* **128:**89.

Braford, M. R., Jr., 1972, Ascending efferent tectal projections in the South American spectacled caiman, *Anat. Rec.* **172:**275.

Campbell, C. B. G., and Hodos, W., 1970, The concept of homology and the evolution of the nervous system, *Brain Behav. Evol.* **3:**353.

Carey, C. L., and Webster, D. B., 1971, Ascending and descending projections of the inferior colliculus in the kangaroo rat (*Dipodomys merriami*), *Brain Behav. Evol.* **4:**401.

Fink, R. P., and Heimer, L., 1967, Two methods for selective silver impregnation of degenerating axons and their synaptic endings in the central nervous system, *Brain Res.* **4:**369.

Foster, R. E., 1974, The ascending brainstem auditory pathways in a reptile, *Iguana iguana, Anat. Rec.* **178:**357.

Foster, R. E., and Peele, T. L., 1975, Thalamotelencephalic auditory pathways in the lizard (*Iguana iguana*), *Anat. Rec.* **181:**530.

Glendenning, K. K., Hall, J. A., Diamond, I. T., and Hall, W. C., 1975, The pulvinar nucleus of *Galago senegalensis, J. Comp. Neurol.* **161:**419.

Hall, W. C., and Ebner, F. F., 1970*a*, Thalamotelencephalic projections in the turtle (*Pseudemys scripta*), *J. Comp. Neurol.* **140:**101.

Hall, W. C., and Ebner, F. F., 1970*b*, Parallels in the visual afferent projections of the thalamus in the hedgehog (*Paraechinus hypomelas*) and the turtle (*Pseudemys scripta*), *Brain Behav. Evol.* **3:**135.

Harting, J. K., Diamond, I. T., and Hall, W. C., 1973*a*, Anterograde degeneration study of the cortical projections of the lateral geniculate and pulvinar nuclei in the tree shrew (*Tupaia glis*), *J. Comp. Neurol.* **150:**393.

Harting, J. K., Hall, W. C., Diamond, I. T., and Martin, G. F., 1973*b*, Anterograde degeneration study of the superior colliculus in *Tupaia glis*: Evidence for a subdivision between superficial and deep layers, *J. Comp. Neurol.* **148:**361.

Heric, T. M., and Kruger, L., 1965, Organization of the visual projection upon the optic tectum of a reptile (*Alligator mississippiensis*), *J. Comp. Neurol.* **124:**101.

Hunt, S. P., and Webster, K. E., 1972, Thalamo-hyperstriate interrelations in the pigeon, *Brain Res.* **44:**647.

Karten, H. J., 1967, The organization of the ascending auditory pathway in the pigeon (*Columba livia*). I. Diencephalic projections of the inferior colliculus (nucleus mesencephali lateralis, pars dorsalis), *Brain Res.* **6:**409.

Karten, H. J., 1968, The ascending auditory pathway in the pigeon (*Columba livia*). II. Telencephalic projections of the nucleus ovoidalis thalami, *Brain Res.* **11:**134.

Karten, H. J., and Hodos, W., 1970, Telencephalic projections of the nucleus rotundus in the pigeon (*Columba livia*), *J. Comp. Neurol.* **140:**35.

Karten, H. J., and Revzin, A. M., 1966, The afferent connections of the nucleus rotundus in the pigeon, *Brain Res.* **2:**368.

Karten, H. J., Hodos, W., Nauta, W. J. H., and Revzin, A. M., 1973, Neural connections of the "visual Wulst" of the avian telencephalon. Experimental studies in the pigeon (*Columba livia*) and owl (*Speotyto cunicularia*), *J. Comp. Neurol.* **150:**253.

Manley, J. A., 1971, Single unit studies in the midbrain auditory area of *Caiman, Z. Vergl. Physiol.* **71:**255.

Meier, R. E., Mihailovic, J., and Cuénod, M., 1974, Thalamic organization of the retino-thalamo-hyperstriatal pathway in the pigeon (*Columba livia*), *Exp. Brain Res.* **19:**351.

Mesulam, M.-M., and Pandya, D. N., 1973, The projections of the medial geniculate complex within the Sylvian fissure of the rhesus monkey, *Brain Res.* **60:**315.

Moore, R. Y., and Goldberg, J. M., 1963, Ascending projections of the inferior colliculus in the cat, *J. Comp. Neurol.* **121:**109.

Moore, R. Y., and Goldberg, J. M., 1966, Projections of the inferior colliculus in the monkey, *Exp. Neurol.* **14:**429.

Morest, D. K., 1964, The neuronal architecture of the medial geniculate body of the cat, *J. Anat.* **98:**611.

Niimi, K., and Naito, F., 1974, Cortical projections of the medial geniculate body in the cat, *Exp. Brain Res.* **19:**326.

Northcutt, R. G., 1969, Discussion of the preceding paper, *Ann. N.Y. Acad. Sci.* **167:**180.

Powell, E. W., and Hatton, J. B., 1969, Projections of the inferior colliculus in cat, *J. Comp. Neurol.* **136:**183.

Pritz, M. B., 1974*a*, Ascending connections of a midbrain auditory area in a crocodile, *Caiman crocodilus, J. Comp. Neurol.* **153:**179.

Pritz, M. B., 1974*b*, Ascending connections of a thalamic auditory area in a crocodile, *Caiman crocodilus, J. Comp. Neurol.* **153:**199.

Pritz, M. B., 1975, Anatomical identification of a telencephalic visual area in crocodiles: Ascending connections of nucleus rotundus in *Caiman crocodilus, J. Comp. Neurol.* **164:**323.

Ramón y Cajal, S., 1966, *Studies on the Diencephalon,* Thomas, Springfield, Ill.

Repérant, J., Raffin, J.-P., and Miceli, D., 1974, La voie rétino-thalamo-hyperstriatale chez le Poussin (*Gallus domesticus* L.), *C. R. Acad. Sci. (Paris)* **279:**279.

Rezak, M., and Benevento, L. A., 1975, Some cortical projections of the inferior pulvinar in the rhesus monkey (*Macaca mulatta*), *Anat. Rec.* **181.**461.

Romer, A. S., 1966, *Vertebrate Paleontology,* University of Chicago Press, Chicago.

Ryugo, D. K., and Killackey, H. P., 1974, Differential telencephalic projections of the medial and ventral divisions of the medial geniculate body of the rat, *Brain Res.* **82:**173.

Sanides, F., 1970, Functional architecture of motor and sensory cortices in primates in the light of a new concept of neocortex evolution, in: *Advances in Primatology* (C. R. Noback and W. Montagna, eds.), pp. 137–208, Appleton-Century-Crofts, New York.

Tarlov, E. C., and Moore, R. Y., 1966, The tecto-thalamic connections in the brain of the rabbit, *J. Comp. Neurol.* **126:**403.

van Noort, J., 1969, *The Structure and Connections of the Inferior Colliculus,* Van Gorcum, Assen.

Wilson, M. E., and Cragg, B. G., 1969, Projections from the medial geniculate body to the cerebral cortex in the cat, *Brain Res.* **13:**462.

Woolsey, C. N., and Fairman, D., 1946, Contralateral, ipsilateral, and bilateral representation of cutaneous receptors in somatic areas I and II of the cerebral cortex of pig, sheep, and other mammals, *Surgery* **19:**684.

12

Behavioral Studies of Telencephalic Function in Reptiles

ELLENGENE PETERSON

I. Introduction

Within the past two decades there has been a growing appreciation of the role of behavior in the ecology and evolution of populations. Behavior, we now recognize, plays a pivotal role in those organism–environment interactions—such as food gathering, niche differentiation, and social organization—which together help to define each population and provide the raw material of selection (Mayr, 1969, 1970, 1974; Moynihan, 1973). Indeed, the behavioral complexes of the various taxa are as distinctive as their morphology. What, then, are the neural substrates of these behaviors which delineate taxa and act, through selection, to shape the course of evolution?

To some investigators it has seemed reasonable to search for the neural mechanisms underlying interspecies behavioral variability within the telencephalon. Anatomically, interspecies variation is greater in the forebrain, especially in the telencephalon, than in more caudal divisions of the neuraxis (Romer, 1970). Recognition of this has led to the intuitive notion that the telencephalon—more so than, although not irrespective of, the brainstem—may provide the key to understanding those distinctive behaviors by which taxa may be differentiated.

Historically, then, students of comparative neurology and brain evolution have focused on understanding telencephalic function. Progress has been slow, especially with regard to the Reptilia—the ancient and successful group which stands at the origin of the amniote radiation. Within the last 10 years, however, two independent

ELLENGENE PETERSON • Department of Anatomy, The University of Chicago, Chicago, Illinois 60637. *Present address*: School of Anatomy, The University of New South Wales, Kensington, New South Wales, Australia 2033.

trends have emerged which, together, have aroused new interest in understanding forebrain function in reptiles and which have given us reason to hope that future progress in these studies will be more rapid than it has been in the past.

The first trend is the recent growth of comparative neuroanatomy, triggered by the advent of experimental techniques such as improved silver stains and methods for tracing intra-axonally transported substances (Ebbesson, 1970; Ebbesson *et al.*, 1975; Lasek, 1975). The resulting increase in anatomical data has begun to have an impact on behavioral investigators since—as we begin to understand the structural organization of the reptile telencephalon—it is natural to inquire into the functions subserved by these newly elucidated pathways.

The second trend has been an increasing sophistication in the behavioral testing of reptiles. Two lines of behavioral research have emerged, both shaped by the growing body of literature on the behavioral ecology of reptiles. On the one hand, psychologists have continued their efforts at laboratory analyses of reptile behavior, but with a new appreciation of the need for ecologically relevant cues and reinforcers (Burghardt, 1977; Brattstrom, 1978). As a result, the number of successful studies of reptile learning and discrimination behavior has increased rapidly over the past 10 years. On the other hand, investigators with a background in zoology have begun to develop techniques for experimental behavioral analyses in the field or in "naturalistic" settings (e.g., Brattstrom, 1974; Burghardt, 1970; Carpenter, 1967). A few studies now exist which use these newer behavioral methods in attempting to understand telencephalic function in reptiles.

The present chapter is intended to provide—with certain qualifications—a comprehensive review of behavioral studies on reptile telencephalic function published since 1916. In addition, this chapter presents related data from some recent, heretofore unpublished, experiments. Certain segments of the reptile brain–behavior literature are not represented here: (1) Studies published prior to 1916. These have been reviewed in detail by Ten Cate (1937). The year 1916 was chosen as a starting point because that is the year when Johnston published his influential paper on the "motor pallium" in reptiles (Johnston, 1916). (2) Studies originating from Russian research groups, such as those at Leningrad (Sechenov Institute) and Moscow. Much of this literature is difficult to understand without a substantial background in Russian psychological and physiological literature, something well outside the scope of this chapter. Furthermore, most of these studies are not available in English translation. As a result, a fair and comprehensive treatment of the Russian literature on reptile brain–behavior relations is not possible here. Much of this work has been reviewed by Belekhova (1979). (3) Studies on reptile EEG patterns which may include observations on behavioral correlates of certain EEG states. Some of these experiments are dealt with in Belekhova's review.

Behavioral studies of reptile telencephalic function have been reviewed previously by several authors. Ten Cate's paper (1937) is by far the most useful treatment of the early literature. More recently, Goldby and Gamble (1957) included a brief section on "Functional Investigations" in their comprehensive review of the literature on the reptile cerebral hemispheres, and Aronson (1970) has published a selected review of this same literature. No review exists which is both detailed and comprehensive. The present chapter is intended to fill that gap: to assess our progress in these studies and to provide a framework for future investigations of telencephalic function in reptiles.

For convenience, the studies to be reviewed will be grouped into those dealing with the pallium and those dealing with the subpallium.

II. Subpallium

A. Introduction

Behavioral studies of subpallial function can conveniently be divided into two groups: those which antedate and those which follow the advent of the "new" comparative neuroanatomy in the late 1960s (Ebbesson, 1970).

Early behavioral investigations into the function of subpallial structures consisted primarily of lesion experiments, and the results of these studies were "often equivocal and difficult to interpret" (Goldby and Gamble, 1957, p. 408). These early experiments were marred by two procedural weaknesses. First, investigators tended to approach this part of the telencephalon as an undifferentiated mass. Little effort was made to restrict lesion sites to specific cellular aggregates and, consequently, it was impossible to relate observed behavioral effects to any particular nucleus or nuclear complex. Second, the behavioral tests used usually consisted of nothing more than recording the experimental animal's postural reflexes, its response to painful stimuli, and the presence or absence of voluntary movement and feeding. Thus they were too crude to uncover any but the most gross sensory or motor aspects of subpallial function.

Within the last decade, however, behavioral investigators have begun to focus their attention on the function of specific cellular aggregates within the subpallium and to use a more sophisticated array of behavioral tests to assess the effects of telencephalic lesions. The resulting experiments have begun to yield new insights into the function of the reptile subpallium.

In addition to these lesion studies, there have been a few reports regarding the behavioral effects of electrically stimulating various subpallial structures. As was true of the early lesion experiments, stimulation sites were not verified histologically or specified in terms of cytoarchitectural boundaries. Within the last 10 years, a small number of stimulation studies have appeared which focus on the behavioral effects of stimulating specific subpallial structures.

B. Terminology

In neurological studies on reptiles the term "pallium" has been understood to include those cellular and fiber aggregates which lie dorsal to the lateral ventricles. "Subpallium," then, refers to all those forebrain structures which lie below the pallium (Senn and Northcutt, 1973). Various divisions of this subpallial area have been recognized by different workers. However, as a rough guide to the organization of the subpallium, Goldby and Gamble's (1957) classic description is still useful. For the most part, it will be adhered to in this chapter, primarily because it is simple and because their nomenclature has been the most widely used by those behavioral workers whose experiments are reviewed here. The anatomy of the reptile telencephalon has been reviewed in Chapters 9 and 10 of this volume and by Northcutt (1978).

In Goldby and Gamble's terminology the subpallium of each hemisphere can be divided into medial and lateral parts by the lateral ventricle. The medial subdivision is the septum; the lateral subdivision is the strio-amygdaloid complex. Approximately the posterior one-third of the strio-amygdaloid complex is called the amygdala or amygdaloid group by Goldby and Gamble. This region corresponds to the basal dorsal ventricular ridge in some recent anatomical descriptions (Balaban, 1978; Peterson and Ulinski, 1980). The anterior two-thirds is called the striatum. It includes, dorsally, the hypopallium and, ventral to this, the paleostriatum. The area designated hypopallium by Goldby and Gamble has recently become the subject of much speculation, and at present it is better understood, hodologically, than perhaps any other part of the subpallium (e.g. Lohman and van Woerden-Verkley, 1978). Virtually all modern workers now refer to this area as the anterior dorsal ventricular ridge (ADVR) and that term will be adopted here, in lieu of Goldby and Gamble's "hypopallium." Northcutt (1978) reviews the evidence that this area may be derived, embryologically, from the pallium. The paleostriatum of Goldby and Gamble lies ventral to ADVR. It corresponds to the striatum of some anatomists (Peterson and Ulinski, 1980).

In reading the following account it is important to keep in mind that although many of Goldby and Gamble's terms are also used in descriptions of the mammalian brain (e.g., amygdala, septum), one cannot therefore infer that like-named structures in reptilian and mammalian brains are necessarily homologous. To be sure, such names often derived originally from a supposed resemblance between certain reptilian and eutherian nuclear groups. However, evidence for homology (*sensu* Simpson, 1961) is often weak or entirely lacking.

C. Lesion Studies of Subpallial Function: 1823 to 1967

Ablation studies published through approximately the turn of the century have been reviewed by Ten Cate (1937). Those data will be summarized briefly here for the sake of completeness. Ten Cate mentions seven studies conducted between 1823 and 1905 which included work on several squamate and chelonian species. In each of the studies both hemispheres were extirpated, with or without varying amounts of the diencephalon and midbrain. All but two (Schrader, 1892; Sergi, 1905*a,b)* of these workers reported that spontaneous activity was reduced in their animals but that such movements as occurred (usually as the result of some applied irritant) appeared to be completely normal. Also reported were lack of ability to avoid obstacles (Fano, 1884; Bickel, 1901), absence of "fear" and "rage" responses (Schrader, 1892), absence of spontaneous feeding (Bickel, 1901), normal reaction to light (Bickel, 1901), normal head withdrawal to threat in turtles (Bickel, 1901), and increased "reflex" excitation (Sergi, 1905*a,b)*.

The last lesion experiment cited in Ten Cate's review was published in 1905. No new ablation studies of forebrain function in reptiles appeared until over 20 years later with the publication of a brief report by Bagley and Langworthy (1926) concerning the effects of bilateral hemispherectomy in alligators (species not given).

This paper was one of two which dealt primarily with electrical stimulation of the pallium. However, in an unspecified number of animals the authors removed the telencephalon, taking care not to injure the thalamus (although no histology is reported) and to "avoid troublesome bleeding." Motor activity in these animals was not much different from that of intact alligators. Voluntary locomotion was observed, although Bagley and Langworthy did not report whether the frequency of voluntary movement was decreased, as suggested by earlier workers.

Perhaps the most careful of the lesion studies of this period is that of Goldby (1937). In each lizard (*Lacerta viridis*) the extent of tissue destruction was verified histologically and reported in detail together with—in some cases—appropriate illustrations. Two animals (XXV and XXIV) sustained bilateral cortical damage without bilateral involvement of the subpallium, thus, in theory, allowing assessment of any pallial contribution to the total hemispherectomy syndrome reported by earlier workers.

Several lizards which sustained partial lesions of one hemisphere appeared essentially normal within a few hours after surgery. In another lizard (XXXII) the "antero-dorsal" hemispheres were removed (probably including the ADVR), sparing the paleostriatium and amygdala, although the latter were "much damaged by hemmorrhages." This lizard likewise appeared normal in most respects, although it was not seen to feed until its death 22 days later. The remaining four lizards (XXV,XX,XXI,XXIV) sustained varying amounts of bilateral damage to the telencephalon. All four animals showed essentially the same pattern of behavior: (1) They were sluggish, exhibiting reduced voluntary movement. (2) Movements, when they did occur, were normal. (3) Response to mechanical (usually noxious) stimulation was normal. (4) There was slight hypertonus, especially of the neck muscles. (5) None of the lizards were seen to eat, although two animals (XXI and XXV) snapped at a worm within their field of vision.

One problem with Goldby's study is that the range and complexity of behavioral tests he used were quite limited. Diebschlag (1938) sought to remedy this in a more ambitious study using several species of *Lacerta* and the snake *Tropidonotus natrix*. He states that surgery was performed with great care to prevent bleeding and that the extent of his lesions was checked histologically, although no details or illustrations are given.

Diebschlag confirmed earlier reports that decerebrate reptiles show loss of spontaneous movement and feeding. However, after extirpating progressively larger and larger amounts of telencephalon, he concluded that such spontaneity seems to depend on the basal part of the posterior third of the hemispheres (presumably the amygdaloid group). When this latter area was removed, animals spent most of the time lying on the floor of the cage with their eyes closed. When pinched with forceps, they would open their eyes for brief periods and sometimes move, such movements always being perfectly normal. However, they soon subsided into the previous "somnolent" condition. These animals did not feed, nor did they show the flight or "panic" reactions characteristic of intact subjects. Also, unlike normal controls, they did not seek their usual hiding places or attempt to bask. Diebschlag found that optomotor responses to a rotating striped cylinder were present, although difficult to measure since the lesioned animals tended to keep their eyes closed. Agonistic behavior and visual discriminations were not examined in totally decerebrate lizards since these animals were rarely active. One animal which had the critical posterior basal third of the telencephalon spared was apparently deficient in the retention of a color discrimination, although no data are given. There was no mention of the hypertonus described by Goldby. Diebschlag's results are in general agreement with those of Goldby and several earlier workers who reported that cerebrumless lizards are extremely sluggish. Unlike Goldby, Diebschlag states this effect occurs only when the posterior basal third of the telencephalon is removed.

Three other reports should be mentioned which belong to this early group of ablation studies because the lesions in these experiments were large and, in some cases, the behavioral tests were nonspecific. Abbie (1948) reported neck hypertonus in the lizard *Trachysaurus rugosus* following total hemispherectomy. Northcutt (1967) reports briefly that *Caiman sclerops* shows no loss of spontaneity or ability to feed when part of the pallium (dorsal cortex) and ADVR are removed. There was, however, "a change in the nature of spontaneous activity to sensory threshold levels."

Spiegel and Ellis (1966) studied the effect of large cerebral lesions on passive avoidance learning in the turtle *Chrysemys*. Their experimental paradigm was as follows. When confined in an upright cylinder, turtles normally attempt to climb out. If a shock is delivered each time the animal attempts to climb, it will eventually cease such escape efforts. The cessation of this climbing response was operationally defined by the authors as passive avoidance. Although under some conditions (30 V) lesioned turtles stopped climbing significantly faster than controls, this same difference occurred when no shock was administered (0 V), suggesting that their lesions affected the tendency to climb *per se* (which the authors interpret as an emotional response) rather than passive avoidance acquisition. Unfortunately, their lesions are such that these data are impossible to interpret. It is difficult to tell just what structures were damaged (apparently very different areas were lesioned in different animals), whether the lesions in a given subject were bilaterally symmetrical, and to what extent the observed effects result from the pallial destruction which occurred in all cases.

D. Lesion Studies of Subpallial Function: 1968 to the Present

In contrast to earlier work, lesion studies conducted during the last decade have been concerned with the function of relatively restricted portions of the reptile subpallium. Therefore, the studies included in this section will be grouped according to their primary anatomical focus rather than treated chronologically.

1. Anterior Dorsal Ventricular Ridge (ADVR)

The ADVR has attracted more attention in recent years than any other division of the subpallium—in the anatomical literature at least. There have been several reports that the ADVR in reptiles receives a major ascending projection from sensory nuclei in the dorsal thalamus (see reviews by Northcutt, 1978, and Chapter 10 of this volume). As a result, there has been widespread speculation that the ADVR may represent a homologue of sensory neocortex in mammals (e.g., Ebbesson, 1972; Northcutt, 1978; see also Karten, 1969). Such speculations were the basis of the study by Bass *et al.* (1973) on the effects of ADVR lesions on visual discrimination in the turtle *Podocnemis unifilis.* Using a two-choice simultaneous presentation procedure (Pritz *et al.,* 1973), Bass and his co-workers trained four turtles to choose between horizontal and vertical stripes, following which they ablated dorsal cortex (a subdivision of the pallium; see Section III), together with varying amounts of ADVR. As a control for the effects of pallial destruction, three turtles sustained lesions of dorsal cortex alone. In postsurgical testing three out of four ADVR-lesioned animals reached criterion in the same or fewer trials than were required to learn the task preoperatively, suggesting to these investigators that the ADVR may not be necessary for this type of visual discrimination. It is worth pointing out, however, that there are at least three difficulties with this experiment which may have contributed to the negative results. First, as the authors point out, the ADVR lesions may not have been optimal. Histology for one case is illustrated, PV-2, which sustained "one of the largest telecephalic ablations." From this figure it appears that little of ADVR was destroyed bilaterally, suggesting that all four turtles may have received substantially subtotal lesions. Second, a very modest criterion was set (three out of four correct choices for four consecutive days). Third, in the absence of appropriate controls, it is impossible to tell whether their lesions may have reduced some potential postoperative savings on the behavioral task. In intact animals, or when lesions are truly without effect, many species may show considerable savings in trials or errors to criterion when exposed to a task for the second time, as, for example, when subjects undergo preoperative and then postoperative acquisition. Unfortunately, no behavioral data are reported for intact or sham surgical controls which would allow us to judge whether the ADVR lesions affected savings on the postoperative stripe discrimination.

Data regarding the effects of ADVR lesions have been reported from three other laboratories (Greenberg *et al.*, 1976; Greenberg, 1977, 1978; Tarr, 1975, 1977; Keating *et al.,* 1970). However, these experiments were concerned primarily with other divisions of the subpallium. Their data on ADVR lesions will be described in the appropriate sections below.

2. Paleostriatum

In recent years, only one laboratory has been concerned with the behavioral effects of lesions in reptile paleostriatum (Greenberg *et al.,* 1976; Greenberg, 1977; 1978). This work is especially interesting because it represents one of the few attempts to study the effects of brain lesions on "natural" agonistic behavior. Greenberg and his colleagues first developed a detailed behavioral inventory (ethogram) for the lizard *Anolis carolinensis,* based on observations of these animals in large naturalistic enclosures and on field behavior. As with many other lizard species, agonistic behavior in *A. carolinensis* involves a complicated series of displays (e.g., head bobbing, "pushups") which are thought to act as signals between conspecifics (Rand, 1967; Carpenter, 1967; Greenberg and MacLean, 1978). Two types of display commonly recognized in adult males are (1) an "assertion" or "arousal" display which does not require the presence of a conspecific and may occur at any time during the lizard's activity period, e.g., when moving from one perch to another, and (2) a "challenge" display which is said to be more intense than the assertion display and is elicited only by an appropriate conspecific, e.g., by an adult male intruding on a resident male's territory (Carpenter, 1967; Crews, 1975; Jenssen, 1971). In Greenberg's study, adult males were allowed to establish territories and then the paleostriatum was lesioned unilaterally. The experimenters tested the reaction of these animals to the intrusion of a conspecific adult male and, in addition, recorded their normal home cage activity. A within-subjects design allowed each animal to serve as its own control, i.e., each lesioned lizard was tested both (1) with the eye contralateral to the lesion occluded and (2) with the ipsilateral eye occluded. In this way the experimenters could control whether visual input reached primarily the lesioned or the intact hemisphere. The rationale behind such a control procedure is that retinal efferents in reptiles are primarily contralateral. In fact, there is a distinct ipsilateral retinal projection in *A. carolinensis* (Butler and Northcutt, 1971) as in all other squamates which have been examined (Chapter 10, this volume). Nevertheless, data from Greenberg's work suggest that this ipsilateral pathway, if it reaches the telencephalon, is not sufficient to sustain the types of agonistic behavior measured in this experiment.

Paleostriatum-lesioned lizards showed a significant decrease in the incidence of challenge displays, but, in contrast, the assertion display was unaffected. This effect was seen when subjects were tested with the eye contralateral to the lesion. When tested with the ipsilateral eye, the lizards behaved entirely normally, indicating that their lesion did not destroy the capacity to emit a challenge display (i.e., there was no motor impairment *per se*). The authors suggest that the experimental lizards were "unable to perceive the 'conspecificity' of their antagonist." These animals were not blind on the lesioned side as they were able to track prey with the eye contralateral to the lesion. The authors compare their results with earlier work (MacLean, 1973, 1975) which reports that the pallidum in mammals may mediate certain species-specific display behaviors. Control lesions of the ADVR had no effect on display activity as measured in this experiment.

3. Amygdala

Within the past decade, two laboratories have been concerned with understanding the functions of the reptilian amygdaloid complex. The behavioral tests used in these two experiments were suggested by data from studies of the mammalian amygdala which implicate this nuclear group in the regulation of affective behavior ("rage" and "fear") and intraspecific agonistic interactions (Clemente and Chase, 1973).

Keating *et al.* (1970) studied the effects of amygdala ablations in 32 South American caimans (*C. sclerops*). Fifteen animals received bilateral amygdalectomies, and 17 control animals sustained unilateral lesions or bilateral craniotomies only. The experimenters kept detailed notes on the animals' general behavior and, in addition, scored their responses to various noxious stimuli on 5-point "attack" and "retreat" scales which had previously been tested for interexperimenter reliability. All scoring was done blind. Each animal was tested before and after surgical intervention and thus served as its own control. A comparison of pre- and postoperative scores indicates that animals with bilateral amygdalectomies became significantly less reactive following surgery than did controls. Both attack and retreat behaviors were affected by the lesions. The authors emphasize that their experimental animals were otherwise normal; they were active, struggled when handled, and, when sufficiently provoked, showed normal attack and retreat responses. However, the thresholds for these reactions were elevated and responses tended to be shorter in duration and less vigorous than prior to surgery. Furthermore, the affective components of these behaviors—pupillary and respiratory changes, vocalization, etc.—were absent. There was a significant correlation between the amount of ventromedial nucleus involvement (VMN; *sensu* Crosby, 1917) and the extent of behavioral deficit. On the other hand, lesions of the anterior dorsolateral area (DLA of Crosby, corresponding approximately to ADVR) had no measurable effect on the behavior tested in this experiment.

Tarr (1975, 1977*a*) has taken a somewhat different approach to understanding the reptilian amygdaloid complex. Like Greenberg, Tarr studied the effect of forebrain lesions on the social behavior of iguanid lizards (*Sceloporous occidentalis)* in a "naturalistic" setting. Several groups of six to eight lizards were allowed to establish normal dominance hierarchies in large, appropriately equipped, enclosures.* For each lizard, detailed notes were made as to its status in the group, "territory" or favored perch, and habitual behavior toward conspecifics. One or two lizards from each group were then removed, subjected to one of three experimental treatments, returned to the group within 24–48 hr, and observed for 2 weeks. The three treatments were: (1) bilateral amygdala lesions ($N = 10$), (2) bilateral ADVR lesions ($N = 10$), (3) surgical controls ($N = 25$).

Lizards with amygdala lesions showed two types of behavioral changes: decreased spontaneous activity and loss of social responsiveness. Decreased spontaneity involved periods of "somnolence" (eyes closed, no movement) and periods of reduced alertness (eyes open, some movement, but less attentive than controls to surroundings). These episodes of decreased spontaneity alternated with normal periods in which the behavior of the lesioned animals was—in all respects but one (see below)—undistinguishable from that of controls.

All lizards sustaining amygdala lesions exhibited abnormal social behavior. This included lack of appropriate response (e.g., flight, challenge) to displays of conspecifics, aberrant displays (assertion displays emitted in an inappropriate context), and adoption of new location preferences without regard to the position of other (dominant) members of the group. All lesioned animals, even previous alpha males, became nonagressive. Tarr points out that this lack of reponsiveness to social signals is not simply a manifestation of decreased arousal since the lesioned animals showed periods of normal spontaneity during which they easily caught insects and apparently attended to activity within their enclosures. During these same periods, however, they never responded to assertion displays by conspecifics. At no time did these animals evidence any sensory or motor impairment. Moreover, they were capable of emitting displays since they occasionally were seen to give random assertion displays, although never in an aggressive context. In contrast to the results of Keating *et al.* (1970), these lesion effects did not appear to depend on the involvement of VMN.

* Carpenter (1961, 1967) and others (e.g., Brattstrom, 1971; Bustard, 1965) have demonstrated that many lizard species, when kept in such large "naturalistic" enclosures, will quickly develop a form of social organization best described as a loose hierarchical or dominance relationship. The exact form of this organization will depend on the species and the characteristics of the enclosure.

Of lizards sustaining lesions of ADVR, a majority showed decreases in spontaneity similar to that seen in amygdalectomized animals. Most, however, showed no change in social behavior and resumed their presurgical positions in the dominance hierarchy. This is a critical point. Iguanid dominance hierarchies in such enclosures are subject to disruption when one member of the group is removed (Carpenter and Grubits, 1960; Evans, 1953). Under the conditions of this experiment, change in dominance position is not, by itself, evidence for brain dysfunction since some alteration of the hierarchy might be expected merely as a result of removing a lizard from the group for 1 or 2 days. The fact that ADVR- and sham-lesioned animals resumed their preoperative dominance positions indicates that the behavioral effects observed in amygdala-lesioned lizards were not simply a result of disrupting the hierarchy. Two animals in this group also became unresponsive to social signals, but both of these lizards were unusual in that they "rarely moved" for 2 weeks following surgery, and so data from these animals are impossible to interpret (Tarr, personal communication).

4. Medial Wall

Two final studies should be mentioned in this section on the behavioral effects of basal telencephalic lesions. One study, by Berk and Heath (1975), grew out of the now extensive body of literature on behavioral thermoregulation in reptiles. In their experiment Berk and Heath made large lesions in the ventromedial wall of the telencephalon of lizards *(Dipsosaurus dorsalis)*, including septum, medial cortex, and medial forebrain bundle (MFB), which in squamates is thought to carry information from medial wall structures to the hypothalamus (Ulinski, 1976; Chapters 9 and 10, this volume). Behavioral thermoregulation, as measured by shuttling in a thermal gradient and adoption of "thermal" postures, was disrupted by these lesions as well as by damage to the medial preoptic area and parts of the hypothalamus. The lizards tended to let their body temperature drop to levels not tolerated by intact individuals during their activity periods. The authors point out that these large lesions provide little information about the role of specific telencephalic structures in behavioral thermoregulation in reptiles. They note, however, that one reason for the often reported decrease in activity following large telencephalic lesions may be that these animals do not maintain body temperatures at levels sufficient to support normal acitivity.

A second study (Tarr, 1977*b*) examined the effects of septal lesions on reactivity to mild stimulation and intraspecific agonistic behavior in *Sceloporous occidentalis.* Lesioned animals showed no increase in emotionality and no evidence of a "septal syndrome" (DeFrance, 1976). Similarly, septal lesions had no consistent effect on social signaling (e.g., challenge and assertion displays) when animals were tested under naturalistic conditions (described in Tarr, 1977*a*).

E. Stimulation Studies of Subpallial Function

Prior to the late 1960s stimulation studies of telencephalic function in reptiles were primarily concerned with trying to find a "motor cortex" in the pallium. These studies will be described in some detail in Section III.B. There were, however, occasional reports on the effects of stimulating subpallial structures, and those data will be summarized here.

The earliest and most influential of the stimulation studies was that of Johnston (1916). Johnston had identified a cytoarchitecturally distinct area in the turtle pallium (the pallial thickening, Johnston, 1915) which he believed might "correspond to the motor cortical area in the mammalian brain" (Johnston, 1916, p. 475). The stimulation study which followed (Johnston, 1916) was designed to test that hypothesis, and thus most of Johnston's data deal with movements following stimulation of the pallial thickening. However, he also reported that—under deep anesthesia—monopolar or bipolar stimulation of the striatal area (apparently comparable to Goldby and Gamble's paleostriatum) in turtles (*Chelydra serpentia, Cistudo carolina, Chrysemys marginata)* and the lizard *Gerrhonotus* led to movements in head, neck, body, and limbs. These responses he ascribed to stimulation of descending fibers in the lateral forebrain bundle (LFB, i.e., pallial thickening efferents). After pallial removal the surface of the ADVR was stimulated. Some head and limb muscle contractions were obtained, but Johnston attributed this to spread of current to the pallial thickening or to the LFB. Likewise, movements elicited by stimulation of the "amygdaloid eminence" seemed to Johnston to be due to current spread to the thalamus.

Virtually all the subsequent stimulation studies of this early period were inspired by Johnston's claim to have discovered a "motor cortex" in reptiles. As such, they dealt primarily with the pallium, but corollary observations on the effects of subpallial stimulation were often included in these studies. Bagley and Langworthy (1926) reported that while pallial stimulation in alligators produced a variety of head and body movements, no motor responses could be obtained from stimulation of any part of the subpallium. On the other hand, Koppányi and Pearcy (1925) reported coordinated swimming movements in turtles (species not given) following bipolar stimulation of the "striatum," at a current intensity "just detectable to the tongue." The same response was elicited from the cerebral peduncles at lower current intensities, and sectioning of the peduncles abolished the response to striatal stimulation. In alligators, however, no motor responses were obtained from forebrain stimulation.

Goldby (1937), using bipolar electrodes and deep anesthesia, was unable to elicit movements from stimulating any part of the telencephalon with a current sufficiently strong to produce movements from the tectum or to activate muscles directly. Abbie (1948) reported similar results in the lizard (*Trachysaurus rugosus).* Distel (1978*a,b)* and others (e.g., Sugerman, 1974; Sugarman and Demski, 1978) have observed, however, that more current is required to produce a response from telencephalic structures than from the tectum. It is possible, then, that Goldby and Abbie used currents which were somewhat too low.

In a much quoted study Bremer *et al.* (1939) were able to produce neck, jaw, and feet movements in unanesthetized turtles (species not given) using either bipolar or monopolar stimulation of the telencephalic surface. They attributed these effects to an electrically excitable area in the subpallium since cocainization of the pallium failed to abolish these responses. The authors did not, however, adduce any independent evidence that the application of cocaine effectively "shut down" the pallium.

Within the past decade a small number of stimulation studies have appeared which focus specifically on the electrical excitability of various subpallial structures. Keating *et al.* (1970) investigated the behavioral effects of electrically stimulating the amygdaloid complex, defined by the authors as (1) the nucleus of the lateral olfactory tract, (2) the ventromedial nucleus, and (3) the posterolateral part of the dorsolateral area (nomenclature of Crosby, 1917). Small-diameter unipolar electrodes were chronically implanted in the telencephalon of 25 animals, 14 of which were later found to have been positioned in the amygdala. In three of these 14 animals stimulation was ineffective, but at the other 11 sites electrical stimulation (60 Hz, 0.05–60 mA for 5–15 sec) elicited sharp ipsilateral turning followed by "flight." This was not simply a motor response since the animals reacted appropriately to obstacles placed in their path, e.g., by climbing over or crawling under barriers or retracing their steps when necessary. Affective components (respiratory changes, micturition, vocalization) were sometimes present. Stimulation of sites in the ADVR produced somewhat different responses which were similar to those reported by Schapiro and Goodman (1969; see below), i.e., movements of jaw and eyes and "deliberate pacing" which could be distinguished from the flight response by its intensity and direction.

Schapiro and Goodman (1969) reported the behavioral effects of stimulating the ADVR in 29 caimans (*C. sclerops*). Current (60 Hz, 0.2–0.6 mA for 10 sec) was delivered via chronically implanted monopolar electrodes (60–90 μm diameter). At low current intensities, stimulation produced eye and head movement and occasional "affective" behaviors (respiratory changes, vocalization, retching). At slightly higher current strengths the animals showed a characteristic ipsilateral turning. This response was flexible and "goal directed," i.e., the animals would modify their movements appropriately when confronted with obstacles. The authors contrast this behavior with that elicited by tectal stimulation, the latter being characterized by rapid "acute" circling movements which were stereotyped, i.e., not modified by the environment.

Recently, a more ambitious stimulation study has been reported by Distel (1978*a,b*). Like Greenberg (1977, 1978), Distel first compiled a normal behavioral inventory for his lizards (*Iguana iguana).* Subsequently, he investigated the electrical excitability of the brains of 21 unrestrained, unanesthetized iguanas with a device (Distel, 1976) by which the (130 μm diameter) monopolar electrodes could be advanced during testing of the awake animal. Using 60-sec stimulus trains (1-msec biphasic square waves, 30 Hz at 25–450 μA), he explored a total of 518 sites, of which 164 were in the telencephalon. Location of the electrode tracts was verified histologically. Behavioral testing was conducted in a small enclosure maintained at 33–38°C and equipped with food, water, and a conspecific.

Behaviors elicited by electrical stimulation of the telencephalon tended to involve nondirected head movements or "exploratory" behaviors. For example, the majority of sites in the ADVR and the "ventrolateral" portion of the telencephalon either were ineffective or yielded only head movements and nonspecific alerting responses. Stimulation of medial wall structures (e.g., medial cortex, septum, n. accumbens, olfactory tubercle) resulted in locomotion and tongue flicking which resembled exploratory behavior seen in normal lizards. In the septum stimulation sometimes yielded "pre-escape behavior" (ipsilateral turning, head lowering, backward movements), but this was seldom followed by fully developed escape responses of the type elicited from mesencephalic and medullary sites. Interestingly, display response sequences (dewlapping, head bobbing, and defensive behaviors such as lateral compression, hissing, engorged tongue, and tail lashing) were almost impossible to elicit from telencephalic sites. Similarly, feeding, drinking, copulation, and fighting were never elicited by telencephalon stimulation. Distel points out that responses elicited from telencephalic sites were "more integrated and natural" than responses derived from more caudal regions such as the ventral thalamus, tectum, and tegmentum.

One final experiment of this group is that of Sugerman (1974; Sugerman and Demski, 1978) who studied agonistic behavior in the iguanid lizard *Crotaphytus collaris* following electrical stimulation of several sites within the telencephalon. Using both anesthetized and free-ranging animals with monopolar stimulation (2-ms biphasic square waves, 50Hz, 10 to 750 μA), he elicited "defensive or agressive behavior" (e.g., gular extension) from the septum and nucleus sphaericus. A third site in the olfactory tubercle (cf. their Figure 3, site #1) probably involved afferent fibers to n. sphaericus from the accessory olfactory bulb (Peterson and Ulinski, 1980). Like Distel, Sugerman reported that higher current intensities were required to elicit such responses from telencephalic sites than from the brainstem.

F. Summary

The most common result of subpallial lesions in reptiles is a decrease in "arousal" levels or loss of spontaneity. However, such data are difficult to interpret since decreased activity is reported to follow lesions of widely different telencephalic areas such as cortex (Goldby, 1937), ADVR (Tarr, 1977*a*), and the amygdaloid group (Diebschlag, 1938; Tarr, 1977*a*). Since no pattern is apparent in the reports of arousal deficits, it is likely that these effects may be due to some nonspecific consequences of surgery (see Section IV).

It does seem reasonably clear that the telencephalon in reptiles is not required for normal movement. Cerebrumless reptiles exhibit normal posture (excluding occasional reports of slight cervical hypertonus), gait, and coordination of axial and appendicular musculature. From early stimulation studies it is apparent that some movements of the head, neck, and limbs may be elicited by electrical stimulation of certain (unspecified) subpallial structures, suggesting some telencephalic influence over more caudal motor areas. This is hardly surprising, but it is impossible to interpret in the absence of specific information about stimulation sites and current parameters.

Although few in number, recent studies of subpallial function have provided some new insight into brain–behavior relationships in reptiles. Experiments by Keating *et al.* and by Tarr suggest that the amygdaloid complex may be involved in affective behaviors and intraspecific aggression. Lesions of the amygdala produce animals which are unreactive toward noxious or threatening stimuli and toward aggressive displays by conspecifics, an effect which can be dissociated from the general activity deficits sometimes produced by such lesions. Stimulation of this area, on the other hand, may produce goal-directed "flight," some autonomiclike responses, and perhaps some agonistic behavior (Keating *et al.*, 1970; Distel, 1978*a,b;* Sugerman, 1974; Sugerman and Demski, 1978).

Lesions of the paleostriatum produce effects on intraspecific aggression similar to the effects of amygdalectomy, e.g., a significant decrease in challenge displays (but not in the assertion display) and in postural attitudes which normally attend aggressive encounters (Greenberg, 1977). Finally, work by Berk and Heath (1975) suggests that medial wall structures and the MFB system may be involved in behavioral thermoregulation in reptiles.

Although anatomically the best understood of all the subpallial structures, the ADVR has, to date, yielded almost nothing to behavioral investigators. Stimulation of this area produces only some eye and head movement as well as ipsilateral turning of a flexible (goal-directed) sort (Keating *et al.*, 1970; Schapiro and Goodman, 1969; Distel, 1978*a,b*). Social behavior, as measured in Tarr's and Greenberg's experiments, is apparently undisturbed by ADVR lesions, and at least some pattern vision may be equally unaffected (Bass *et al.,* 1973).

III. Pallium

A. Introduction

The term "pallium" (Latin) means mantle. By it we denote the thin sheet of fibers and cells which overlies the lateral ventricle of each hemisphere, i.e., the roof of the telencephalon. The neuronal constituents of the pallium are said to be arranged in three layers, oriented parallel to the pial surface: (1) a fiber layer subadjacent to the pia, (2) a more or less compact layer of cell somata, and (3) a fiber layer bordering the ventricular ependyma (Goldby and Gamble, 1957). This is a useful oversimplification. In fact, the number of recognizable layers in the reptile pallium varies with the species and the subarea under consideration and even with the tendency of a given investigator to be a "lumper" or a "splitter." Detailed accounts of pallial cytoarchitecture of several reptile species have been published (see Chapters 9 and 10 of this volume and Northcutt, 1978) including some information on its ultrastructure (e.g., Ulinski, 1974; Ebner and Colonnier, 1975). The reptile pallium is thought to qualify as a "true" cortex (Latin for bark, i.e., the outer covering) in the sense that the cell somata in this area no longer line the ventricles as in amniotes but are located more superficially, closer to the pial surface.

By the early part of this century it had become traditional to recognize three principal cellular aggregrates within the reptile pallium (Ariëns Kappers *et al.*, 1936). Seen in cross section these are: (1) medial cortex, (2) lateral cortex, and (3) between them, dorsal (general) cortex. The evolution of ideas concerning the significance of these three cell groups and their various subdivisions constitutes an instructive chapter in the history of comparative neurology. For present purposes it is important only to realize that certain of the hypotheses adduced by early comparative anatomists (e.g., Herrick, 1926; Johnston, 1915, 1923; Smith, 1919; Crosby, 1917) concerning the connections and evolutionary significance of these three cell fields have endured until recently with surprisingly little change, and it is these conceptions of pallial organization which have—for better or worse—shaped the course of behavioral investigations into cortical function in reptiles.

These traditional lines of thought about each of the three cortical groups can be summarized here, although such brief accounts can in no sense do justice to the long controversy which has surrounded these three cell fields for much of this century and which continues to the present (Kruger, 1969). The earlier literature on this subject has been summarized by Ariëns Kappers *et al.* (1936) and by Goldby and Gamble (1957). Northcutt (1978), Halpern (Chapter 9), and Butler (Chapter 10) review the recent literature on the reptile telencephalon.

1. Medial Cortex

This cell field was identified as "hippocampus" by Spitzka in 1880 (Ariëns Kappers *et al.,* 1936), and it has widely been referred to as hippocampal cortex ever since (but see Riss *et al.,* 1969, and Ebbesson and Voneida, 1969, for recent, alternate terminologies). The early comparative anatomists believed that it differentiated primarily under the influence of secondary and tertiary olfactory projections, and this, together with its position in the dorsomedial wall of the hemisphere, suggested to them the homology with the mammalian hippocampal complex (Humphrey, 1967). Since 1892 (Meyer, 1892), two principal subdivisions of this cell field have been recognized: (1) a medial, small-celled component and (2) a dorsal, large-celled component. Further subdivisions of medial cortex have been suggested by some authors (Northcutt, 1978).

2. Lateral Cortex

Early investigators believed that the lateral cortex received direct projections from the olfactory bulb and thus compared it with mammalian pyriform cortex. Direct olfactory bulb projections to lateral cortex have recently been confirmed with experimental anatomical methods (e.g., Heimer, 1969; Scalia *et al.,* 1969; Rainey, 1976; Peterson and Ulinski, 1980).

3. Dorsal (General) Cortex

Herrick, Johnston, Crosby, and certain of their contemporaries believed that the dorsal cortex received somatic projections from the dorsal thalamus and thus differentiated as a correlation center for exteroceptive (nonolfactory) input to the telencephalon, in contrast to "pyriform" and "hippocampal" cortices, which were thought to develop primarily under the influence of olfactory input. In this and in its position between presumptive hippocampus and pyriform cortex it was reminiscent of mammalian neocortex. Thus they proposed that the reptile dorsal cortex may be homologous with mammalian neocortex. As Crosby put it, "the whole of the general cortex . . . is a step toward the differentiation of a [mammalian] neopallial area" (Crosby, 1917, p. 358).

Reptile neuroanatomists now recognize at least two major subdivisions of dorsal cortex (Northcutt, 1978; Butler, Chapter 10). However, the differential connections of these two divisions are as yet poorly understood, and this distinction between portions of dorsal cortex has not been recognized by behavioral workers. In this chapter, therefore, the term "dorsal cortex" is meant in the most general sense, i.e., those cell groups lying between medial and lateral cortices.

From the beginning, behavioral studies of cortical function in reptiles have focused on only one of the three pallial fields, the dorsal (general) cortex. Inspired by early suggestions that this tissue might be homologous with mammalian neocortex, behavioral investigators have hoped to find in dorsal cortex a simplified version of the neopallium, one more amenable to investigation than its putative mammalian counterpart. Ironically, this "simple" tissue has proved almost totally refractory to our understanding, and there is still little behavioral evidence that this cell group in any way resembles mammalian neocortex.

B. Stimulation Studies

The first and most influential experiment on the electrical excitability of the reptile cortex was that of Johnston (1916). Like many of the early comparative neurologists, Johnston believed that the brains of reptiles, especially turtles, stood in "an intermediate position between fishes and mammals" (Johnston, 1915, p. 427) and that, consequently, the forerunners of many mammalian neural systems were to be found in reptile brains. Johnston had earlier (Johnston, 1915) described a highly specialized rostro-lateral subdivision of general cortex, the pallial thickening, which he believed to be an important source of fibers descending via the lateral forebrain bundle (LFB) to the brain stem. This, together with its topographic position, led Johnston to suggest that the pallial thickening "may correspond to the motor cortical area in the mammalian brain" (Johnston, 1916, p. 475). The stimulation study which he published in 1916 was an attempt to test this hypothesis.

Johnston worked with anesthetized turtles (*Chelydra serpentina, Cistudo carolina,* and *Crysemys marginata)* using both mono- and bipolar stimulation at unspecified current intensities. He emphasized that clear responses (movements of eyes, jaw, neck, and extremities) could be obtained only under very deep levels of anesthesia. Less deeply anesthetized animals showed widespread muscular responses similar to those elicited by direct stimulation of the dura and adjacent head muscles, and these movements obscured the more discrete, short-duration responses to pallial stimulation. This latter, "specific" type of movement could be elicited only from the dorsal surface of the olfactory bulb, from the part of dorsal cortex corresponding to the pallial thickening, and from the "striatum" (probably the paleostriatum). Responses to olfactory bulb stimulation he attributed to current spread over the closely adjacent pallial thickening; striatal responses resulted, Johnston believed, from involvement of descending fibers in the LFB (i.e., pallial thickening efferents). Similar results were obtained from lizards (*Gerrhonotus)* and one alligator. Johnston interpreted his data as evidence for a motor pallium in the reptile forebrain "comparable to the mammalian motor cortex" (Johnston, 1916, p. 475).

Some years later, Bagley and Richter (1924) and Bagley and Langworthy (1926) reported data which, superficially, appeared to support Johnston's contention. Using bipolar electrodes and "mild" current, Bagley and his co-workers mapped the surface of the pallium in awake, unrestrained alligators (species not given). They obtained mass movements of head, body, and extremities in response to stimulation of a restricted area in the rostral pallium, an area which included not only dorsal cortex but medial ("hippocampal") cortex and lateral cortex as well. Thus the positive area included, but was not limited to, Johnston's pallial thickening.* To control for the possibility of current spread to underlying striatum, a knife cut was made along the rostral, lateral, and caudal borders of the responsive area, and the resulting flap of tissue was reflected medially and electrically isolated (with a sheet of mica) from the contralateral hemisphere. Stimulation of the exposed underside of the flap produced the aforementioned gross movements, as did stimulation of the medial wall following removal of the "striatum" (probably ADVR). In contrast, when the positive area was left attached to the pallium at its lateral border only, no motor responses could be elicited. Bagley and his co-workers concluded that this "motor cortex" in the alligator sends efferents down the medial wall of the hemisphere in the medial forebrain bundle, presumably to the hypothalamus. In this it differs from Johnston's turtles, and, as Bagley and Langworthy point out, "The arrangement has nothing in common with the direct corticosegmental or pyramidal path of the mammals" (Bagley and Langworthy, 1926, p. 158).

Like Bagley and his co-workers, Koppányi and Pearcy (1925) were stimulated by Johnston's (1916) work to look for a motor area in the pallium of reptiles. Using fine bipolar electrodes and a current "just detectable to the tongue," they were unable to obtain any motor responses to pallial stimulation in unanesthetized turtles or alligators (species not given), although these same procedures elicited swimminglike movements when the "striatum" (probably ADVR) or LFB was stimulated. They attributed Johnston's results to current spread from the pallial thickening to the underlying "striatum."

The only other stimulation experiment to report positive results was that of Tuge and Yazaki (1934). Using both mono- and bipolar stimulation and "weak" currents, they mapped discrete areas in the pallium for head retraction, lifting the head, and opening the jaws in anesthetized turtles (*Clemmys japonica*). From their figures it appears that these positive areas lay within the dorsal cortex (perhaps including some medial cortex). They do not correspond to Johnston's positive area, and the authors state that they were unable to obtain motor responses from stimulation of this latter site.

In the succeeding years several other investigators attempted to localize a "motor" area within the reptile pallium, all with negative results. Goldby (1937), using bipolar electrodes and currents above threshold for evoking movement from the tectum, was unable to elicit responses from the pallium of anesthetized lizards (*Lacerta viridis*). The author notes that "Movements resulted from stimulation of the forebrain only after the use of a stimulus so strong that it spread even to the adjacent temporal muscle and must have effected the whole brain at least" (Goldby, 1937, p. 346). About the same period, Diebschlag (1938) reported that he was unable to elicit movements in the same species by electrical stimulation of the hemispheres, although no details of the experiment are given. Similarly, Abbie (1948) was unable to evoke movements from any part of the pallium of ether-anesthetized lizards (*Trachysaurus rugosus*), using either mono- or bipolar stimula-

* Johnston described the pallial thickening from chelonian material. A similar area in crocodilians was identified by Crosby (1917) and named the "primordium general cortex." Johnston's terminology has been more widely accepted, however, and is now used to denote this segment of cortex in most reptile species, e.g., Goldby and Gamble (1957), Riss *et al.* (1969).

tion and a current sufficient to evoke a response when applied to the tectum or directly to a muscle.

Bremer *et al.* (1939) evoked movements of neck, jaw, and feet from the pallium in unanesthetized turtles (species not given) using both mono- and bipolar stimulation and a current adequate to evoke a response from the masticatory area of the cortex in rabbits. However, these responses were not abolished by a 5-min application of 2% cocaine to the pallium, leading the authors to conclude that the obtained movements were subcortical in origin. As pointed out earlier, it is unfortunate that these workers had no independent measure of the effectiveness of their cocainization.

Recently, Schapiro and Goodman (1969; Schapiro, 1965) briefly reopened the question of a motor area in the pallium. They used 15 unanesthetized, unrestrained alligators (*Caiman sklerops*) in which small-diameter (60–90 μm) monopolar electrodes had been chronically implanted. Constant current stimulation (60 Hz) of 20 sites in dorsal cortex (up to 0.6 mA for 10 sec) produced no motor responses, although the same or lower current intensities elicited movements from tectum and "striatum" (DLA, *sensu* Crosby, 1917). The authors conclude that earlier reports of positive loci in the pallium reflected the results of current spread to the adjacent "striatum."

On balance, stimulation studies of pallial function suggest that reptile cortex contains nothing that could be considered a "motor" area and certainly no area comparable to motor cortex in mammals. A majority of studies have reported negative results, and although some of these experiments can be criticized on procedural grounds (e.g., inadequate current, too deep anesthesia) other studies (e..g, Schapiro and Goodman, 1969) seem to have answered most of these objections.

It is more difficult to interpret those studies reporting positive results. Very deep levels of anesthesia were required in Johnston's study to suppress the mass movements and struggling which accompanied cortical stimulation and always masked the more discrete evoked muscular contractions. This suggests that an extensive current spread may have occurred (e.g., to the meninges), and thus it is possible that the responses he obtained were not pallial in origin. In this and all the other stimulation studies except that of Schapiro, no current parameters are given, making it extremely difficult to interpret and compare results. Tuge and Yazaki (1934) reported positive results, but they did not control for current spread. The work of Bremer *et al.* (1939) is often quoted as the most compelling evidence against the idea of a motor cortex in reptiles. However, as mentioned earlier, their data are difficult to interpret in the absence of independent evidence that their cocainization of the pallium was effective.

The most difficult data to reconcile are those of Bagley and his co-workers with those of Schapiro. Bagley reported positive results of pallial stimulation and included specific and careful controls for current spread to subcortical structures. According to these workers, no motor responses could be elicited from the underlying striatum. However, Schapiro and Goodman (1969), also working with crocodilians, reported exactly opposite results, i.e., stimulation of the "striatum" produced movement but pallial stimulation did not. Species differences seems an unlikely explanation for so fundamental a difference between two representatives of the same order, nor is there any other obvious way to account for the discrepancy between these two sets of data.

C. Ablation Studies

As noted earlier, most of the early behavioral work on telencephalic function in reptiles involved total or near total removal of the cerebral hemispheres. A few experiments, however, attempted to remove the pallium only.

Goldby (1937) reported that lizards (*Lacerta viridis)* which had sustained bilateral pallial ablations were sluggish and refused to feed, although one animal (XXV) was seen to snap at a worm. Qualitatively, these animals resembled hemispherectomized animals, although their symptoms were somewhat less severe. Diebschlag (1938), on the other hand, believed that pallial ablations in lizards (*Lacerta*) and the snake *Tropidonotus natrix* did not reduce spontaneity. He reported, however, that pallial-ablated lizards were somewhat less likely than intact animals to hide or bask in the usual way. Ablated males, furthermore, no longer reacted appropriately to conspecific males (i.e., appropriate to their position in the dominance hierarchy) and did not attempt to mate. Finally, pallial lesions tended not to affect retention of a color discrimination.

Some 30 years later, Hertzler and Hayes published a series of papers (Hertzler and Hayes, 1967; Hayes and Hertzler, 1967; reviewed in Hertzler, 1972) which dealt with the role of dorsal cortex in visual discrimination behavior. The primary rationale for these experiments was the notion that reptile general cortex might represent a stage in the development of mammalian neocortex. In addition, several studies published in the early 1960s (Kruger and Berkowitz, 1960; Orrego, 1961; Orrego and Lisenby, 1962; Moore and Tschirgi, 1962) had reported that visually evoked population responses could be recorded from an area on the surface of the pallium roughly coincident with dorsal cortex. These electrophysiological data suggested to Hertzler and Hayes that the reptile dorsal cortex might indeed play a role in visual discrimination behavior, in spite of earlier work by Goldby, Diebschlag, and others which indicated that visually guided behavior was unimpaired following pallial lesions or even total hemispherectomy.

Hertzler and Hayes (1967) first tested turtles (*Terrapene carolina)* on a visual cliff task. There were three experimental groups: (1) turtles with bilateral ablation of dorsal cortex, (2) those with bilateral tectal ablation, and (3) those with bilateral ablation of both dorsal cortex and tectum. Pre- and postoperative performance of the turtles was compared, and the extent of lesions was verified histologically. In this, as in other such ablation experiments, there was always some minimal involvement of adjacent medial and lateral cortices. The authors report that lesions of either cortex or tectum alone had no effect on visual cliff choices; i.e., like intact turtles, experimental animals chose the shallow side significantly more often than the deep side. The choice latencies of these operated turtles were significantly increased, although this increase appears to reflect primarily the scores of a single animal in each of the two experimental groups (Hertzler, 1972) and thus is probably spurious. In contrast, turtles with combined cortical-tectal lesions showed no increase in choice latencies but chose the shallow and deep sides equally often, suggesting to the authors that these turtles were capable of little visually guided behavior. Unfortunately, Hertzler and Hayes give no information about the behavior of these turtles outside the testing situation, e.g., about their ability to feed or avoid obstacles.

The authors (Hertzler and Hayes, 1967) also tested turtles (*T. carolina* and *Pseudemys scripta)* in an optokinetic drum. Neither cortical nor tectal ablations alone affected the frequence of optokinetic nystagmus (OKN), whereas combined lesions of cortex and tectum led to a significant reduction in this type of eye movement. The absence of cortical lesion effects on OKR was confirmed in a subsequent study (Hayes and Hertzler, 1967), leading these investigators to conclude that the dorsal cortex "is not of particular functional importance" (Hertzler, 1972), at least in the kinds of visual discrimination capabilities they tested. They point out, however, that the cortex may play some role in visual behavior since combined cortical-tectal lesions produced more severe deficits than did tectal lesions alone.

A similar study was reported by Bass *et al.* (1973). Using the turtle *Podocnemis unifilis*, in which dorsal cortex is highly developed (Riss *et al.*, 1969), they compared the effects of cortical and tectal lesions (histologically verified) on discrimination of horizontal from vertical stripes. Like Hertzler and Hayes, Bass and his co-workers elected to investigate visual discrimination behavior because of electrophysiological studies indicating that the dorsal cortex is visually responsive and anatomical experiments (Hall and Ebner, 1970; Knapp and Kang, 1968) which reported a visual projection to the general cortex via a retinorecipient nucleus in the dorsal thalamus. Bass *et al.* found that turtles sustaining large bilateral lesions of the dorsal cortex reached criterion on the stripe discrimination in approximately the same number of trials as were required to learn the problem preoperatively, whereas tectal-lesioned animals were unable to relearn the task. The authors note that dorsal cortex–lesioned turtles behaved essentially like intact animals within the test situation, and they conclude that dorsal cortex may not be involved in this type of discrimination. As pointed out earlier (Section II.D), a subtotal deficit probably would not have been revealed by their design since (1) an undemanding criterion was set and (2) post- vs. preoperative "savings" scores, if any, were not reported or compared with similar scores from controls.

A further attempt to elucidate the function of dorsal cortex was made by Morlock (1972), who tested turtles on two kinds of general activity measures and on a learning task. For all tests, there were three experimental groups: (1) turtles sustaining bilateral ablation of dorsal cortex, (2) sham operates, and (3) intact controls. All scoring was done blind, and the extent of lesions was verified histologically. The first test measured open-field activity: turtles were placed in an enclosure, the floor of which was lined with a grid of squares, and the number of squares entered in two 10-min testing sessions was counted. No differences in open-field activity were noted between ablated turtles (*Pseudemys scripta* and *Chrysemys picta)* and either of the control groups. As Morlock points out, these data indicate that dorsal cortex lesions do not reliably affect spontaneity. Activity deficits of the sort reported by Goldby (1937) and other earlier workers were sometimes noted in both ablated and sham operates, suggesting that nonspecific effects of surgery might have been involved. In a second experiment the animals were food deprived 24 hr and then food was introduced and the number of seconds until the first strike was counted for each animal. Dorsal cortex ablation did not affect latency to eat in either species.

Finally, subjects (*C. picta* only) were tested for their ability to learn a spatial discrimination task. Turtles were trained, against their preference, to choose one arm of a modified T maze for a food reward. Five trials were given every other day with an intertrial interval of 1 min. Criterion was set at nine out of ten correct choices within 100 trials. Four out of five ablated turtles reached criterion; the fifth animal was unable to break its initial position preference. Unfortunately we have no independent measure of the strength of these initial position preferences since Morlock used only one pretraining trial per subject to establish its position habit. Ablated subjects took more trials to reach criterion than did controls (75.5 vs. 60.5 trials), although apparently this difference was not significant. Data for individual subjects were not given so that intragroup variability cannot be assessed.

One of the few experiments which has reported a clear deficit following dorsal cortex ablation was that of Killackey *et al.* (1972), who studied habituation of the head withdrawal reflex in turtles (*Pseudemys scripta).* Turtles were restrained and positioned so that they faced a 2-inch styrofoam ball which was held on a moving arm and which, when released. moved toward the turtle's head at a rate of 55 cm/sec. In intact animals the initial presentation of this stimulus elicits head withdrawal but with repeated stimulus presentations the response habituates. Habituation was defined according to (some of) the criteria of Thompson and Spencer (1966); that is, the response (1) decreases in amplitude with repeated stimulus presentations (habituation), (2) shows spontaneous recovery, (3) decreases progressively faster across daily test sessions, (4) habituates more rapidly with higher stimulation rates, and (5) habituates more rapidly with weaker stimuli. A strain gauge attached to the turtle's head allowed quantitative specification of response strength (amplitude) and latency. Performance of dorsal cortex–ablated turtles differed from that of intact and sham surgical controls in that they exhibited a smaller progressive decrement of response amplitude both within and across daily test sessions. The authors conclude that dorsal cortex "participates in the control of response levels to visual stimuli."

1. Experiments with *Dipsosaurus dorsalis*

I first became interested in the role of dorsal cortex in reptile behavior several years ago while working as a graduate student in the laboratory of Dr. Ann Richardson. Like other workers in the field, we were intrigued by the then prevailing notion that this tissue might represent a neocortical homologue. A review of the literature indicated, however, that few behavioral investigations into reptile cortical function had been conducted and that those few studies had all reported essentially negative results. We decided on a somewhat different approach to the problem.

In the early years of this century, when mammalian neocortex was very poorly understood, Karl Lashley undertook a series of experiments designed to elucidate neocortical function in mammals (Lashley, 1929). One group of these studies dealt with the performance of cortically ablated rats on complex spatial learning. Taking our cue from Lashley, we decided to investigate the effects of dorsal cortex ablation on spatial (maze) learning in the lizard *Dipsosaurus dorsalis*. *Dipsosaurus* was chosen because previous behavioral studies of reptile pallial function had dealt almost exclusively with representatives of the Chelonia and because we already knew that *Dipsosaurus* could master a series of maze problems of progressively increasing difficulty (Julian and Richardson, 1968).

D. dorsalis is well suited for behavioral studies in the laboratory. It is hardy and, with proper care, can be maintained in excellent health for the long periods of time required for many behavioral studies. Unlike most lizards (Burghardt, 1977) it responds well to handling, quickly becoming docile and apparently undisturbed by the presence of the experimenter. *Dipsosaurus* is a diurnal iguanid, largely herbivorous, with unusually high heat requirements. It has, in fact, the highest preferred body temperature of any North American reptile (Norris, 1953; DeWitt *et al.*, 1967). As a result, *Dipsosaurus* will readily learn a variety of tasks when rewarded with the opportunity to sit on a hotplate for 2–3 min.

a. Maze Learning. In our first experiment we used two mazes (Fig. 1) chosen to represent two levels of difficulty in terms of the number of cul-de-sacs and the number of errors required to learn the maze by both reptiles and mammals (Lashley, 1929; Julian and Richardson, 1968). Twenty-four lizards (12 on each maze) were trained to a criterion of 12 consecutive correct choices (i.e., 2 perfect days in succession, at six trials per day), which is significant ($p < 0.01$) if reached

8

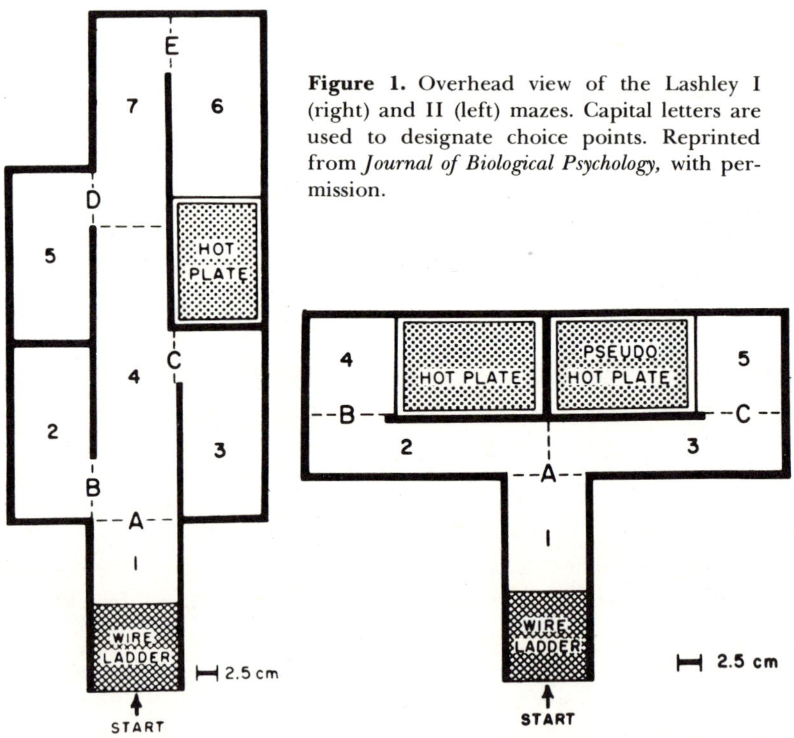

Figure 1. Overhead view of the Lashley I (right) and II (left) mazes. Capital letters are used to designate choice points. Reprinted from *Journal of Biological Psychology*, with permission.

within 252 or fewer trials (Bogartz, 1965). In this and the succeeding experiments, training trials were conducted in the morning, to conform to the normal activity period of this species (Norris, 1953; Minnich and Schoemaker, 1970; Gelderloos, 1976). Between trials animals were maintained at 32°C since, under the conditions of our experiment, learning is optimal when subjects are maintained at this temperature (Krekorian *et al.*, 1968).

The initial training of the 24 lizards was conducted at varying times throughout the year and required a wide range of trials, with the result that some lizards had long ago completed training when others were finishing their original learning. To control for any possible seasonal effects of learning or response to surgery, all 24 animals were simultaneously brought to criterion a second time and then divided into experimental groups. For each maze five lizards sustained bilateral lesions of dorsal cortex (group I); four lizards underwent sham surgery, i.e., craniotomy and incision of the dura (group II); and three lizards served as intact controls (group III). Surgery for groups I and II was performed within 24 hr of the animals having reached criterion for the second time (postcriterion day 1), and the animals were allowed 4 days to recover. For all three groups testing was begun on the sixth postcriterion day. At the completion of testing the extent of all lesions was verified histologically.

The results on initial learning (Fig. 2A,B) were consistent with earlier reports of maze learning in *Dipsosaurus* (Julian and Richardson, 1968). The lizards learned maze I with a mean of 48 trials and maze II with a mean of 94 trials, a difference which was significant (t = 4.299, df = 22, p = 0.01). Both groups showed savings on the second learning (31.5 trials and 48.9 trials, respectively), although an average of 1–2 months intervened between first and second training phases.

Our postsurgical test results (Fig. 2C) indicate that dorsal-cortex-ablated lizards lost the ability to perform on both maze I and maze II and, furthermore, they could not relearn. For both mazes all sham surgical and intact controls reached criterion with considerable savings in errors when compared with original learning. In contrast, none of the ablated lizards reached criterion even though they were allowed twice as many trials as required by controls.

For purposes of statistical analysis the average number of errorless goals (perfect runs) made per day during the test phase was calculated for each animal. A two-way analysis of variance (treatment by maze) indicated that there was a significant treatment effect: ablated animals made fewer perfect runs per day than controls ($p < 0.001$, df = 2.18). Small effects of sham surgery were consistently seen on both mazes (Fig. 2C), but these differences were not significant. There was no differential effect of the lesions on performance of the two mazes.

Histological analysis of the lesioned brains indicated that, in all cases, destruction of dorsal cortex was incomplete: the caudal one-quarter to one-third of this cell group was usually spared. In some cases there was slight damage to adjacent large-celled medial cortex. None of the lesions encroached on the underlying ADVR.

It must be emphasized that these ablated lizards appeared to be completely normal in all other respects. When tested on a variety of simple motor tasks (righting, placing, climbing an inclined screen), they were indistinguishable from normals. They were active and ate well in their home cages. On the apparatus, by contrast, ablated lizards showed a characteristic behavior which effectively precluded solution of the maze. They no longer exhibited the relaxed but alert exploratory behavior typical of intact *Dipsosaurus.* Instead, each animal adopted an idiosyncratic response pattern from which it seldom varied. Usually this consisted of wandering into one of the various cul-de-sacs or other deadends in the maze and remaining there until the time allotted for a trial (180 sec) had elapsed. This behavior became increasingly rigid over days, resembling the "fixation response" exhibited by rats and other mammals when confronted by an insoluble problem (e.g., Maier *et al.,* 1940).

The results of our maze study were encouraging in that they provided the first—at that time—unequivocal evidence of behavioral dysfunction following destruction of dorsal cortex in reptiles. However, failure to perform successfully on a maze may be due to a variety of factors. It may reflect an inability to learn or remember, a sensory or attentional deficit, or a reduction in the incentive value of the reward. Thus the experiments which followed were an attempt to eliminate some of these alternatives and to provide further information about the kinds of behaviors which might be mediated by reptile dorsal cortex.

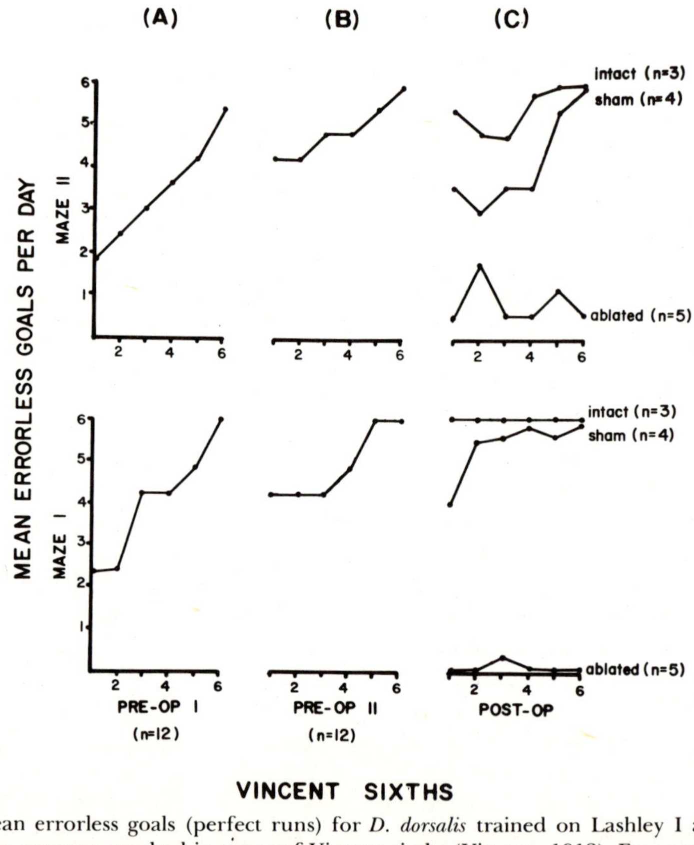

Figure 2. Mean errorless goals (perfect runs) for *D. dorsalis* trained on Lashley I and II mazes. Performance curves are graphed in terms of Vincent sixths (Vincent, 1912). For example, the first Vincent sixth represents mean daily errorless goals for the first sixth of all trials; i.e., on maze II the 12 lizards averaged slightly less than two perfect runs per day during the first sixth of their total trials.

b. Brightness Difference Thresholds. Perhaps the most persistent suggestion related to reptile dorsal cortex is that it is homologous, in part, to visual neocortex of mammals (see Section IV). As pointed out earlier, this idea appeared to receive support from electrophysiological studies which reported that dorsal cortex is responsive to both photic and optic tract stimulation (see review by Belekhova, 1979). Furthermore, in turtles at least, dorsal cortex receives a projection from retinorecipient areas in the dorsal thalamus (Hall and Ebner, 1970; Foster *et al.*, 1976), a projection reminiscent of the mammalian geniculocortical system. Surprisingly, then, Hertzler and Hayes (1967) failed to show an effect of dorsal cortex ablation on simple visual–motor or pattern discrimination behaviors. However, no data have been available as to the possible role of dorsal cortex in brightness discrimination. Since Hodos had reported increases in brightness difference thresholds following ablation of the visual wulst in pigeons (Hodos and Bonbright, 1974), and brightness discrimination deficits may follow striate lesions in mammals (e.g., Bekoff *et al.*, 1973), I decided to test the effects of dorsal cortex ablation on brightness difference thresholds in *D. dorsalis.*

In this and the succeeding experiment the apparatus was a modified T-maze (Fig. 3). The interchangeable arms of the apparatus (shaded) were identical except that a hotplate, used to deliver reinforcement, was embedded under the floor of one arm. This hotplate was maintained at 40°C (Krekorian *et al.*, 1968), and heat conduction from the hotplate into the choice area (B) was controlled with asbestos insulation and the presence of an air gap between the choice area and each arm of the apparatus. [In control experiments detailed elsewhere (Peterson, 1976) I have determined that *D. dorsalis* is unable to detect the location of this hotplate from the choice area.] In the brightness difference thresholds problem the luminance of each maze arm could be varied by use of interchangeable linings with reflectance values of 0.92 (white), 0.52, 0.26, 0.16, 0.109, and 0.04 (black).

Six *D. dorsalis,* three intact control and three ablated (bilateral dorsal cortex) lizards, were first trained on a white$^+$–black$^-$ discrimination (luminance ratio of 22.5 : 1). They then began the second phase of the experiment in which five different stimulus pairs were used: white vs. each of the five lower-reflectance stimuli. Thus the lumiance ratios of the five stimulus pairs were 22.5 : 1; 11 : 1; 5.6 : 1; 3.5 : 1, 1.8 : 1. On each day of this second phase of training all subjects were presented with each of the five stimulus pairs in a random order. White continued to be the positive stimulus. This procedure was continued for 60 days, i.e., until all animals had received 60 presentations of each of the five stimulus pairs, at which time scores for every animal were plotted in terms of percent correct responses to the five stimulus pairs (Fig. 4).

There was no significant difference in the speed with which ablated and intact

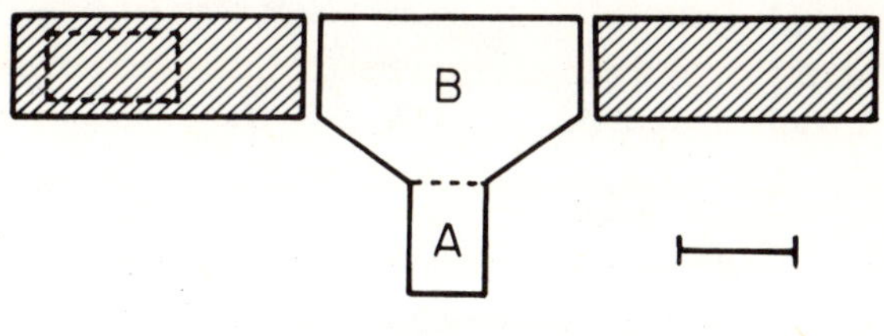

Figure 3. Overhead view of training apparatus used on brightness difference discrimination and successive spatial reversal training. Goal arms (shaded) are interchangeable. A hot plate (dashed box) is embedded under the floor at one goal arm. All walls are 18 cm high. Scale 12 cm.

lizards learned the original white^{+}–black^{-} problem (criterion: 80% for 3 successive days or 90% across 2 days, five trials a day). Ablated subjects achieved criterion with a mean of 24.0 errors (range 3–57) and controls with an average of 49.33 errors (range 9–88). These scores are similar to those reported for black–white discrimination in *Dipsosaurus* by Garzanit and Richardson (1974). In the second stage of training, in which the lizards were required to discriminate between white and each of five different shades of gray, correct responses for all animals increased over the first 20 days and appeared to stabilize thereafter. Consequently the following analyses were carried out on the last 40 days of training.

There was little variation in the scores for the four easiest stimulus pairs (Fig. 4). On the most difficult problem, however, i.e., on the white vs. "lightest-gray" discrimination (luminance ratio of 1.8 : 1), performance levels dropped significantly. A two-factor analysis of variance for repeated measures (luminance ratio by treatment group) indicates that performance on the most difficult problem was lower than performance on the other four stimulus pairs ($F = 4.79$, df $= 4.16$, $p < 0.01$); thus percent correct responses showed the expected decrease with increase in problem difficulty. The animals were, nevertheless, performing above chance on the most difficult problem ($t = 2.28$, df $= 5.00$, $p < 0.05$).

Bilateral ablation of dorsal cortex appeared to have no effect on the brightness difference thresholds of *Dipsosaurus;* there was no significant difference between the control and the lesioned groups (Fig. 4). Furthermore, there was no interaction between experimental group and problem difficulty, suggesting that the lesion had no differential effect on the more difficult discrimination. As with intact lizards, performance of the ablated animals decreased only on the most difficult of the five stimulus pairs (Figs. 4 and 5).

Histological analysis of lesioned animals (Fig. 5) revealed that all three lizards had sustained bilateral destruction of the rostral three-quarters of dorsal cortex (primarily dorsal cortex, *sensu* Ebbesson and Voneida, 1969). In most cases there was also extensive damage to the large-celled portion of medial cortex (dorsomedial cortex of Ebbesson and Voneida, 1969). Animal DDBT-6A, in addition, sustained significant unilateral damage to the dorsalmost ADVR. The lesions in all three cases involved the pallial area (dorsal cortex and adjacent dorsomedial cortex, *sensu* Ebbesson and Voneida, 1969), which is a primary cortical target of afferents from

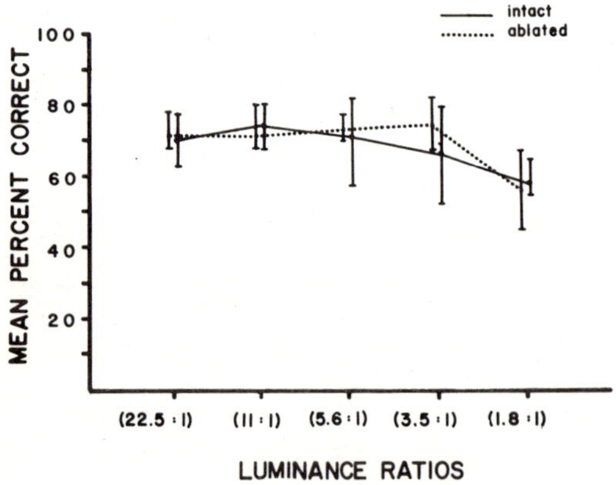

Figure 4. Percent correct choice on the five stimulus pairs used in the brightness difference threshold experiment. On the abscissa the stimulus pairs are represented, from left to right, in order of decreasing luminance difference, beginning with the white vs. black (1:22.5) discrimination. Bars represent the range of scores for the ablated ($N = 3$) and intact ($N = 3$) animals.

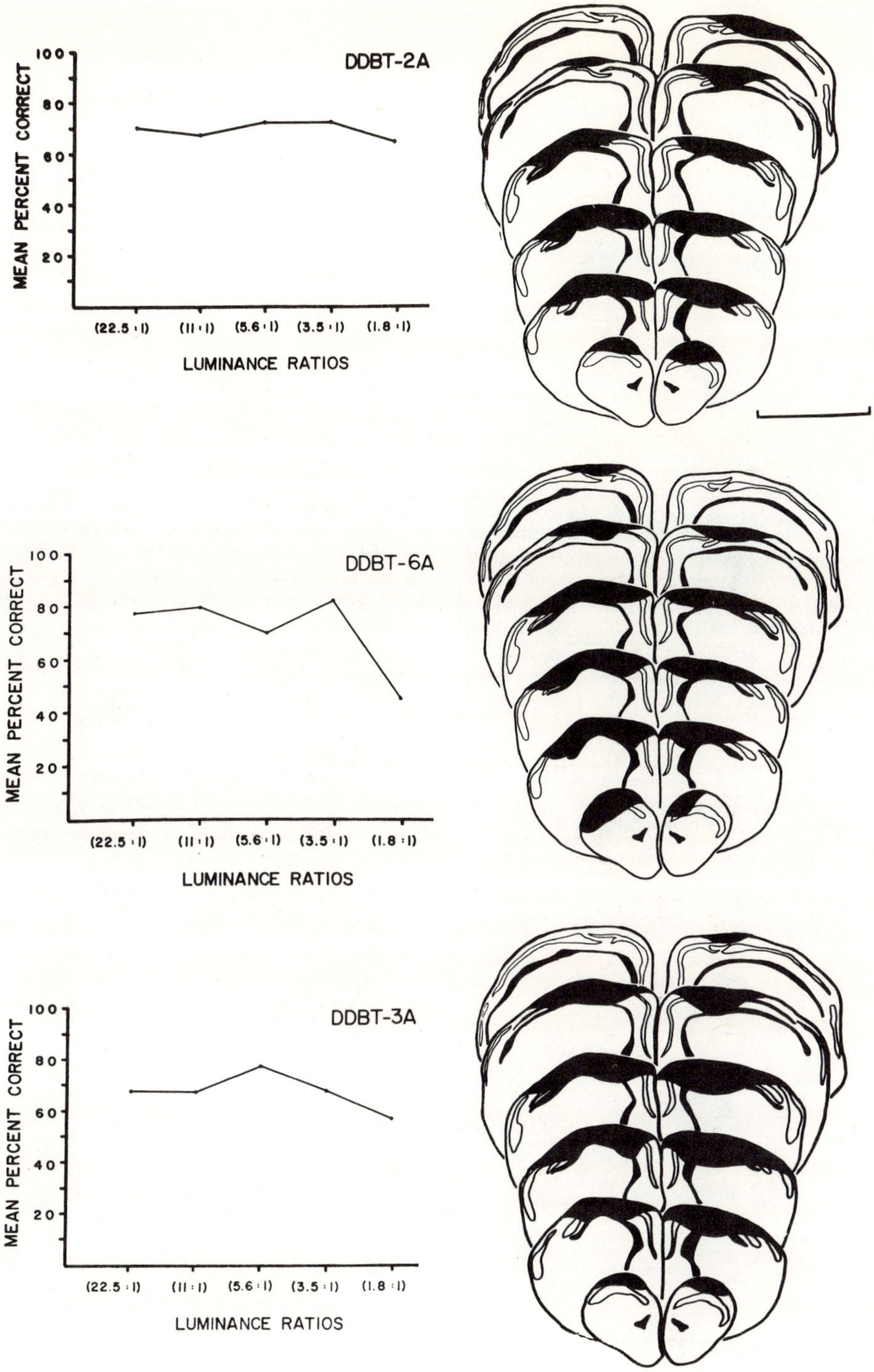

Figure 5. Performance curves and histological results for the three lesioned *D. dorsalis* whose combined scores are shown in Fig. 4. The extent of the lesion (ablated area plus surround of heavy gliosis) is indicated by shading on six representative anterior to posterior levels through the telencephalon. See Fig. 4 for explanation of coordinates. Scale: 2 mm.

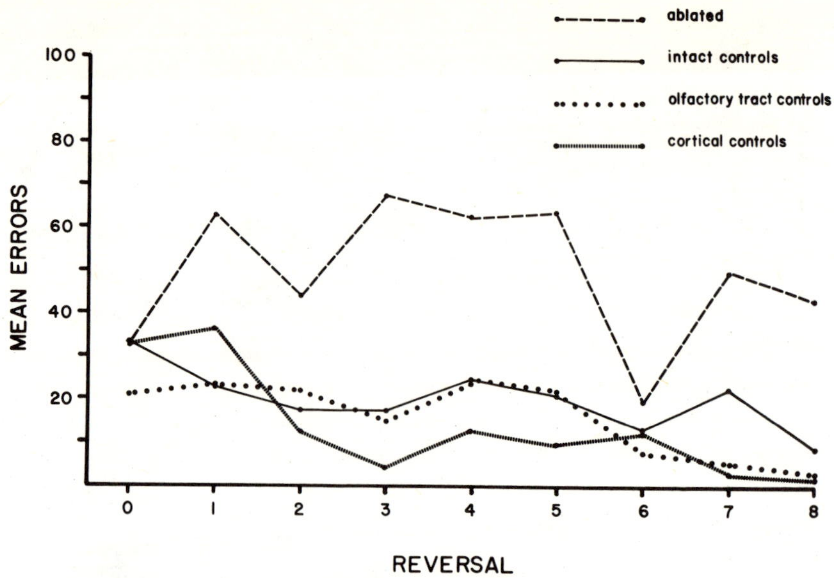

Figure 6. Mean errors per reversal for three control groups and one dorsal cortex–lesioned group of *D. dorsalis* trained on the successive spatial reversal task. Reversal zero indicates initial acquisition. Cortical controls: DDPR-11A and DDPR-13A.

the dorsal thalamus in lizards (Butler and Ebner, 1972; Distel and Ebbesson, 1975; Lohman and van Woerden-Verkley, 1978).

The results of the brightness difference threshold experiment indicate that dorsal cortex and the adjacent pallial areas which receive dorsal thalamic projections are not required for normal brightness discrimination in lizards. It is possible, of

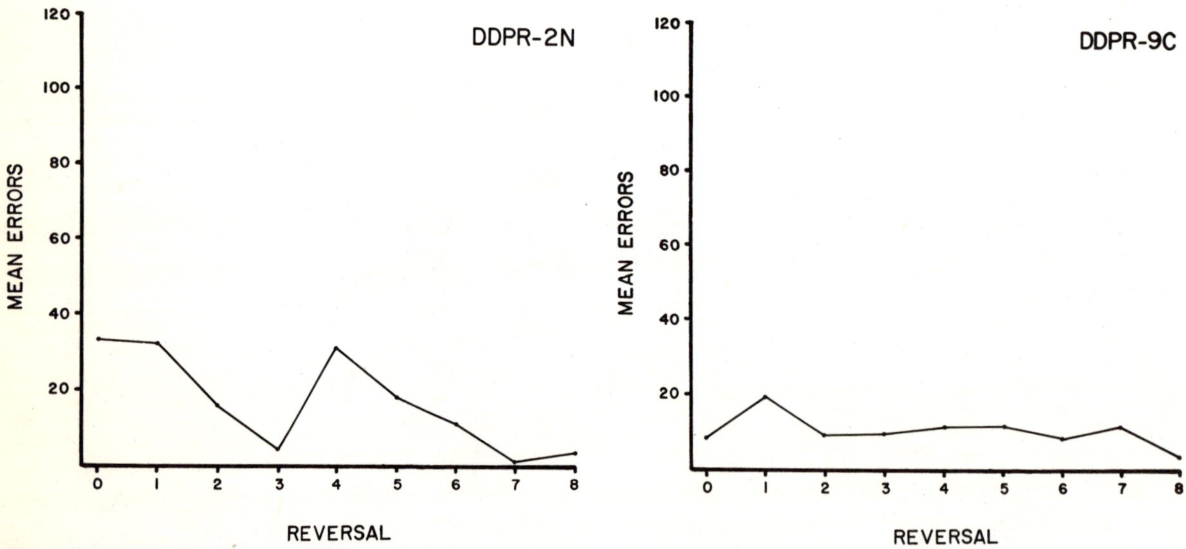

Figure 7. Mean errors per reversal on the successive spatial reversal task for representative intact (DDPR-2N) and olfactory tract (DDPR-9C) controls.

course, that the small amount of dorsal cortex remaining in the caudal fourth of the telencephalon was sufficient to sustain normal luminance discriminations. However, it seems likely that some degree of dysfunction should have been observed—given the near total lesions in this experiment and the demonstrably difficult nature of the behavioral task—if dorsal cortex is indeed necessary for brightness discrimination in this species.

It is clear from this experiment that bilateral destruction of dorsal cortex (plus large-celled medial cortex) does not result in a generalized inability to learn or remember. Ablated animals performed at least as well as or better than controls both on acquisition of the original black–white discrimination and on the subsequent test of asymptotic brightness discrimination performance. Neither does this lesion decrease the efficacy (incentive value) of the heat reward. This is an important point since there is some evidence that the medial wall of the telencephalon—i.e., medial cortex, the principal intracortical target of dorsal cortex efferents in squamates (Ulinski, 1976; Halpern, Chapter 9)—may be involved in behavioral thermoregulation in this species (Berk and Heath, 1975).

c. Reversal Learning. The initial idea for the reversal learning experiment grew out of observations of dorsal-cortex-ablated lizards on the Lashley mazes used in our original study. I had been struck by the apparent inflexibility exhibited by these animals. Observed informally, their behavior had an automatic, predictable quality which was different from the relaxed and "curious" behavior characteristic of intact *Dipsosaurus* on a maze. Since performance on a serial reversal problem may be considered a measure of behavioral flexibility, and since I needed additional information about the effects of dorsal cortex lesions on spatial ability, I decided to investigate the effects of dorsal cortex ablation on successive spatial reversal learning in *Dipsosaurus*.

Eleven *Dipsosaurus* were randomly divided into three groups: group I (N = 3), intact controls; group II (N = 2), surgical controls sustaining bilateral section of the olfactory peduncles including the olfactory tracts, accessory olfactory tracts, and perhaps the anterior olfactory nucleus together with certain of its connections (Heimer, 1969; Halpern, Chapter 9; Peterson and Ulinski, 1980); and group III (N = 6), lizards with bilateral ablation of dorsal cortex. Operated animals (groups I and II) appeared to behave normally within 24 hr of surgery, and training was begun on postoperative day 4. The method and apparatus used were the same as those described for the brightness difference threshold experiment (Fig. 3) except that, for the reversal study, the apparatus was painted flat black throughout. The lizards were trained against their preference (Peterson, 1976) to choose one arm of the apparatus to a criterion of 80% for 3 successive days or 90% across 2 days (five trials a day). As each subject reached criterion, the position of the positive arm was reversed and the subject was again trained to criterion. This procedure was continued for a total of eight reversals.

The results for group I (intact controls) and group II (olfactory stalk controls) were similar (Figs. 6 and 7). Both groups showed a decrease in errors to criterion across reversals, reaching an average of 6.8 errors (range 1–21) on the eighth

Figure 8. Mean errors per reversal and histological results for the six ablated *D. dorsalis*. The extent of the lesion (ablated area plus surround of heavy gliosis) is indicated by shading on six representative anterior to posterior levels through the telencephalon. Scale: 2 mm.

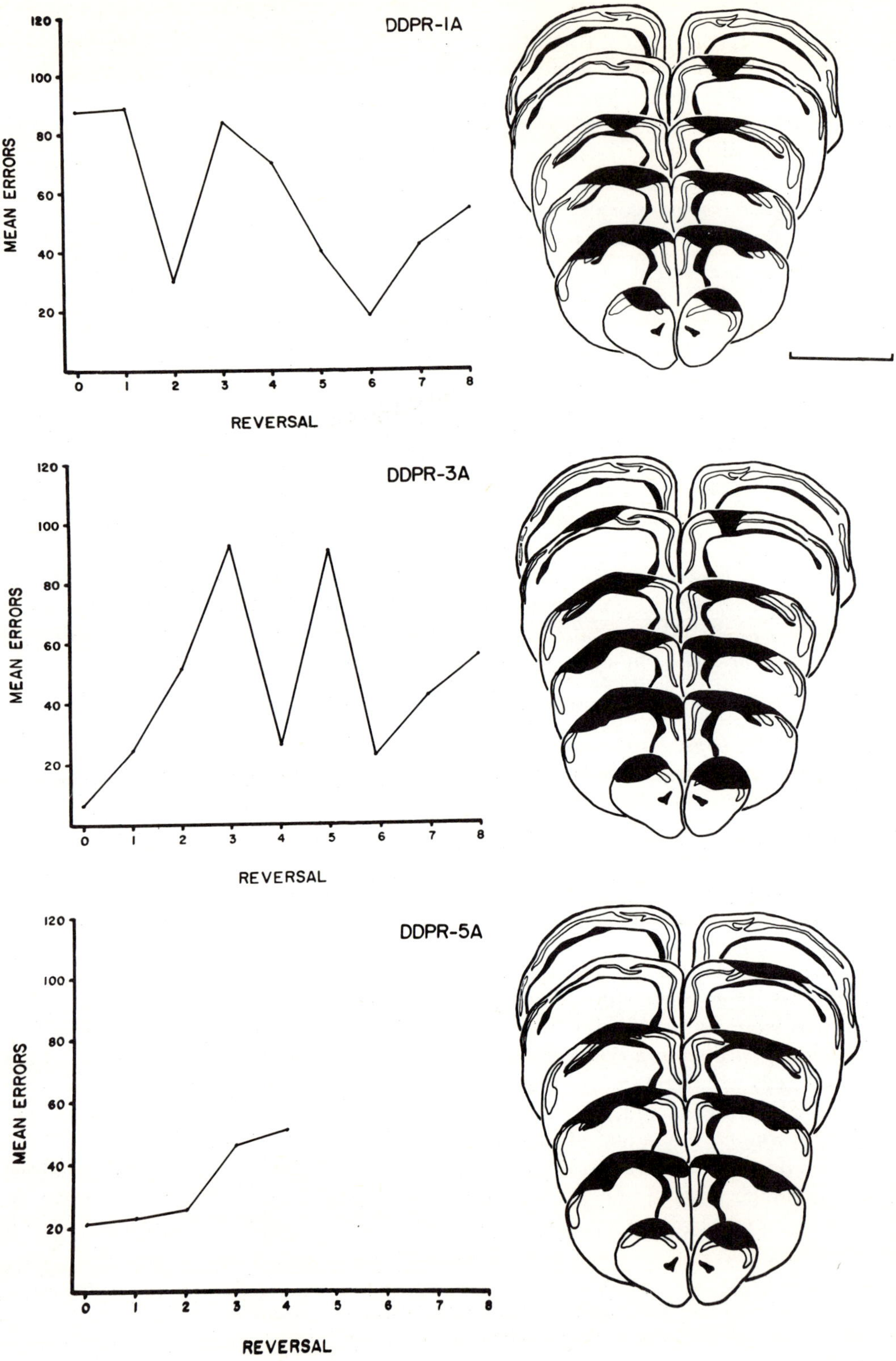
DDPR-1A
MEAN ERRORS
120
100
80
60
40
20
0
1
2
3
4
5
6
7
8
REVERSAL
DDPR-3A
MEAN ERRORS
120
100
80
60
40
20
0
1
2
3
4
5
6
7
8
REVERSAL
DDPR-5A
MEAN ERRORS
120
100
80
60
40
20
0
1
2
3
4
5
6
7
8
REVERSAL

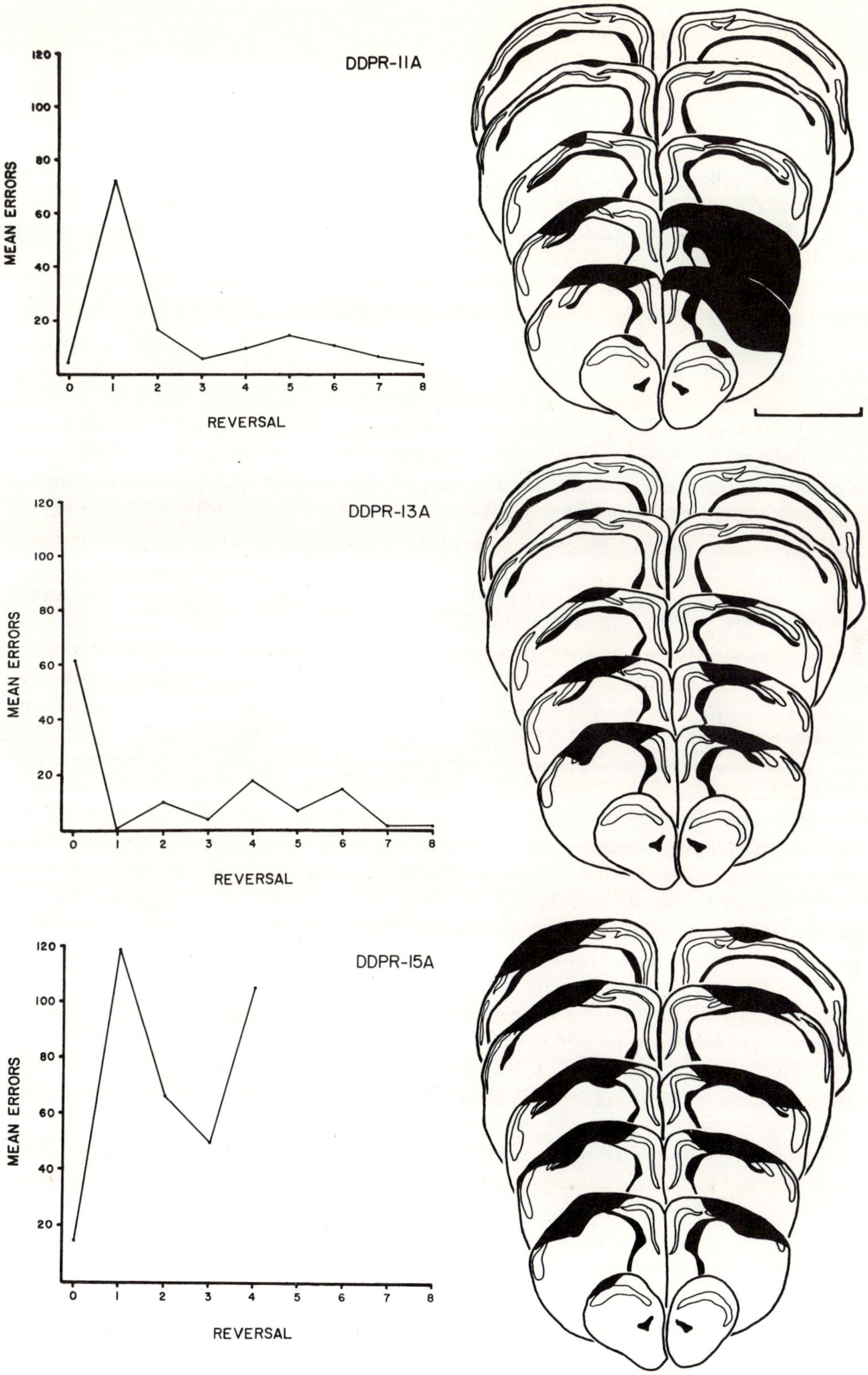
DDPR-11A
MEAN ERRORS
REVERSAL
DDPR-13A
MEAN ERRORS
REVERSAL
DDPR-15A
MEAN ERRORS
REVERSAL

reversal. The curves for these two groups are typical of curves generated on serial reversal problems by a wide range of mammals, birds, and reptiles (Bitterman, 1975; Stettner, 1974; Mackintosh and Holgate, 1969).

Although the two lizards with olfactory stalk transections experienced no more difficulty than normals in reversing a position habit, it is interesting to note that their behavior was distinctly unlike that of intact controls. These animals were extremely irritable. They appeared "fearful" or "watchful" when placed on the apparatus, never really becoming accustomed to the presence of the experimenter. Their behavior was, in fact, reminiscent of that shown by birds and mammals with similar lesions (see Cain, 1974; Hilger and Rowe, 1975).

The performance of individual ablated animals is shown in Fig. 8; their data are summarized in Fig. 6. For four animals (DDPR-1A, DDPR-3A, DDPR-5A, DDPR-15A) the number of errors per reversal never declined to levels characteristic of controls. Average errors per reversal were significantly greater for these animals than for groups I and II ($t = 3.51$, df $= 7.00$, $p < 0.01$). In fact, for three of these four lizards, errors progressively increased across reversals rather than decreased. One animal (DDPR-5A) died and one (DDPR-15A) was accidentally injured before completing the fifth reversal. By the end of R4, however, both of these animals were showing a steady increase in errors per reversal (when compared with original learning; Fig. 8), a trend which was never seen in any of the intact or surgical controls (Fig. 7).

Two ablated lizards (DDPR-11A and DDPR-13A) yielded curves essentially indistinguishable from that of control animals (Fig. 8). DDPR-11A experienced considerable difficulty on the first reversal, but on subsequent reversals it averaged 0–20 errors, as did DDPR-13A. An analysis of variance for repeated measures on data from these two animals plus intact and surgical controls reveals a significant decrease in errors across reversals ($F = 2.6$, df $= 8.48$, $p < 0.05$).

Histological analysis of the lesioned brains indicates that the severity of the deficit appeared to correlate with the degree to which the caudal half of the pallium was damaged. In animals DDPR-11A and DDPR-13A, which showed essentially no behavioral deficit, damage was restricted to approximately the rostral half of the telencephalon (Fig. 8). The absence of a behavioral effect in DDPR-11A, which sustained massive unilateral damage to the rostral telencephalon, suggests that the amount of tissue destruction *per se* does not predict the degree of behavioral deficit observed. Rather, difficulty in reversing apparently depends on destruction of dorsal cortex (dorsal cortex and probably dorsolateral cortex, *sensu* Ebbesson and Voneida, 1969) throughout its rostro-caudal extent. Animal DDPR-15A, which showed the most severe deficit (Fig. 8), was the only animal in which the lesion extended bilaterally into the caudalmost quarter of the hemispheres. In contrast, the smallest behavioral effect was seen in DDPR-1A (Fig. 8). Both in the degree of caudal pallial destruction and in the severity of its behavioral deficit, DDPR-1A is intermediate between DDPR-3A, DDPR-5A, DDPR-15A (which experienced striking difficulty with reversals) and DDPR-11A and DDPR-13A (which were essentially indistinguishable from normals).

All six of the lesioned animals sustained some degree of damage to medial cortex, especially the large-celled part. The amount of destruction to this latter area did not appear to correlate with the degree of behavioral deficit. For example,

DDPR-15A, which experienced the most difficulty with reversals, sustained only minor bilateral damage to large-celled medial cortex.

2. Interpreting the Results of Experiments on *Dipsosarus*

A number of problems inevitably arise in any attempt to interpret the effects of dorsal cortex lesions. One source of difficulty has to do with the large-celled portion of medial cortex (dorsomedial cortex, *sensu* Ebbesson and Voneida, 1969). In *D. dorsalis*, as in most reptiles (Goldby and Gamble, 1957; Northcutt, 1978), this tissue consists of a few large cells which, in cross section, overlap the medial edge of dorsal cortex. As a result, these cells must be destroyed to achieve a complete lesion of general cortex.

A second and more fundamental problem has to do with the terminal distribution of afferents from the brainstem. Present evidence suggests that it is precisely the area of overlap between dorsal and medial cortices (dorsomedial cortex and dorsal cortex, Ebbesson and Voneida, 1969), which is a primary target of projections from the dorsal thalamus and portions of the neuraxis caudal to the diencephalon—in lizards at least (Butler and Ebner, 1972; Butler, Chapter 10; Distel and Ebbesson, 1975). The functional significance of this pattern of fiber distribution is not known, and we cannot be certain—in the absence of electron microscopy data—whether fibers from a given locus in the brainstem synapse on cells of medial cortex, or dorsal cortex, or both. Nevertheless, it is possible that certain functional systems cannot be disrupted unless both dorsal and dorsomedial cortices are destroyed.

A third set of problems involves the route by which fibers from the brainstem reach the cortex in lizards. There is some experimental evidence (Butler and Ebner, 1972; Butler, Chapter 10) that many of these fibers course up over the caudal pole of the telencephalon and pass rostrally in the superficial fiber layer, synapsing en route with somata and processes of cortical cells. Consequently, dorsal cortex lesions will disrupt this pathway, eliminating its input to any cells rostral to the lesion.

For all these reasons behavioral effects of dorsal cortex lesions must be interpreted with extreme care. For example, it appears that on the position reversal task the greatest behavioral deficits are produced in animals with the most caudal pallial lesions. However, it is impossible to state whether this effect of lesion placement is due to the destruction of a critical cell group in the more caudal pallium or simply to the deafferentation of a larger number of equipotential cells. Since there was no difference between ablated and control groups in acquisition of the initial problem (reversal zero, Fig. 6), these data suggest that dorsal cortex lesions do not interfere with simple position learning.

Similarly, the results on reversal zero provide further evidence, along with data from the brightness difference threshold experiment, that the deficits observed were not due to some generalized inability to perform within the experimental situation or to a reduction in the incentive value of the reward. Like the animals in our initial maze experiment, all the lizards used in both the brightness difference threshold and the position reversal studies (except DDPR-5A) remained healthy and, from informal observations, appeared indistinguishable from normals in their home cage. Animal DDPR-15A, which showed a very striking behavioral deficit on the testing apparatus, was nevertheless the dominant male in one colony, reacting entirely normally to conspecific males (assertion and challenge displays, fighting, chasing).

3. Summary

Virtually all the information we have regarding pallial function in reptiles has become available within the last 10 years. In all of these recent experiments the focus of attention has been on dorsal (general) cortex, one of the three principal cell groups of the pallium. Essentially nothing is known from behavioral studies about the function of either the medial or lateral cortices.

To date, data from dorsal cortex ablation studies have yielded more negative than positive results. It appears that destruction of this tissue does not impair the ability to learn or remember simple spatial (Morlock, 1972; Peterson, this chapter) or visual problems (Bass *et al.*, 1973; Peterson, this chapter). Neither is dorsal cortex necessary for discrimination of color (Diebschlag, 1938) or brightness (Peterson, this chapter), for normal optokinetic or visual cliff behavior (Hertzler and Hayes, 1967; Hayes and Hertzler, 1967), or for certain types of pattern vision (Bass *et al.*, 1973).

The effects of dorsal cortex ablation on more "naturalistic" behaviors have been less systematically studied, but it appears that neither spontaneity, activity levels, nor feeding behavior is reliably effected by dorsal cortex lesions (Morlock, 1972; Peterson, this chapter). Diebschlag's (1938) data provide a possible exception, but they are difficult to interpret since he removed the entire pallium. On the other hand, Killackey *et al.* (1972) have demonstrated that dorsal cortex ablations do interfere with normal habituation of a reflex response (head withdrawal) in turtles. Similar lesions in lizards (Peterson, this chapter) produce animals which experience great difficulty in reversing a learned position habit and are rendered totally incapable of remembering or relearning relatively complex mazes which are easily mastered by normal conspecifics.

IV. Discussion

Most of the studies reviewed here must be described as somewhat crude. To a great extent, this reflects the meager amount of information which has been available regarding both the anatomy of the reptile telencephalon and the best methods for the behavioral testing of reptiles. Within the last decade, however, definable advances have been made in both these fields (see Section I), and as a result the design and the success of behavioral studies of telencephalic function have begun to change.

There has been little change, however, in the kinds of questions being addressed by behavioral investigators. With one important exception—i.e., the recent studies on subpallial mediation of iguanid social behavior—most of the behavioral experiments reviewed here have focused on a limited number of issues. The remainder of this section will deal with these questions and the progress which has been made in answering them.

A. Telencephalon as an Arousal System

The most common result of many telencephalic lesions in reptiles (as in other vertebrates, Aronson, 1970) is a decrease in spontaneity or loss of responsiveness to the environment. Such data are difficult to interpret for a number of reasons. First, this is not a constant finding. For example, Fano (1884; cited in Ten Cate, 1937) stated that activity levels were decreased in some decerebrate turtles but unaffected in others, and neither Keating *et al.* (1970) nor Greenberg (1977) reported decreases in activity or attentiveness in their lesioned animals. Second, such effects, when they do occur, cannot be referred reliably to any subdivision of the telencephalon. Diebschlag's data, for example, suggest that arousal levels are disrupted only when there is damage to the amygdaloid group, but in Goldby's experiments the same sluggishness was obtained in cases (after pallial lesions) where this area was spared, and Tarr (1977*a*) has recently reported decreased activity levels in both amygdala and ADVR-lesioned lizards. Indeed, Morlock (1972) reports that decreased activity was sometimes observed both in dorsal-cortex-lesioned turtles and in sham-surgical controls. Similar "arousal" deficits following destruction of widely different telencephalic sites have been reported in mammals (see Kling and Steklis, 1976) and birds (Benowitz, Chapter 13).

Even if the behavioral effects were reproducible, there is a second and more serious problem in interpreting reports of arousal deficits following telencephalic lesions. Reports of "sluggishness" are difficult to evaluate without specific tests of behavioral dysfunction. Apparent arousal deficits may result from sensory or motor dysfunction, or from disruption of the system by which behaviors acquire incentive value ("motivation" deficits). Furthermore, such "sluggishness" may result from incidental damage to *extratelencephalic* structures, via hemorrhage, pressure changes, or infection. This is especially likely in the early group of experiments in which lesions typically were very large. Goldby (1937), the only investigator of that period to give histological details, reported that such extralesion damage was common in his lizards. Indeed, the occasional reports of cervical hypertonus in telencephalic-lesioned reptiles suggest a possible involvement of motor nuclei in the caudal brain stem. Finally, it is important to note that activity levels in reptiles are now known to depend on factors such as diet, temperature, humidity, illumination levels, season, the availability of space, and the presence of conspecifics (e.g., Benes, 1969; Boycott and Robbins, 1961; Crews, 1975; Gourley, 1972; Moehn, 1974). Typically, these parameters have not been controlled for or even reported.

To some investigators (e.g., Aronson, 1970), the changes in activity levels which sometimes follow telencephalic lesions have suggested that these forebrain structures may be involved in an "arousal system." The hypothesis that the vertebrate telencephalon may act to "arouse" or "facilitate" activity in more caudal divisions of the neuraxis has been discussed in detail by Flood *et al.* (1976). As these authors point out, such a hypothesis is (1) inconsistent with much of the available behavioral data and (2) inadequate as a theory because "either excitatory or inhibitory lower centers may be facilitated . . . and these may influence behaviors which are either compatible or incompatible with that required in a task. Thus, the arousal hypothesis can explain anything, but predict nothing, *a priori.*"

B. Visual Telencephalon

There is now a considerable body of both anatomical (cf. Butler, Chapter 10; Northcutt, 1978) and physiological (Peterson and Rowe, 1976; Andry and Northcutt, 1976; Bass *et al.,* 1977; and review by Belekhova, 1979) evidence that visual input reaches at least two areas of the reptile telencephalon: (1) the dorsal—and perhaps medial—cortex and (2) a restricted portion of the ADVR. These data have prompted a number of lesion experiments designed to assess the role of reptilian telencephalic structures in visual information processing. Curiously, all of these experiments have produced essentially negative results and, as yet, we have little information as to how the telencephalon might mediate visual behavior in reptiles.

1. Pallium

Behavioral tests following lesions of dorsal cortex—with or without adjoining (large-celled) medial cortex—indicate that this tissue is not necessary for color (Diebschlag, 1938), brightness (Peterson, this chapter), depth (Hertzler and Hayes, 1967), and pattern (i.e., stripe; Hertzler and Hayes, 1967; Hayes and Hertzler, 1967; Bass *et al.,* 1973) vision. These results are consistent with evidence from more informal observations (Morlock, 1972; Goldby, 1937; Peterson, this chapter; Bass *et al.,* 1973; Tarr, 1977*a*) that dorsal-cortex-lesioned animals show no apparent deficits in visually guided behavior either on the testing apparatus or in a more "natural" setting such as the home cage (including large enclosures which simulate the experimental animal's environment in the wild).

One possible interpretation of these data is that the lesions spared significant amounts of visual pallium. This might be especially likely in experiments with lizards since, in squamates, the exact terminations of visual thalamic afferents to the cortex are not known (see Section IV.C). It is possible, for example, that these projections involve medial cortex (Butler, Chapter 10). However, Diebschlag reported no deficit in color vision after removal of the entire pallium of *Lacerta,* and data reported in this chapter indicate that *Dipsosaurus* experiences no elevation of brightness difference thresholds even after lesions which involve (at least the rostral two-thirds of) dorsal and large-celled medial cortex. In experiments with turtles (Morlock, 1972; Hertzler and Hayes, 1967; Hayes and Hertzler, 1967; Bass *et al.,* 1973) the lesions appear to have destroyed, bilaterally, most of dorsal cortex (the primary target of afferents from the retinorecipient thalamus in Chelonia: Hall and Ebner, 1970; Foster *et al.,* 1976; Hall *et al.,* 1977). Thus it is unlikely that subtotal lesions could account for the reported negative results.

A second possible interpretation of these data is that dorsal cortex lesions produce a "real" impairment of one or more visual capacities, but the behavioral tests used to date have been inappropriate or too insensitive to reveal the deficit. No such judgment is possible in the case of Diebschlag's experiment since details of his procedure were not given. The various "pattern" experiments quoted in this chapter all involved a stripe discrimination, and, since the stripes were quite wide in each case, these experiments cannot be considered to have tested acuity. The most that can be said is that they involved a form of simple "edge" detection. It remains possible that use of a more complex pattern (Zusne, 1970) or a legitimate test of stereopsis or acuity might reveal a deficit following lesions of the visual pallium. Finally, it is unlikely that the negative results reported for the brightness thresholds experiment (Peterson, this chapter) can be attributed to a too insensitive test since the training procedure used clearly taxed the ability of the intact animals (Fig. 4).

The fact that retinal input reaches the pallium says nothing, in itself, about the possible role this tissue might play in visual information processing. The notion that the pallium might act as a primary sensory analyzer (i.e., a "feature extractor") derived originally from the purported homology between dorsal cortex and striate cortex in mammals (Section IV.C), and an implicit assumption: that the visual input to reptile cortex is analogous to striate layer IV input in (many) mammals. To date, there is no behavioral evidence in reptiles to support this position, and much of the available anatomical and physiological evidence suggests, instead, an analogy with either lemniscal or extralemniscal layer I input in mammals (Benevento and Rezak, 1976; Hubel and Wiesel, 1972; Jones and Burton, 1976; Rosenquist *et al.*, 1974). For example, projections from the retinorecipient thalamus in turtles terminate just below the pial surface of dorsal cortex, on the tips of the apical dendrites (Hall and Ebner, 1970; Ebner and Colonnier, 1975). Furthermore, electrophysiological experiments suggest that many visually responsive cortical cells are "nonspecific" in the sense that they (1) have very large receptive fields, (2) are polysensory, (3) have long latencies, (4) are highly susceptible to barbiturate anesthesia, and (5) fatigue readily with repeated stimulus presentation (Moore and Tschirgi, 1962; Kruger and Berkowitz, 1960; Belekhova, 1979).

The significance of these data for behavior research on visual cortex function in reptiles is not clear. One possibility is that behavioral deficits following pallial lesions might prove similar to effects produced in mammals by lesions of the molecular layer of visual cortex in the sense that they may involve a disruption of (selective) visual attention (Levey and Jane, 1975). A related idea has been proposed by Killackey *et al.* (1972) that dorsal cortex "participates in the control of response levels to visual stimuli." Both of these suggestions have in common the notion that the visual pallium of reptiles may be involved not so much in feature extraction as in the modulation of responses to visual stimulation (see Section IV.C). This is a somewhat troublesome idea, given the notorious difficulties involved in defining just what is meant by "response modulation" and in designing experiments to test it (e.g., see Nadel *et al.*, 1975). Yet on balance, the available anatomical, physiological, and behavioral data appear to favor such a hypothesis.

2. Anterior Dorsal Ventricular Ridge

Far less attention has been devoted to the possible role of the ADVR in visual information processing. Diebschlag (1938) mentions briefly that lizards sustaining lesions of the anterior two-thirds of the hemisphere (i.e., including ADVR) were impaired in color discrimination, but it is difficult to interpret this statement since his lesions were very large and no experimental details are given. Tarr (1977*a*) and Greenberg (1977, 1978) made control lesions in ADVR, and their data are in agreement with earlier reports (Ten Cate, 1937; Goldby, 1937) that lesions of (or including) ADVR produce no obvious deficits in visually guided behavior. For example, ADVR-lesioned sceloporine lizards feed readily and resume their presurgical position in a dominance hierarchy. Bass *et al.* (1973) reported no deficit on a stripe discrimination in ADVR-lesioned turtles, although, as mentioned earlier, a subtotal deficit probably would not have been detected by their experiment (see Section II.D). If their lesions destroyed significant amounts of visual ADVR bilaterally and if, as claimed, ADVR animals also sustained bilateral destruction of dorsal cortex, we can infer that neither of the two known visual areas of the turtle telencephalon is necessary either for stripe discrimination or for visually guided behavior as (informally) measured in this experiment. This is a curious finding in light of recent data on the dramatic effects of similar lesions (i.e., lesions which include the telencephalic target of both the thalamofugal and tectofugal visual systems) in elasmobranchs (Graeber *et al.,* 1972), birds (Benowitz, Chapter 13), and mammals (Snyder and Diamond, 1968). Further, their experiment illustrates the fact that lesion studies which focus on the sensory projection areas of ADVR offer considerable problems of interpretation since, in the absence of cytoarchitectural boundaries (e.g., of the visual or auditory projection areas), it is impossible to judge the effective extent of a given lesion with any degree of precision.

C. Function of Dorsal Cortex

For more than 60 years the single most influential idea among behavioral investigators interested in reptile telencephalic function has been the notion that reptile dorsal cortex might represent a homologue of mammalian neocortex. The question being asked is this: by studying the pallium of reptiles, can we reconstruct the earliest, and presumably the simplest, stage in the evolution of neocortex?

In attempting to determine just what this most fundamental level of neocortical organization might be, a majority of behavioral investigators have been led to ask whether dorsal cortex is necessary for either simple sensory discriminations or the initiation of discrete movements. Three factors have dictated this approach. First, certain of the available anatomical and physiological data appeared to be consistent with the notion that dorsal cortex might be organized like primary sensory or motor cortices in mammals (see Section III). Second, it is relatively easy to test for the presence of "motor cortex" using either ablation or stimulation procedures. Similarly, deficits in simple sensory discriminations (intensity and pattern) can readily be assessed even in traditionally "difficult" behavioral subjects such as reptiles. Third, since the beginning of this century, the dominant conception of primitive mammalian neocortex has been that it consisted of contiguous, primary projection areas plus a motor cortex without the intervening "association" areas characteristic of many Recent mammals (Smith, 1910). A reasonable corollary to this notion is that reptilian dorsal cortex should exhibit a similar (although less elaborate) organization, if indeed it reflects an immediately "premammalian" stage in the evolution of neocortex.

Whatever the reasons for the focus on simple sensory or motor behaviors, it is apparent that this approach has failed to yield a coherent picture of dorsal cortex function. What is required is that we (1) reassess the extent to which reptile dorsal cortex resembles mammalian neocortex and (2) determine whether alternative conceptions of dorsal cortex function emerge from a consideration of the available anatomical and behavioral literature.

The connections of reptile dorsal cortex are not well understood. One of the perplexing questions to arise out of the recent body of work on this cell group is whether there are significant differences between the first-order afferent and efferent connections of dorsal cortex in chelonians and in squamates. Dorsal cortex in turtles is known to receive input from the retinorecipient thalamus, i.e., from the so-called dorsal geniculate—as well as from the anterior dorsal thalamus (DLA) and from n. ventralis (Foster *et al.*, 1976; Hall *et al.*, 1977). The extratelencephalic efferents of turtle dorsal cortex project to the visual thalamus (DGN and rotundus), to the midline "reuniens," and to the mesencephalic tegmentum, but apparently not to the hypothalamus (Hall *et al.*, 1977). Experimental data on the intrahemispheric connections of dorsal cortex in turtles have not been reported. We do not know, for example, whether dorsal cortex in turtles has a major output to medial cortex—and thus perhaps to the hypothalamus (Hall *et al.*, 1977)—as it does in squamates. Northcutt has suggested such a projection on the basis of his Golgi material (Northcutt, 1970).

In squamates we know that large lesions of the dorsal thalamus produce terminal degeneration over the cells of dorsal cortex (Butler and Ebner, 1972) and that this projection includes a component from DLA (Distel and Ebbesson, 1975; Lohman and van Woerden-Verkley, 1978), but apparently not from the dorsal geniculate (see Hall *et al.*, 1977). The output of dorsal cortex in squamates includes a major projection to medial cortex, to the septum, to the hypothalamus, and perhaps to the anterior thalamus (Northcutt, 1978; Halpern, Chapter 9; Butler, Chapter 10; Ulinski, 1976). No projections to the visual thalamus have been reported (Hall *et al.*, 1977). Thus to date there is no direct anatomical evidence for either limb of the closed loop linking visual thalamus and dorsal cortex which has been reported in turtles.

If confirmed, these data on the connections of dorsal cortex would appear to have at least two implications for behavioral investigators interested in the function of dorsal cortex. First, they suggest that dorsal cortex may be expected to play a somewhat different role in the visual behavior of turtles and squamates. Second, the available data on dorsal cortex connections suggest that while this cell group resembles mammalian sensory neocortex in its connections with the visual thalamus, it also resembles certain "limbic" structures in the sense that it (1) receives input from the anterior thalamus and (2) sends an extrapallial projection (both directly and indirectly via medial cortex) to the septum and hypothalamus. Such a statement implies that the reptile septum, hypothalamus, and anterior thalamus can be meaningfully compared with like-named structures in mammals, something which is far from certain given our limited knowledge of the connections and embryological derivation of these cell groups and the fact that CNS phylogeny is, in the final analysis, unknowable.

What information is available from behavioral studies which might help us to assess the function of reptile dorsal cortex? Superficially, at least, the existing behavioral data suggest that dorsal cortex is more closely analogous to the mammalian "limbic" system, specifically the hippocampus and septum, than it is to motor or sensory neocortex. We have already seen that dorsal cortex is apparently not necessary for the initiation of discrete movements or for those elemental forms of information processing (color, pattern, and brightness thresholds) commonly associated with mammalian visual cortex. Indeed, only three behavioral experiments on dorsal cortex function have yielded positive results. All three deal with phenomena which have figured more or less prominently in the literature on "limbic" (hippocampal) lesions in mammals: spatial learning, habituation, and discrimination reversal. The following brief description of certain effects of hippocampal lesions in mammals is taken from recent reviews by McCleary (1966), Douglas (1967), Kimble (1968), Thomas *et al.* (1968), Isaacson and Kimble (1972), Altman *et al.* (1973), Hirsch (1974), Nadel and O'Keefe (1974), and Nadel *et al.* (1975).

First, hippocampal lesions in mammals result in impaired acquisition and retention of complex (multiple-choice) but not simple (single-choice) spatial discriminations. Performance of hippocampally lesioned mammals on mazes is characterized by perseverative reentry into blind alleys, lack of flexibility in the choice of pathways to the goal, absence of spontaneous alternation, and increased tendency to develop a fixation response. Second, several investigators have reported that habituation in hippocampectomized mammals is not as rapid as it is in controls. Third, hippocampectomized animals are reported to learn simultaneous discriminations of spatial, visual, and tactile stimuli at least as rapidly as (and sometimes more rapidly than) intact animals. However, they are significantly impaired in the reversal of such discriminations. In other words, they are able to master the reversed discrimination, but at a much slower rate than normal controls.

There is a clear similarity between the behavior of hippocampectomized mammals and that of reptiles with lesions of dorsal cortex. Both are impaired in performance on multiple-choice but not on single-choice spatial discriminations. In each case the behavior of these experimental animals can be characterized as "rigid" (e.g., perseverative errors and response fixation). Both habituate more slowly than normal controls. Both show no deficit in acquisition of simultaneous visual (brightness and pattern) discriminations. Both are severely impaired in performance of spatial reversal.

Just what mechanism(s) might underlie this behavioral syndrome is unknown. The voluminous literature on the behavioral effects of limbic lesions in mammals has prompted several authors to suggest theories of limbic system function, but, as yet, no consensus has been reached. Nor can we assume that the mechanisms underlying these behaviors are the same in mammals and in reptiles. Nevertheless, the available behavioral data suggest that reptile dorsal cortex and parts of the mammalian limbic system are functionally similar.

At this point a caveat is in order. The pattern of behavioral results, especially when considered in conjunction with the available anatomical data, suggests a relationship between reptile dorsal cortex and the mammalian hippocampal complex. However, inferences based on such data must be drawn with care, i.e., with due regard for alternative interpretations. (For example, there are a number of similarities—both anatomical and functional—between reptile dorsal cortex and mammalian frontal cortex.) Nor should the foregoing account be taken to preclude the possibility that dorsal cortex is analogous, in some respects, to mammalian striate cortex. Indeed, there is behavioral evidence that, in some mammals, primary visual cortex may not be necessary for pattern vision (e.g., Sprague *et al.*, 1977) or may be involved more in the focus and shift of visual attention than in feature detection (Killackey and Diamond, 1971). Such a possibility has never been tested in reptiles. Furthermore, there is now anatomical evidence in mammals that primary sensory cortices project to the hippocampal fields via relays in secondary sensory areas and entorhinal cortex (Van Hoesen *et al.*, 1971). Thus mammals and reptiles appear to share a sensorimotor loop through the forebrain in which lemniscal input is relayed indirectly to the (hippocampal–hypothalamic) visceral effector system. In reptiles, dorsal cortex occupies a pivotal point in this circuit since it receives sensory input from the dorsal thalamus and projects to septum and hypothalamus both directly and indirectly via media cortex. Thus it may be meaningless to compare dorsal cortex with either neo- or limbic cortex alone. The point here is that the dominant conception of dorsal cortex—as "motor cortex" and "striate cortex"—has proved less than fruitful. Behavioral investigators could, with profit, enlarge their perspective on this little-understood cell group.

V. References

Abbie, A. A., 1948, The prosencephalization of motor control: A preliminary note, in: *Essays in Biology Presented to Arthur Neville Burkitt,* pp. 85–100, Australasia Medical Publishing Co., Glebe, N.S.W.

Altman, J., Brunner, R. L., and Hayer, S. A., 1973, The hippocampus and behavioral maturation, *Behav. Biol.* **8:**557.

Andry, M. L., and Northcutt, R. G., 1976, Telencephalic visual responses in the lizard *Gekko gecko, Neurosci, Abstr.* **2:**176.

Ariëns Kappers, S. U., Huber, G. C., and Crosby, E. C., 1936, *The Comparative Anatomy of the Nervous System of Vertebrates, Including Man,* Macmillan, New York.

Aronson, L. R., 1970, Functional evolution of the forebrain in lower vertebrates, in: *Development and Evolution of Behavior* (L. R. Aronson, E. Tobach, D. S. Lehrman, and J. S. Rosenblatt, eds.), Freeman, pp. 75-107, San Francisco.

Bagley, C., and Langworthy, O. R., 1926, The forebrain and midbrain of the alligator with experimental transections of the brain stem, *Arch. Neurol. Psychiat.* **16:**154.

Bagley, C., and Richter, C. P., 1924, Electrically excitable region of the forebrain of the alligator, *Arch. Neurol. Psychiat.* **11:**257.

Balaban, C. D., 1978, Structure of anterior dorsal ventricular ridge in a turtle (*Pseudemys scripta elegans*), *J. Morphol.* **158:**291.

Bass, A. H., Pritz, M. B., and Northcutt, R. G., 1973, Effects of telencephalic and tectal ablations on visual behavior in the side-necked turtle, *Podocnemis unifilis, Brain Res.* **55:**455.

Bass, A. H., Andry, M. L., and Northcutt, R. G., 1977, Telencephalic visual responses in the painted turtle, *Chrysemys picta, Neurosci. Abstr.* **3:**89.

Bekoff, M., Lockwood, A., and Meikle, T. H., 1973, Effects of serial lesions in cat visual cortex on a brightness discrimination, *Brain Res.* **49:**190.

Belekhova, M. G., 1979, Neurophysiology of the forebrain, in: *Biology of the Reptilia,* Vol. 10 (C. Gans, R. G. Northcutt, and P. S. Ulinski, eds.), pp. 287–359, Academic Press, London.

Benes, E. S., 1969, Behavioral evidence for color discrimination by the whiptail lizard, *Cnemidophorus tigris, Copeia* **4:**707.

Benevento, L. A., and Rezak, M., 1976, The cortical projections of the inferior pulvinar and adjacent lateral pulvinar in the rhesus monkey (*Macaca mulatta*): An autoradiographic study, *Brain Res.* **106:**1.

Berk, M. L., and Heath, J. E, 1975, Effects of preoptic, hypothalamic, and telencephalic lesions on thermoregulation in the lizard, *Dipsosaurus dorsalis, J. Thermal Biol.* **1:**65.

Bickel, A., 1901, Beiträge zur Gehirnphysiologie der Schildkröte, *Arch. Anat. Physiol. Physiol. Abt.* **25:**52.

Bitterman, M. E., 1975, The comparative analysis of learning, *Science* **188:**699.

Bogartz, R. S., 1965, The criterion method; some analyses and remarks, *Psychol. Bull.* **64:**1.

Boycott, B. B., and Robbins, M. W., 1961, The care of young red-eared terrapins (*Pseudemys scripta elegans*), *Br. J. Herpetol.* **1:**206.

Brattstrom, B. H., 1971, Social and thermoregulatory behavior of the bearded dragon, *Amphibolurus barbatus, Copeia* **3:**484.

Brattstrom, B. H., 1974, The evolution of reptilian social behavior, *Am. Zool.* **14:**35.

Brattstrom, B. H., 1978, Learning studies in lizards, in: *Behavior and Neurology of Lizards* (N. Greenberg and P. D. MacLean, eds.), pp. 173–181, NIMH, Rockville, Md.

Bremer, F., Dow, R. S., and Moruzzi, G., 1939, Physiological analysis of the general cortex in reptiles and birds, *J. Neurophysiol.* **2:**473.

Burghardt, G. M., 1970, Chemical perception in reptiles, in: *Advances in Chemoreception,* Vol. 1 (J. W. Johnston, D. G. Moulton, and A. Turk, eds.) pp. 241–308, Appleton-Century-Crofts, New York.

Burghardt, G. M., 1977, Learning processes in reptiles, in: *Biology of the Reptilia,* Vol. 7 (C. Gans and D. Tinkle, eds.), pp. 555–681, Academic Press, New York.

Bustard, H. R., 1965, Observations on the life history and behavior of *Chamaeleo hohnelii* (Steindachner), *Copeia* **4:**401.

Butler, A. B., and Ebner, F. F., 1972, Thalamotelencephalic projections in the lizard *Iguana iguana, Anat. Rec.* **172:**282.

Butler, A. B., and Northcutt, R. G., 1971, Retinal projections in *Iguana iguana* and *Anolis carolinensis, Brain Res.* **26:**1.

Cain, D. P., 1974, The role of the olfactory bulb in limbic mechanisms, *Psychol. Bull.* **81:**654.

Carpenter, C. C., 1961, Patterns of social behavior in the desert iguana, *Dipsosaurus dorsalis, Copeia* **4:**396.

Carpenter, C. C., 1967, Aggression and social structure in iguanid lizards, in: *Lizard Ecology: A Symposium* (W. W. Milstead, ed.), pp. 87–105, University of Missouri Press, Columbia, Mo.

Carpenter, C. C., and Grubits, G., 1960, Dominance shifts in the tree lizard (*Urosaurus ornatus*—Iguanidae), *Southwest. Nat.* **5:**123.

Clemente, C. D., and Chase, M. H., 1973, Neurological substrates of aggressive behavior, *Annu. Rev. Physiol.* **35:**329.

Crews, D., 1975, Inter- and intraindividual variation in display patterns in the lizard, *Anolis carolinensis, Herpetologica* **31:**37.

Crosby, E. C., 1917, The forebrain of *Alligator mississippiensis, J. Comp. Neurol.* **27:**325.

DeFrance, J. F. (ed.), 1976, *The Septal Nuclei,* Plenum Press, New York.

DeWitt, C. B., McGinnis, S. M., and Dickson, L. L., 1967, Behavioral thermoregulation in the desert iguana, *Science* **158:**809.

Diebschlag, V. E., 1938, Beobachtungen und Versuche an intakten und grasshirnlosen Eidechsen und Ringlnathern, *Zool. Anz.* **124:**30.

Distel, H., 1976, Behavior and electrical brain stimulation in the green iguana, *Iguana iguana* L. I. Schematic brain atlas and stimulation device, *Brain Behav. Evol.* **13:**421.

Distel, H., 1978*a*, Behavioural response to the electrical stimulation of the brain in the green iguana, in: *Behavior and Neurology of Lizards* (N. Greenberg and P. D. MacLean, eds.), pp. 135–147, NIMH, Rockville, Md.

Distel, H., 1978*b*, Behavior and electrical stimulation in the green iguana, *Iguana iguana* L. II. Stimulation effects, *Exp. Brain Res.* **31:**353.

Distel, H., and Ebbesson, S. O. E., 1975, Connections of the thalamus in the monitor lizard, *Neurosci. Abstr.* **1:**559.

Douglas, R. J., 1967, The hippocampus and behavior, *Psychol. Bull.* **67:**416.

Ebbesson, S. O. E., 1970, The selective silver-impregnation of degenerating axons and their synaptic endings in non-mammalian species, in: *Contemporary Research Methods in Neuroanatomy* (W. J. H. Nauta and S. O. E. Ebbesson, eds.), pp. 132–161, Springer-Verlag, New York.

Ebbesson, S. O. E., 1972, A proposal for a common nomenclature for some optic nuclei in vertebrates and the evidence for a common origin of two such cell groups, *Brain Behav. Evol.* **6:**75.

Ebbesson, S. O. E., and Voneida, T. J., 1969, The cytoarchitecture of the pallium of the tegu lizard (*Tupinambis nigropunctatus*), *Brain Behav. Evol.* **2:**431.

Ebbesson, S. O. E., Schroeder, D. M., and Butler, A. B., 1975, The Golgi method and the revival of comparative neurology, in: *Golgi Centennial Symposium* (M. Santini, ed.), pp. 153–160, Raven Press, New York.

Ebner, F. F., and Colonnier, M., 1975, Synaptic patterns in the visual cortex of turtle: An electron microscopic study, *J. Comp. Neurol.* **160:**51.

Evans, L. T., 1953, Tail display in an iguanid lizard, *Liocephalus carinatus coryi, Copeia* **1:**50.

Fano, G., 1884, *Saggio Sperimentale dul Meccanismo dei Movimenti Volontari nella Testuggine palustre (Emys europaea),* Pubbl. Ist. Stud. Super. Firenze.

Flood, N. C., Overmier, J. B., and Savage, G. E., 1976, Teleost telencephalon and learning: An interpretive review of data and hypotheses, *Physiol. Behav.* **16:**783.

Foster, R. E., Hall, J. A., and Ebner, F. F., 1976, Visual cortex in the turtle (*Pseudemys scripta* and *Chrysemys picta*), *Anat. Rec.* **184:**405.

Garzanit, F. S., and Richardson, A. M., 1974, Black–white discrimination and orienting behavior in the desert iguana (*Dipsosaurus dorsalis*), *Anim. Learn. Behav.* **2:**126.

Gelderloos, O. G., 1976, Circadian activity patterns in the desert iguana, *Dipsosaurus dorsalis, Zoology* **49:**100.

Goldby, F., 1937, An experimental investigation of the cerebral hemispheres of *Lacerta viridis, J. Anat.* **71:**332.

Goldby, F., and Gamble, H. J., 1957, The reptilian cerebral hemispheres, *Biol. Rev.* **32:**383.

Gourley, E. V., 1972, Circadian activity rhythm of the gopher tortoise *Gopherus polyphemus, Anim. Behav.* **20:**13.

Graeber, R. C., Schroeder, D. M., Jane, J. A., and Ebbesson, S. O. E., 1972, The importance of telencephalic structures in visual learning in nurse sharks, paper presented at Second Annual Meeting of Society for Neuroscience, Houston, Tex.

Greenberg, N., 1977, A neuroethological study of display behavior in the lizard *Anolis carolinensis* (Reptilia, Lacertilia, Iguanidae), *Am. Zool.* **17:**191.

Greenberg, N., 1978, Ethological considerations in the experimental study of lizard behavior, in: *Behavior and Neurology of Lizards* (N. Greenberg and P. D. MacLean, eds.), pp. 203–224, NIMH, Rockville, Md.

Greenberg, N., Ferguson, L. F., and MacLean, P. D., 1976, A neuroethological study of display behavior in lizards, *Neurosci. Abstr.* **2:**689.

Greenberg, N., and MacLean, P. D. (eds.), 1978, *Behavior and Neurology of Lizards*, NIMH, Rockville, Md.

Hall, J. A., Foster, R. E., Ebner, F. F., and Hall, W. C., 1977, Visual cortex in a reptile, the turtle (*Pseudemys scripta* and *Chrysemys picta*), *Brain Res.* **130:**197.

Hall, W. C., 1972, Visual pathways to the telencephalon in reptiles and mammals, *Brain Behav. Evol.* **5:**95.

Hall, W. C., and Ebner, F. F., 1970, Thalamotelencephalic projections in a turtle (*Pseudemys scripta*), *J. Comp. Neurol.* **140:**101.

Hayes, W. N., and Hertzler, D. R., 1967, Role of the optic tectum and general cortex in reptilian vision, *Psychon. Sci.* **9:**521.

Heimer, L., 1969, The secondary olfactory connections in mammals, reptiles and sharks, *Ann. N.Y. Acad. Sci.* **167:**129.

Herrick, C. J., 1926, *Brains of Rats and Men,* University of Chicago Press, Chicago.

Hetzler, D. R., 1972, Tectal integration of visual input in the turtle, *Brain Behav. Evol.* **5:**240.

Hetzler, D. R., and Hayes, W. N., 1967, Cortical and tectal function in visually guided behavior of turtles, *J. Comp. Physiol. Psychol.* **63:**444.

Hilger, W. N., and Rowe, F. A., 1975, Olfactory bulb ablation: Effects on handling reactivity, open-field behavior, and agonistic behavior in male and female hamsters, *Physiol. Psychol.* **3:**162.

Hirsch, R., 1974, The hippocampus and contextual retrieval of information from memory: A theory, *Behav. Biol.* **12:**421.

Hodos, W., and Bonbright, J. C., 1974, Intensity difference thresholds in pigeons after lesions of the tectofugal and thalamofugal visual pathways, *J. Comp. Physiol. Psychol.* **87:**1013.

Hubel, D. H., and Wiesel, T. N., 1972, Laminar and columnar distribution of geniculo-cortical fibers in the macaque monkey, *J. Comp. Neurol.* **146:**421.

Humphrey, T., 1967, The development of the human hippocampal formation correlated with some aspects of its phylogenetic history, in: *Evolution of the Forebrain* (R. Hassler and H. Stephan, eds.), pp. 104–116, Plenum Press, New York.

Isaacson, R. L., and Kimble, D. P., 1972, Lesions of the limbic system: Their effects upon hypotheses and frustration, *Behav. Biol.* **7:**767.

Jenssen, T. A., 1971, Display analysis of *Anolis nebulosus* (Sauria, Iguanidae), *Copeia* **2:**197.

Johnston, J. B., 1915, The cell masses in the forebrain of the turtle *Cistudo carolina, J. Comp. Neurol.* **25:**393.

Johnston, J. B., 1916, Evidence of a motor pallium in the forebrain of reptiles, *J. Comp. Neurol.* **26:**475.

Johnston, J. B., 1923, Further contributions to the study of the evolution of the forebrain, *J. Comp. Neurol.* **36:**143.

Jones, E. G., and Burton, H., 1976, Areal differences in the laminar distribution of thalamic afferents in cortical fields of the insular, parietal and temporal regions of primates, *J. Comp. Neurol.* **168:**197.

Julian, B., and Richardson, A. M., 1968, Maze learning in the lizard *Dipsosaurus dorsalis, J. Biol. Psychol.* **10:**4.

Karten, H. J., 1969, The organization of the avian telencephalon and some speculations on the phylogeny of the amniote telencephalon, *Ann. N.Y. Acad. Sci.* **167:**164.

Keating, E. G., Kormann, L. A., and Horel, J. A., 1970, The behavioral effects of stimulating and ablating the reptilian amygdala (*Caiman sklerops*), *Physiol. Behav.* **5:**55.

Killackey, H., and Diamond, I. T., 1971, Visual attention in the tree shrew: An ablation study of the striate and extrastriate visual cortex, *Science* **171:**696.

Killackey, H., Pellmar, T., and Ebner, F., 1972, The effects of general cortex ablation on habituation in the turtle, *Fed. Proc.* **31:**819.

Kimble, D. P., 1968, Hippocampus and internal inhibition, *Psychol. Bull.* **69:**285.

Kling, A., and Steklis, H. D., 1976, A neural substrate for affiliative behavior in non-human primates, *Brain Behav. Evol.* **13:**216.

Knapp, H., and Kang, D. S., 1968, The retinal projections of the sidenecked turtle (*Podocnemis unifilis*) with some notes on the possible origin of the pars dorsalis of the LGN, *Brain Behav. Evol.* **1:**369.

Koppányi, T., and Pearcy, J. F., 1925, Comparative studies on the excitability of the forebrain, *Am. J. Physiol.* **71:**339.

Krekorian, C. O'N., Vance, V., and Richardson, A. M., 1968, Temperature-dependent maze learning in the desert iguana, *Dipsosaurus dorsalis, Anim. Behav.* **16:**429.

Kruger, L., 1969, Experimental analysis of the reptilian nervous system, *Ann. N.Y. Acad. Sci.* **167:**102.

Kruger, L., and Berkowitz, E. C., 1960, The main afferent connections of the reptilian telencephalon as determined by degeneration and electrophysiological methods, *J. Comp. Neurol.* **115:**125.

Lasek, R. J., 1975, Axonal transport and the use of intracellular markers in neuroanatomical investigations, *Fed. Proc.* **34:**1603.

Lashley, K. S., 1929, *Brain Mechanisms and Intelligence*, University of Chicago Press, Chicago.

Levey, N. H., and Jane, J. A., 1975, Laminar thermocoagulation of the visual cortex of the rat. II. Visual pattern discrimination, *Brain Behav. Evol.* **11:**275.

Lohman, A. H. M., and van Woerden-Verkley, I., 1978, Ascending connections to the forebrain in the tegu lizard, *J. Comp. Neurol.* **182:**555.

Mackintosh, N. J., and Holgate, V., 1969, Serial reversal training and nonreversal shift learning, *J. Comp. Physiol. Psychol.* **67:**89.

MacLean, P. D., 1973, Effects of pallidal lesions on species-typical display behavior of squirrel monkey, *Fed. Proc.* **32:**384.

MacLean, P. D., 1975, Role of pallidal projections in species-typical display behavior of squirrel monkey, *Tr. Am. Neurol. Assoc.* **100:**25.

Maier, N. R. F., Glaser, N. H., and Klee, J. B., 1940, Studies of abnormal behavior in the rat. III. The development of behavior fixations through frustration, *J. Exp. Psychol.* **26:**521.

Mayr, E., 1969, *Principles of Systematic Zoology,* McGraw-Hill, New York.

Mayr, E., 1970, *Populations, Species, and Evolution,* Harvard University Press, Cambridge, Mass.

Mayr, E., 1974, Behavior programs and evolutionary strategies, *Am. Sci.* **62:**650.

McCleary, R. A., 1966, Response-modulating functions of the limbic system: Initiation and suppression, in: *Progress in Physiological Psychology,* Vol. 1 (E. Stellar and J. M. Sprague, eds.), pp. 209–272, Academic Press, New York.

Meyer, A., 1892, Über das Vorderhirn einiger Reptilien, *Z. Wis. Zool.* **55:**63.

Minnich, J. E., and Shoemaker, V. H., 1970, Diet, behavior and water turnover in the desert iguana, *Dipsosaurus dorsalis, Am. Midl. Nat.* **84:**496.

Moehn, L. D., 1974, The effect of quality of light on agonistic behavior of iguanid and agamid lizards, *J. Herpetol.* **8:**175.

Moore, G. P., and Tschirgi, R. D., 1962, Nonspecific responses of reptilian cortex to sensory stimuli, *Exp. Neurol.* **5:**196.

Morlock, H. C., 1972, Behavior following ablation of the dorsal cortex of turtles, *Brain Behav. Evol.* **5:**256.

Moynihan, M., 1973, The evolution of behavior and the role of behavior in evolution, *Breviora,* No. 415, pp. 1-29.

Nadel, L., and O'Keefe, J., 1974, The hippocampus in pieces and patches: an essay on modes of explanation in physiological psychology, in: *Essays on the Nervous System: A Festschrift for Professor J. Z. Young* (R. Bellairs and E. G. Gray, eds.), pp. 367–390, Clarendon Press, Oxford.

Nadel, L., O'Keefe, J., and Black, A., 1975, Slam on the brakes: A critique of Altman, Brunner, and Bayer's response-inhibition model of hippocampal function, *Behav. Biol.* **14:**151.

Norris, K. S., 1953, The ecology of the desert iguana, *Dipsosaurus dorsalis, Ecology* **34:**265.

Northcutt, R. G., 1967, Architectonic studies of the telencephalon of *Iguana iguana, J. Comp. Neurol.* **130:**109.

Northcutt, R. G., 1970, *The Telencephalon of the Western Painted Turtle (Chrysemys picta belli),* Illinois Biological Monographs, University of Illinois Press, Chicago.

Northcutt, R. G., 1978, Forebrain and midbrain organization in lizards and its phylogenetic significance, in: *Behavior and Neurology of Lizards* (N. Greenberg and P. D. MacLean, eds.), pp. 11–64, NIMH, Rockville, Md.

Orrego, F., 1961, The reptilian forebrain. I. The olfactory pathways and cortical areas in the turtle, *Arch. Ital. Biol.* **99:**425.

Orrego, F., and Lisenby, D., 1962, The reptilian forebrain. IV. Electrical activity in the turtle cortex, *Arch. Ital. Biol.* **100:**17.

Peterson, E., 1976, Behavioral studies of visual discrimination in the lizard, *Dipsosaurus dorsalis,* Ph. D. dissertation, University of California, Riverside

Peterson, E., and Rowe, M., 1976, Electrophysiological evidence for a visual projection to the dorsal ventricular ridge in a lizard, *Dipsosaurus dorsalis, Anat. Rec.* **184:**500.

Peterson, E. H., and Ulinski, P. S., 1980, Olfactory projections in the desert iguana, *Dipsosaurus dorsalis.* In preparation.

Pritz, M. B., Andrew, H. B., and Northcutt, R. G., 1973, A simple apparatus and training techniques for teaching turtles to perform a visual discrimination task, *Copeia* **1:**181.

Rainey, W. T., 1976, Organization of lateral cortex in snakes, *Anat. Rec.* **184:**507.

Rand, A. S., 1967, The adaptive significance of territoriality in iguanid lizards, in: *Lizard Ecology: A Symposium* (W. W. Milstead, ed.), pp. 106–115, University of Missouri Press, Columbia, Mo.

Riss, W., Halpern, M., and Scalia, F., 1969, The quest for clues to forebrain evolution—The study of reptiles, *Brain Behav. Evol.* **2:**1.

Romer, A. S., 1970, *The Vertebrate Body,* 4th ed., Saunders, Philadelphia.

Rosenquist, A. C., Edwards, S. B., and Palmer, L. A., 1974, An autoradiographic study of the projections of the dorsal lateral geniculate nucleus and the posterior nucleus in the cat, *Brain Res.* **80:**71.

Scalia, F., Halpern, M., and Riss, W., 1969, Olfactory bulb projections in the South American caiman, *Brain Behav. Evol.* **2:**238.

Schapiro, H., 1965, Motor functions and their anatomical basis in the forebrain and tectum of the alligator, *Diss. Abstr.* **25:**5492.

Schapiro, H., and Goodman, D. C., 1969, Motor functions and their anatomical basis in the forebrain and tectum of the alligator, *Exp. Neurol.* **24:**187.

Schrader, M. E. G., 1892, Über die Stellung des Grosshirns im Reflexmechanismus des zentralen Nervensystems des Wirbeltiere, *Arch. Exp. Pathol.* **29:**55.

Senn, D. G., and Northcutt, R. G., 1973, The forebrain and midbrain of some squamates and their bearing on the origin of snakes, *J. Morphol.* **140:**135.

Sergi, S., 1905*a*, Sull'attivita muscolare volontaria nelia testudo graeca, *Arch. Farmacol. Sper.* **3:**179.

Sergi, S., 1905*b*, Il sistema nervoso centrale nei movimenti della testudo graeca, *Arch Farmacol. Sper.* **4:**474.

Simpson, G. G., 1961, *Principles of Animal Taxonomy,* Columbia University Press, New York.

Smith, G. E., 1910, Some problems relating to the evolution of the brain, *Lancet* **1:**147, 221.

Smith, G. E., 1919, A preliminary note on the morphology of the corpus striatum and the origin of the neopallium, *J. Anat.* **53:**271.

Snyder, M., and Diamond, I. T., 1968, The organization and function of the visual cortex in the tree shrew, *Brain Behav. Evol.* **1**:244.

Spiegel, I. M., and Ellis, K. R., 1966, Cerebral lesions and climbing suppression in the turtle, *Psychon. Sci.* **5**:211.

Sprague, J. M., Levy, J., DiBerardino, A., and Berlucchi, G., 1977, Visual cortical areas mediating form discrimination in the cat, *J. Comp. Neurol.* **172**:441.

Stettner, L. J., 1974, The neural basis of avian discrimination and reversal learning, in: *Birds: Brain and Behavior* (I. J. Goodman and M. W. Schein, eds.), pp. 165–201, Academic Press, New York.

Sugerman, R. A., 1974, Gular extension evoked by electrical stimulation in collared lizards (*Crotaphythus collaris*), *Am. Zool.* **14**:1282.

Sugerman, R. A., and Demski, L. S., 1978, Agonistic behavior elicited by electrical stimulation of the brain in western collared lizards, *Crotaphytus collaris, Brain Behav. Evol.* **15**:446.

Tarr, R., 1975, Effects of telencephalic lesions on the social behavior of the western fence lizard, *Sceloporus occidentalis, Neurosci. Abstr.* **1**:560.

Tarr, R., 1977*a*, Role of the amygdala in the interspecies aggressive behavior of the iguanid lizard, *Sceloporus occidentalis, Physiol. Behav.* **18**:1153.

Tarr, R., 1977*b*, Effects of septal lesions on the aggressive behavior of the western fence lizard, *Sceloporus occidentalis, Neurosci. Abstr.* **3**:95.

Ten Cate, J., 1937, Physiologie des Zentralnervensystems der Reptilien, *Ergeb. Biol.* **14**:225.

Thomas, G. J., Hostetter, G., and Barker, D. J., 1968, Behavioral functions of the limbic system, in: *Progress in Physiological Psychology,* Vol. 2 (E. Stellar and J. M. Sprague, eds.), pp. 229–311, Academic Press, New York.

Thompson, R. F., and Spencer, W. A., 1966, Habituation: A model phenomenon for the study of neuronal substrates of behavior, *Psychol. Rev.* **73**:16.

Tuge, H., and Yazaki, M., 1934, Experimental note on the presence of electrically excitable areas in the reptilian cerebral hemisphere: *Clemmys japonica, Tohoku Univ. Sci. Rep. Ser. 4* **9**:79.

Ulinski, P. S., 1974, Cytoarchitecture of the cerebral cortex in snakes, *J. Comp. Neurol.* **158**:243.

Ulinski, P. S., 1976, Intracortical connections in the snakes *Natrix sipedon* and *Thamnophis sirtalis, J. Morphol.* **150**:463.

Van Hoesen, G. W., Pandya, D. N., and Butters, N., 1971, Cortical afferents to the entorhinal cortex of the rhesus monkey, *Science* **175**:1471.

Vincent, S. B., 1912, The function of the vibrissae in the behavior of the white rat, *Behav. Monogr.* **1(5)**:1.

Zusne, L., 1970, *Visual Perception of Form,* Academic Press, New York.

13

Functional Organization of the Avian Telencephalon

LARRY BENOWITZ

I. Introduction

The brain mechanisms which underlie birds' remarkable behavioral capacities have been a subject of interest since the early nineteenth century. Beginning with the pioneering work of Rolando and Flourens, numerous investigators have used brain lesions to explore the functional significance of various elements in the avian central nervous system (for review, see Pearson, 1972; Ten Cate, 1965). From this research emerged the idea that, as in mammals, birds' cerebral hemispheres play a critical role in the organization of complex behavioral patterns, particularly those which involve learning (see especially Rogers, 1922). Consistent with such notions, comparative morphological studies have indicated a strong correlation between a species' behavioral complexity and plasticity and the relative size of its forebrain hemispheres (Portmann and Stingelin, 1961; Stettner, 1974). Yet, at a more fundamental level, the mechanisms by which the telencephalon might participate in various behavioral capacities had remained unfathomable. Until fairly recently, standard anatomical descriptions included both correct and incorrect notions generously mixed together, a situation which precluded any understanding of the brain's functional organization or any interpretation of brain lesion studies. Within the past 15 years, however, specific connections, general organizational principles, and mammalian homologies for much of the avian cerebrum have been established through the use of modern neuroanatomical tracing techniques. From this work has emerged a picture showing clearly delineated sensory-specific projection areas,

LARRY BENOWITZ • Department of Psychiatry, Harvard Medical School, and Lowell Laboratories, McLean Hospital, Belmont, Massachusetts 02178.

skeletal and autonomic effector zones, and interposed associative networks. Together with the attendant insights gained from brain lesion and electrophysiological studies, these advances have not only revolutionized our understanding of the avian telencephalon but also helped shed light on certain basic issues concerning general vertebrate brain–behavior relationships.

II. Development and Organization

In contrast to the laminar organization of the mammalian cortical mantle, the avian telencephalon is characterized by broad fields of cells, some nuclear clusters, and a thin overlying laminated zone. Yet despite the morphological dissimilarities, comparative embryological, anatomical, and histochemical studies all suggest that most of the bird's telencephalon is comparable with elements of the mammalian cortex.

In both vertebrate classes the telencephalon develops as a set of lateral evagi-

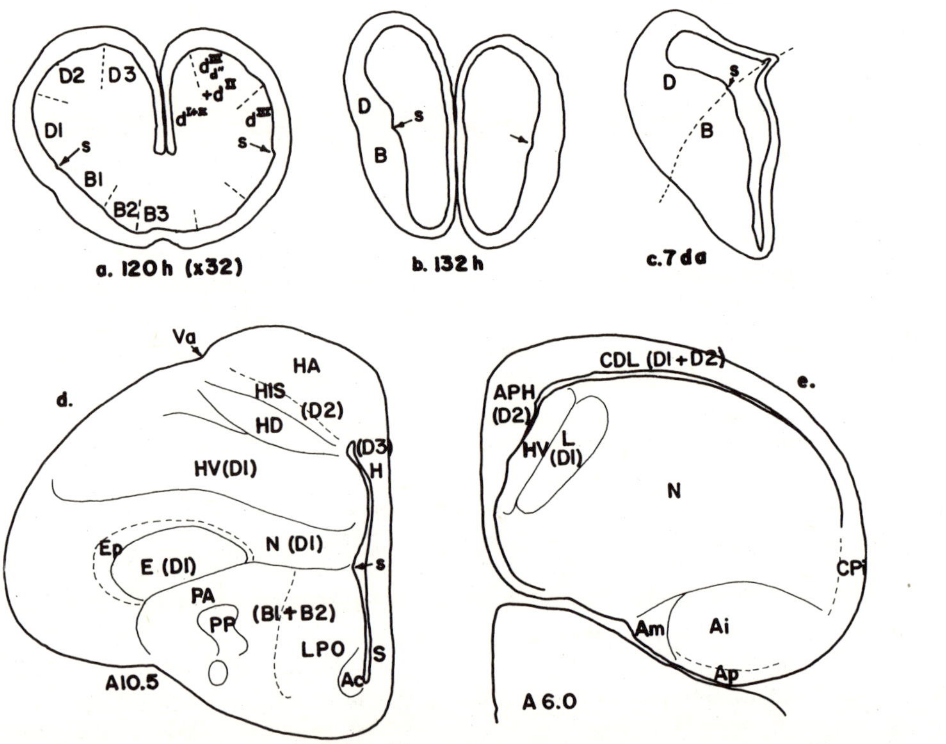

Figure 1. a,b,c: Cross sections through the telencephalon of the developing chick. Redrawn from Kuhlenbeck (1938). The sulcus (s) separates zones giving rise to pallial (D) and basal (B) telencephalic structures. The right-hand side of (a) shows the same regions according to the system of Källén (1962). d,e: Cross sections through the adult pigeon brain indicating some major structures and their embryological zones of origin (in parentheses). Abbreviations are explained in Table I. Table II more fully reviews the embryogenesis of avian telencephalic structures based on the studies of Kuhlenbeck and Källén, along with proposed mammalian homologies.

nations from the rostral end of the neural tube. Each evagination closes back upon itself, forming the tubular precursors of the two cerebral hemispheres (Fig. 1b). On the lateral wall of each tube an important sulcus (s, Fig. 1a–c) can be discerned very early. (See Table I for abbreviations used in the text.) In mammals all tissue arising from the zone dorsal to this sulcus becomes part of the cortical mantle (Källén, 1951). The avian structures which have a comparable embryological origin include not only the dorsalmost portions of the telencephalon, which are laminar in appearance (i.e., the corticoid, parahippocampal, and wulst regions), but also the nonlaminar cell masses of the hyperstriatum ventrale (HV), neostriatum (N), ectostriatum (E), and portions of the archistriatum (A). The embryological origin of these latter regions would suggest that they may have a common phyletic ancestry, and thus be homologous, with portions of the mammalian neocortex (Table II). This notion is supported by comparative anatomical and histochemical data (Karten, 1969; Karten *et al.*, 1973; Karten and Dubbeldam, 1973).

Based primarily on morphological considerations, Ariëns Kappers *et al.* (1936) regarded nonlaminar regions of the telencephalon to be elaborations of the basal ganglia, and thus their use of the suffix "-striatum." Although we will continue to

Table I. List of Abbreviations

A	Archistriatum	L	Field L, auditory projection zone
Aa	—— anterior	LFS	Lamina frontalis superior
Ai	—— intermedium	LMD	—— medullaris dorsalis
Aid	—— —— dorsalis	LPO	Lobus parolfactorius
Am	—— mediale	MFB	Medial forebrain bundle
Ap	—— posterior	MLd	N. mesencephali lateralis pars dorsalis (inferior colliculus)
APH	Area parahippocampalis		
B	Telencephalic zones of basal origin	N	Neostriatum
		OM	Tractus occipitomesencephalicus
Bas	N. basalis prosencephali	OPT	Regio opticus principalis thalami
CA	Anterior commissure	Ov	N. ovoidalis thalami
Cd	Caudate	PA	Paleostriatum augmentatum
CDL	Dorsolateral corticoid region	POA	Preoptic area
CPi	Pyriform cortex	PP	Paleostriatum primitivum
D	Pallial telencephalic zones	Pu	Putamen
DA	Tractus dorsoarchistriaticus	QFT	Tractus quinto-frontalis
DLL	N. dorsolateralis lateralis	RA	N. robustus archistriaticus
DLLd	—— pars dorsalis	Rt	N. rotundus thalami
DLLv	—— pars ventralis	S	Septal region
DVR	Dorsal ventricular ridge	s	Ventricular sulcus separating basal and pallial forebrain
E	Ectostriatum		
Ep	Periectostriatal belt	SGC	Stratum griseum centrale of tectum
GLv	N. geniculatis lateralis pars ventralis thalami		
		Tn	N. taeniae
GP	Globus pallidus	TPO	Temporo-parieto-occipital zone
H	Hippocampal region	TSM	Tractus septo-mesencephalicus
HA	Hyperstriatum accessorium	Va	Vallecula
HD	Hyperstriatum dorsale	X	Area X in LPO/PA
HIS	—— intercalatus superior		
HOM	Tractus occipitomesencephalicus pars hypothalami		
HV	—— ventrale		
HVc	—— —— caudale		

use the nomenclature of Ariëns Kappers, it should be emphasized that the only portion of the avian telencephalon now thought to be truly comparable with the mammalian striatum in terms of phyletic ancestry, anatomical connections, and neurochemistry is the paleostriatal complex (Källén, 1962; Karten and Dubbeldam, 1973).

The prominent bulge on the dorsal and anterior aspect of the avian telencephalon is known as the wulst. This region originates from the D2 zone of Fig. 1 and includes the hyperstriatum dorsale (HD), hyperstriatum intercalatus superior (HIS), and hyperstriatum accessorium (HA). A major portion of the wulst is a visual projection area related to the striate cortex of mammals (Cuénod, 1974; Karten *et al.,* 1973; Revzin, 1969; Pettigrew and Konishi, 1976). Ascending projections to this area arise from a nuclear complex of the anterior dorsolateral thalamus, a region comparable to the dorsal lateral geniculate nucleus of mammals. Projections from the visual wulst descend down the medial hemispheric wall as a component of the tractus septo-mesencephalicus (TSM), terminating in a variety of brainstem visual nuclei. While the mammalian equivalents of the nonvisual wulst are uncertain, it would appear that both "limbic" and somato-motor components exist (Karten *et al.,* 1973). Inputs to these latter regions arise from medial and

Table II. Proposed Origins and Mammalian Homologies of Some Avian Forebrain Nuclei

Structure (Ariëns Kappers)	Embryological derivatives: System of Kuhlenbeck	Embryological derivatives: System of Källén	Presumed mammalian homologies	
N. lateralis septi	{B3 + B4}	a }	Septal nuclei	Basal forebrain
N. medialis septi		bm + cm }		
N. accumbens	B2	$b^{I} + b^{II} + c_v^{II}$	N. accumbens	
N. basalis	D1	c^{I}ext	VPM (thalamus)	
Paleostriatum primitivum	B2 + hypothalamus	c^{I}int	Globus pallidus	
Paleostriatum augmentatum	B1 + B2	{c^{I}ext + c^{II}d}	Caudate–putamen	
Archistriatum mediale, posterior + n. taeniae			Amygdala	
Ectostriatum	D1	{d_1^{III}}	?Layer IV cells, extrastriate cortex	Neocortex
Archistriatum anterior, intermediale, dorsale	D1		?Layer V cortical efferents	
Neostriatum	D1	d_v^{III}	?Layer IV cells, auditory cortex	
Field L	D1	d_v^{III}		
Hyperstriatum ventrale	D1	$d_{d'}^{III}$		
Hyperstriatum dorsale	D1 }	$d_{d''}^{III}$ }	Parts of striate cortex; also somatomotor + limbic elements	
Hyperstriatum intercalatus superior	D2 }			
Hyperstriatum accessorium	D2 }	$d^{I} + d^{II}$	Presubiculum, cingulate + ?	Paleocortex
Area parahippocampalis	D3 }			
Hippocampal region	D2 }		Fascia dentata + cornu ammonis	

caudal nuclei of the dorsal thalamus (Powell and Cowan, 1961; Karten, 1965*a*; Hunt and Webster, 1972). Descending projections from nonvisual wulst also course down the medial hemispheric wall, forming in the brainstem a medial division of the bird's pyramidal tract (Fig. 2a) (Karten *et al.*, 1973).

Pallial structures below the wulst derive from the D1 zone of Fig. 1. Certain nuclei of this complex receive sensory-specific projections from the thalamus (E, L), while another portion projects out of the telencephalon (A). Interposed between the sensory and motor areas is a complex region (N, HV) whose connections are

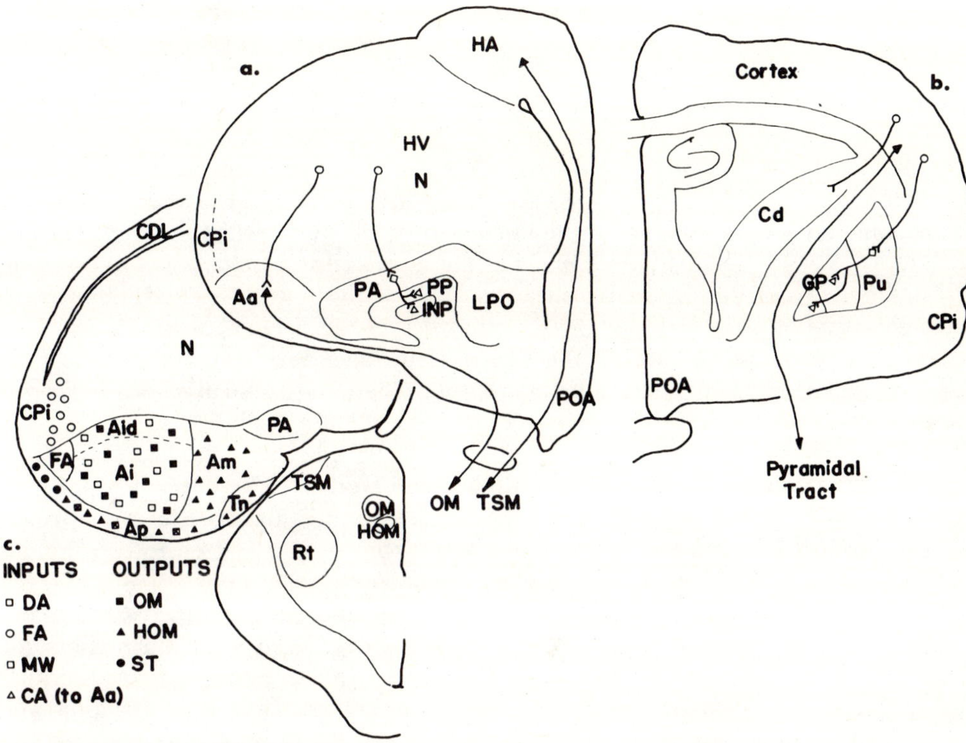

Figure 2. a,b: Origins of somatomotor efferents in birds and mammals. a: In birds the hyperstriatum ventrale (HV) and neostriatum (N) project on two efferent zones: the paleostriatum augmentatum (PA) and the archistriatum (anterior division, Aa, shown in figure). PA projects on the paleostriatum primitivum (PP) and the intrapeduncular nucleus (INP), a projection equivalent to the projection in mammals (b) from caudate-putamen (Pu) to the globus pallidus (GP). Birds' PP-INP and mammals' GP give rise to the descending "extrapyramidal" pathway, the ansa lenticularis. Pyramidal tract efferents in mammals (b) arise from layer V cells in neocortex; the comparable efferent pathway in birds arises from two sources: the hyperstriatum accessorium (HA), which projects out by way of the tractus septomesencephalicus (TSM), and the archistriatum, which sends its efferents out by way of the occipitomesencephalic tract (OM). From Karten and Dubbeldam (1973). c: Subdivisions of the archistriatum. Am, Ap, and Tn project to the hypothalamus by way of the tr. occipitomesencephalicus pars hypothalami (HOM); these regions appear to be equivalent to the mammalian amygdala. Aa (not shown), Ai, and Aid are the somatomotor portions of the archistriatum. Their input comes from the contralateral archistriatum via the anterior commissure (CA), from the medial hemispheric wall (MW), and from overlying N and HV via the tractus dorsoarchistriaticus (DA). OM, the lateral portion of birds' pyramidal tract, originates only in somatomotor portions of the archistriatum. From Zeier and Karten (1971).

all intrinsic to the telencephalon. Nauta and Karten (1970) have suggested that, in the development of mammalian neocortex, the different zones of D1 origin might become laminated with each other to become the various layers of a cortical region associated with thalamic input, extratelencephalic output, and intrinsic connections.

One portion of birds' nonlaminar pallium, the ectostriatum, is the telencephalic projection zone of the elaborate visual pathway which arises in the optic tectum (Karten and Hodos, 1970). Visual information from deep tectal neurons projects on the nucleus rotundus thalami (Rt), which in turn projects on the ectostriatum. The organization and physiology of this system suggest that it is comparable with the pathway in mammals from retina to superior colliculus to the latero-posterior-pulvinar complex of the thalamus and then on to extrastriate cortex (Karten, 1969; Nauta and Karten, 1970; Revzin, 1970). On this basis the ectostriatum would seem to be homologous with the thalamorecipient cells in layer IV of extrastriate cortex.

The anatomical organization of birds' auditory system in many respects parallels that of the tectofugal visual pathway. Ascending auditory information from the cochlear nuclei terminates primarily on the nucleus mesencephali lateralis pars dorsalis (MLd), the birds' inferior colliculus (Karten, 1967). MLd then projects to a thalamic nucleus medial to Rt, the nucleus ovoidalis (Ov), which in turn sends its efferents to field L (Karten, 1968). Like the ectostriatum, field L is a deep-lying, differentiated portion of the neostriatum. The equivalence of field L neurons to thalamorecipient cells in layer IV of auditory cortex has been proposed (Karten, 1969). Tactile responses within the neostriatum have also been reported (Delius and Bennetto, 1972; Erulkar, 1955), although ascending tactocutaneous pathways to the telencephalon have not been demonstrated anatomically.

The sensory-specific zones send their outputs into the complex web of the surrounding neo- and hyperstriatum (Karten and Hodos, 1970; L. Leibler, personal communication). These latter two areas neither receive inputs from, nor project out to, lower brain centers. Instead, efferents from N and HV go to two regions of the telencephalon which do give rise to major extratelencephalic pathways: the archistriatum and the paleostriatal complex (Zeier and Karten, 1971; Karten and Dubbeldam, 1973). The paleostriatal complex is organized very much the same way as the basal ganglia of mammals. Efferents from this region form the ansa lenticularis, an "extrapyramidal" pathway projecting to a variety of thalamic and subthalamic nuclei (Karten and Dubbeldam, 1973). Pathways arising from certain areas of the archistriatum, on the other hand, resemble a portion of the mammalian pyramidal tract. Efferents from archistriatum anterior (Aa), archistriatum intermedium (Ai), and archistriatum intermedium dorsalis (Aid) form the occipitomesencephalic tract (OM) (Fig. 2b), a pathway projecting to a variety of di- and mesencephalic centers, motor nuclei, and the medial reticular formation down through spinal levels. Figure 2 summarizes the proposed relationship between the pyramidal tracts of mammals and birds. In mammals the pyramidal tract arises from layer V cells in neocortex, while in birds the comparable pathway originates in cells in the wulst (via the TSM) and from portions of the archistriatum (via OM).

Medial and posterior components of the archistriatum (Am, Ap) are equivalent to the amygdala of mammals. These regions, perhaps together with the nucleus taeniae, project directly to lateral hypothalamus by way of the tractus occipitomesencephalicus pars hypothalami (Zeier and Karten, 1971) (Fig. 2b). Another pathway to hypothalamus arises in the lobus paralfactorius (LPO), a medial "limbic" portion of the paleostriatal complex (Karten and Dubbeldam, 1973).

Considerable differences in the degree of telencephalic development exist among avian species. As shown in the studies of Stingelin, the index of telencephalization, the ratio between the weights of the cerebral hemispheres and the brain stem (minus cerebellum and optic tectum), varies among birds by a factor of 10, being equal to 3 in the chicken and 28 in parrots (Portmann and Stingelin, 1961). In general, this ratio appears to roughly correlate with informal notions about species' relative behavioral complexity and plasticity, as well as with their performances on certain formalized problem-solving tasks (Stettner, 1974). Tremendous species variability also exists in the relative development of the different telencephalic cell masses. The owl shows an enormous dorsal and frontal expansion of the wulst; cross sections through this structure in the owl reveal a pattern of lamination which resembles mammalian neocortex; in the chick or pigeon this region is only weakly differentiated (Karten *et al.,* 1973). The parrot, on the other hand, shows a marked proliferation of neostriatum and hyperstriatum ventrale. The owl and the parrot are thought to reflect extremes in two divergent lines of avian brain evolution (Fig. 3) (Portmann and Stingelin, 1961).

Before proceeding with the behavioral effects of various telencephalic lesions, a cautionary note would seem to be in order. The general objectives of lesion studies are to discover the functional contributions of specific brain structures "by subtraction," and to elucidate the constituent subroutines of behavior. It must be remembered, however, that normal functioning reflects an intricate set of feedback loops, summations, facilitations, and inhibitions among brain elements. While it is tempting to assign a function to a region whose ablation results in the loss of that capacity, this must be viewed with caution. Even for sensory or motor pathways, interpretation of the behavioral losses which result from lesions is not straightforward. For example, studies in both cat (Sprague, 1966) and pigeon (Hodos and Bonbright, 1975) have shown that while lesions in one element of the visual system may result in a very severe behavioral deficit, a second lesion elsewhere can nearly restore normal function. Such results indicate that one effect of a lesion can be to enhance the inhibition on some remote center, which might subsequently be alle-

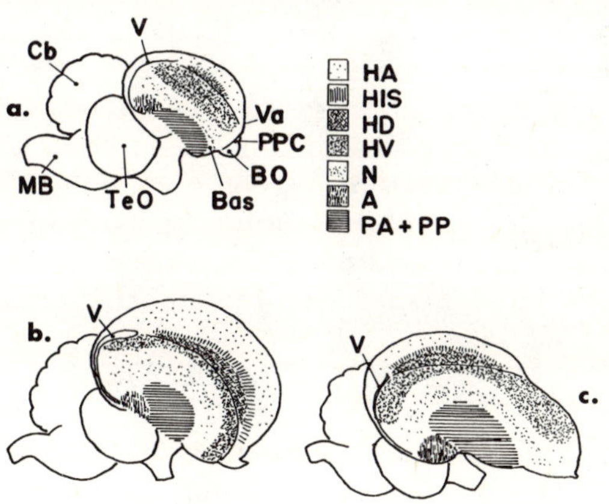

Figure 3. Parasagittal sections through (a) a primitive avian hemisphere (pigeon) and (b,c) two evolved avian hemispheres (owl and parakeet). Sections show the structural evolution of the forebrain and the two possible types of front formation: dorsal front formation in b (increased sagittal elevation) and basal front formation in c (increased frontal neostriatum, N, and hyperstriatum ventrale, HV). A, archistriatum; Bas, n. basalis; BO, olfactory bulb; Cb, cerebellum; HA, hyperstriatum accessorium; HD, hyperstriatum dorsale; HIS, hyperstriatum intercalatus superior; MB, medullary bulb; PPC, prepyriform cortex; TeO, optic tectum; Va, vallecula; V, ventricle. From Portmann and Stingelin (1961).

viated by an appropriate second lesion (Sprague, 1966; Hodos and Bonbright, 1975). In such a case it would have been erroneous to assume that the function lost after the first lesion was "controlled" by that structure.

For those structures having highly complex and still undefined connections, behavioral effects of lesions are even more difficult to interpret. In addition to the aforementioned considerations, a great multiplicity of other factors could account for an observed behavioral deficit: e.g., motivational changes, loss of proper context for information processing, loss of proper affective concomitants, or loss of access to appropriate skeletal and motor centers. Experimentation is often done in a very narrow context, and we are frequently left to determine the nature of a deficit from an animal's performance on one particular task.

Yet, despite these problems, it is probably fair to say that some of our most fundamental notions on the significance of various brain structures derive from lesion studies. When properly combined with neuroanatomical and neurophysiological knowledge, such studies provide an invaluable tool for understanding brain–behavior relationships.

III. Bilateral Hemispherectomy

If one views each telencephalic nucleus as a distinct, specialized entity, total removal of the forebrain hemispheres might then seem to be a rather crude and fruitless approach to understanding the functional organization of the brain. Yet if the various cell groups represent constituent elements subserving some more global capacity, decerebration might then provide insight into holistic properties of the telencephalon. Bilateral hemispherectomies were performed by numerous investigators of the nineteenth and early twentieth centuries, and to some extent this did help contribute to the formulation of coherent notions about telencephalic function.

While reflexive behaviors survive decerebration, spontaneous activity level and responsiveness to external stimuli are depressed. Bilateral hemispherectomy in the pigeon initially results in a sleeplike state. After a short recovery period, the animal, when forced to walk about, exhibits normal equilibrium, guides itself tactually and visually, and can even fly about without hitting obstacles if thrown in the air (Åkerman *et al.,* 1962; Ten Cate, 1965). Eating and drinking are diminished, although reflexive swallowing of food placed in the back of the beak remains. Loud noises cause flinching, but less intense ones do not. Foot shock does not elicit an orienting reaction except when presented repeatedly. Diencephalic stimulation, normally capable of eliciting various well-organized motivated behavioral sequences, also produces activation in the decerebrate bird; however, such behavior is never directed toward appropriate objects, and consummatory acts do not occur (Åkerman *et al.,* 1962).

Studies by Rogers (1922) most clearly demonstrate the effects of bilateral hemispherectomy on behavioral patterns that require learning. Following such surgery, isolated elements in the chain of behaviors connected with mating might still appear, but these are improperly put together and are elicited by inappropriate cues. Courtship displays or the movement of the hen preparing to lay an egg will occur out of context. A hen might ignore the egg she has just laid, and a sexually excited male will ignore a receptive female. Rogers points out that the proper performance of these behaviors requires a learned association between environmental cues and appropriate behavioral acts. The reliance of associative capacities on the integrity of the telencephalon is further suggested by two hallucinatory behaviors displayed by the decerebrate pigeon: these birds will feed at nonexistent objects in the air, and will also stop suddenly, look around, and then begin to "run for dear life." However, fear and aggressivity toward appropriate objects are lost. A comparable dissociation of behavioral elements is seen in the decerebrate falcon: such birds will pounce on a mouse, hold it, but not eat it (Schrader, cited in Pearson, 1972). Decerebrate chicks and pigeons peck at stationary objects but will not seize or swallow food (Martin and Rich, 1918; Tuge and Yueh, 1962; Rogers, 1922).

These studies indicate that while many behavioral capacities are organized at subtelencephalic levels, the proper coordination of such acts, their elicitation by appropriate environmental stimuli, and perhaps even the ability to form new associations may all require the cerebral hemispheres.

The control that the telencephalon exerts over lower centers would appear to be both a maturational and an evolutionary phenomenon. In neonatal chicks decortication does not have nearly so devastating an effect as in adults; more spontaneous activity is seen and reactivity levels are less impaired (Martin and Rich, 1918). In pigeons decortication in the neonate allows classical conditioning still to take place, a capacity that is lost following comparable surgery in the adult (Tuge and Yueh, 1962). Thus corticalization of function may develop only with time, with early behavioral patterns perhaps being carried out autonomously at lower levels. And, in comparing different species, hemispherectomy or archistriatal lesions in parrots result in much more severe deficits than does similar surgery in ducks, chickens, or pigeons (Kalischer, 1905; Phillips, 1968). These results imply that the degree to which lower centers rely on descending telencephalic control for their functioning may increase with the evolution of the forebrain hemispheres.

IV. Lesions of the Tectofugal Visual Pathway

Much of avian behavior is visually dominated, and the central pathways associated with visual function are correspondingly extremely elaborate. The retina projects to many portions of the di- and mesencephalon, including nucleus geniculatis lateralis pars ventralis (Glv), nucleus lentiformis mesencephali, the pretectal region, nucleus ectomammillaris, hypothalamus, the OPT complex of the anterior dorsolateral thalamus, and the optic tectum. The last two regions receive the most massive retinal inputs and give rise, in turn, to two major, anatomically distinct visual pathways which ascend to the telencephalon: the thalamofugal pathway to the wulst and the tectofugal pathway to the ectostriatum.

The bird's optic tectum is an enormously elaborate structure. Cells in the superifical tectal layers receive the retinal input, while cells lying at various depths within the stratum griseum centrale (SGC) give rise to several efferent channels. Subdivisions of nucleus rotundus thalami (Rt) and the adjacent nucleus triangularis receive input from the different tectofugal channels; these various subdivisions of

Rt in turn project to their own characteristic regions of the ectostriatum (E) (Benowitz and Karten, 1976*a*; Karten and Hodos, 1970; Karten and Revzin, 1966). Cells in the tectal SGC, in Rt, and in E have highly complex response characteristics (Granda and Yazulla, 1971; Revzin, 1970), indicating that visual information in the tectofugal system has already undergone a good deal of transformation prior to

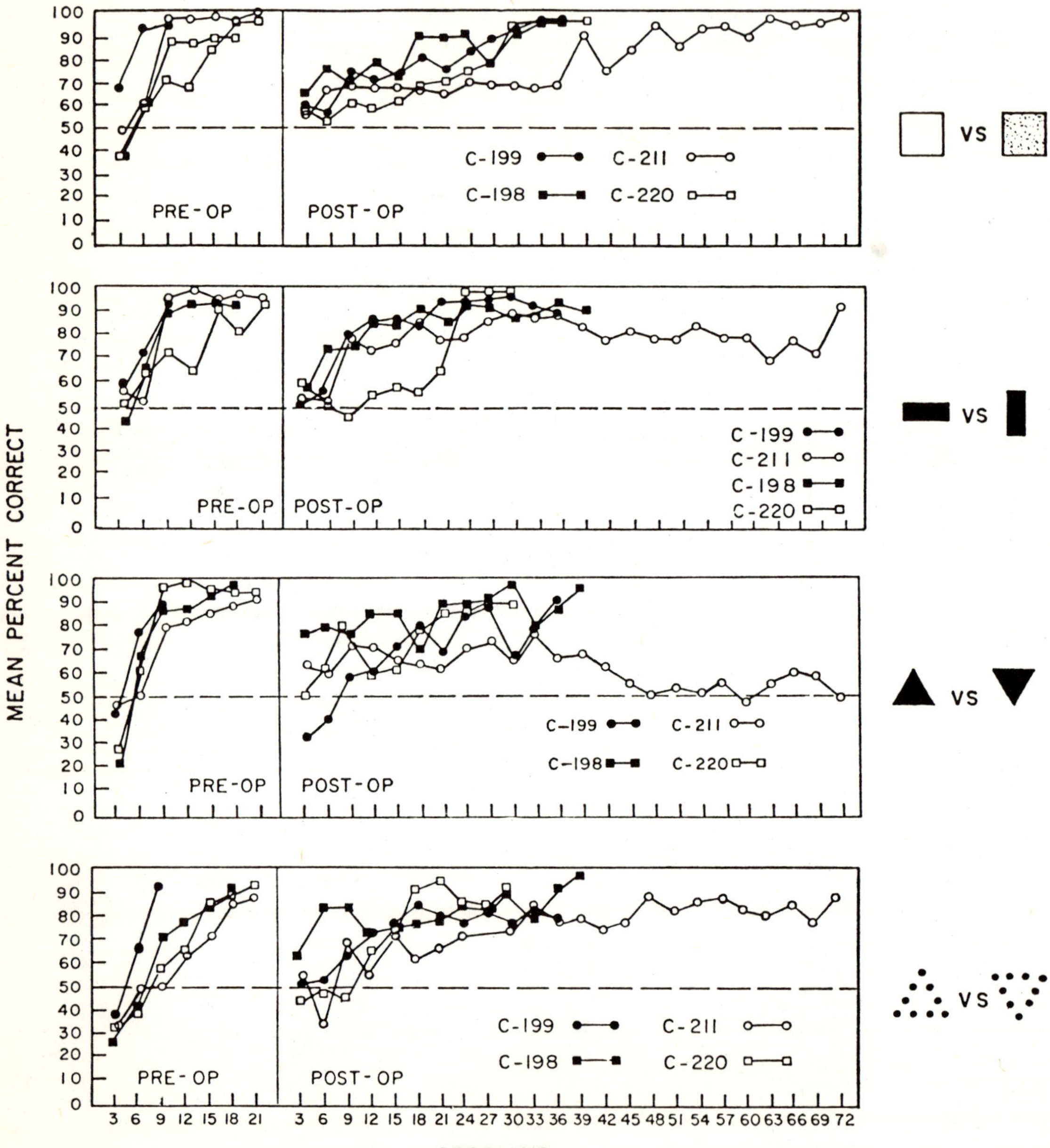

Figure 4. Effects of ectostriatal lesions on four different discrimination tasks. Percent correct responses are plotted against the session number (24 trials per session) for four pigeons suffering extensive ectostriatal damage. From Hodos and Karten (1970).

attaining the telencephalic level. Subsequent processing beyond the ectostriatum and its surrounding belt zone may occur in the complex associative web of the overlying hyperstriatal structures (Karten and Hodos, 1970).

Lesions of the ectostriatum severely disrupt pigeons' capacity for visual learning. Even the simplest of visual discriminations are lost, and subsequent relearning takes up to twice as long as the initial acquisition (Hodos and Karten, 1970). Both intensity and pattern discriminations suffer (Fig. 4), with the severity of the deficit varying with the amount of ectostriatum removed. Comparable deficits result from lesions of the tectofugal visual pathway at the diencephalic level. Acquisition of new tasks is severely affected (Hodos and Fletcher, 1974); brightness and pattern discriminations that had been learned prior to surgery are completely lost following destruction of Rt, with relearning taking up to 2–3 times as long as the initial acquisition (Hodos and Karten, 1966). Although presurgically acquired color discriminations are also lost following Rt damage, relearning proceeds as rapidly as the initial preoperative acquisition (Hodos, 1969).

While these results clearly demonstrate the importance of tectofugal visual structures, the nature of the observed deficits is not obvious. The fact that the animal continues to peck at the response keys, to drink, and to eat after surgery, all indicate that a good deal of behavior governed by learned visual associations remains intact. Why the pigeon's differentiation of the discriminanda used in the formal experiment should be particularly disrupted is hard to understand. Perhaps the deficit is related to the complexity of the operant training procedure rather than to a visual loss *per se*: conceivably, the deficits might appear less severe if differential cardiac conditioning were used instead of an operant situation to assess the effect of the lesion. Cohen and Trauner (1969) in fact report that classical conditioning to whole-field illumination is not impaired after ectostriatal damage; unfortunately, however, these authors were unable to obtain a differential conditioned response in either control or ectostriate birds.

The eventual mastery of discriminations which takes place after tectofugal damage can be accelerated by also lesioning the nucleus GLv (Hodos and Bonbright, 1975). This suggests that Rt lesions may be increasing the inhibitory influences on other important visual structures, an effect that can be reversed (i.e., disinhibited) by lesioning the GLv as well. This observation serves as a reminder that the various elements of the visual system interact with each other in a complex fashion, and that the deficits which result from a given lesion do not necessarily lead one to correctly conclude the functional contributions of that structure. Lesions of GLv alone produce no noticeable visual defects, nor do lesions of several other brain stem visual structures: nucleus lentiformis mesencephali, area pretectalis, and nucleus ectomammillaris. Damage to the OPT complex, does, however, result in visual deficits to be described in the next section.

V. Thalamofugal Visual Pathway and Wulst

The second principal terminus of retinal fibers in the brain stem is a complex of nuclei in the anterior dorsolateral thalamus, an area collectively called the regio opticus principalis thalami (OPT). The nuclei lateralis anterior and dorsolateralis anterior pars dorsolateralis (DLLd) receive the heaviest retinal input, with a more modest one going to dorsolateralis anterior pars magnocellularis and dorsolateralis anterior pars ventrolateralis (DLLv) (Karten *et al.,* 1973; Cowan *et al.,* 1961; Mihailovic *et al.,* 1974; Meier *et al.,* 1974). DLLv projects on a particular lamina of the ipsilateral wulst, while DLLd sends its afferents by way of the dorsal supraoptic decussation (DSOD) to a different layer of the contralateral wulst (Perisic *et al.,* 1971; Karten *et al.,* 1973; Meier *et al.,* 1974). Unit recordings show that cells in the wulst have tuning characteristics extremely similar to those of the cat's striate cortex (Pettigrew and Konishi, 1976; Revzin, 1970).

Lesion studies generally show the pigeon's thalamofugal visual pathway to be much less critical than the tectofugal pathway for the performance of discriminative conditioning. Simple brightness or pattern discriminations acquired presurgically show almost no losses after lesions of the wulst or OPT (Hodos *et al.,* 1973; Fig. 5). Pritz *et al.* (1970) report no losses for a presurgically acquired color discrimination task following wulst damage, although these authors do report deficits for certain brightness and pattern discriminations. The brightness stimuli used in the latter study differed by a value approaching the operated animal's postsurgical threshold of discriminability (0.40 log unit, cf. 0.86 in Hodos *et al.,* 1973; see also Hodos and Bonbright, 1974), and the pattern discrimination (× vs. +), although not appearing particularly difficult, actually does require a large number of trials to master in the normal pigeon. Thus, while relatively simple discriminations are not affected by wulst damage, more subtle discriminations are impaired. This observation is supported by studies combining unilateral lesions of the wulst or OPT with transection of the supraoptic decussation (DSO). Because the DSO is the only pathway which

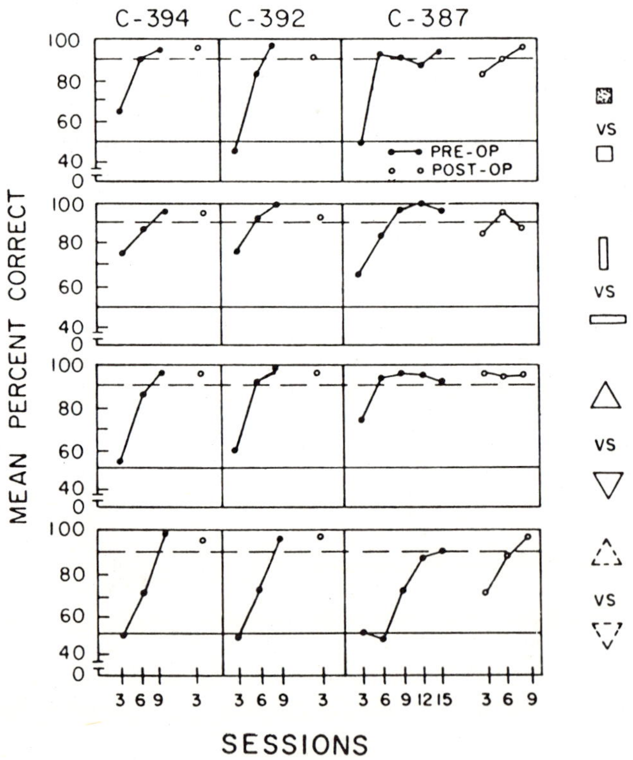

Figure 5. Effects of extensive wulst lesions on retention and relearning of visual discrimination problems. In contrast to the effects of ectostriatal lesions (Fig. 4), little impairment is seen here using the same patterns. From Hodos *et al.* (1973).

mediates bilateral visual representation in pigeon (Meier, 1971), cutting it produces a "split-brain" preparation in which monocularly presented information remains lateralized. When the wulst or OPT is destroyed on one side of the brain and the animal is trained through the contralateral eye, little impariment is seen for a simple visual discrimination (||| vs. ≡). However, using a more difficult pattern (× vs. +), Maier (1974) reports large deficits, a result fully consistent with the results of the two studies which used bilateral OPT or wulst lesions (Fig 6).

VI. Combined Lesions of Tectofugal and Thalamofugal Visual Structures

While damage to either the tectofugal or the thalamofugal pathway alone allows for a good deal of residual visual functioning, lesions which include both produce very extreme deficits. At the thalamic level, lesions of OPT + Rt result in

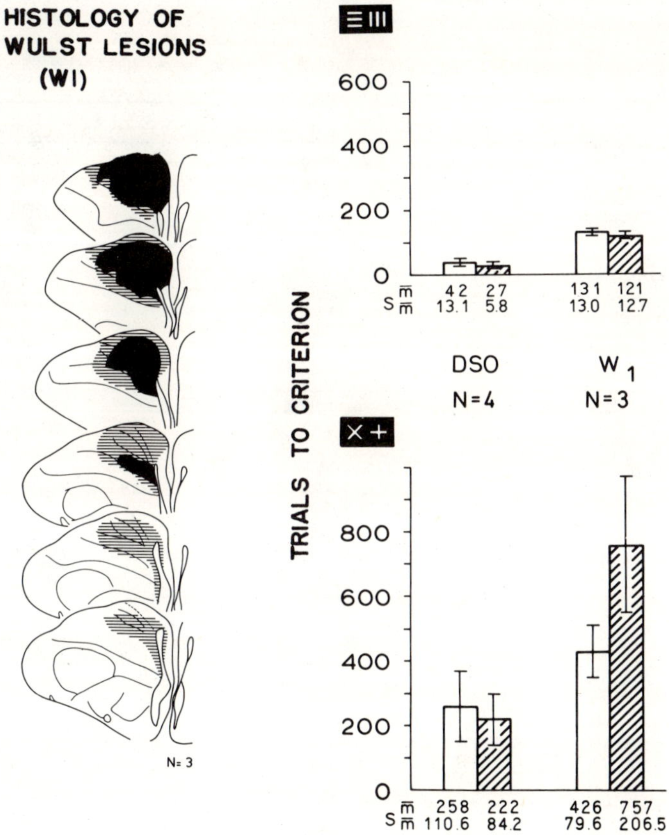

Figure 6. Effects of large unilateral wulst lesions (W1) on the monocular performance of a simple (||| vs. ≡) and a more difficult (× vs. +) pattern discrimination task in split-brain pigeons. While the pattern that is readily acquired presurgically shows no postoperative deficit, the one that had required more trials to acquire preoperatively shows greater postoperative losses. DSO pigeons have dorsal supraoptic decussation cut but no wulst lesions. Mean trials to criterion ($\bar{m}$) and standard errors ($S_{\bar{m}}$) are indicated below bars.

learning impairments far greater than those caused by an equivalent amount of damage to either nucleus alone. In a study by Hodos *et al.* (1973), pigeons suffering extensive OPT + Rt lesions required 60–90 sessions to relearn problems that presurgically had required fewer than 9 (Fig. 7); also, an interference among successively performed discriminations was found. This is in striking contrast to birds with either extensive lesions of the wulst (Fig. 5), which showed almost no impairments on the same problems, or birds with E lesions (Fig. 4), whose deficits, although considerable, were still far less severe. It would seem, then, that each visual pathway alone is functionally adequate for certain visual tasks but that damage to both is devastating. In the study by Hodos *et al.* (1973) the animals were eventually able to reach criterion, a phenomenon attributed to either nontelence-

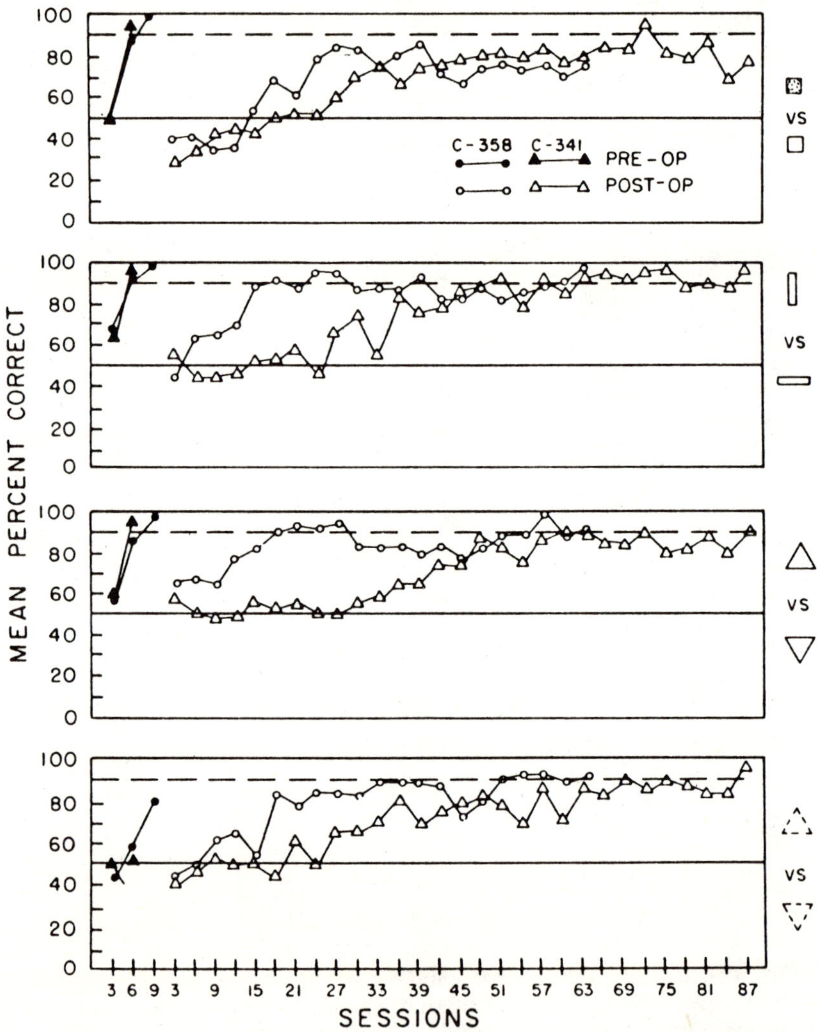

Figure 7. Effects of combined OPT + Rt lesions on retention and relearning. Although mastery of the four discrimination problems is prolonged, it eventually does occur. From Hodos *et al.* (1973).

phalic learning or residual functioning of intact visual structures. In contrast, the studies of Maier (1974) indicate no residual learning capacity in OPT + Rt pigeons. In this case "split-brain" animals with DSO transections and unilateral OPT + Rt destruction were tested monocularly through the eye contralateral to the lesion. Discrimination of the patterns × vs. + and ||| vs. ≡ was never achieved, whereas in split-brain preparations having Rt or OPT damaged alone, learning was always possible (Fig. 8).

Similarly, combined damage of E + wulst obliterates pigeons' capacity to establish a conditioned aversive reaction to a flash of light (Cohen, 1974). Transmission of the conditioned stimulus (the light flash) to the telencephalon can occur adequately via either visual pathway: lesions of either E or the wulst alone have no effect on the conditioning (Fig. 9a,b). However, the loss of even the simplest of visual learning following combined tectofugal + tectofugal visual pathway damage suggests that sensory representation on the telencephalon may be an essential requirement for any associative processes requiring the given modality to take place.

Suprisingly, combined lesions of OPT + Rt do not have the same devastating effects on cardiac conditioning to a light flash (Fig. 9d) as E + wulst lesions. Cohen (1974) suggests that this may indicate some visual inputs into E or wulst from sources other than Rt and OPT. However, none has been demonstrated anatomically. The greater impairments resulting from the telencephalic lesions might instead reflect some additional properties of the higher centers, such as maintaining the activation of other brain processes necessary for the associations to take place. In such a case, while any small amount of visual information from the thalamic nuclei might still allow the telencephalic centers to continue functioning in both specific and nonspecific capacities, destruction of E + wulst would be more serious.

The tectofugal and thalamofugal visual pathways show great dissimilarities in anatomical organization. Tuning properties of cells in the two systems are very different (Revzin, 1969, 1970), as are the behavioral effects resulting from lesions of the two. Yet the functional specializations of each system have remained hard to define. To study this issue further, Hodos and Bonbright (1974) used psycho-

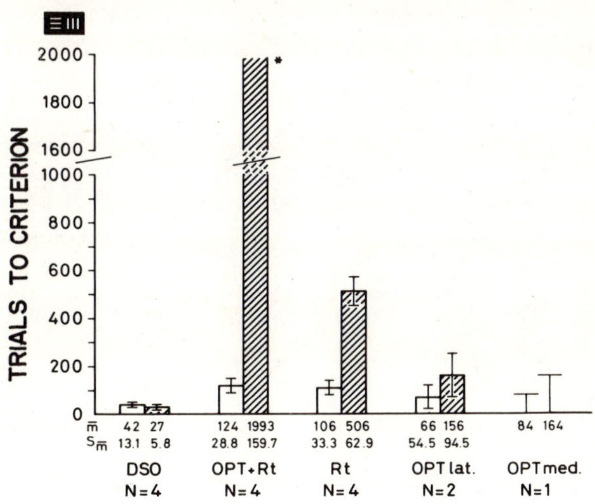

Figure 8. Effects of unilateral thalamic lesions on a pattern discrimination problem in split-brain pigeons. Section of DSO results in no noticeable deficit, nor does destruction of medial or lateral OPT. Rt lesions result in a severe deficit. OPT + Rt lesions render learning impossible. Mean number of trials ($\bar{m}$) and standard errors ($S_{\bar{m}}$) are indicated below bars. From Maier (1974).

physical techniques to examine changes in intensity discrimination thresholds resulting from lesions of OPT vs. Rt. Rt lesions were found to damage the animal's performance on even the coarsest discriminations, yet after extensive retraining the threshold of discriminability returned to preoperative levels. OPT lesions, on the other hand, greatly increased the pigeons' minimal detectable difference threshold, although birds took little time to achieve a new stable performance. One interpretation of these results would be that while the thalamofugal system might include finely tuned detectors for recognizing various stimulus qualities, the orientation of subtle visual properties in a complex behavioral situation might more intimately require tectofugal mechanisms. In contrast to the deficits resulting from OPT lesions, however, Pasternak and Hodos (1977) have recently shown that wulst lesions do allow the pigeon to eventually recover brightness discriminability to near preoperative thresholds. The authors suggest that the greater deficit resulting from the OPT lesions may reflect a more complete damage to the ascending thalamofugal pathway, or perhaps even a destruction of visual structures whose telencephalic targets are other than in the wulst.

VII. Wulst Lesions and Reversal Learning

Although removal of the dorsalmost telencephalon does not greatly impair simple visual discriminations, reversal learning and related tasks have consistently been shown to suffer. In bobwhite quail, lesions of HA, HIS, HD, APH, and CDL have no noticeable effect on the initial acquisition of a simple pattern discrimination, yet when the significance of the stimuli is reversed (i.e., the previously unrewarded choice now becomes the reinforced one), these birds make up to twice the normal

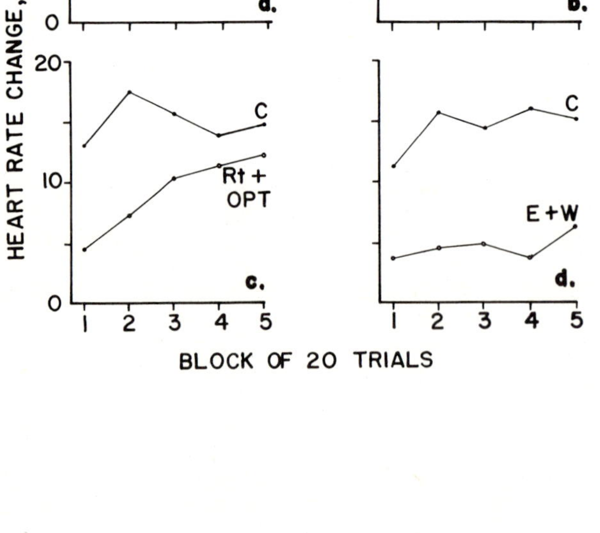

Figure 9. Classical cardiac conditioning to a flash of light paired with footshock: effects of visual system lesions. a,b: Lesions of either the wulst (W) or ectostriatum (E) allow conditioning to proceed normally (C, controls). c: Combined damage to tectofugal and thalamofugal pathways at the thalamic level (Rt + OPT) causes an initially depressed conditioning. However, with repeated pairings, cardiac changes approach the level of controls, d: Combined ectostriatal + wulst (E + W) render learning impossible; after 100 pairings, conditioned cardiac changes attain only one-third the level of controls. From Cohen (1974).

number of errors in learning the new problem. This impairment persists for all subsequent reversals (Fig. 10). Examination of the histology suggests that the severity of the deficit varies with the damage to the "corticoid" regions APH and CDL (Stettner and Schultz, 1967). Deficits specific to reversal learning after dorsal hyperstriatal lesions have also been reported for pattern discrimination in baby chicks (Benowitz and Lee-Teng, 1973) and position learning in pigeons (MacPhail, 1971). These impairments might be viewed as a decreased capacity to alter a prior response tendency or an inability to reinterpret a stimulus once a context has been established. Other behavioral deficits in hyperstriate birds are consistent with these notions. Following wulst lesions, baby chicks' capacity to suppress their innate pecking tendency is diminished despite strong negative reinforcement. Yet if the passive avoidance has been acquired prior to surgery, it is retained postoperatively (Benowitz, 1972; Lee-Teng and Sherman, 1969).

Zeigler (1963) reports that although hyperstriate pigeons show losses in their overall movement, they display a more sustained pattern of activity in an unchanging environment. They move about or explore continuously, showing less habituation than controls. A diminished habituation of defensive vocalization is reported to follow hyperstriatal lesions in the lovebird (Phillips, 1968). And in chickens comparable surgery causes a decreased habituation of head orientation to repeated presentations of an auditory stimulus (Adamo and Bennett, 1967).

Although the neurological basis for these losses is completely unknown, it is interesting to note that phenomenologically they all resemble deficits which follow hippocampal lesions in mammals (Benowitz and Lee-Teng, 1973; MacPhail, 1975). Douglas (1967) and Kimble (1968) have both remarked on hippocampectomized mammals' losses in reversal learning, passive avoidance, and other tasks involving response inhibition or the reinterpretation of a stimulus in the context of prior associations. The importance of the hippocampus for habituation is also well doc-

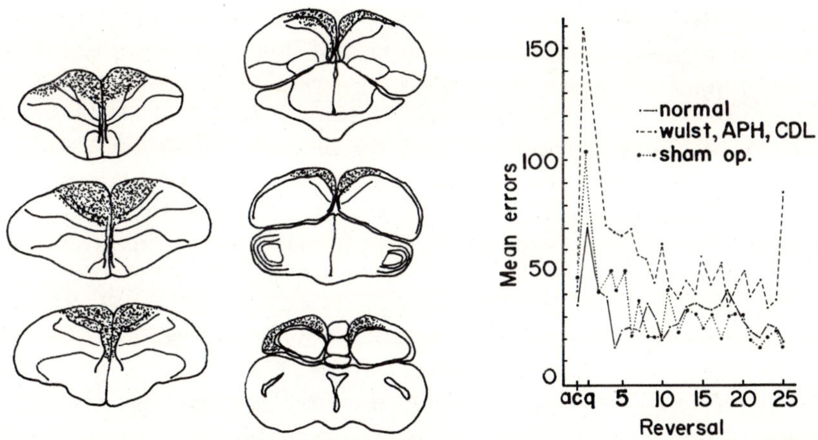

Figure 10. Effects of dorsal telencephalic lesions on reversal learning in the quail. Histology for one case is shown on the left. Following destruction of the wulst, area parahippocampalis (APH), dorsolateral corticoid zone (CDL), and hippocampal region, birds show a dramatic loss in reversal learning; the initial acquisition of the discrimination is not affected, however. Mean errors to criterion for acquisition and for each of 25 successive reversals of the response are shown on the right. From Stettner and Schultz (1967).

umented (Vinogradova, 1975). Yet in the avian studies the hippocampus proper is generally not extensively damaged, although the surgery does include paleocortical and limbic structures which may be connected with the hippocampus (Ariëns Kappers *et al.,* 1936; Benowitz and Karten, 1976*b*; Kuhlenbeck, 1938). The ablated regions also include the visual projection zone in the wulst along with tissue presumed comparable to elements of somatomotor cortex (Karten *et al.,* 1973). The role that each of these cellular populations plays in producing the deficits has not been systemically explored.

Another dramatic deficit seen after wulst lesions is in a delayed matching to sample task (DMTS) (Pasternak, 1977). Here, a stimulus is first presented; after some time interval the animal is given a choice between two stimuli, one of which matches the initial pattern. This can be considered a conditional discrimination, in contrast to conventional pattern discriminations in which the significance of the two stimuli is invariant. Prior to surgery DMTS performance varies as a function of delay time, with some subjects scoring as high as 80% correct for an 8-sec separation between presentations of the initial and the two choice stimuli. After surgery, performance drops to a chance level. While extensive retraining allows for eventual recovery of simultaneous and "0-sec" delay conditions, no recovery is seen for delays of 1 sec or more in subjects suffering substantial wulst losses.

Insofar as these impairments are a function of temporal rather than visual qualities of the stimuli, it seems unlikely that the deficit can be attributed to loss of visual representation alone. Other information-processing capacities of the wulst are likely to be involved, perhaps, as suggested by Pasternak, akin to those important for discrimination reversal.

VIII. Extensive Hyperstriatal Lesions

Lesions which include the hyperstriatum ventrale produce deficits considerably more severe than those resulting from removal of the wulst alone. Although HV contains no primary visual projection areas, incorporation of it in surgery impairs all visual associations that have been examined. In pigeons Zeigler (1963) has shown such lesions to be highly disruptive to both the new acquisition and postoperative retention of even the simplest discriminations. Brightness and pattern problems both suffer, and in some instances discriminations are never mastered. In newly hatched chicks damage to HV greatly augments the deficits caused by more restricted dorsal telencephalic lesions (Benowitz, 1972; Greif, 1976).

In the studies of Rogers (1922) inappropriate patterns of mating and parental behavior could be brought about by lesions of the hyperstriatum. Some birds attempted to mate with inanimate objects, others showed improper courtship. Mothers did not feed their young adequately. However, as long as some of the hyperstriatal complex remained intact, normal behavior could eventually be restored. Rogers suggests that the hyperstriatum is involved in learning to coordinate complex behavioral sequences and in triggering these in response to appropriate stimuli. In the absence of properly learned associations, elements of behavior presumed to be genetic and organized at lower levels are exhibited out of context. This is further seen in hyperstriate pigeons' hallucinatory pecking and escape behaviors that are elicited by, or directed toward, inappropriate objects (Rogers, 1922).

As mentioned earlier, the hyperstriatum ventrale, the region whose inclusion in surgery so severely disrupts learned associations, neither receives direct ascending sensory information from the brain stem nor projects out of the telencephalon (Zeier and Karten, 1971; Karten, 1969 and personal communication). Instead, HV would appear to be a polysensory, nonlemniscal integrative center interposed between the sensory and motor zones of the telencephalon. One might well imagine a region having such properties to be well suited for associative processes. However, whether this region is actually the principal site of plastic mechanisms is not known.

Several studies indicate that the hyperstriatal region may not be essential for forming associations between a light flash and footshock in a classical conditioning situation. Fairly extensive dorsal telencephalic lesions still allow heart rate conditioning to proceed normally, although the respiratory component of the conditioned response (CR) lags behind (Cohen, 1967). Tuge and Shima (1959) report a loss only to the skeletal component of the CR after hyperstriatal lesions. However, both studies found that a differential conditioned response cannot be established in the absence of the hyperstriatum. Thus, while the lesions may damage the capacity for visual recognition, the neural machinery to form associations *per se* is not necessarily confined to the hyperstriatum. It is not until the neostriatum and paleostriatum are also included in surgery that conditioning disappears altogether (Tuge and Shima, 1959). Yet if surgery is done early enough in life, conditioning and even differentiation between two tonal stimuli can take place in the absence of all dorsal telencephalic structures (Tuge and Yueh, 1962).

IX. Interhemispheric Relations

Little communication of learned information appears to take place between the bird's two cerebral hemispheres. In certain instances information that is learned through one eye cannot be retrieved through the other eye, and conflicting behavioral tendencies can be established on the two sides of the brain (Benowitz, 1974; Zeier, 1975). This has been observed in pigeons trained in an appetitive discrimination task through the superior visual field (Levine, 1945) and in chicks trained monocularly either to suppress their aversion to the deep end of a visual cliff apparatus (Zeier, 1970) or to extinguish their learned fear of an aversive lure (Benowitz, 1974). In this latter instance the initial acquisition of the aversive reaction does show interocular transfer (Cherkin, 1970), yet the subsequent monocular extinction conditioning does not. Correspondingly, studies using central brain lesions indicate that while a memory trace for the initial monocularly perceived aversive experience gets laid down in both hemispheres, memory for the subsequent extinction conditioning may be formed only in the hemisphere contralateral to the eye exposed to the unreinforced trials (Benowitz, 1974; Greif, 1976). These results imply that in those cases when interocular transfer does occur, it may be predicated on the formation of bilateral engrams for the monocular experience; when memory for a monocular experience is stored unilaterally this cannot be retrieved on the untrained side. The factors which govern the lateralization of memory are not yet clear, but they may depend on associative or motivational aspects of the experience.

Positive interocular transfer seems to require the supraoptic decussation (Meier, 1971; Cuénod, 1974). The dorsal part of this pathway (DSOD) conveys visual information from the OPT complex to the contralateral wulst (Karten *et al.*, 1973; Meier *et al.*, 1974), while the ventral part (DSOV) projects from the optic tectum to the contralateral GLv and Rt (Benowitz and Karten, 1976; Karten, 1965*b*). Transection of the telencephalic commissures alone does not affect transfer, but cutting the DSO while leaving the forebrain commissures intact abolishes it (Meier, 1971).

X. Archistriatum and Agonistic Behavior

On the basis of neuroanatomical connections, Zeier and Karten (1971) have shown the medial and posterior portions of the archistriatal complex (Am, Ap) to be the bird's equivalent of the mammalian amygdala. Further support for this comparison comes from embryological and physiological investigations (Källén, 1962; Kuhlenbeck, 1938; MacDonald and Cohen, 1973).

The avian amygdala appears to be the prime telencephalic effector of agonistic responses. Stimulation of the medial archistriatum induces escape behavior in mallards, while destroying this area drastically reduces fearfulness (Phillips, 1964). Quite unlike controls, the amygdalectomized animals can be approached and even touched. Similar effects have been obtained from Am lesions in the peach-faced lovebird (Phillips, 1968). In contrast to birds suffering a variety of other brain lesions, medial archistriate lovebirds will continue to eat in the presence of aversive stimuli; they will approach, nibble, and even sit on a waving rod that is normally avoided. A similar "tameness" following archistriatal lesions has also been noted in pigeons (Zeier, 1968, 1971). These results suggest that the archistriatal bird is unable to organize the appropriate agonistic response and/or is simply not "perceiving" the proper significance of the aversive stimuli. Alternatively, the effects of amygdalectomy have been described as an inability to suppress approach responses. Zeier (1971) has shown Am lesions to increase the response rate in a food-motivated key-pecking situation even when this results in a lowered rate of reinforcement.

The recent studies of Cohen (1975) provide the most graphic illustration of the rôle of the "limbic" archistriatum in agonistic behavior. Normal pigeons establish a strong conditioned aversive reaction (CAR) to a light flash associated with foot-shock within 20 pairings. Control lesions, including damage to Ai, Aid, and Aa, produce no deficits. However, pigeons suffering damage to Am and Ap show a very severe performance deficit (Fig. 11a), and transection of the fiber tract issuing from the archistriatum prevents pigeons from ever attaining one-fourth the heart rate change of controls (Fig. 11b). Even the pigeon's initial orienting reaction to light is eliminated by Am/Ap lesions, suggesting that perhaps primitive autonomic responses to external stimuli may also require these structures.

Chicks with ventral posterior lesions of the hemispheres are completely unable to refrain from pecking at an aversive stimulus (Benowitz, 1972). Despite repeated negative reinforcements, the chicks continue to peck as if untrained. While the lesions in these studies were not restricted to one nucleus, destruction of chicks' medial archistriatum alone has since been found to cause the same passive avoidance losses (Benowitz, unpublished).

As in mammals, birds' amygdala projects heavily on the lateral hypothalmus, which, by way of a polysynaptic chain of neurons, ultimately exercises control on sympathetic centers of the medulla (Cohen, 1974; MacDonald and Cohen, 1973). However, the telencephalic pathways by which information about the stimulus reach the amygdala remain undetermined. Furthermore, the initial registration of an aversive experience at the telencephalic level might likewise involve the amygdala, but pathways which might mediate this are also unknown. Our own preliminary retrograde tracing studies indicate that telencephalic projections to the amygdala arise from adjacent archistriatal neurons and from the area parahippocampalis. Ascending projections to Am/Tn arise from the locus coeruleus and ventral tegmental nucleus of Gudden (Benowitz and Karten, unpublished).

In conformity with the conditioning deficits, electrophysiological studies show the medial and posterior archistriatum to be the most cardioactive centers of the telencephalon (MacDonald and Cohen, 1973). Low-level stimulation of these re-

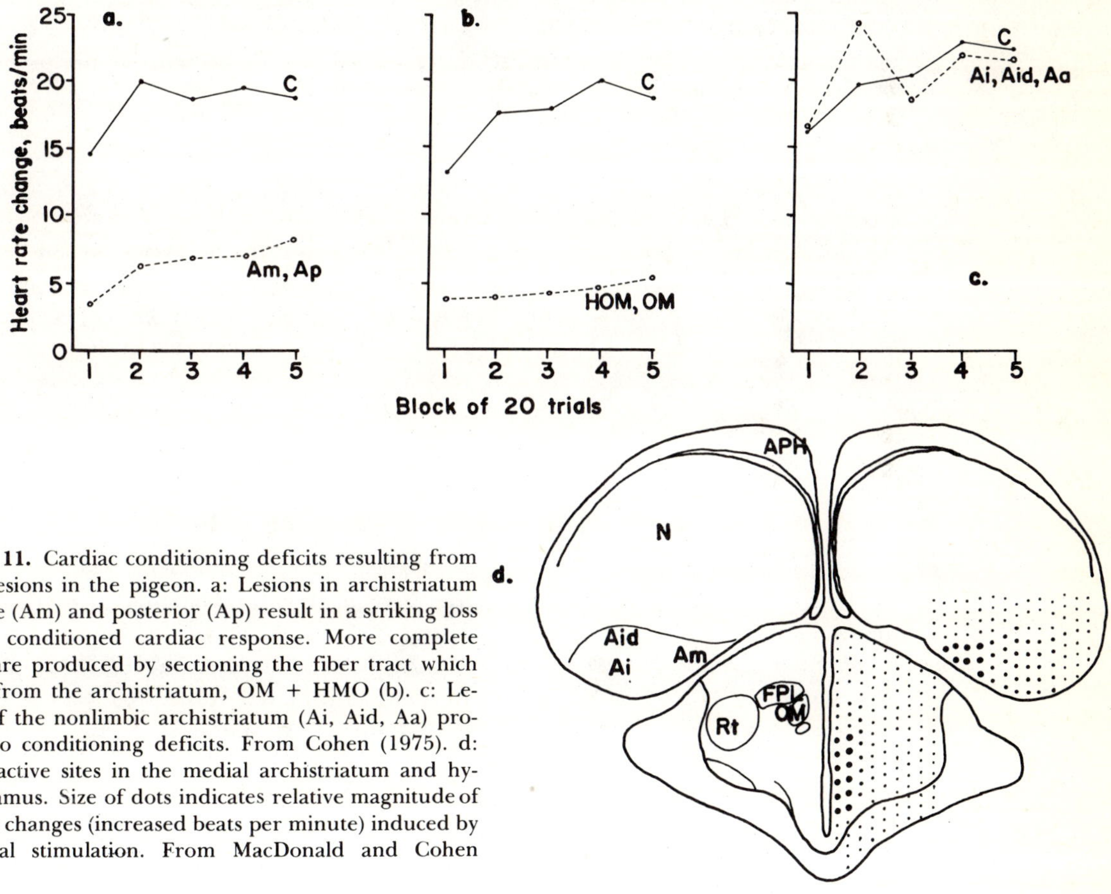

Figure 11. Cardiac conditioning deficits resulting from brain lesions in the pigeon. a: Lesions in archistriatum mediale (Am) and posterior (Ap) result in a striking loss of the conditioned cardiac response. More complete losses are produced by sectioning the fiber tract which issues from the archistriatum, OM + HMO (b). c: Lesions of the nonlimbic archistriatum (Ai, Aid, Aa) produce no conditioning deficits. From Cohen (1975). d: Cardioactive sites in the medial archistriatum and hypothalamus. Size of dots indicates relative magnitude of cardiac changes (increased beats per minute) induced by electrical stimulation. From MacDonald and Cohen (1973).

gions causes hypertension, hyperpnea, and heart rate changes of up to 100–200 beats per minute. Other basal "limbic" centers (i.e., septum, LPO, preoptic area) and the hippocampal–parahippocampal regions also exert some influence on autonomic responses. However, the latter are much less active than the amygdala, requiring higher stimulation currents and producing responses with longer onset latencies and weaker magnitudes.

It is clear from these studies that the medial and posterior archistriatum of birds plays a role essentially identical to that of its mammalian equivalent, the amygdala. In both vertebrate classes this region would appear to be essential for the organization of agonistic reactions in response to external stimuli (Goddard, 1964). Its destruction precludes the proper performance of any aversive reactions, learned or genetic.

In contrast, the anterior, intermediate, and dorsal portions of the archistriatum do not seem to play any significant role in controlling autonomic or emotional responses. These regions are not particularly cardioactive (MacDonald and Cohen, 1973), and their destruction has little effect on autonomic conditioning (Fig. 11c) (Cohen, 1975) or fear-mediated reactions (Phillips, 1964, 1968). In fact, Zeier (1971) reports that destruction of Ai/Aid/Aa actually increases fear and aggressivity.

As mentioned earlier, the nonlimbic archistriatum is derived from embryological tissue whose presumed equivalent in mammals becomes incorporated into neocortex (Källén, 1962; Kuhlenbeck, 1938). Inputs to this region arise from the overlying neo- and hyperstriatum; its efferents, via the tractus occipitomesencephalicus, resemble those of a portion of the mammalian pyramidal tract. On these grounds, the cells in Ai/Aid/Aa have been considered homologous with certain neurons in layer V of mammalian neocortex (Zeier and Karten, 1971; Karten and Dubbeldam, 1973). In parrots (Kalischer, 1905; Phillips, 1968) and canaries (Nottebohm *et al.,* 1976) damage to portions of nonlimbic archistriatum leads to vocalization deficits. Motoric feeding deficits also result from lesions to this region, although motivation for food reinforcment remains (Zeier, 1971; Zeigler *et al.,* 1969 and personal communication). The latter motoric impairment reflects damage to one link in the chain of brain centers controlling feeding behavior to be described next.

XI. Nucleus Basalis and Feeding Behavior

In birds, feeding requires pecking, holding the food at the tip of the beak, manipulating it back with the tongue, and then swallowing it. While the last stage is reflexive, the others have long been known to involve portions of the telencephalon (Rogers, 1922; Flourens, 1824). Recent studies have shown that it is the higher brain centers related to the trigeminal system that are required for feeding behavior.

The principal nucleus of the trigeminal nerve (PrV) receives its innervation from the oral region by way of the Gasserian ganglion. Sensory information from the beak and mouth is then relayed monosynaptically to a distinct region of the anteroventral forebrain, the nucleus basalis (Wallenberg, 1903; Zeigler and Karten, 1973*a*). A severe aphagia is produced by lesioning Pr V, the pathway from Pr V to Bas (QFT, Fig. 12a), Bas itself, and areas which receive the subsequent projections from Bas (Zeigler *et al.*, 1969; Zeigler and Karten, 1973*a,b*). Ascending components of this circuit are illustrated in Fig. 12a.

In the first week or so after Bas lesions in the pigeon, the amount of pecking at grains is greatly diminished. However, in an operant conditioning situation the birds will peck more vigorously for water reinforcement than for food. This differential responsiveness to food vs. water illustrates that it is not pecking *per se* which is suffering most strongly from the lesions but rather the motivation for food. Within 2 weeks, pecking returns to a normal level, but food intake nevertheless remains low. This reflects a deficiency in the bird's ability to manipulate food from the tip of the beak to the back of the throat. Presumably, sensorial representation of the food position is needed for proper coordination of the manipulatory responses. As shown in Fig. 12b, the ratio of grains consumed per grains pecked is equal to unity in controls but remains low in birds suffering Bas lesions.

Thus the aphagia resulting from lesions of Bas (or QFT or Pr V) reflects a transitory motivational deficit together with a more persistent sensorimotor impairment. These deficits closely resemble the so-called lateral hypothalamic syndrome (Epstein, 1967; Teitelbaum and Epstein, 1963). Zeigler and Karten point out, however, that lesions in pigeons' lateral hypothalamus which avoid hitting the ascending trigeminal lemniscus (i.e., QFT) do not produce any aphagia. On the basis of this and parallel experiments done in rats, Zeigler (1974) has suggested that the "hypothalamic syndrome" might in part be a sensory trigeminal deficit.

Bas in turn projects on the "temporo-parieto-occipital" (TPO) region of the caudolateral telencephalon (Zeier and Karten, 1971). The subsequent projections from TPO are still undetermined; yet if its connections parallel those of the adjacent caudal neostriatal cell fields, TPO might be expected to project upon the archistriatum. Lesions of the archistriatum or its efferent pathway, OM, result in an aphagia (Zeier, 1971; Zeigler *et al.*, 1969; Zeigler, personal communication). In contrast to Bas lesions, however, archistriatal lesions only damage the sensorimotor control of feeding behavior without producing any motivational deficits (Zeier, 1971). These birds will perform normally on an operant task for food reinforcement but will still exhibit an inability to properly manipulate the grains of food in the beak. Thus those neurological mechanisms which control goal-oriented behavior appear to involve efferents from Bas other than those projecting to the archistriatum, a seemingly pure motor zone. Another elegant illustration of the motoric functions of the archistriatum comes from studies on the pathways controlling vocalization in the canary (Nottebohm *et al.*, 1976) described in the next section.

In mammals the cells which receive the second order trigeminal input are found in the ventral diencephalon, in nucleus ventralis posterior medialis (VPM). Whether the cells in VPM and Bas have a common phyletic ancestry is unknown. If this were the case, it would indicate a very different migration pattern for the second-order trigeminal projection cells during the embryogenesis of mammals and birds. Also undetermined is the relationship between cells receiving the third-order trigeminal projections in the avian TPO and the cellular populations in somatosensory neocortex receiving a comparable input in mammals.

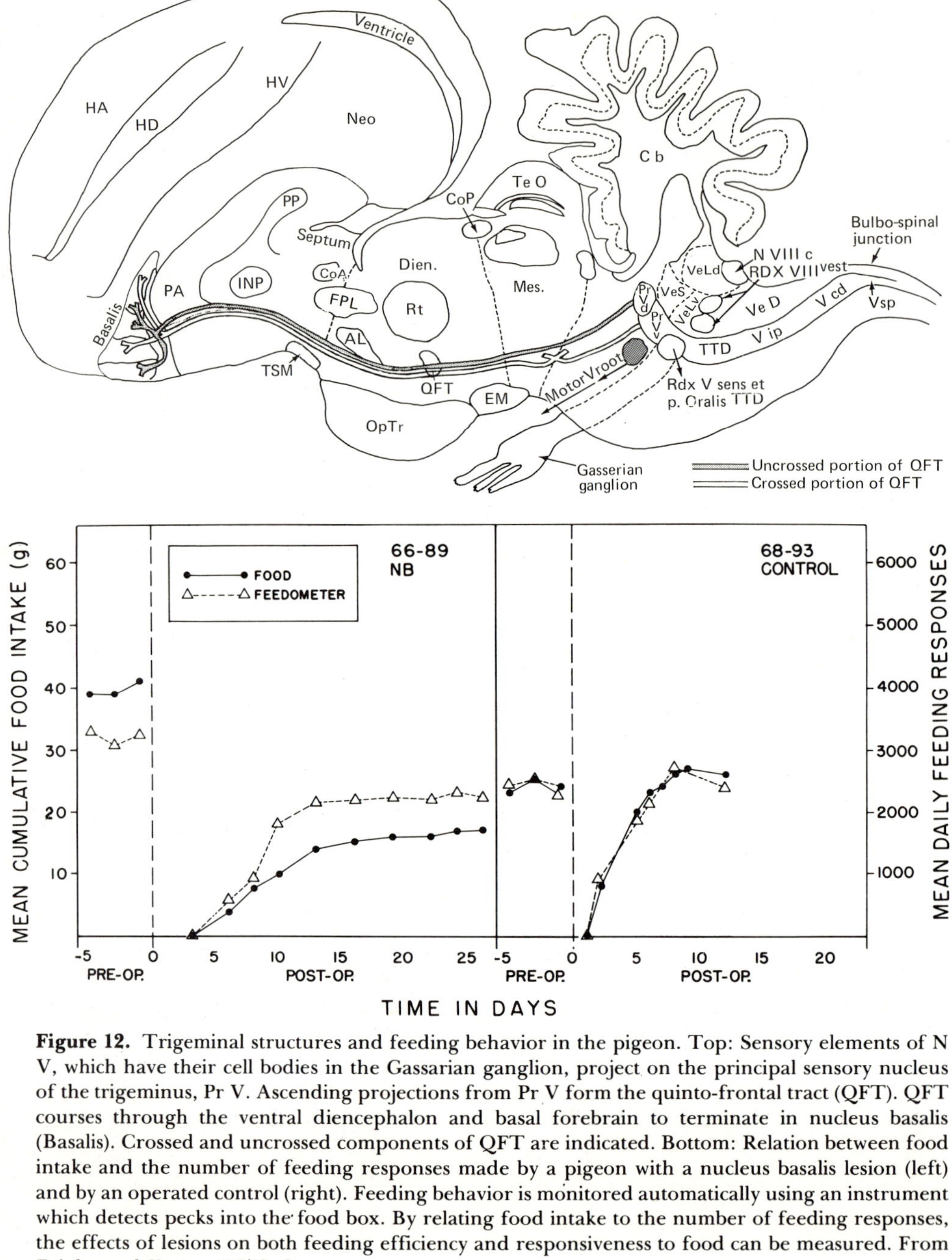

Figure 12. Trigeminal structures and feeding behavior in the pigeon. Top: Sensory elements of N V, which have their cell bodies in the Gassarian ganglion, project on the principal sensory nucleus of the trigeminus, Pr V. Ascending projections from Pr V form the quinto-frontal tract (QFT). QFT courses through the ventral diencephalon and basal forebrain to terminate in nucleus basalis (Basalis). Crossed and uncrossed components of QFT are indicated. Bottom: Relation between food intake and the number of feeding responses made by a pigeon with a nucleus basalis lesion (left) and by an operated control (right). Feeding behavior is monitored automatically using an instrument which detects pecks into the food box. By relating food intake to the number of feeding responses, the effects of lesions on both feeding efficiency and responsiveness to food can be measured. From Zeigler and Karten (1973*a,b*).

As with all other complex, learned behavioral patterns, birds' song production appears to depend on telencephalic mechanisms. The pathways which convey ascending auditory information from the cochlear nuclei to field L in the telencephalon have been described by Karten (1967, 1968) and Boord (1969). By combining anatomical tracing techniques with behavioral testing after brain lesions, Nottebohm *et al.* (1976) have now also delineated specific telencephalic centers which mediate the production of song.

Destruction of a distinct field of cells in the caudal hyperstriatum ventrale (HVc) completely abolishes singing in the canary. As illustrated in the frequency spectrographs of Fig. 13b, bilateral HVc lesions abolish all components of the bird's vocalization. However, postures associated with singing remain intact and can be elicited by the appropriate stimuli.

In earlier studies a bilateral asymmetry in motor control of song had been found: lesions of the left tracheosyringeal branch of the hypoglossal nerve (N XII ts) produce far more serious vocalization deficits than comparable damage on the right side (Nottebohm, 1971). This asymmetry has now been found to also exist at the telencephalic level. In the cases shown in Fig. 13c,d a lesion of the right HVc destroyed only three out of 25 original syllables, slightly modified 13, and left phrase structure intact; a left HVc lesion, on the other hand, destroyed 18 out of 20 syllables and severely upset the phrase structure.

Tracing of the anterograde degeneration which resulted from the HVc lesions showed that this nucleus projects on two other telencephalic areas. One of these is a subnucleus of the archistriatum termed RA, the other a distinct field termed "area X" in the medial "limbic" portion of the paleostriatal complex, LPO. Lesions of area X do not produce any noticeable behavioral changes. Lesions of RA, on the other hand, produce deficits as severe as those resulting from HVc lesions: bilateral destruction abolishes song, and left RA lesions produce far more serious deficits than comparable damage on the right.

RA directly innervates the motor nucleus of song production, n. N XII ts. Other descending projections from RA terminate in the nucleus intercollicularis, the optic tectum, and the medial reticular formation through spinal levels. Area X projects to RA and to a medial thalamic nucleus of unknown associations.

A recent finding of interest is that field L in the canary sends projections directly to HVc and RA, thus providing a direct link between sensory and motor control areas of the telencephalon (Kelley and Nottebohm, 1976).

The connections described by Nottebohm *et al.* (1976) are consistent with a previously noted pattern of telencephalic organization. Earlier studies had shown that HV does not project out of the telencephalon but rather acts on lower centers by way of their connections with two other areas: the paleostriatal complex, which gives rise to the descending "extrapyramidal" pathway, the ansa lenticularis, and the archistriatum, which projects out by way of the "pyramidal" OM (Karten and Dubbeldam, 1973; Zeier and Karten, 1971). The projections from HVc to RA and area X appear to be a subsystem of this general class of neural associations. It would be interesting to explore whether other motoric patterning systems of the telencephalon are also organized in a fashion parallel to the vocalization pathways.

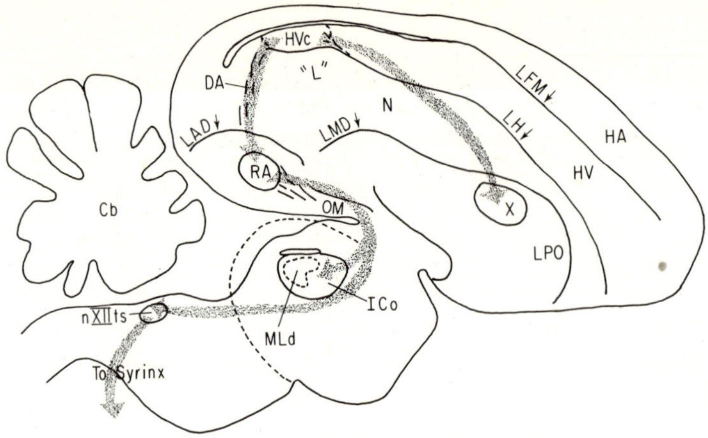
HVc
"L"
DA
LFM
N
LAD
LMD
LH
HA
RA
HV
X
OM
Cb
LPO
ICo
nXIIts
MLd
To Syrinx

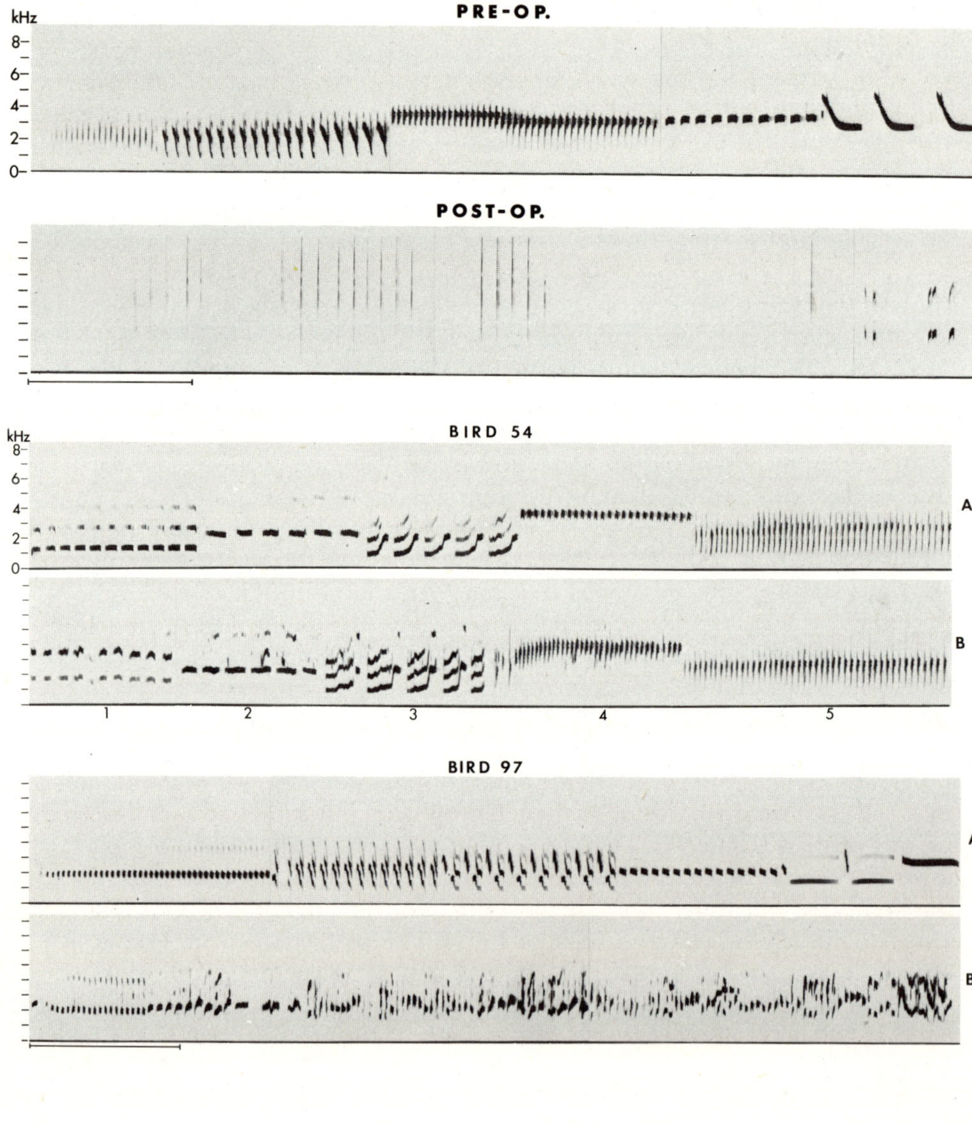
PRE-OP.
kHz
8
6
4
2
0
POST-OP.
BIRD 54
kHz
8
6
4
2
0
A
B
1
2
3
4
5
BIRD 97
A
B

Despite its critical involvement in song production, HVc does not appear to be the "highest" command center controlling singing behavior. First, although all vocal components are lost after HVc or RA lesions, appropriate stimuli may still elicit other postural components characteristic of the canary's singing behavior. Second, while it is apparent that the two halves of the brain act in concert to produce the bird's normal song, no commissural pathways from either RA or HVc appear to exist to account for such coordination. Therefore, while HVc and RA might well be organizers of vocalization patterns, some "higher" control center seems to coordinate the activity of these nuclei on the two sides of the brain and effect vocalization as part of a complex behavioral response to an appropriate stimulus.

XIII. Summary and Conclusions

Studies done more than 50 years ago had suggested that birds' telencephalon mediates complex, well-organized behavioral patterns, particularly those involving learning. While not refuting this basic notion, modern studies have greatly clarified how various neural systems contribute toward the overall pattern of cerebral functioning.

Sensorial representation at the telencephalic level may be essential for associative processes involving a given modality. Combined lesions of the tectofugal plus thalamofugal pathways (i.e., E + wulst) result in complete losses to visual discriminative conditioning. Damage to either pathway alone allows residual functioning to continue, and destruction of both still allows for visual guidance in locomotion and pecking. However, the formation or retrieval of any complex behavioral associations based on vision is lost after destruction of both pathways, an effect resembling "cortical blindness."

Removal of trigeminal representation at the telencephalic level interferes with motivation for food and with performance of the coordinated mandibulatory response needed to feed properly. Whether this sensorimotor association requires any learning would be interesting to know. It would also be worthwhile to examine whether associative behaviors involving other sensory modalities would likewise be lost following the appropriate telencephalic lesions. However, the effects of field L

←

Figure 13. Central control of song in the canary. Top: Schematic sagittal section of the canary brain showing structures and pathways implicated in song control. Hyperstriatum ventrale p. caudale (HVc), the highest structure whose destruction results in loss of song, projects on two other telencephalic centers: n. robustus archistriaticus (RA) and area X in the lobus parolfactorius (LPO). RA projects to nucleus intercollicularis (ICo), a nucleus previously implicated in vocalization, and to the motor nucleus innervating the syrinx, n. N XII ts. Below: Partial segments of song before and after destruction of HVc. Spectrographs show frequency of vocalizations (kiloherz) plotted against time (bar equals 1 sec). Bilateral HVc lesion in bird 48 completely disrupted all aspects of song production. Postoperative recording done 9 months after surgery. In canary 54 destruction of the right HVc allowed good retention of phrase structure: syllables 1, 2, 3, and 5 closely resembled their preoperative versions; syllable 2 was accompanied at times by a second, unrelated sound; syllable 4 was completely altered. Destruction of the left HVc in bird 97 severely disrupted phrase structure; most of the sounds produced were highly variable, and two unrelated sounds occurred frequently. From Nottebohm *et al.* (1976).

lesions on, for example, song learning or auditory discrimination have not yet been studied.

Efferent regions of the telencephalon are critical for effecting certain organized behavioral patterns in response to appropriate stimuli. Lesions of the anterior and intermediate archistriatum damage the performance of certain highly coordinated motoric patterns: Complex vocalizations and mandibulation in feeding suffer, although key-pecking in the performance of an operant task proceeds normally. The limbic portion of the archistriatum, on the other hand, seems to be essential for the organization of agonistic reactions. Following lesions of this region, animals seem tamer and no longer avoid stimuli that normally induce fear. Yet appetitively motivated behaviors proceed normally.

Interposed between sensory and motor regions is the complex, nonlemniscal network of the neostriatum and hyperstriatum ventrale. The neural organization of these regions would suggest that they may be sites of polysensory integration and perhaps even associative plasticity. Lesions which include these areas damage all behaviors based on learned associations: proper coordination of mating, courtship, and discriminative conditioning. While animals can still display many elements of behavior (fleeing, feeding, components of mating), these acts are frequently performed out of context and directed at inappropriate stimuli. Biochemical studies show the principal metabolic changes associated with imprinting in the baby chick to fall in a region which includes HV (Bateson *et al.,* 1973). And comparative morphological studies show that birds having the most diverse behavioral repertoire and greatest associative capacities (i.e., crows, parrots), possess a particularly well-developed HV and N (Portmann and Stingelin, 1961).

All of these observations suggest that it may indeed be valid to speak about general functions which are characteristically telencephalic: While these would not necessarily include motor sequences or responsiveness to stimuli *per se,* the functions of the cerebral hemispheres would seem to encompass complex sensorimotor associations and the adaptive reorganization of behavioral patterns. Toward these themes, sensory, motor, and intermediate components of the telencephalon all seem to be subordinate elements.

The similarity in deficits which result from destroying comparable brain structures in birds and mammals is very striking. (1) Studies in tree shrew (Diamond and Hall, 1969) show that lesions of the striate cortex do not impair simple discriminations, only more complex ones (e.g., embedded patterns); it is not until extrastriate areas (areas 18, 19, inferotemporal) are damaged that general visual learning capacity suffers greatly. Studies in the pigeon reveal comparable relative losses from lesions of the wulst (related to striate cortex) and ectostriatum (presumed equivalent with layer IV cells of extrastriate cortices). (2) With regard to the limbic archistriatum (Am/Ap/Tn), the losses to fearfulness and conditioned aversive reactions are identical to the effects produced by amygdalectomy in mammals (Goddard, 1964). (3) Zeigler (1974) has presented evidence that the feeding deficits which result from sensory trigeminal lesions may account for a good deal of the so-called lateral hypothalamic syndrome in mammals as well as in birds. Such observations suggest that homologous neural populations in the two classes' forebrains may subserve similar functions. For these mechanisms to have been conserved through 300,000,000 years of divergent evolution may well indicate their being essential components of higher functioning.

The advances that have been made toward understanding the functional organization of the avian telencephalon have been considerable. Nevertheless, phenomena such as hierarchically organized patterning of behavior, associative plasticity, and affectivity remain beyond our grasp, both in birds and in mammals. Comparative studies can be a fruitful approach toward understanding these phenomena. While there are many similarities between birds and mammals, there are also great differences, i.e., the dissimilar behavioral repertories and the different intrinsic organization of telencephalic neural populations. Continued comparisons between the two classes promise to reveal general principles of telencephalic functional organization as well as the significance of the two classes' specializations.

ACKNOWLEDGMENTS. I am grateful to Dr. William Hodos for critically reviewing the manuscript, to Mrs. M. A. Taleas for help in preparation, and to the Medical Foundation of Boston for support during the period in which this was written. I wish to thank the following for permission to reproduce figures used in the text: Dr. Hartwig Kuhlenbeck and The Wistar Institute Press (Fig. 1); Drs. Hans Zeier and Harvey Karten, The Wistar Institute Press, and Elsevier Publishing Company (Fig. 2); Academic Press (Fig. 3); Dr. William Hodos and The Wistar Institute Press (Figs. 4, 5, and 7); Dr. Verena Maier (Fig. 6 and 8); Dr. David Cohen, Plenum Press, and The Wistar Institute Press (Figs. 9 and 11); Dr. Lawrence Stettner and *Science* (Copyright, 1967, AAAS) (Fig. 10); Dr. H. Phillip Zeigler and The Wistar Institute Press (Fig. 12); and Dr. Fernando Nottebohm and The Wistar Institute Press (Fig. 13).

XIV. References

Adamo, N. J., and Bennett, T. L., 1967, The effect of hyperstriatal lesions on head orientation to a sound stimulus in chickens, *Exp. Neurol.* **19:**166.

Åkerman, B., Fabricius, E., Larsson, B., and Steen, L., 1962, Observations on pigeons with prethalamic radiolesions in the nervous pathway from the telencephalon, *Acta Physiol. Scand.* **56:**286.

Ariëns Kappers, C. U., Huber, C., and Crosby, E. C., 1936, *The Comparative Anatomy of the Nervous System of Vertebrates, including Man,* Macmillan, New York.

Bateson, P. P. G., Rose, S. P. R., and Horn, G., 1973, Imprinting: Lasting effects on uracil incorporation into chick brain, *Science* **181:**576.

Benowitz, L., 1972, Effects of forebrain ablations on avoidance learning in chicks, *Physiol. Behav.* **9:**601.

Benowitz, L., 1974, Conditions for the bilateral transfer of monocular learning in chicks, *Brain Res.* **65:**203.

Benowitz, L. I., and Karten, H. J., 1976*a*, Organization of the tectofugal visual pathway in the pigeon: A retrograde transport study, *J. Comp. Neurol.* **167:**503.

Benowitz, L. I., and Karten, H. J., 1976*b*, The tractus infundibuli and other afferents to the parahippocampal region of the pigeon, *Brain Res.* **102:**174.

Benowitz, L., and Lee-Teng, E., 1973, Contrasting effects of three forebrain ablations on discrimination learning and reversal in chicks, *J. Comp. Physiol. Psychol.* **84:**391.

Beritov, J. S., 1965, *Neural Mechanisms of Higher Vertebrate Behavior,* transl. and ed. by W. T. Liberson, Little, Brown, Boston.

Boord, R. L., 1969, The anatomy of the avian auditory system, *Ann. N.Y. Acad. Sci.* **167:**186 (Art. 1).

Cherkin, A., 1970, Eye-to-eye transfer of an early response modification in chicks, *Nature* (*London*) **227:**1153.

Cohen, D. H., 1967, The hyperstriatal region of the avian forebrain: A lesion study of possible functions, including its role in cardiac and respiratory conditioning, *J. Comp. Neurol.* **131:**559.

Cohen, D. H., 1974, The neural pathways and informational flow mediating a conditioned autonomic response, in: *Limbic and Autonomic Nervous Systems Research* (L. V. DiCara, ed.), pp. 223–275, Plenum Press, New York.

Cohen, D. H., 1975, Involvement of the avian amygdalar homologue (archistriatum posterior and mediale) in defensively conditioned heart rate change, *J. Comp. Neurol.* **160:**13.

Cohen, D. H., and Trauner, D. A., 1969, Studies of avian visual pathways involved in cardiac conditioning: Nucleus rotundus and ectostriatum, *Exp. Brain Res.* **7:**133.

Cowan, W. M., Adamson, L., and Powell, T. P. S., 1961, An experimental study of the avian visual system, *J. Anat.* **95:**545.

Cuénod, M., 1974, Commissural pathways in interhemispheric transfer of visual information in the pigeon, in *The Neurosciences, Third Study Program* (F. O. Schmitt and F. G. Worden, eds.), pp. 21–29, MIT Press, Cambridge, Mass.

Delius, J. D., and Bennetto, L., 1972, Cutaneous sensory projections to the avian forebrain, *Brain Res.* **37:**205.

Diamond, I. T., and Hall, W. C., 1969, Evolution of neocortex, *Science* **164:**251.

Douglas, R. J., 1967, The hippocampus and behavior, *Psychol. Bull.* **67:**416.

Epstein, A. N., 1967, Oropharyngeal factors in feeding and drinking, in: *Handbook of Physiology*, Sect. 61, Vol. 1: *Alimentary Canal: Control of Food and Water Intake* (C. E. Code, ed.), American Physiological Society, Washington, D.C.

Erulkar, S. D., 1955, Tactile and auditory areas in the brain of the pigeon, *J. Comp. Neurol.* **103:**421.

Flourens, P., 1824, *Recherches Expérimentales sur les Propriétés et les Fonctions du Système Nerveux dans les Animaux Vertébrés,* Vol. 1, Baillière, Paris.

Goddard, G. V., 1964, Functions of the amygdala, *Psychol. Bull.* **62:**89.

Granda, S. M., and Yazulla, S., 1971, The spectral sensitivity of single units in the nucleus rotundus of pigeon (*Columba livia*), *J. Gen. Physiol.* **57:**363.

Greif, K. F., 1976, Bilateral memory for monocular one-trial passive avoidance in chicks, *Behav. Biol.* **16:**453.

Hodos, W., 1969, Color discrimination deficits after lesions of the nucleus rotundus in pigeons, *Brain Behav. Evol.* **2:**185.

Hodos, W., and Bonbright, J. C., Jr., 1974, Intensity difference thresholds in pigeons after lesions of the tectofugal and thalamofugal visual pathways, *J. Comp. Physiol. Psychol.* **87:**1013.

Hodos, W., and Bonbright, J. C., Jr., 1975, Intensity and pattern discrimination after lesions of the pretectal complex, accessory optic nucleus and ventral geniculate in pigeons, *J. Comp. Neurol.* **161:**1.

Hodos, W., and Fletcher, G. V., 1974, Acquisition of visual discriminations after nucleus rotundus lesions in pigeons, *Physiol. Behav.* **13:**501.

Hodos, W., and Karten, H. J., 1966, Brightness and pattern discrimination deficits in the pigeon after lesions in the nucleus rotundus, *Exp. Brain Res.* **2:**151.

Hodos, W., and Karten, H. J., 1970, Visual intensity and pattern discrimination deficits after lesions of ectostriatum in pigeons, *J. Comp. Neurol.* **140:**53.

Hodos, W., Karten, H. J., and Bonbright, J. C., Jr., 1973, Visual intensity and pattern discrimination after lesions of the thalamofugal visual pathway in pigeons, *J. Comp. Neurol.* **148:**447.

Hunt, S. P., and Webster, K. E., 1972, Thalamo-hyperstriate interrelations in the pigeon, *Brain Res.* **44:**647.

Kalischer, O., 1905, Das Grosshirn der Papageien in anatomischer und physiologischer Beziehung, *Abh. Kon. Preuss. Akad. Wiss.* **4(1):**1.

Källén, B., 1951, Embryological studies on the nuclei and their homologization in the vertebrate forebrain, *Kungl. Fysiograf. Sallskapets Handl. N.F.* **62:**1.

Källén, B., 1962, Embryogenesis of brain nuclei in the chick telencephalon, *Ergebn. Anat. Entwicklungsgesch.* **36:**62.

Karten, H. J., 1965*a*, Organization of afferent connections to the thalamus of the pigeon, paper presented at Cajal Club Meeting, Miami Beach, Fla.

Karten, H. J., 1965*b*, Projections of the optic tectum of the pigeon (*Columba livia*), *Anat. Rec.* **151:**369.

Karten, H. J., 1967, The organization of the ascending auditory pathway in the pigeon (*Columba *livia*). I. Diencephalic projections of the inferior colliculus (nucleus mesencephali lateralis, pars dorsalis), *Brain Res.* **6:**409.

Karten, H. J., 1968, The ascending auditory pathway in the pigeon. II. Telencephalic projections of the nucleus ovoidalis thalami, *Brain Res.* **11:**134.

Karten, H. J., 1969, The organization of the avian telencephalon and some speculations on the phylogeny of the amniote telencephalon, *Ann. N.Y. Acad. Sci.* **167:**164 (Art. 1).

Karten, H. J., and Dubbeldam, J. L., 1973, The organization and projections of the paleostriatal complex in the pigeon (*Columba livia*), *J. Comp. Neurol.* **148:**61.

Karten, H. J., and Hodos, W., 1970, Telencephalic projections of the nucleus rotundus in the pigeon (*Columba livia*), *J. Comp. Neurol.* **140:**35.

Karten, H. J., and Revzin, A. M., 1966, The afferent connections of the nucleus rotundus in the pigeon, *Brain Res.* **2:**268.

Karten, H. J., Hodos, W., Nauta, W. J. H., and Revzin, A. M., 1973, Neural connections of the "visual wulst" of the avian telencephalon: Experimental studies in the pigeon and owl, *J. Comp. Neurol.* **150:**253.

Kelley, D. B., and Nottebohm, F., 1976, Projections of field L in the canary, *Serinus canarius, Neurosci. Abstr.* **2:**21 (Society for Neuroscience, 6th Annu. Meet., Toronto).

Kimble, D. P., 1968, Hippocampus and internal inhibition, *Psychol. Bull.* **70:**285.

Kuhlenbeck, H., 1938, The ontogenetic development and phylogenetic significance of the cortex telencephali in the chick, *J. Comp. Neurol.* **68:**273.

Lee-Teng, E., and Sherman, S. M., 1969, Effects of forebrain lesions on acquisition and retention of one-trial learning in chicks, *Proc. 77th Annu. Conv. APA,* pp. 203–204.

Levine, J., 1945, Studies in the interrelations of central nervous structures in binocular vision. I. The lack of binocular transfer of visual discrimination habits acquired monocularly by the pigeon, *J. Genet. Psychol.* **67:**105.

MacDonald, R. L., and Cohen, D. H., 1973, Heart rate and blood pressure responses to electrical stimulation of the central nervous system in the pigeon, *J. Comp. Neurol.* **150:**109.

MacPhail, E. M., 1971, Hyperstriatal lesions in pigeons: Effects on response inhibition, behavioral contrast and reversal learning, *J. Comp. Physiol. Psychol.* **75:**500.

MacPhail, E. M., 1975, The role of the avian hyperstriatal complex in learning, in: *Neural and Endocrine Aspects of Behavior in Birds* (P. Wright, P. G. Caryl, and D. M. Vowles, eds.), pp. 139–162, Elsevier, Amsterdam.

Maier, V., 1974, Effekte unilateraler telencephaler und thalamischer Läsionen auf die monokulare Musterdiskriminations Fahigkeit kammissurotomiertier Tauben, inaugural dissertation, University of Zurich.

Maier, V., Tanaka, M., and Cuénod, M., 1974, Visual deficits in pigeons after unilateral forebrain lesions, *Experientia* **30:**681.

Martin, E. G., and Rich, W. H., 1918, The activities of decerebrate and decerebellate chicks, *Am. J. Physiol.* **46:**396.

Meier, R. E., 1971, Interhemispheric transfer of two-choice discrimination in commissurotomized pigeons, *Psychol. Forsch.* **34:**220.

Meier, R. E., Mihailovic, J., and Cuénod, M., 1974, Thalamic organization of the retino-thalamo-hyperstriatal pathway in the pigeon (*Columba livia*), *Exp. Brain Res.* **19:**351.

Mihailovic, J., Perisic, M., Bergoni, R., and Meier, R. E., 1974, Dorsolateral thalamus as a relay in the retino-wulst pathway in pigeon (*Columba livia*): An electrophysiological study, *Exp. Brain Res.* **21:**229.

Nauta, W. J. H., and Karten, H. J., 1970, A general profile of the vertebrate brain, with sidelights on the ancestry of cerebral cortex, in: *The Neurosciences: Second Study Program* (F. O. Schmitt, ed.), pp. 7–26, Rockefeller University Press, New York.

Nottebohm, F., 1971, Neural lateralization of vocal control in a passerine bird. I. Song, *J. Exp. Zool.* **177:**229.

Nottebohm, F., Stokes, T. M., and Leonard, C. M., 1976, Central control of song in the canary, *Serinus canarius, J. Comp. Neurol.* **165:**457.

Pasternak, T., 1977, Delayed matching performance after visual wulst lesions in pigeons, *J. Comp. Physiol. Psychol.* **91:**472.

Pasternak, T., and Hodos, W., 1977, Intensity difference thresholds after visual wulst lesions in pigeons, *J. Comp. Physiol. Psychol.* **91:**485.

Pearson, R., 1972, *The Avian Brain,* Academic Press, London.

Perisic, M., Mihailovic, J., and Cuénod, M., 1971, Electrophysiology of contralateral and ipsilateral visual projections to the wulst in pigeon (*Columba livia*), *Int. J. Neurosci.* **2:**7.

Pettigrew, J. D., and Konishi, M., 1976, Neurons selective for orientation and binocular disparity in the visual wulst of the barn owl (*Tyto alba*), *Science* **193:**675.

Phillips, R. E., 1964, "Wildness" in the mallard duck: Effects of brain lesions and stimulation on escape behavior and reproduction, *J. Comp. Neurol.* **122:**139.

Phillips, R. E., 1968, Approach–withdrawal behavior of peach-faced lovebirds, *Agapornis roseicolis,* and its modification by brain lesions, *Behavior* **31:**163.

Portmann, A., and Stingelin, W., 1961, The central nervous system, in: *The Biology and Comparative Physiology of Birds,* Vol. 2 (A. J. Marshall, ed.), pp. 1–36, Academic Press, New York.

Powell, T. P. S., and Cowan, W. M., 1961, The thalamic projection upon the telencephalon in the pigeon (*Columba livia*), *J. Anat.* **95:**78.

Pritz, M. B., Mead, W. R., and Northcutt, R. G., 1970, The effects of wulst ablation on color, brightness and pattern discrimination in pigeons (*Columba livia*), *J. Comp. Neurol.* **140:**81.

Revzin, A. M., 1969, A specific visual projection area in the hyperstriatum of the pigeon, *Brain Res.* **3:**246.

Revzin, A. M., 1970, Some characteristics of wide-field units in the brain of the pigeon, *Brain Behav. Evol.* **3:**195.

Rogers, F. T., 1922, Studies of the brain stem. VI. An experimental study of the corpus striatum of the pigeon as related to various types of behavior, *J. Comp. Neurol.* **35:**21.

Sprague, J. M., 1966, Interaction of cortex and superior colliculus in the mediation of visually guided behavior, *Science* **153:**1544.

Stettner, L. J., 1974, The neural basis of avian discrimination and reversal learning, in: *Birds, Brain and Behavior* (I. J. Goodman and M. W. Schein, eds.), pp. 165–201, Academic Press, New York.

Stettner, L. J., and Schultz, W. J., 1967, Brain lesions in birds: Effects on discrimination acquisition and reversal, *Science* **155:**1689.

Teitelbaum, P., and Epstein, A. N., 1963, The role of taste and smell in the regulation of food and water intake, in: *Olfaction and Taste* (Y. Zotterman, ed.), Pergamon Press, London.

Ten Cate, J., 1965, The nervous system of birds, in: *Avian Physiology,* 2nd ed. (P. D. Sturkie, ed.), Comstock Publishing Associates, Ithaca, N.Y.

Tuge, H., and Shima, I., 1959, Defensive conditioned reflex after destruction of the forebrain in pigeons, *J. Comp. Neurol.* **111:**427.

Tuge, H., and Yueh, C. H., 1962, Functional compensation of the somatic and visceral components of the defensive conditioned reflexes after decerebration in young pigeons, *Activitas Nervosa Superior* **4:**275.

Vinogradova, O. S., 1975, The hippocampus and the orienting reflex, in: *Neuronal Mechanisms of the Orienting Reflex* (E. N. Sokolov and O. S. Vinogradova, eds.), pp. 128–154, Lawrence Erlbaum Associates, Hillsdale, N.J.

Wallenberg, A., 1903, Die Ursprung des Tractus isthmo-striatus der Taube, *Neurol. Centr.* **22:**98.

Zeier, H., 1968, Changes in operant behavior of pigeons following bilateral forebrain lesions, *J. Comp. Physiol. Psychol.* **66:**198.

Zeier, H., 1970, Lack of eye to eye transfer of an early response modification, *Nature* (*London*) **225:**708.

Zeier, H., 1971, Archistriatal lesions and response inhibition in the pigeon, *Brain Res.* **13:**327.

Zeier, H., 1975, Interhemispheric interactions, in: *Neural and Endocrine Aspects of Behavior in Birds* (P. Wright, P. G. Caryl, and D. M. Vowles, eds.), pp. 163–180, Elsevier, Amsterdam.

Zeier, H., and Karten, H. J., 1971, The archistriatum of the pigeon: Organization of afferent and efferent connections, *Brain Res.* **31:**313.

Zeigler, H. P., 1963, Effects of endbrain lesions upon visual discrimination learning in pigeons, *J. Comp. Neurol.* **120:**161.

Zeigler, H. P., 1974, Feeding behavior in the pigeon: A neurobehavioral analysis, in: *Birds: Brain and Behavior* (I. Goodman and M. Schein, eds.), Academic Press, New York.

Zeigler, H. P., and Karten, H. J., 1973*a*, Brain mechanisms and feeding behavior in the pigeon (*Columba livia*). I. Quinto-frontal structures, *J. Comp. Neurol.* **152:**59.

Zeigler, H. P., and Karten, H. J., 1973*b*, Brain mechanisms and feeding behavior in the pigeon (*Columba livia*). II. Analysis of feeding behavior deficits after lesions of quinto-frontal structures, *J. Comp. Neurol.* **152:**83.

Zeigler, H. P., and Karten, H. J., 1974, Central trigeminal structures and the lateral hypothalamic syndrome in the rat, *Science* **186:**636.

Zeigler, H. P., Green, H. L., and Karten, H. J., 1969, Neural control of feeding behavior in the pigeon, *Psychon. Sci.* **15:**156.

14

Morphological Correlates of Specialized Elaborations in Somatic Sensory Cerebral Neocortex

JOHN IRWIN JOHNSON, Jr.

I. Introduction

More engaging and frivolous titles for this review might be "Bumps and Barrels, Brains and Behaviors" or "The New Phrenology." As with the Old Phrenology, the subject matter here is the correlation of morphological characters—growth and bumps—with "mental faculties and traits of character," behavioral character, the probabilities of occurrence of specific kinds of actions. The Old Phrenology restricted its concern to humans, and failed because of its flawed premise that brain growths could be detected through faithfully correlated protuberances in the overlying bone. Our New Phrenology looks at the brain directly, and, by widening its attention to consider all mammals, it succeeds in discovering correlations between the observed morphology and the predictive probabilities of behavior.

The germinal study of raccoon cerebral cortex by W. Welker and Seidenstein (1959) can be considered as marking the birth of the New Phrenology. This allows for a considerable preceding gestation period in the laboratory and mind of Clinton Woolsey (1959) and others, such as Adrian (1943) and Papez and Hunter (1929), who shrewdly surmised that the morphology was behavior related in much the way that it turned out to be.

A chief method used to establish this relationship between behavioral specialization and cerebral morphology was that of electrophysiological mapping of sensory projections as elaborated in the Woolsey laboratory. Somatic sensory receptors

JOHN IRWIN JOHNSON, Jr. • Departments of Biophysics, Psychology, and Zoology, Michigan State University, East Lansing, Michigan 48824.

are mechanically stimulated, and the resulting neural activity is recorded at specific locations in the brain. The receptive fields on the body which activate each cerebral locus are plotted, and the resulting map of sensory projections shows that they are organized, as a general rule, in several brain regions in all mammals studied, into a somatotopic representation of the entire body surface. The topological relationships of the receptors to each other are maintained in register in the brain regions activated by receptor response. Figure 1 illustrates some of these representations as found in sensory cerebral cortex, along with some current notions of the pathways from receptors to somatic sensory cortex.

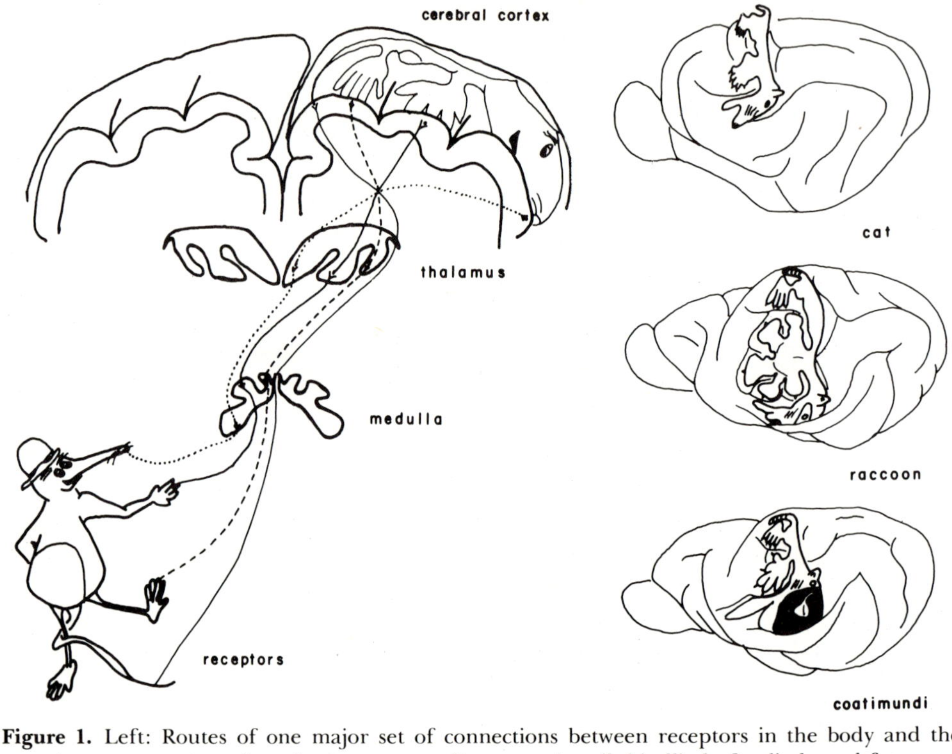

Figure 1. Left: Routes of one major set of connections between receptors in the body and the somatic sensory region of cerebral neocortex. Receptors in tail, hindlimb, forelimb, and face send processes to distinct lobules in the cuneate-gracile and spinal trigeminal cell groups in the medulla, such that the shape of the body surface is reflected in the morphology of the nuclear regions (see Figs. 9 and 11). Cells in these medullary regions send processes to the sensory region in the ventrobasal thalamus, where the body shape again has correlates in cytoarchitecture (Fig. 8). Cells in this thalamic region provide input to sensory neocortex, where one correlate of body morphology is the pattern of sulcal folds (Figs. 2, 5, 6, 7, and 14). Cells at each of these levels have many other connections, both afferent and efferent, as well as internuncial connections with one another. Right: The relative extent of the amount of neocortex associated with the projections from a given part of the body is proportional to the use of a body part in tactile exploratory activity, and probably to the density of receptors in that part of the body. Cats have a slight preponderance of projections from the head (Rubel, 1971); raccoons have most projections from the forepaw (W. Welker and Seidenstein, 1959); and coatimundis have a large set of projections from the glabrous rhinarium (W. Welker and Campos, 1963). Distinctive sulci and gyri mark the specialized regions in the cerebral "representations" of forelimb in raccoons and nose in coatimundis. Drawings by Doug Green.

II. Gyral Configuration in Somatic Sensory Cerebral Cortex Related to Behavioral Specialization

A. Proposed from Procyonids

Welker and Seidenstein found that in the region of somatic sensory projections to the cerebral cortex of raccoons there was an extraordinarily large representation of the forepaw which could be correlated with the prominent use of the member in behavior. Furthermore, sulci separated the forepaw projection region from those of the hindlimb and head, and individual gyral crowns marked the representation of each of the different digits of the forepaw (Fig. 1).

These sulci separating representations of the limbs and head were also seen in other members of the raccoon's family, Procyonidae (W. Welker and Campos, 1963). An additional sulcus appears in another member of this family, the coatimundi, which shows a behavioral propensity for tactile investigation with its mobile nose. This sulcus marks the separation of lateral from medial, and dorsal from ventral, rims of the nostril as it appears in the cortical sensory representation.

Figure 2 shows a photomicrograph of a section through the sensory neocortex of this most specialized region in the forepaw representation of the raccoon. The convolutions involve variations in intracortical architecture; they are not simple foldings of a uniformly laminated cortical sheet.

The sulcus dividing forelimb from face representations is seen in cats and is known as the coronal sulcus. Many cats also show a small sulcal formation known as the postcruciate dimple, which has been termed an analogue of the central sulcus of primates since it separates motor cortex anteriorly from sensory cortex posteriorly; however, it also separates the sensory representation of the hindlimb medially from that of the forelimb laterally. With these two sulci cats follow the basic principle of sulcal divisions corresponding to the representation of body parts in the cerebral cortex.

B. Tested in Marsupial Wombats

To test whether this phenomenon is a general feature of mammalian brain development or is a specialization of the Carnivora (it is not seen in Primates, for example), we turned to marsupials. Marsupials have a phylogenetic history greatly different from that of the carnivores (Fig. 3), yet many have developed convoluted neocortices. One family in particular—the wombats, Vombatidae (Fig. 4)—show a well-developed neocortex with a number of sulci in what could be expected to be the somatic sensory region (much as Papez and Hunter had noticed in raccoons). Figure 5 presents our map of the sensory projections to this cortex (Johnson *et al.*, 1973), and Fig. 6 is a photomicrograph of a section through the sensory representation. These afford a striking confirmation of the hypothesis: Sulci have formed between the representations of the major separated tactile surfaces of the body, hindfeet, forepaws, and face, and there are additional sulci marking the representations of the lips and, as in coatimundis, of the nostril.

Sensible naming of neuroanatomical features has always been a problem, and

I hope we are minimizing rather than adding to such problems by applying a new set of names to sulci based on sensory projections. The new names have the advantage that they can be applied validly to all mammals, as shall be seen. The sulcus separating the projections of the fore- and hindlimbs we call the *interbrachial* sulcus; that between the forelimb and face representations locates the "neck" of the somatotopic representation, so we have termed it the *jugular* sulcus; that which marks (but does not seem to separate) the representations of the lips is the *labial* sulcus; and the *narial* sulcus locates the representation of the nostril. The application of these names to distantly related species is illustrated in Fig. 7.

There is impressive support from distantly related animals that cortical evolution has proceeded along parallel courses to produce, in each of several cases, gyral accretions separated by sulcal divisions, each of which corresponds to a specialized receptor surface of the body. Animals with rhinarial tactile specialization show a narial sulcus (coatimundis, wombats, pigs); those with tactile specializations

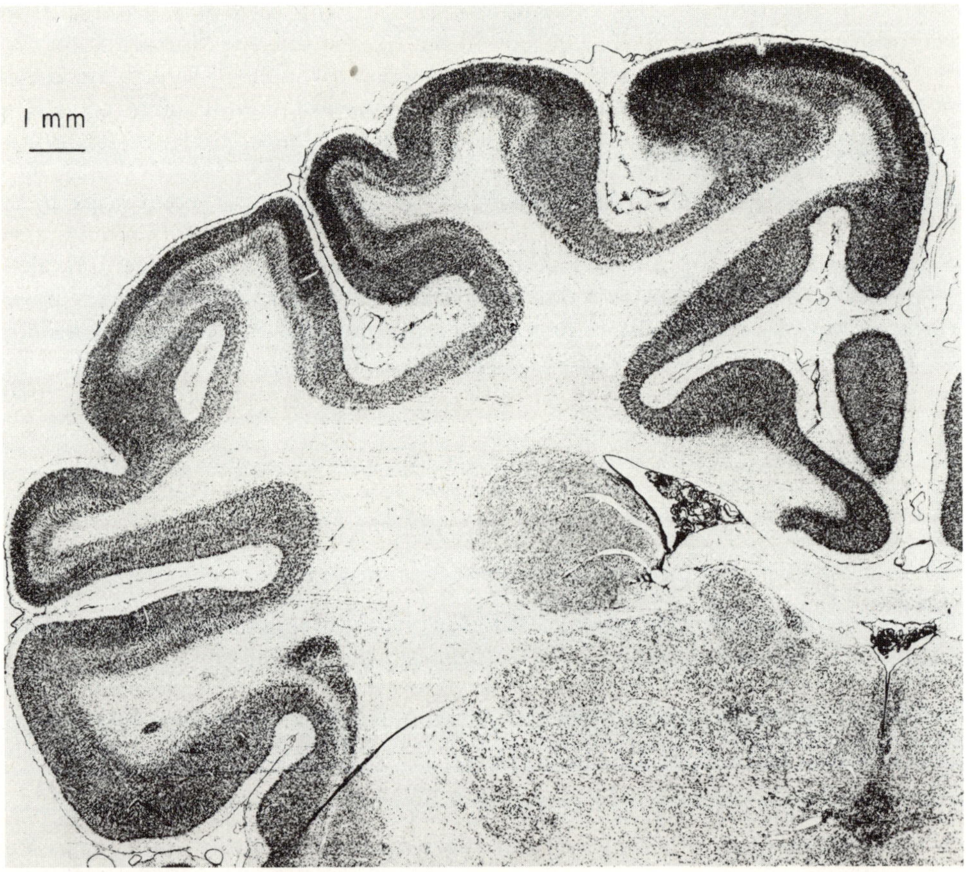

Figure 2. Coronal section 180 through the somatic sensory region of cerebral neocortex of raccoon 566, stained with thionin to show cell bodies (courtesy of Paul Herron). The cytoarchitecture of the cortical mantle is not homogeneous; many features seen in gyral crowns, such as the broad white band representing the outer stripe of Baillarger, are absent in the much thinner cortex found at certain locations in the sulcal depths.

of the lips often have labial sulci (wombats, sheep, llamas); interbrachial sulci are found in animals which gather mechanosensory information with the limbs (raccoons, coatimundis, cats, wombats, agoutis); and the most frequently found is the jugular sulcus marking the limit of face-receptor projections (all, except agoutis, of the animals shown in Fig. 7). Sensory specialization does not always result in corresponding cortical folding: many small animals have no cortical folds yet show pronounced specializations (e.g., the rats and mice to be described below); and primates do not show much folding, perhaps because of the "stretching" of the cortical sensory surface by the great expansion of other regions of the brain. (This might be expressed better by saying that the cortical surface of the sensory region is large enough because of overall brain size that folding has not been necessary to accommodate special sensory input.) Studies of relative thickness of cortex and of

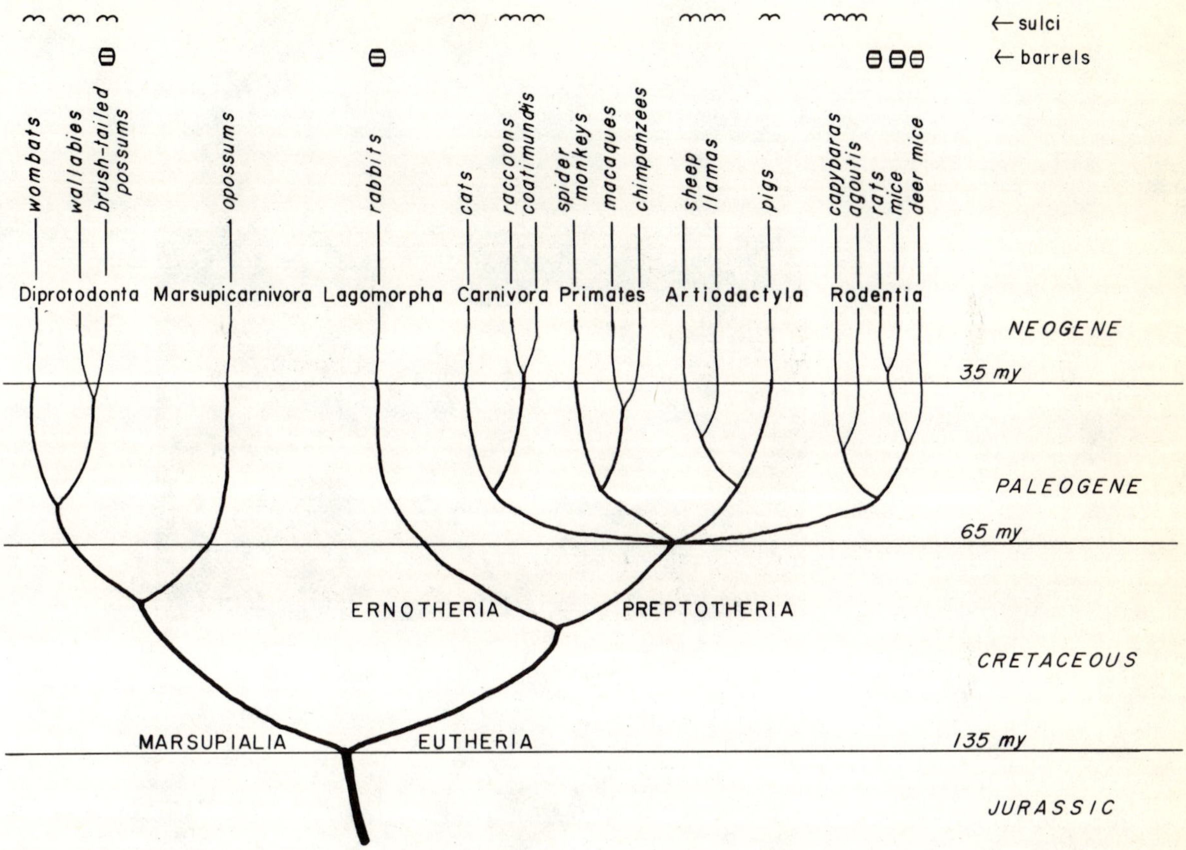

Figure 3. One current view of the possible phylogenetic relationships of the mammals mentioned in this chapter. This scheme is based on a recent attempt to construct a phylogeny on cladistic principles (McKenna, 1975). Some additional details are from Simpson (1961) and Kirsch (1976), and others are more or less fabricated out of whole cloth, as any such scheme must be in large part, given the lack of critical data. For example, most of the data of divergence will probably be pushed back to considerably earlier dates as more paleontological data become available. my, Millions of years ago. Symbols at the top indicate the species showing boundary sulci and barrels in somatic sensory neocortex. Neither of these features is restricted to any given phylogenetic grouping, and both features may thus be regarded as examples of convergence. More probably, however, they are general mammalian features which become apparent at a certain stage of cerebral cortical development.

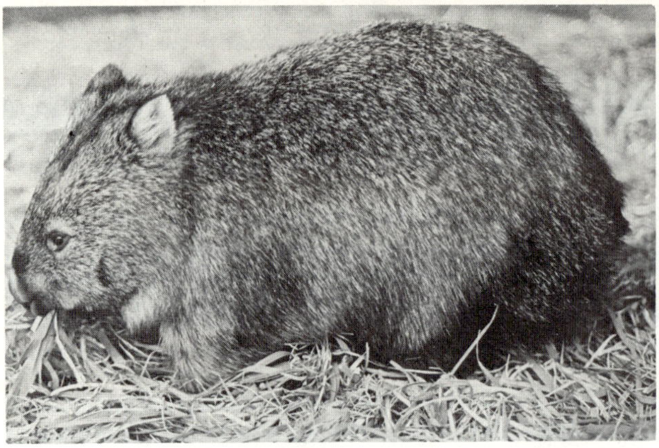

Figure 4. A wombat (*Vombatus ursinus*), a large (up to 30 kg adult body weight), herbivorous, burrowing Australian marsupial with a well-developed somatic sensory neocortex.

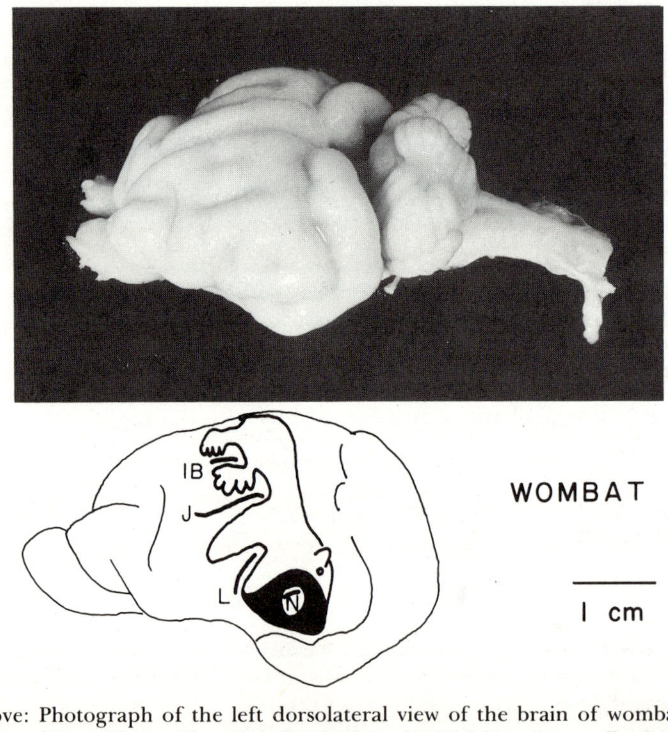

Figure 5. Above: Photograph of the left dorsolateral view of the brain of wombat 14. Specimen numbers in this and later figures identify individuals in the Michigan State collection. Below: Sketch of projections from body receptive fields as determined by electrophysiological mapping (Johnson *et al.*, 1973). Letters denote sulci related to projections of body parts: IB, interbrachial sulcus, between projections from fore- and hindlimbs; J, jugular sulcus, at the representation of the neck between projections from forelimb and those from the face; L, labial sulcus, marking projections from the lips; N, narial sulcus, locating the cortical representation of the nostril.

"cellular condensations" in layer IV (see below) in primate sensory cortex will be of great interest. [In one unusual spider monkey an anteroposterior sulcus did appear in the postcentral sensory cortex. This sulcus was found electrophysiologically to separate hindlimb from forelimb projections, and was thus an interbrachial sulcus (Pubols and Pubols, 1980).]

III. Subcortical Correlates of Gyral Formations: Lobules

To examine correlates of these neocortical specializations in other parts of the nervous system, W. Welker undertook a systematic analysis of sensory projections and neuromorphology at the sites of synaptic interaction in the major input pathway to the sensory cortex, using raccoons since they show a most pronounced set of gyral divisions in sensory cortex (W. Welker *et al.,* 1964). Using normal and experimental anatomical techniques to complement electrophysiological mapping, nuclear morphology and sensory projections were analyzed in the ventrobasal

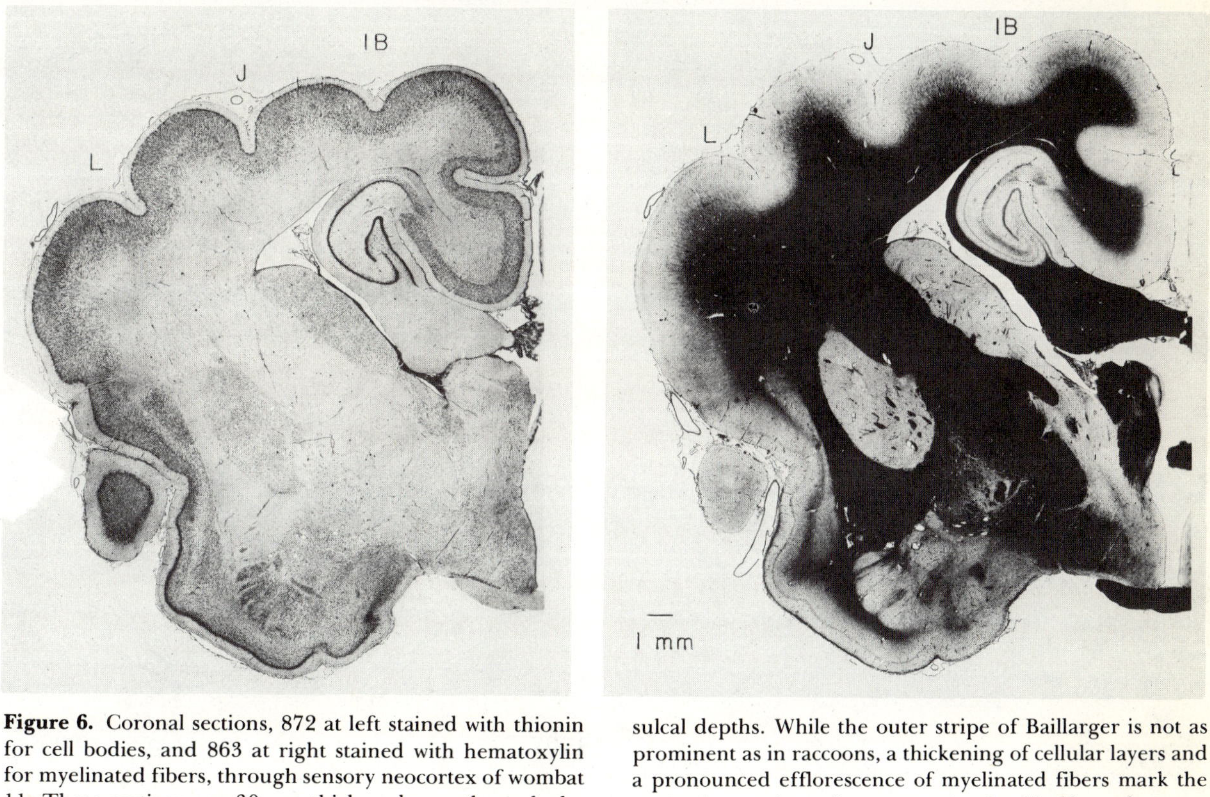

Figure 6. Coronal sections, 872 at left stained with thionin for cell bodies, and 863 at right stained with hematoxylin for myelinated fibers, through sensory neocortex of wombat 11. These sections are 30 μm thick and pass through the interbrachial (IB), jugular (J), and labial (L) sulci. As in raccoons (Fig. 2), both cyto- and myeloarchitecture show features present in gyral crowns which are not found in sulcal depths. While the outer stripe of Baillarger is not as prominent as in raccoons, a thickening of cellular layers and a pronounced efflorescence of myelinated fibers mark the projection region of receptors in the hindfoot, forepaw, mandibular, and maxillary regions in the separate gyral crowns.

nuclear complex of the dorsal thalamus (W. Welker and Johnson, 1965) and the cuneate–gracile nuclear complex of the medulla (Johnson *et al.,* 1968). These were then related to the segregation of input in the dorsal spinal roots (Pubols *et al.,* 1965).

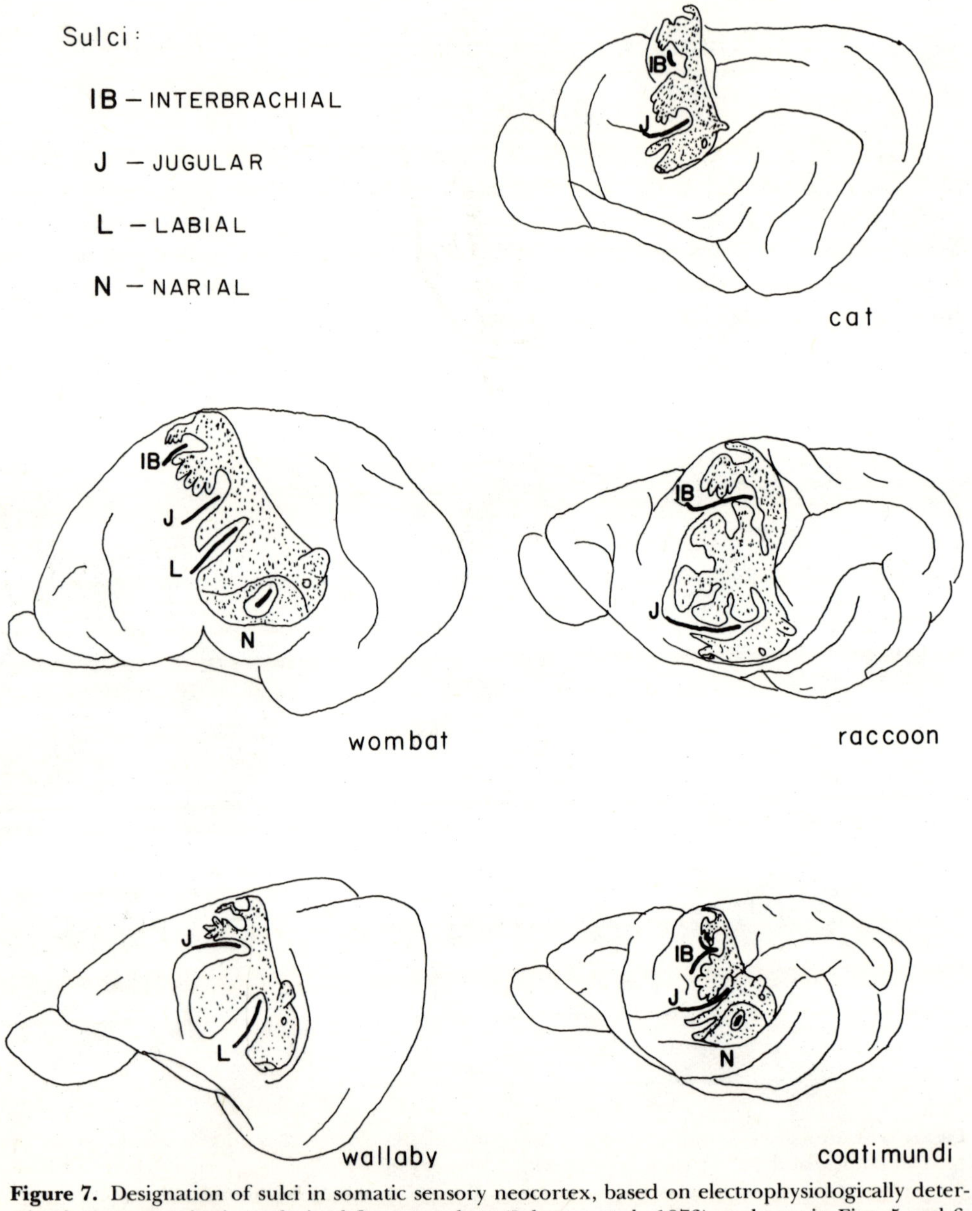

Figure 7. Designation of sulci in somatic sensory neocortex, based on electrophysiologically determined sensory projections, derived from wombats (Johnson *et al.,* 1973) as shown in Figs. 5 and 6, can be applied to other mammals as shown. Data for wallaby are from Lende (1963), cat from Rubel (1971), raccoon from W. Welker and Seidenstein (1959), coatimundi from W. Welker and Campos (1963), sheep from Johnson *et al.* (1974), llama from W. Welker *et al.* (1976), pig from C. Woolsey

A. Ventrobasal (Somatic Sensory) Nucleus of Thalamus

Somatotopic representation of the body surface in this sensory thalamic nuclear region was again found to have striking morphological correlates, paralleling those seen in sensory cortex (Fig. 8). The representations of the face, the hindlimbs, and

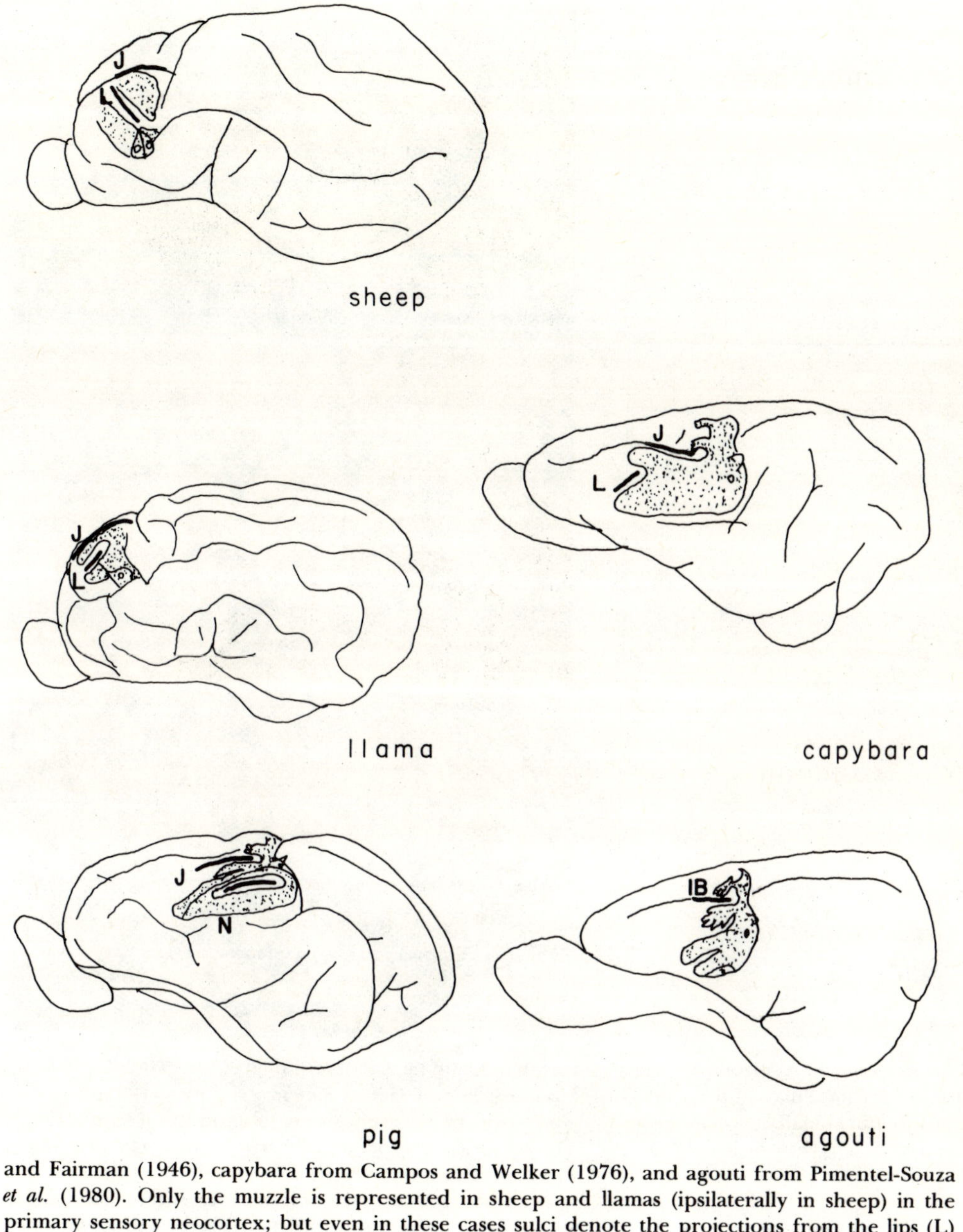

and Fairman (1946), capybara from Campos and Welker (1976), and agouti from Pimentel-Souza *et al.* (1980). Only the muzzle is represented in sheep and llamas (ipsilaterally in sheep) in the primary sensory neocortex; but even in these cases sulci denote the projections from the lips (L) and demarcate the limit of projections from the chin (J).

each of the forelimb digits correspond to discrete groupings of cell bodies (and therefore, presumably, of synaptic contacts). These groupings we term *lobules* of the nuclear formation. In raccoons they are outlined vividly by bands or capsules of myelinated fibers running between them.

The principle of lobulation corresponding to sensory representation in ven-

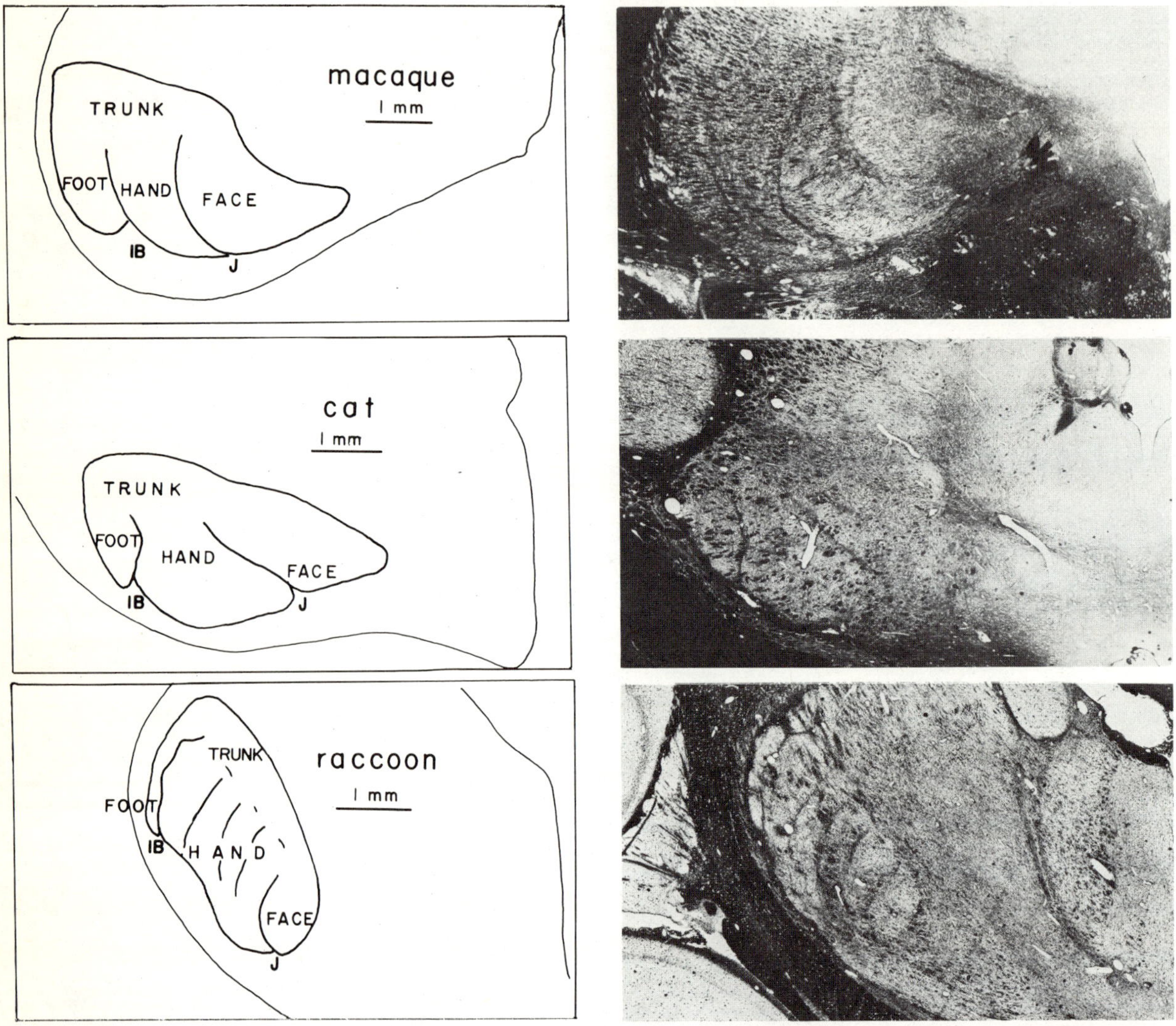

Figure 8. Coronal sections through the ventrobasal thalamus, stained with hematoxylin for myelinated fibers, showing lobular subdivisions in three mammalian species. Top: Section 1511 from *Macaca mulatta* (courtesy of R. L. Raisler and H. F. Harlow). Center: Section 659 from *Felis catus* 324B (courtesy of J. R. Haight and E. G. Haight). Bottom: Section 750 from *Procyon lotor* 58-128 (courtesy of W. I. Welker and T. P. Stewart). Lobules can be seen in each species representing projection fields of receptors in hindfoot, hand, and face as determined electrophysiologically by Mountcastle and Henneman in macaques (1952) and cats (1949) and by W. Welker and Johnson in raccoons (1965). The lobules are separated by bands of myelinated fibers which correspond to the interbrachial (IB) and jugular (J) sulci of the somatic sensory cerebral cortex. Additional bands and lobules within the hand region in raccoons demarcate the projection fields of individual digits.

trobasal thalamus had long been "latently" recognized in other mammals by subdivision into separate nuclei which were later shown to receive projections from separate body parts. Thus nucleus ventralis posterolateralis (VPL, Walker, 1938) in primates and pars externa of nucleus ventrobasalis (Rioch, 1929) in cats and dogs receive projections from the body and limbs (Mountcastle and Henneman, 1949, 1952; Rose and Mountcastle, 1952), and are separated by a band of myelinated fibers from the corresponding regions of facial projections, VPM, and pars arcuata, respectively. Additional but unnamed subdivisions can be located in both primates (Krishnamurti *et al.,* 1972) and carnivores (Fig. 8) which are coextensive with the projections from the hindlimbs.

B. Cuneate–Gracile Nuclear Complex of the Medulla

A major source of input to the ventrobasal thalamus are the cells whose perikarya lie at the rostral end of the dorsal columns of the spinal cord and their neighbors in the trigeminal nuclear complex. The "nuclei of the dorsal columns" have long been regarded as separate nuclei: the cuneate nucleus, which receives input from the forelimb; the gracile nucleus, which receives its projections from the hindlimb, and, in animals with sensory development of the tail, the "median accessory nucleus," identified by Bischoff (1899), who hypothesized that its degree of development signified the importance of tactile sensation from the tail for a particular animal. Rather than separate nuclei, the cuneate, gracile, and Bischoff's nuclei are probably better considered as lobules of a single cuneate-gracile nuclear complex. The principle of lobulation related to projections from different body parts can then be seen to have been long recognized in the taxonomy of these cell groupings.

Raccoons again show an extreme case of elaboration of lobulation (Fig. 9); in the cuneate nucleus separate lobules of cell bodies, separated by bands of myelinated fibers, contain the projections of each of the separate digits of the forepaw. Chimpanzees show similar lobulation in both the cuneate and gracile nuclei, presumably related to their special development of the digits of both fore- and hindlimbs for mechanosensory perception (Fig. 9). The relative size of any of these lobules is an index of the behavioral use of a body part in tactile exploration: spider monkeys, with their tactile tail pad, have such an expanded median nucleus that it is as large as the gracile nucleus (Chang and Ruch, 1947); sheep have an extremely small cuneate–gracile complex, in line with their concentration of tactile behavior in the face rather than the body and limbs (Fig. 9).

C. What Are Lobules?

In both ventrobasal thalamus and the cuneate–gracile nuclear complex of the medulla there are lobules which correspond to the sensory projections from various body parts. This correspondence extends to a variation in the size of a given lobule corresponding to the behavioral use of a given part in acquiring mechanosensory information, although precise quantitative documentation of this point is needed.

The lobules further correspond, in both size and topology, to the gyral formations in the somatic sensory neocortex (Fig. 1).

Why do cell bodies receiving projections from a particular body region form a lobule, separated from other lobules? One thing we have noted is that separate lobules represent separated body parts. Facial projections do not show obvious

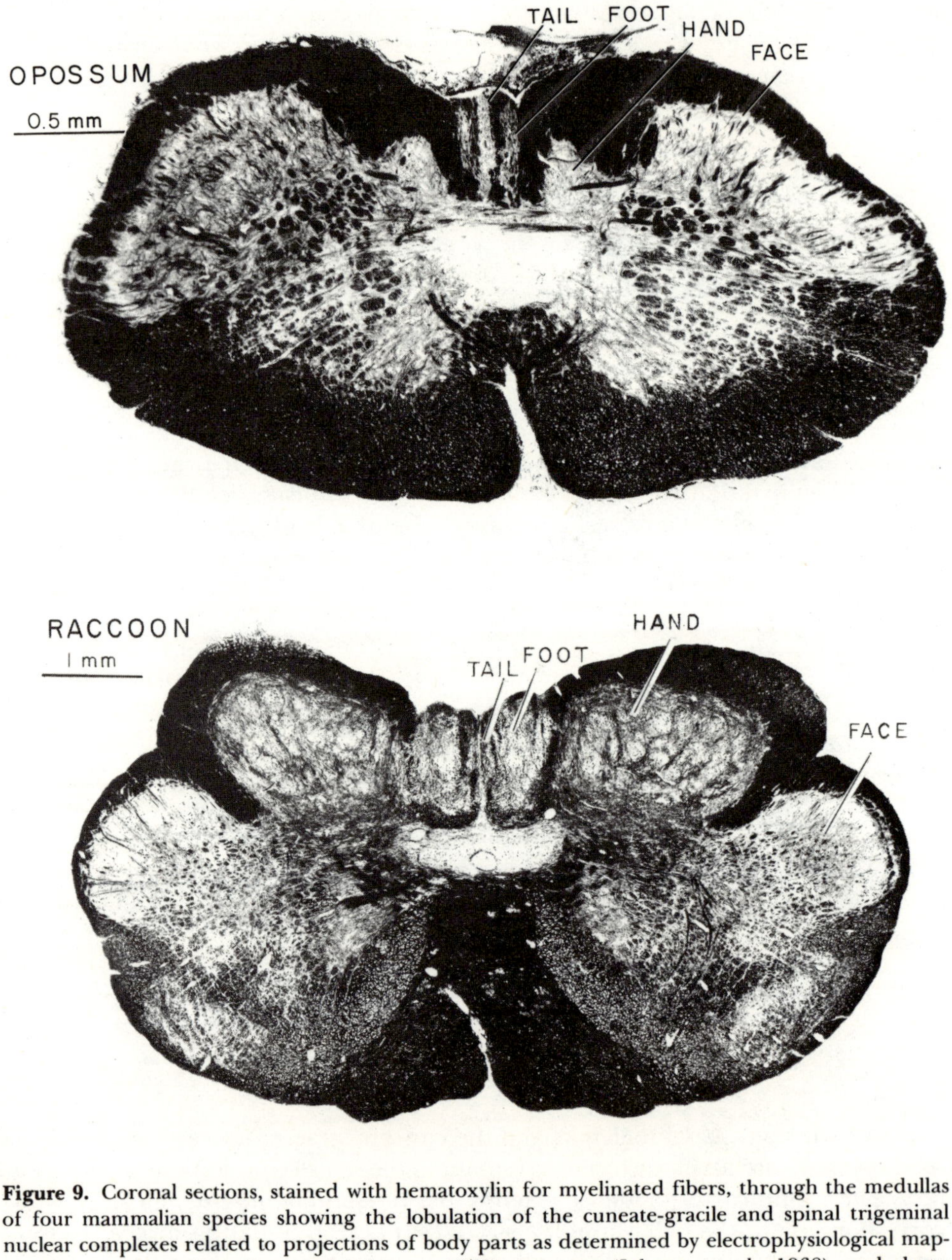

Figure 9. Coronal sections, stained with hematoxylin for myelinated fibers, through the medullas of four mammalian species showing the lobulation of the cuneate-gracile and spinal trigeminal nuclear complexes related to projections of body parts as determined by electrophysiological mapping in opossums (Hamilton and Johnson, 1973), raccoons (Johnson *et al.*, 1968), and sheep

separate lobules. It may well be that projections from continuous receptor surfaces maintain some kind of lateral interaction in successive synaptic regions, requiring close proximity to projections from neighboring receptive fields. But when a break occurs in the receptor surface (e.g., between arm and leg, or between separate digits) a corresponding break in cross-connectivity in the nuclear projections can

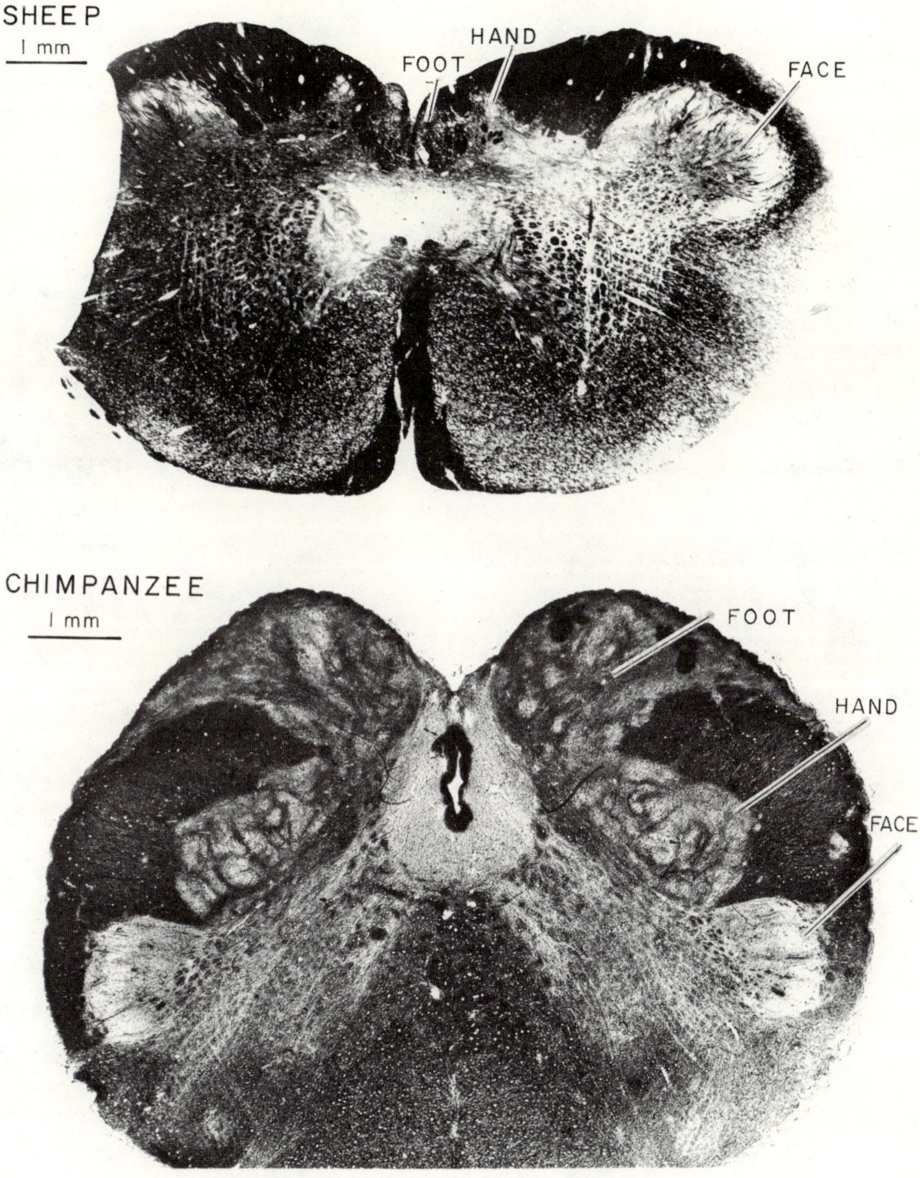

(Woudenberg, 1970). Chimpanzees have not been mapped, but the projections are assumed to be similar to those of other primates (e.g., Chang and Ruch, 1947). Subdivisions within the hand projection region (the cuneate–nucleus) in raccoons and probably also in chimpanzees represent the projection fields of individual digits.

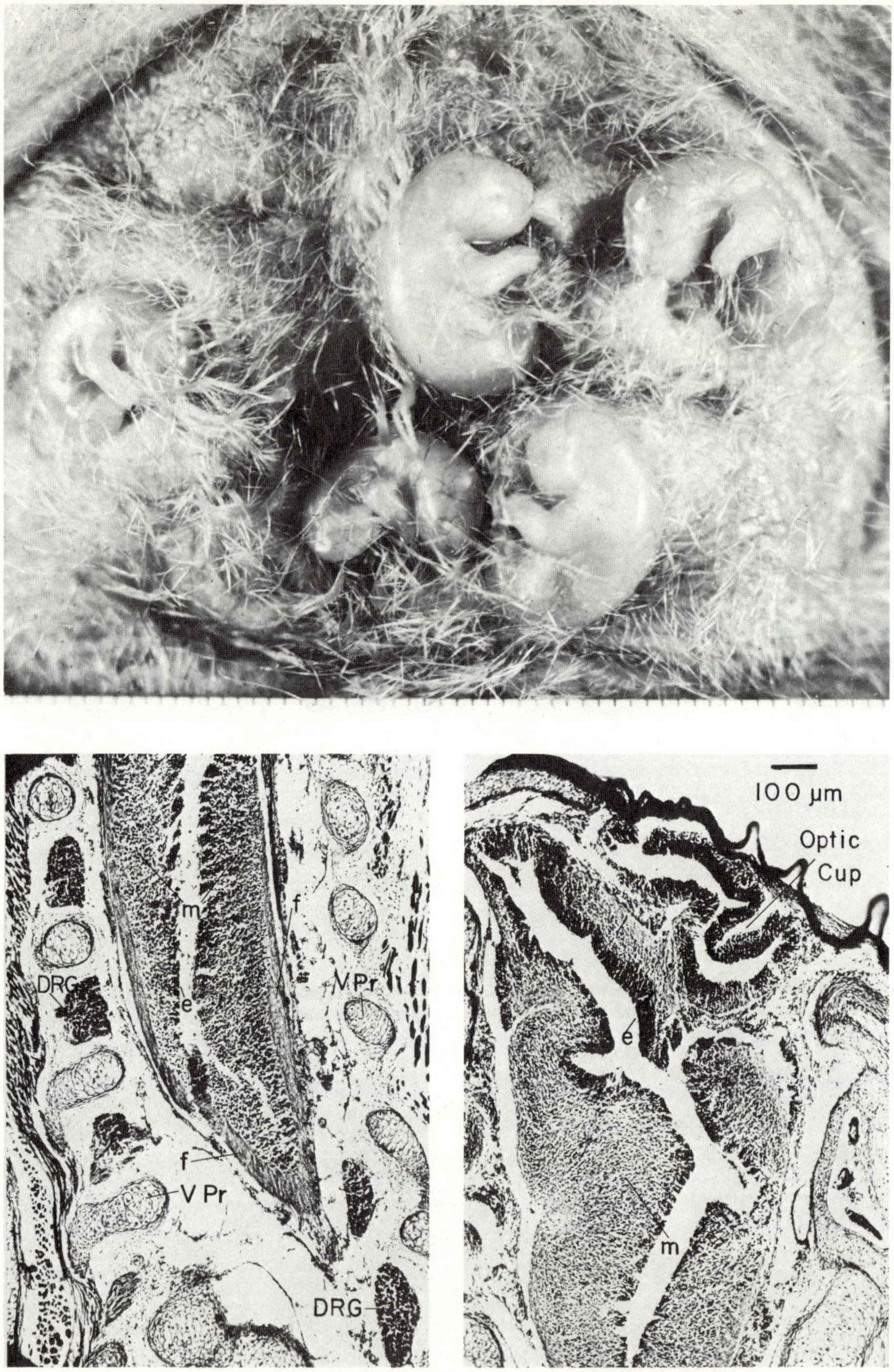

Figure 10. Above: Pouch young opossums in the pouch, 4 days after birth. Forelimbs and mouth are relatively well developed, hindlimbs are rudimentary, the future location of the eyes is marked by pigmented spots. The scale is in mm. Photograph courtesy of R. A. Bombardieri and Neal Brophy. Below: Horizontal sections through the spinal cord (at left) and forebrain (at right), *in situ,*

occur without detriment to sensory function. Passing fibers may then be "forced" into these gaps in the cytoarchitectural network as the only available routes for them to reach their destinations, and in this way the fibrous "boundaries" of the lobules take their shape.

Fibers are apparently relatively free to follow varied paths, within limits, en route to their synaptic destinations. We found fibers from given receptive fields on forepaw digits in raccoons, cats, and coatimundis to enter the central nervous system by any of several different dorsal spinal roots, but their terminals are precisely arranged within the appropriate lobules in the cuneate nucleus (Pubols *et al.,* 1965; Johnson *et al.,* 1968). Similarly, Matzke (1951) found that fibers from the cuneate–gracile complex in cats followed varied routes to the thalamus but terminated appropriately in the ventrobasal complex. Thus the precision of correspondence appears to lie between receptive field and synaptic terminal, and not to fiber tract, dorsal root, or dermatome. Le Gros Clark (1962) characterized this as a general principle of "resorting" of fibers in several neural pathways.

IV. Role of Receptors in the Development of Lobules

A. Relation of Receptor Density to Presence and Volume of Lobules

The precision of correspondence between receptive fields and lobules of nuclear brain regions probably extends to quantitative relationships between numbers of receptors in a receptive field and the number of cell bodies and/or of synapses in the nuclear region. Zollman and Winkelmann (1962) presented qualitative evidence of greater receptor density in the third digit of the raccoon forepaw compared with the analogous locus on the hindpaw, corresponding to the relative size of the central projection regions. Better quantitative data from rat vibrissae support the principle and will be introduced below in relation to the architecture of rat sensory cortex. In general, the principle has been recognized and generally accepted without precise quantitative supporting data. It can be stated as follows: Regions of great receptor density will project to regions of greater cell number and nuclear volume in the brain, and in extreme cases these central regions will show a well-defined organization into separate lobules or subnuclei corresponding to receptor-dense regions which are spatially separated from one another on the body surface.

Such a correspondence between receptors and relative degrees of brain development led us to investigate the possible causal relations underlying this correspondence. In placental mammals, virtually all of the developmental period during which these correspondences are established takes place in intrauterine life, where experimental manipulations usually lead to manifold complications and their productivity is extremely limited as a result. We turned, therefore, to marsupial opossums, which are born at a very early stage of development (Fig. 10); the bulk of brain organization and development takes place well after birth (Ulinski, 1971;

---

of newborn opossum 7043D, Bodian stain. The ependymal (e), mantle (m), and fibrous marginal (f) layers are characteristic of the early embryonic neural tube. Dorsal root ganglia (DRG) are seen between vertebral processes (V Pr). The optic cup is folding to form the primordial retina.

Morest, 1970). The opossum cuneate–gracile complex develops entirely after birth (Ulinski, 1969), and in its caudal regions it shows a distinct lobulation corresponding to receptive fields on tail, hindlimb, and forelimb, respectively, in the standard mammalian topology (Hamilton and Johnson, 1973), as shown in Fig. 11.

B. Absence of Cuneate–Gracile Lobules following Early Receptor Removal

Removal of the receptor tissue projecting to one of these lobules, before 10 days of age in the developing pouch young opossum, results in the adult stage in the absence of the corresponding lobule or portion thereof in the cuneate–gracile complex (Johnson *et al.,* 1972), as shown in Fig. 11. When a hindlimb is completely removed, the lobule constituting the "gracile nucleus" is completely absent; when the distal portion of the hindlimb is removed, the dorsal portion of the lobule is absent; when the distal portion of the forelimb is removed, the dorsal bulge of the "cuneate nucleus," where the hand projections are normally found, is not present. Mapping by early amputation confirms precisely the results obtained by electrophysiological mapping.

Our somewhat reluctant interpretation of these findings is that input of some kind from the receptor tissue during the developmental period is necessary for the organization, maintenance, or survival of the cuneate–gracile projection region. This input may consist in activity of nerve impulses, generation of trophic substance by processes from the receptors, or transfer of materials from receptor processes directly to the cuneate–gracile cells. The influence may be exercised through affecting cell proliferation in the cuneate–gracile complex, by governing the course of cell migration in the process of nuclear formation, or by transneuronal degeneration of already connected cuneate–gracile cells, but most probably it is by regulating the process of normal cell death whereby the great number of nerve cells initially generated is reduced to the number and arrangement found in the adult condition. These questions are currently under active study.

An immediate subsequent question is, of course, whether these transneuronal effects of receptor removal are seen further transsynaptically at higher levels in this sensory pathway. Since opossums do not have clearly defined lobules in the sensory thalamus, nor gyri and sulci in the sensory region of cerebral cortex, we turned again to placental mammals to test this proposition, to animals with still another morphological feature correlated with sensory specialization.

V. Intracortical Correlates of Sensory Specialization: Barrels and Cellular Condensations

A. Barrels in Layer IV of Sensory Neocortex

T. Woolsey and Van der Loos (1970) described as "barrels" a morphological configuration best seen in tangential sections through layer IV of certain regions of somatic sensory neocortex of mice. These are illustrated in Fig. 12 and consist

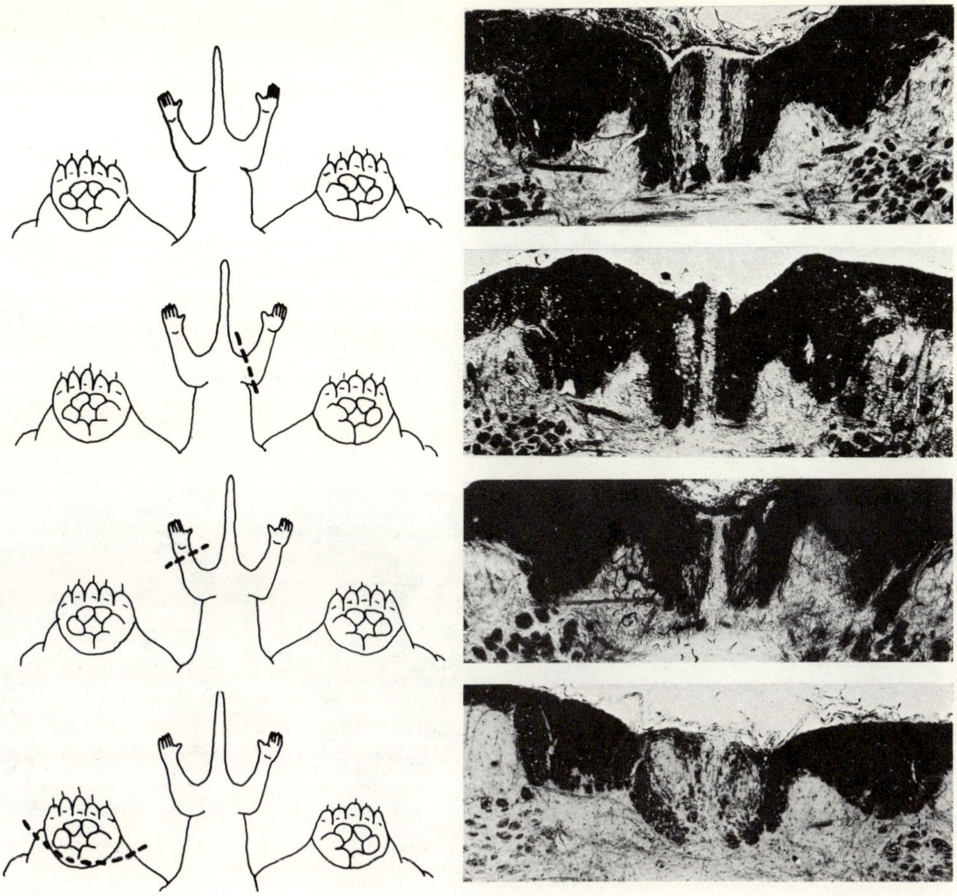

Figure 11. Effects of early amputation on nuclear configuration of the adult cuneate–gracile nuclear complex in opossums (*Didelphis virginiana*). Shown are sections through the caudal part of the nuclear complex which are 25 μm thick and stained with hematoxylin; myelinated fibers are black, cell bodies are neuropil of the nuclear regions are left unstained. At top right is section 207 from normal animal 463, and at top left is a diagram of the projections from body parts as determined by electrophysiological mapping (Hamilton and Johnson, 1973). The column of nuclear tissue at the midline receives projections from the tail in its dorsal part and from the trunk in the ventral part of the column. From either side of this central column (sometimes known as the median accessory nucleus of Bischoff), lobules of nuclear tissue branch out, forming the gracile nuclei of either side, which receive projections from the hindlimb and foot. Lateral to these are the large nuclear clumps forming the cuneate nuclei, which receive projections from the forelimb, largely from the hand. Second from the top is section 157 from opossum 464, from which the right hind limb was amputated 5 days after birth (Johnson *et al.,* 1972). The lobule forming the left gracile nucleus has no counterpart on the right side. Third from the top is section 73 from opossum 42A2, from which the distalmost part of the hindlimb was amputated at 4 days of age; the corresponding dorsal portion of the left gracile nucleus is missing in the adult nuclear formation. At bottom is section 103 from opossum 4403K, from which the distal portion of the left forelimb was removed at 2 days of age. The adult nuclear formation shows a corresponding absence of the dorsal bulge in the left cuneate nuclear lobule; in normal nuclei such as that on the right, the dorsal bulge receives sensory projections from the hand. In each case early amputation of a body part resulted in the absence, in the adult, of the nuclear region normally receiving projections from that body part.

of "condensations" (increases in density) of cell perikarya, forming "barrel sides," separated by perikarya-free zones called "septa" between barrels. In mice the barrels also have "hollows," a region of lowered density of perikarya enclosed by the barrel sides. Woolsey and Van der Loos further noted the correspondence between the size and arrangement of the largest barrels and the size and arrangement of the largest facial vibrissae, as shown in Fig. 12. Electrophysiological mapping studies indicate that each of these large barrels does represent the projection field for sensory information yielded by movement of a single vibrissa (C. Welker, 1971), and the size and number of cells of a barrel correspond well with the number of sensory nerve endings entering a vibrissa follicle (Lee and Woolsey, 1975).

Barrels have been described in a wide variety of rodents, although they are not seen in all rodents (T. Woolsey *et al.,* 1975); they were reported in rabbits (C. Welker and Woolsey, 1974) and in several species of the marsupial families Phalangeridae and Petauridae (Weller, 1972*a*). Among the mammals, according to

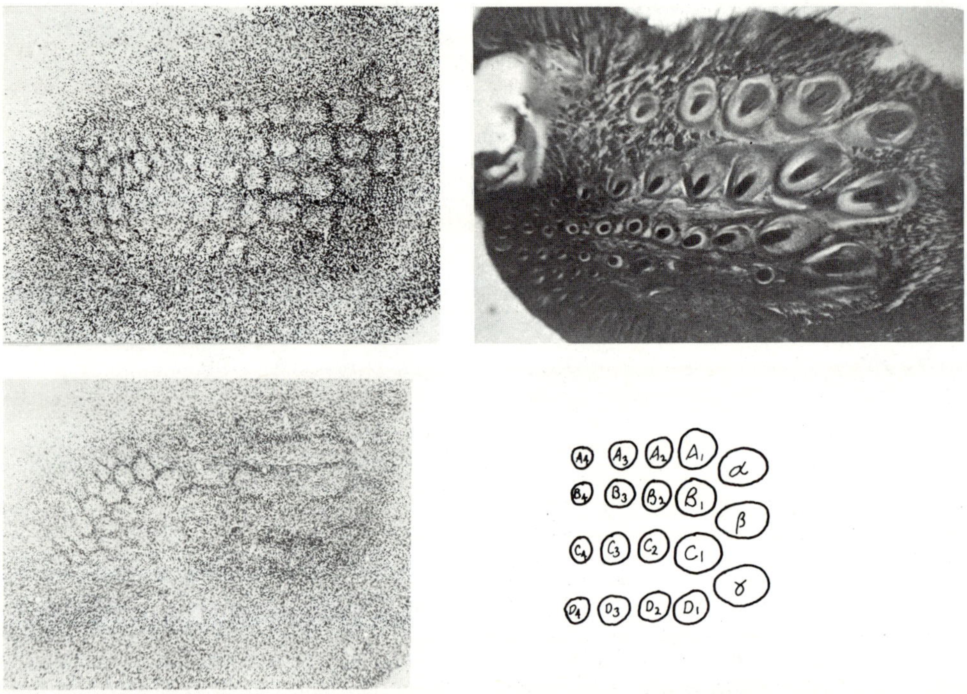

Figure 12. Mystacial vibrissa follicles and the neocortical barrels to which they project, in deer mice (*Peromyscus leucopus*). All sections are stained with thionin. Upper right: Section through vibrissa follicles in the skin. The follicles are arranged in rows, with progressively larger follicles toward the right in this photograph. At the ends of the rows one large follicle is intercalated between each pair of rows. Lower right: Diagram showing the designation of these follicles and their corresponding neocortical barrels. Upper left: tangential section through layer IV of sensory neocortex, showing condensations of cell bodies arranged in "barrel" form. The barrels are arranged in rows with intercalated end-barrels, and in graded size series, replicating the arrangement seen in the follicles which project to these barrels. Lower left: Ablation of the follicles in columns 2, 3, and 4 at birth resulted in the disruption of the pattern of barrels as seen in the mature neocortex: a single long, elliptically shaped formation replaces the normal barrels 1–4 in each of rows A, B, C, and D. Data from Weller and Johnson (1975); photographs courtesy of W. L. Weller.

current views of mammalian phylogeny (Fig. 3), rabbits and marsupials have ancient lineages completely separate from each other and from rodents. Thus, as with the gyral formations described earlier, we seem to be dealing with a general feature of mammalian brain development: At any of several positions on the mammalian family tree, barrels appear with certain degrees and types of sensory specialization. In some species, such as rats among the rodents and the brush-tailed possums among the phalangerid marsupials, the large barrels do not show hollows in the adults (Fig. 14).

B. Role of Receptors in the Development of Barrels

The cell bodies making up a barrel migrate into place during the first 5 days after birth in both murid house mice and cricetid deer mice (Weller, 1972*b*; Rice, 1973, 1974; Rice and Van der Loos, 1977). Destruction of a vibrissa follicle during the first day after birth results in the "disruption of the corresponding barrel in the cortex" (Van der Loos and Woolsey, 1973), but follicle destruction on the fifth day does not affect barrel organization; these results were observed in both the inbred murid and the wild cricetid species (Weller and Johnson, 1975). Thus a transneuronal effect from early receptor removal can be seen across at least three synapses in this system (receptor–trigeminal nuclear complex; trigeminal–thalamus; thalamus–cortex). Similar effects of early follicle removal causing failure of barrel organization were recently observed in the marsupial brush-tailed possum (W. L. Weller, personal communication).

C. Regions of Cellular Condensation and Rarefaction Related to Sensory Maps in Layer IV of Sensory Neocortex

Recent reports of the internal architecture of somatic sensory cerebral cortex in rats (C. Welker, 1976) and in brush-tailed possums (Haight and Weller, 1973; Weller and Haight, 1973) lead to interesting hypotheses concerning the relationships among receptor density, the arrangement of cells in layer IV of sensory cortex, the presence of barrels, the map of sensory projections to cortex, and therefore the patterning of gyral formations in sensory cortex. In both rats and brush-tailed possums, barrels are found within larger patches of what can be termed cellular condensations (regions of increased density of neuronal perikarya) which can be observed in tangential sections through layer IV, as illustrated in Figs. 13 and 14. Barrels appear within condensations where projections are found from regions of particularly high receptor density, not only from vibrissae but also from such regions as the glabrous palmar and plantar surfaces. Receptive fields of not-so-high receptor density project to the regions of cellular condensation not organized into barrels. Separations between peripheral receptive fields show up in the cortical representation as regions of cellular "rarefaction," and in the electrophysiological maps these regions of rarefaction correspond to the separation between representations, for example, of the limbs, or between representations of the forelimb and of the face. This is very reminiscent of the situation with gyral configuration, where sulci mark the location of separations between receptive fields, just as the layer IV rarefactions do.

VI. Possible Relation of Barrels and Other Regions of Cellular Condensation to Gyral Formations

The marsupial brush-tailed possum proves a species of great interest indeed, for while most specimens are lissencephalic, an occasional individual has been observed with some development of gyri and sulci in the cortical sensory region

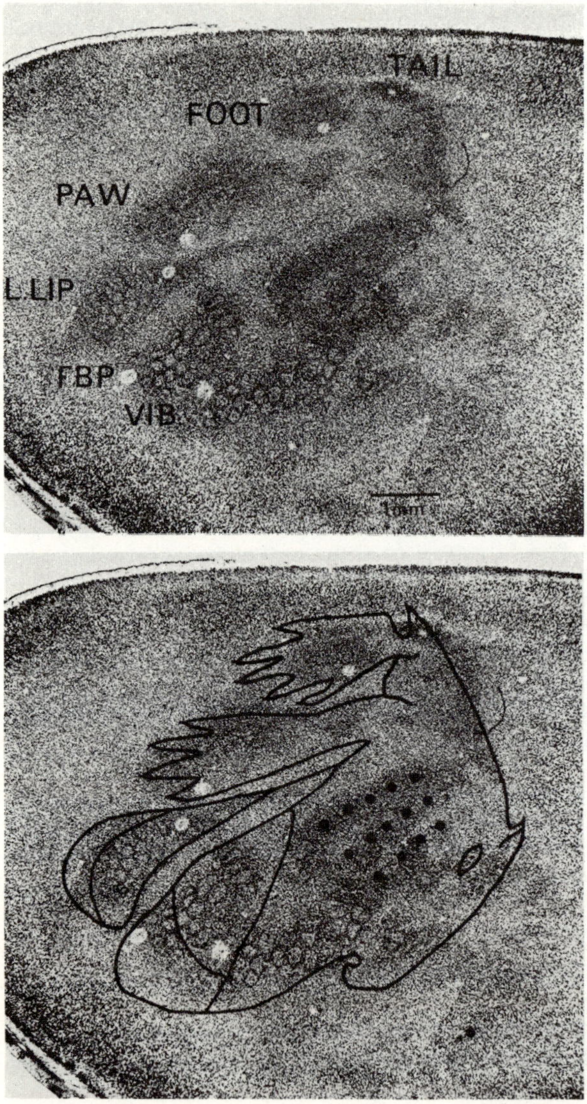

Figure 13. Flattened section through layer IV of sensory neocortex of the rat, stained with thionin. White circular patches are microlesions marking the sites of projections, determined electrophysiologically, from TAIL, hindFOOT, forePAW, Lower LIP, Furry Buccal Pad, and small anterior mystacial VIBrissae. Cellular condensations form morphological counterparts of the body regions projecting to them as seen in the superimposed sketch below. Black dots represent the large posterior mystacial vibrissae which project to "solid" barrels similar to those shown in Fig. 14. Regions of "rarefaction" between condensed projection regions can be labeled interbrachial (IB) between the condensations representing hindFOOT and forePAW, jugular (J) between forePAW and Lower LIP, and labial (L) between Lower LIP and Furry Buccal Pad. Reproduced from C. Welker (1976), through courtesy of C. Welker and the *Journal of Comparative Neurology.*

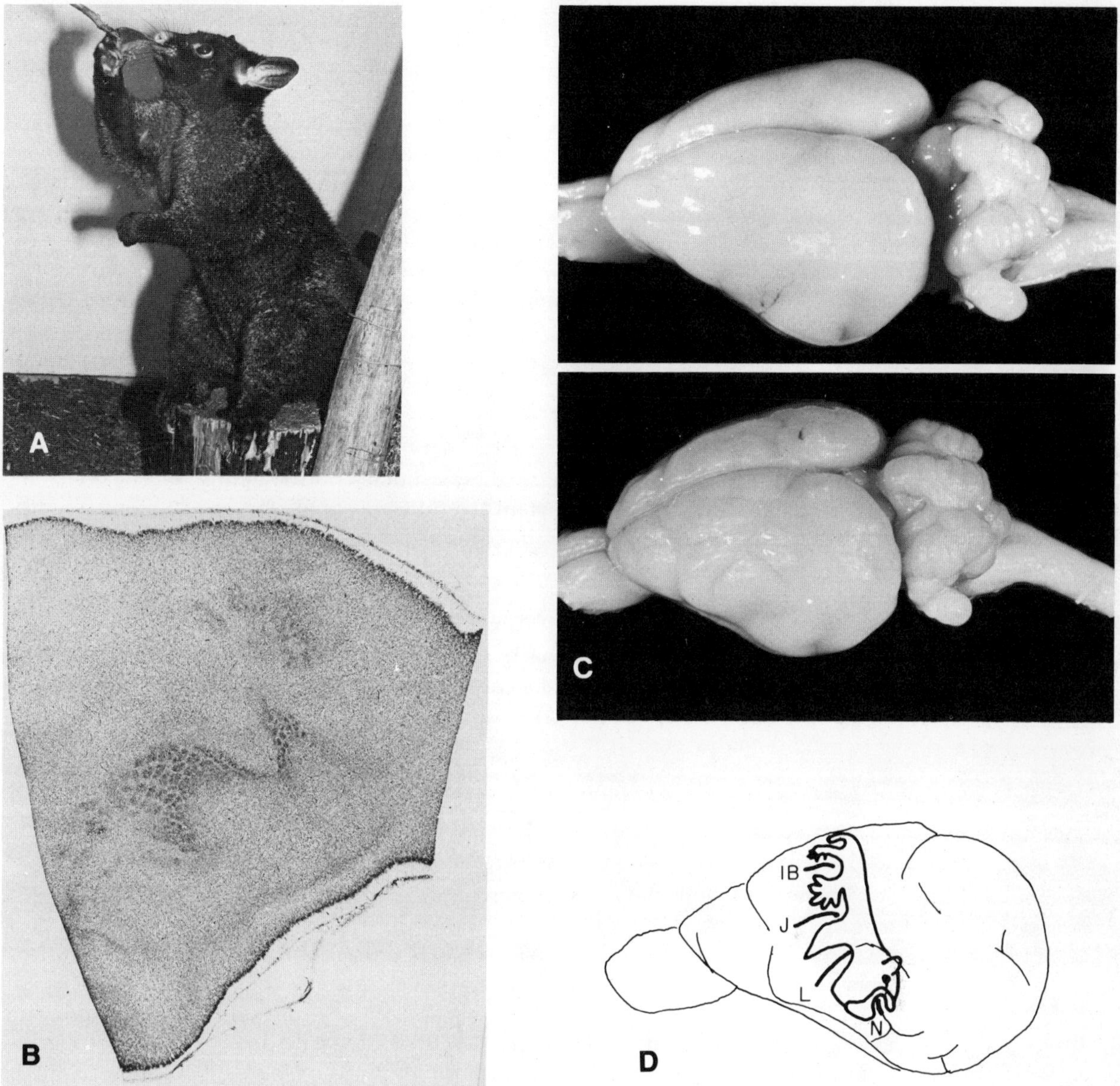

Figure 14. Morphology of somatic sensory neocortex in brush-tailed possums (*Trichosurus vulpecula*). A: A black specimen of the Tasmanian race (other individuals are gray or brown). B: Tangential section through layer IV of sensory neocortex of a 12-cm-long young possum, stained with thionin for cell bodies, showing regions of cellular "condensation" containing barrel formations. Unlike mice barrels, but like the large-vibrissa barrels in rats seen in Fig. 13, the possum barrels do not enclose "hollows"; rather, they are solid clumps of cell bodies separated by spaces of lesser cell density (Weller, 1972*a*). As in the rat in Fig. 13, regions of cell "rarefaction" are seen between regions of "condensation." C: Photographs of the neocortical surfaces of lisssencephalic (above) and gyrencephalic (below) brains of *Trichosurus*; scale is in mm. D: Sketch of sensory projections found in gyrencephalic brains. As in wombats (Fig. 5), sulci appear between projections of body parts: interbrachial (IB), jugular (J), labial (L), and narial (N). Furthermore, these sulci correspond to regions of cellular rarefaction seen in lissencephalic brains (Haight and Weller, 1973; Weller and Haight, 1973). Photographs courtesy of W. L. Weller and J. R. Haight.

(Haight and Weller, 1973), as shown in Fig. 14. These sulci and gyri follow closely in their pattern those seen in marsupial wombats, and partial electrophysiological maps indicate that the sensory projections also follow the pattern seen in wombats, particularly in their relationships to the sulci and gyri. Sulci appear between the representations of separated receptive fields. In lissencephalic specimens, on the other hand, flattened sections can be prepared for the observation of barrels and condensation and rarefaction regions, and here the location of the rarefactions in the sensory map corresponds to the location of the sulci in the gyrencephalic specimens. Condensation regions with their included barrels appear in the map at those locations where gyral crowns occur in gyrencephalic specimens.

We might now speculate that, were rats to develop sulci and gyri, they would occur along the course of the regions of layer IV rarefaction (sulci) and condensation (gyri). Furthermore, we could apply the sulcus names generated from wombats. In fact, we can apply those names to the rarefaction regions themselves, and designate interbrachial, jugular, labial, and perhaps narial patches which can be seen in Welker's photographs (Fig. 13).

Testing the generality of this phenomenon will be difficult, since the tangential and flattened sections necessary to show cellular condensations, rarefactions, and barrels are difficult enough to obtain from lissencephalic brains, let alone attempting to do so in a convoluted brain. The immense good fortune of discovering a species like the brush-tailed possum, which yields individuals with lissencephalic brains for tangential and flattened sections as well as gyrencephalic individuals where sulci can be studied, is not likely to recur with great frequency. It is only through the comparative approach and exploration of new species that such a discovery did come about, with its considerable implications for the fundamentals of general brain organization in mammals.

VII. Summary

Regions of high density of mechanoreceptors in the peripheral body appear to give rise to neural aggregates in the central nervous system, to which these receptors project. These neuronal aggregates represent the successive synaptic beds where information processing and transmission from cell to cell take place. In mammals, the regions of receptor density are often found on hindfeet, hands, lips, vibrissae, and nose, or some partial set of these structures. The corresponding neuronal aggregates in the brain include the lobular nuclear formations in the cuneate–gracile complex of the medulla and the ventrobasal thalamus, cellular condensation regions and barrel formations in layer IV of the somatic sensory cerebral cortex, and gyral efflorescences in this sensory cortex. In each case the size and elaboration of the neuronal aggregate at each level correspond with those seen at each other level, and reflect the specialized behavioral use of the associated receptor surface. Limited evidence thus far suggests a directive role of the receptor surface in the organization and maintenance of its brain correlates at each of these levels.

The separation of aggregates into separate lobules, condensation fields, and gyri may reflect the need for interconnectivity among projections from neighboring receptors; projections from separated body parts are not under this constraint and thus their central projection regions in the brain occur as separate morphological entities. Thus it is that the shape of the body, allowing for the distribution of receptors thereon, is morphologically mimicked by the cellular aggregates at each synaptic level in this system.

ACKNOWLEDGMENTS. The preparation of this chapter (and a good deal of the research reviewed herein) was supported by Research Grants GB 43236 from NSF and NS 05982 from NIH and was assisted by facilities provided by Dr. E. W Rubel and the Psychology Department of Yale University. Where not otherwise indicated, photography was by Neal Brophy and histological preparations were by G. H. Chung Kim, E. G. Haight, and A. B. Harton. Drs. C. Welt and R. W. Dykes provided helpful critical comments.

VIII. References

Adrian, E. D., 1943, Afferent areas in the brain of ungulates, *Brain* **66:**89.

Bischoff, E., 1899, Zur Anatomie der Hinterstrangkerne bei Säugethieren, *Jahrb. Psychiat. Neurol.* **18:**371.

Campos, G. B., and Welker, W. I., 1976, Some physiological and anatomical comparisons between the brains of capybaras (*Hydrochoerus*) and guinea pigs (*Cavia*), *Brain Behav. Evol.* **13:**243.

Chang, H.-T., and Ruch, T. C., 1947, Organization of the dorsal columns of the spinal cord and their nuclei in the spider monkey, *J. Anat.* **81:**140.

Haight, J. R., and Weller, W. L., 1973, Neocortical topography in the brush-tailed possum: Variability and functional significance of sulci, *J. Anat.* **116:**473.

Hamilton, T. C., and Johnson, J. I., 1973, Somatotopic organization related to nuclear morphology in the cuneate–gracile complex of opossums *Didelphis marsupialis virginiana*, *Brain Res.* **51:**125.

Johnson, J. I., Welker, W. I., and Pubols, B. H., 1968, Somatotopic organization of raccoon dorsal column nuclei, *J. Comp. Neurol.* **132:**1.

Johnson, J. I., Hamilton, T. C., Hsung, J.-C., and Ulinski, P. S., 1972, Gracile nucleus absent in adult opossums after leg removal in infancy, *Brain Res.* **38:**421.

Johnson, J. I., Haight, J. R., and Megirian, D., 1973, Convolutions related to sensory projections in cerebral neocortex of marsupial wombats, *J. Anat.* **114:**153.

Johnson, J. I., Rubel, E. W, and Hatton, G. I., 1974, Mechanosensory projections to cerebral cortex of sheep, *J. Comp. Neurol.* **158:**81.

Kirsch, J. A. W., 1976, Classification of marsupials, in: *Biology of Marsupials,* Vol. I (D. Hunsaker, ed.), Academic Press, New York.

Krishnamurti, A., Kanagasuntheram, R., and Wong, W. C., 1972, Functional significance of the fibrous laminae in the ventrobasal complex of the thalamus of slow loris, *J. Comp. Neurol.* **145:**515.

Lee, K. J., and Woolsey, T. A., 1975, A proportional relationship between peripheral innervation density and cortical neuron number in the somatosensory system of the mouse, *Brain Res.* **99:**349.

Le Gros Clark, W. E., 1962, The sorting principle in sensory analysis as illustrated by the visual pathways, *Ann. R. Coll. Surg. Engl. 30:*229.

Lende, R. A., 1963, Cerebral cortex: A sensorimotor amalgam in the Marsupialia, *Science* **141:**730.

Matzke, H. A., 1951, The course of the fibers arising from the nucleus gracilis and cuneatus of the cat, *J. Comp. Neurol.* **94:**439.

McKenna, M. C., 1975, Toward a phylogenetic classification of the mammals, in: *Phylogeny of the Primates* (W. P. Luckett and F. S. Szalay, eds.), pp. 31–46, Plenum Press, New York.

Morest, D. K., 1970, A study of neurogenesis in the forebrain of opossum pouch young, *Z. Anat. Entwicklungsgesch.* **130:**265.

Mountcastle, V. B., and Henneman, E., 1949, Pattern of tactile representation in thalamus of cat, *J. Neurophysiol.* **12:**85.

Mountcastle, V. B., and Henneman, E., 1952, The representation of tactile sensibility in the thalamus of the monkey, *J. Comp. Neurol.* **97:**409.

Papez, J. W., and Hunter, R. P., 1929, Formation of a central sulcus in the brain of the raccoon, *Anat. Rec.* **42:**60.

Pimentel-Souza, F., Cosenza, R. M., Campos, G. B., and Johnson, J. I., 1980, Somatic sensory cortical regions of the agouti, *Dasyprocta aguti,* in preparation.

Pubols, B. H., and Pubols, L. M., 1980, Variation in the fissural pattern of the cerebral neocortex of the spider monkey (*Ateles*), *Brain Behav. Evol.,* in press.

Pubols, B. H., Welker, W. I., and Johnson, J. I., 1965, Somatic sensory representation of forelimb in dorsal root fibers of raccoon, coatimundi, and cat, *J. Neurophysiol.* **28:**312.

Rice, F. L., 1973, Somatosensory cortex of mouse: Development of barrels and of barrel field, *Anat. Rec.* **175:**423.

Rice, F. L., 1974, Somatosensory cortex of the mouse: Time of origin and postnatal migration of neurons in the barrel field. A quantitative autoradiographic study, *Anat. Rec.* **178:**447.

Rice, F. L., and Van der Loos, H., 1977, Development of the barrels and barrel field in the somatosensory cortex of the mouse, *J. Comp. Neurol.* **171:**545.

Rioch, D. M., 1929, Studies on the diencephalon of Carnivora. Part. I. The nuclear configuration of the thalamus, epithalamus, and hypothalamus of the dog and cat, *J. Comp. Neurol.* **49:**1.

Rose, J. E., and Mountcastle, V. B., 1952, The thalamic tactile region in rabbit and cat, *J. Comp. Neurol.* **97:**441.

Rubel, E. W, 1971, A comparison of somatotopic organization in sensory neocortex of newborn kittens and adult cats, *J. Comp. Neurol.* **143:**447.

Simpson, G. G., 1961, *Principles of Animal Taxonomy,* Columbia University Press, New York.

Ulinski, P. S., 1969, Normal development of the cuneate–gracile nuclear complex in pouch young opossums, Ph.D. thesis, zoology, Michigan State University.

Ulinski, P. A., 1971, External morphology of pouch young opossum brains: A profile of opossum neurogenesis, *J. Comp. Neurol.* **142:**33.

Van der Loos, H., and Woolsey, T. A., 1973, Somatosensory cortex: Structural alterations following early injury to sense organs, *Science* **179:**395.

Walker, A. E., 1938, *The Primate Thalamus,* University of Chicago Press, Chicago.

Welker, C., 1971, Microelectrode delineation of fine grain somatotopic organization of SmI cerebral neocortex in albino rat, *Brain Res.* **26:**259.

Welker, C., 1976, Receptive fields of barrels in the somatosensory neocortex of the rat, *J. Comp. Neurol.* **166:**173.

Welker, C., and Woolsey, T. A., 1974, Structure of layer IV in the somatosensory neocortex of the rat: Description and comparison with the mouse, *J. Comp. Neurol.* **158:**437.

Welker, W. I., and Campos, G. B., 1963 Physiological significance of sulci in somatic sensory cortex of mammals of the family Procyonidae, *J. Comp. Neurol.* **120:**19.

Welker, W. I., and Johnson, J. I., 1965, Correlation between nuclear morphology and somatotopic organization in ventro-basal complex of the racoon's thalamus, *J. Anat.* **99:**761.

Welker, W. I., and Seidenstein, S., 1959, Somatic sensory representation in the cerebral cortex of the raccoon (*Procyon lotor*), *J. Comp. Neurol.* **111:**469.

Welker, W. I., Johnson, J. I., and Pubols, B. H., 1964, Some morphological and physiological characteristics of the somatic sensory system in raccoons, *Am. Zool.* **4:**75.

Welker, W. I., Adrian, H. O., Lifschitz, W., Kaulen, R., Caviedes, R., and Gutman, W., 1976, Somatic sensory cortex of llama (*Lama glama*), *Brain Behav. Evol.* **13:**284.

Weller, W. L., 1972*a*, Barrels in somatic sensory neocortex of the marsupial *Trichosurus vulpecula* (brush-tailed possum), *Brain Res.* **43:**11.

Weller, W. L., 1972*b*, Ontogeny of barrels in muroid sensory neocortex: Time course, relation to behavioral development, and dependence upon peripheral input, Ph.D. thesis, biophysics, Michigan State University.

Weller, W. L., and Haight, J. R., 1973, Barrels and somatotopy in SI neocortex of the brush-tailed possum, *J. Anat.* **116:**474.

Weller, W. L., and Johnson, J. I., 1975, Barrels in cerebral cortex altered by receptor disruption in newborn, but not in five-day-old mice (Cricetidae and Muridae), *Brain Res.* **83:**504.

Woolsey, C. N., 1959, Some observations on brain fissurization in relation to cortical localization of function, in: *Structure and Function of the Cerebral Cortex* (D. B. Tower and J. P. Schade, eds.), pp. 64–68, Elsevier, Amsterdam.

Woolsey, C. N., and Fairman, D., 1946, Contralateral, ipsilateral and bilateral representation of cutaneous receptors in somatic areas I and II of the cerebral cortex of pig, sheep and other mammals, *Surgery* **19:**684.

Woolsey, T. A., and Van der Loos, H., 1970, The structural organization of layer IV in the somatosensory region (SI) of mouse cerebral cortex, *Brain Res.* **17:**205.

Woolsey, T. A., Welker, C., and Schwartz, R. H., 1975, Comparative anatomical studies of the SmI face cortex with special reference to the barrels, *J. Comp. Neurol.* **164:**79.

Woudenberg, R. A., 1970, Projections of mechanoreceptive fields to cuneate–gracile and spinal trigeminal nuclear regions in sheep, *Brain Res.* **17:**417.

Zollman, P. E., and Winkelmann, R. K., 1962, The sensory innervation of the common North American Raccoon (*Procyon lotor*), *J. Comp. Neurol.* **119:**149.

15

Thalamocortical Relationships in Echidna (*Tachyglossus aculeatus*)

WALLY WELKER and RICHARD A. LENDE

I. Introduction

Dr. Richard Lende's interest in comparative studies of sensory cortex in mammals led him to examine the somatic sensory, motor, visual, and auditory areas of echidnas (Lende, 1964). This chapter is a direct outcome of Dr. Lende's desire to corroborate his electrophysiological delineation of cortical sensory and motor areas in echidnas by means of retrograde degeneration studies of thalamocortical connections. Striking features of the echidna brain are its relatively large size and fissural complexity, two characteristics which, among others, make these animals of special interest to comparative neurologists (Abbie, 1938).

Echidnas, being monotremes, are traditionally grouped, together with the duck-billed platypus, in the subclass Prototheria of the class Mammalia (Simpson, 1945). The other two great mammalian subclasses are the Metatheria, or marsupials, and the Theria, or placentals. Since little is known about echidnas' ancestral types during the Tertiary period, not much can be said of their evolutionary history or of their degree of affinity to other living mammals (Romer, 1968). There is not yet a consensus whether or not monotremes are related to Mesozoic fossil mammals (Hopson and Crompton, 1969) or represent surviving therapsid reptiles (Van Valen, 1960). Echidnas appear phylogenetically primitive, at least in some anatom-

Portions of this chapter were presented by Dr. J. I. Johnson, Jr., at The Richard A. Lende Memorial Symposium, August 15–16, 1974, The Albany Medical College, Albany, New York. This study was begun in the summer of 1964 at the University of Colorado Medical School in Denver while Dr. Lende was Associate Professor of Neurosurgery.

WALLY WELKER and RICHARD A. LENDE • Department of Neurophysiology, University of Wisconsin, Madison, Wisconsin 53706. Dr. Lende is deceased.

ical and physiological aspects, yet their brain development appears unusually advanced when compared to that of some marsupials or insectivores (Jerison, 1973). For example, discovery of a separate motor area in echidnas indicates greater similarity to the common placental plan than to the apparent sensorimotor overlap or "amalgam" proposed for marsupials (Lende, 1969). However, the echidna brain is different from that of other placentals in the posterolateral displacement of its sensory and motor cortical areas by an unusually large expanse of frontally situated cortex that is unresponsive to cortical stimulation or recording techniques.

It was our purpose in this study to define and describe those thalamic nuclei that contain essential projections to the cerebral neocortex in echidna. We did this by performing a series of selective partial ablations of somatic sensory, auditory, visual, and motor areas, and of several different portions of the unusually large expanse of frontal neocortex. After 2 months' survival time all animals were perfused, the brains were processed histologically, and the location and extent of retrograde degenerative changes in the thalamus were identified microscopically.

We found that the thalamocortical relationships in echidna are similar in most respects to those demonstrated in placental mammals. Most major cortically dependent thalamic nuclear groups were identified. One unusual feature is the large nuclear mass in the dorso-fronto-medial thalamus which projects to the relatively enlarged frontal cortex. We suspect that this large nuclear region is, in part, the mediodorsal nucleus and may be the thalamic component that processes olfactory information destined for the cerebral cortex.

II. Materials and Methods

A. Subjects

Six echidnas were the subjects of this study (Fig. 1). Four were females (body weights 3.1 kg, 3.6 kg, 3.7 kg, and 3.8 kg) and two were males (2.3 kg and 2.9 kg). The females appeared to be adults and the males juveniles. All animals were procured from Avitraders, Inc., Sydney, Australia.

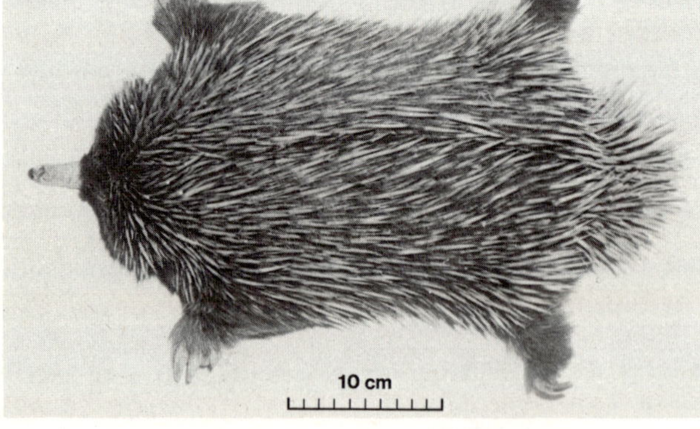

Figure 1. Dorsal view of anesthetized echidna (*Tachyglossus aculeatus*) (cf. Lende, 1964). Reproduced with publisher's permission.

B. Surgical Procedures

All animals were anesthetized with sodium pentobarbital (35 mg/kg body weight). The quills were removed from the head and neck regions with wire cutters, and the body hairs from these regions were clipped short with scissors. The head and neck were then scrubbed with a brush using pHisoHex soap and water, and the scalp was rendered sterile by repeated applications of iodine. Sterile neurosurgical operative procedures were utilized, the scalp being incised at the midline and laterally at locations that would avoid transection of major blood vessels of the skin. The skull was removed, the dura was incised and reflected (and later sutured closed), and selected cerebral neocortical areas were removed by subpial suction (Fig. 8). One aspiration lesion was placed in each hemisphere in every animal (see Section III). All lesions were placed according to fissural and gyral landmarks, which, despite some variability, reliably demarcate different functional cortical areas (Lende, 1964). The several lesions in unresponsive frontal and medial cortex were placed so as to occupy different adjacent portions of this region. Only cellular gray matter was removed on gyral crowns, and care was taken not to extend lesions to the depths of fissures in order to prevent undercutting of fibers to adjacent gyri. However, a few lesions were larger than desired.

C. Histological Preparation

All animals were perfused 60 days postoperatively with 0.9% saline followed by a mixture of formol–saline. The brains were embedded in Celloidin and cut 25 μm thick, and serial sections were stained with thionin and mounted on slides.

D. Identification of Cortical Lesions and Thalamic Degeneration

The adequacy of the cortical lesions was assessed microscopically from serial sections. Retrograde degenerative changes in thalamic nuclei were identified by the presence of patches of gliosis, and by presence of pale, shrunken cell bodies of abnormal shape or that exhibited pyknosis and a displaced nucleus. The severity of these degenerative signs varied with different lesions and appeared positively correlated with the completeness of the cortical lesion.

III. Results

The purpose of this study was to determine whether the echidna thalamus exhibits mammalian thalamocortical dependencies more similar to those found in marsupials or to those in placental mammals. We were particularly concerned with whether there is an enlarged thalamic nucleus sending afferents to the enlarged frontal cortex. Our data reveal that there is. In addition, we hoped to determine whether the projections to the separate motor and somatic sensory cortical areas

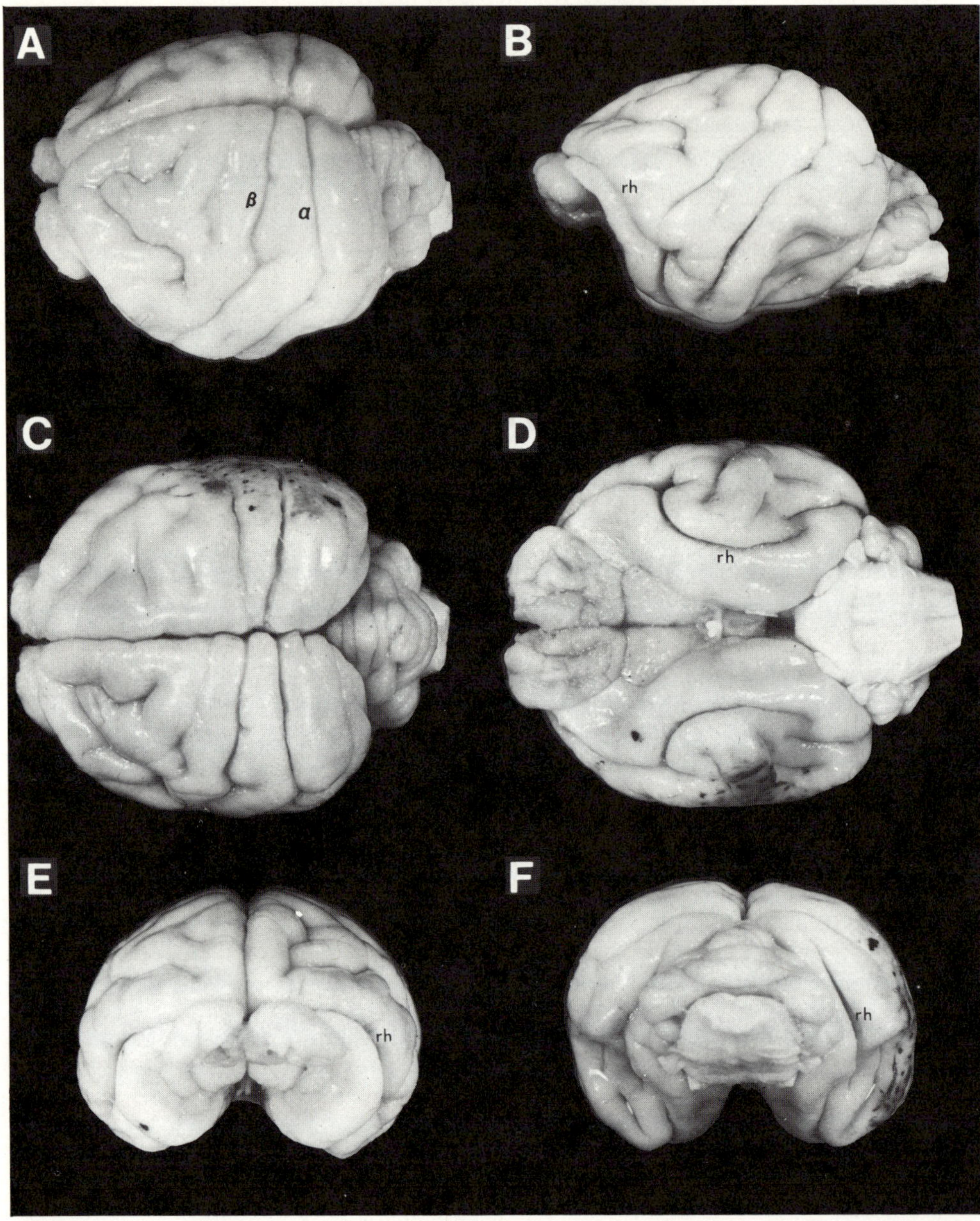

Figure 2. Photographs of brain of adult echidna from left dorsolateral (A), left lateral (B), dorsal (C), ventral (D), rostral (E), and caudal (F) views. Fissures alpha (α) and beta (β) are indicated in A. Rhinal sulcus (rh) is indicated in B, D, E, and F. Millimeter scale at lower right. Black dots visible on right hemisphere indicate recording locations of surface macroelectrodes in an experiment reported by Lende (1964).

from the thalamus are spatially distinct. We found that they are. Data regarding cortex, thalamus, and thalamocortical relationships are presented in that order.

A. Cortical Organization

1. External Morphology

Echidna brains have an unusually extensive and fissured cerebral neocortex (Figs. 2–5). Even the prepyriform cortex exhibits cortical folding (Fig. 5). Indeed, the percent of both area and volume of neocortex buried in fissures is relatively large in the echidna brain (36%) compared to that of a rodent (capybara, 28%), a carnivore (domestic cat, 40%), and a primate (squirrel monkey, 39%) of similar brain size (unpublished volumetric studies from this laboratory).

2. Functional and Architectonic Areas of Cerebral Cortex

Lende's (1964) neurophysiological mapping experiments revealed the locations of somatic sensory, visual, auditory, and motor areas. These areas (Fig. 6) are

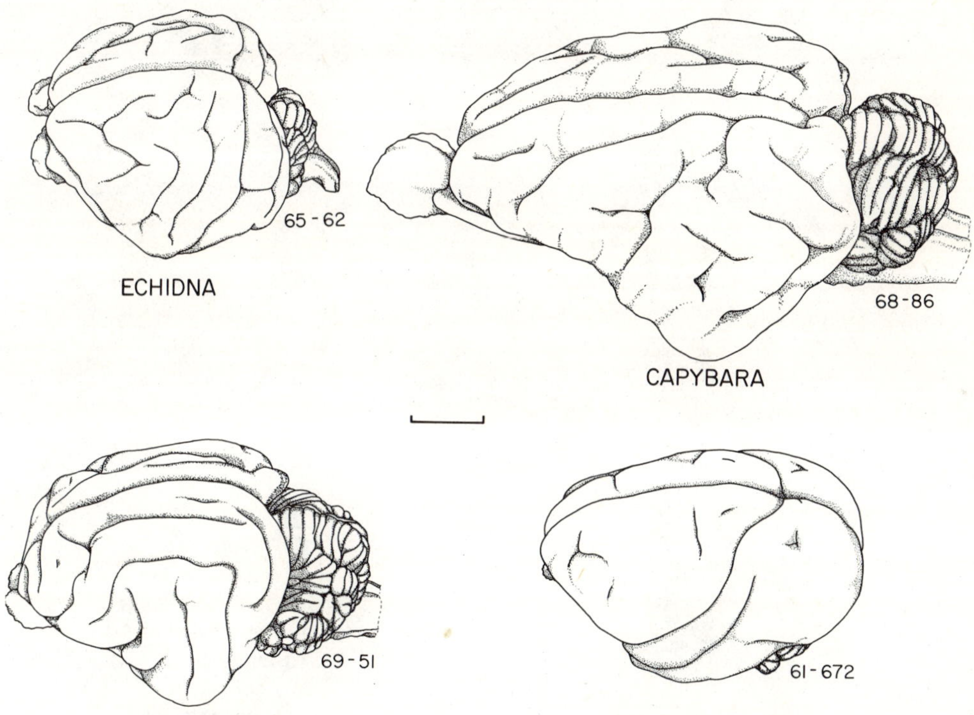

Figure 3. Drawings of brains of four mammals to indicate relatively fissured cerebral neocortex of echidna (monotreme) when compared with that of a rodent (capybara), a felid (domestic cat), and a primate (squirrel monkey). All brains are from adults and drawn to same size (1-cm scale in center).

situated more caudolaterally on the hemispheres of echidnas than are their homologues in placental mammals (Chapter 14, this volume; Woolsey, 1952, 1964, 1971*a,b*) or even marsupials (Chapter 14, this volume; Lende, 1969). Our study of serial sections of echidna cortex through these physiologically defined sensory regions revealed an underlying architecturally distinct laminar pattern with a relatively well-developed granule cell layer IV (cf. Gray, 1924). The striking feature of echidna cortex is, of course, the relatively large expanse of "unresponsive" cortex rostral to the sensory and motor areas (Fig. 6). The surface area of this "frontal" cortex is about 50% of the total neocortical surface of the echidna cerebrum (unpublished data obtained by planimetric methods). One objective of this study was to reveal the thalamic source of afferents to this cortical area. However, before

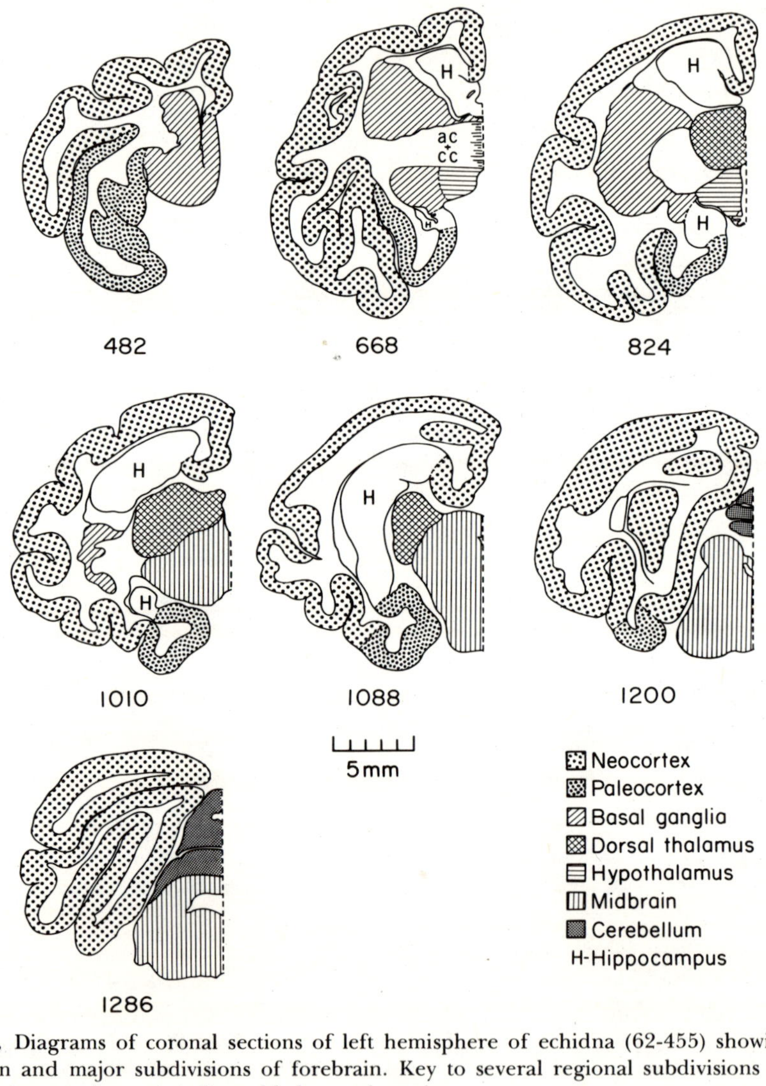

Figure 4. Diagrams of coronal sections of left hemisphere of echidna (62-455) showing cortical fissuration and major subdivisions of forebrain. Key to several regional subdivisions is at lower right. Section numbers are indicated below each section.

reviewing our evidence for thalamocortical relationships, it is useful to examine cytoarchitectonic features of the major thalamic nuclear groups.

B. Thalamic Nuclear Organization

Several thalamic nuclei in echidna exhibit cyto- and myeloarchitectonic features that resemble, to some extent, those found in other mammals (cf. Campbell and Hayhow, 1971). However, they are not all as easily distinguished as they are in opossums (Benevento and Ebner, 1971; Bodian, 1936, 1942; Oswaldo-Cruz and Rocha-Miranda, 1968) or in other commonly used laboratory mammals (Rose, 1942; Rose and Woolsey, 1949). In fact, in our thionin- and hematoxylin-stained specimens the outlines of several nuclei are only faintly discernible, or distinguishable at only certain portions of what we expect to be the total nucleus. Several organizational features of thalamic nuclei of echidna are seen in the 12 normal coronal sections of Fig. 7A–L. Those nuclei that are named in Fig. 7 were identified on the basis of cytoarchitectonic and myeloarchitectonic criteria, on the basis of their relative position, shape, size, and orientation within the thalamus, and on the presence of degeneration following cortical removals as defined in this study (Fig. 8).

Homologues of the paraventricular and some midline and anterior nuclei of the rostral thalamus are definable, as are the reticular nucleus (which is relatively poorly developed), the habenular nuclei, and the pretectal nuclei. The ventrolateral

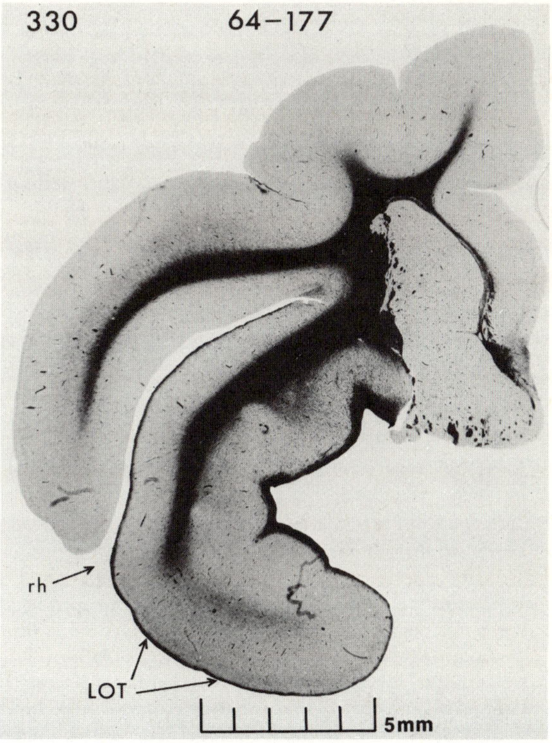

Figure 5. Photomicrograph of coronal section (hematoxylin fiber stain) through frontal region of left hemisphere of echidna 64-177. Note deep rhinal sulcus (rh) and the relatively large folded convolution of prepyriform cortex (lower lobule) with the lateral olfactory tract (LOT, black marginal fiber layer) extending over its entire surface.

and ventrobasal nuclei are relatively easily demarcated, but there are problems in identifying the medial geniculate and portions of the lateral geniculate nuclei, as is discussed further below. Nuclei of the posterior group, dorsolateral group, most other midline nuclei (paracentral, reuniens, central lateral, parafascicular, central, centre median, etc.), and especially the large mediodorsal nuclear region in the rostral half of the thalamus are not easily recognized as discrete nuclei. There are several nuclear and subnuclear groupings in the caudolateral thalamus that are quite distinct in hematoxylin-stained sections, but their architectonic and projectional homologues are uncertain. Most thalamic nuclear regions are not labeled in the illustrations of this chapter because of these uncertainties. One hesitates to use the standard nomenclature for such thalamic regions because of the essential prior importance of defining the specific varieties of functional connectivities of such cell groups.

C. Thalamocortical Relationships*

1. Sensory Nuclei

The nuclear region that degenerated after removal of the somatic sensory area is identified as the ventrobasal (VB) nucleus (Figs. 10A,B and 12C,D). The thalamic loci of retrograde degeneration in animals 64-228 and 64-233, both of which involve visual cortex as defined by Lende (1964), do not correspond exactly with those nuclei found by Campbell and Hayhow (1971) to receive optic tract terminals. In both our cases the large, darkly staining cells of the caudolateral thalamus show clearest degeneration. Their LGN_a (Fig. 7J–L), which receives most optic terminals, does not clearly degenerate in our cases (Figs. 9C and 15J,K), although the region of their LGN_b (Fig. 7G), situated more rostro-laterally but not clearly distinguished in our cases, did seem to degenerate in our animals (Fig. 15J,K). Our data do not suggest an explanation of these basic discrepancies between the two studies. A medial geniculate nucleus was not clearly identified in our cases. The retrograde degeneration following destruction of auditory cortex was not clearly associated with a specific nuclear group. This may be due to the fact that the auditory cortical lesion was minimal and the other lesion of the same hemisphere probably undercut some fibers from somatic sensory and visual cortex (Fig. 15I). Also, the auditory area identified by Lende (1964) may not have been completely defined because the occipital pole is partly inaccessible because of the transverse vascular sinus. Or the medial geniculate may have sustaining projections to other thalamic or basal nuclei (Ebner, 1969). It was our guess on the basis of its relative position, before seeing the data of Campbell and Hayhow, that the medial geniculate was the nucleus (LGN_a) to which they found optic nerve input. Additional physiological and other

* The description of each of the cortical lesions is given in the captions of the figures showing corresponding thalamic degeneration. In these figures all photomicrographs of thalamic retrograde degeneration are paired with normal thalamic pictures of the same region on the opposite side of the same animal. These photomicrographs are shown in Figs. 9–14. Regions of retrograde degeneration and gliosis are encircled by dotted lines. Sections shown are at thalamic level of maximal degeneration following cortical ablation. Thionin stain, 25 μm thick. Abbreviations are the same as for Fig. 7. Location of cortical lesions (black regions) is indicated on small brain diagrams. For most cases, only one rostro-caudal level is shown. The summary diagrams of Fig. 15 show schematically the location and extent of degeneration at 12 standard levels for each case.

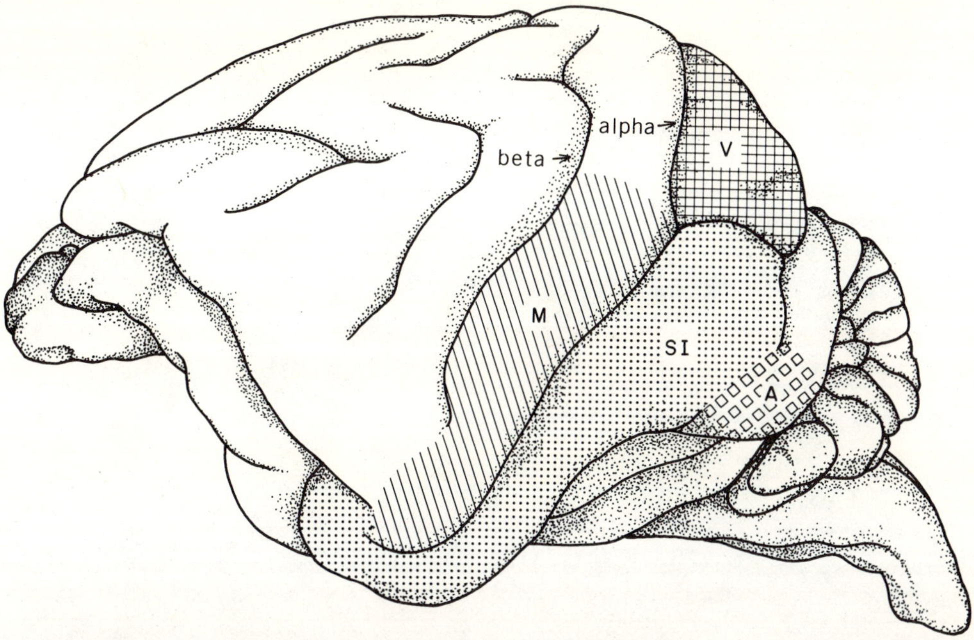

Figure 6. Diagram of left side of echidna brain showing locations of motor and sensory areas defined by Lende (1964). M, Motor area (MI); SI, first somatic sensory area; V, visual area; A, auditory area. Sulci alpha and beta (Elliot-Smith, 1902) are indicated. Note relatively caudal and lateral placement of these areas on the hemisphere and the relatively large frontal cortical region rostral to sulcus beta. Also note "nonsensory" cortex medial to motor (M) area and on occipital pole (see also Fig. 2F) difficult to reach by surface macroelectrodes. Reproduced with publisher's permission.

neuroanatomical studies are required to identify and define these visual and auditory nuclei more accurately.

2. Ventrolateral Nucleus

The ventrolateral nucleus projects to a separate motor cortex in all mammals examined except those with a sensory–motor "amalgam," in which portions or all of the motor and somatic sensory cortices appear to be congruent (Ebner, 1969;

Figure 7. A–L: Photomicrographs of coronal sections of normal echidna thalamus. Sections 772–1102 illustrate 12 bilateral thalamic levels and are ordered from rostral to caudal. Right side of thalamus of each section is at a slightly more caudal level than that of the left side. Magnification is indicated by 1-mm scale, and all sections are at the same enlargement. Only a few thalamic nuclei are indicated by standard abbreviations placed within the confines of each nucleus. Thionin stain. Section thickness is 25 μm. These 12 sections are similar in rostrocaudal level to the 12 diagrams (coronal series only) of Fig. 15 that summarize thalamic degeneration data. AD, Anterior dorsal nucleus; HL, lateral habenula; HM, medial habenula; L, lateral nuclear region; LGN_a, caudoventral lateral geniculate nucleus of Campbell and Hayhow (1971); LGN_b, rostrodorsal lateral geniculate of Campbell and Hayhow (1971); MD, mediodorsal nucleus; OP?, region degenerating after removal of occipital pole; PT, pretectal nucleus; RE, reticular nucleus; SC, superior colliculus; sm, stria medullaris; VB, ventrobasal nucleus; VL, ventrolateral nucleus.

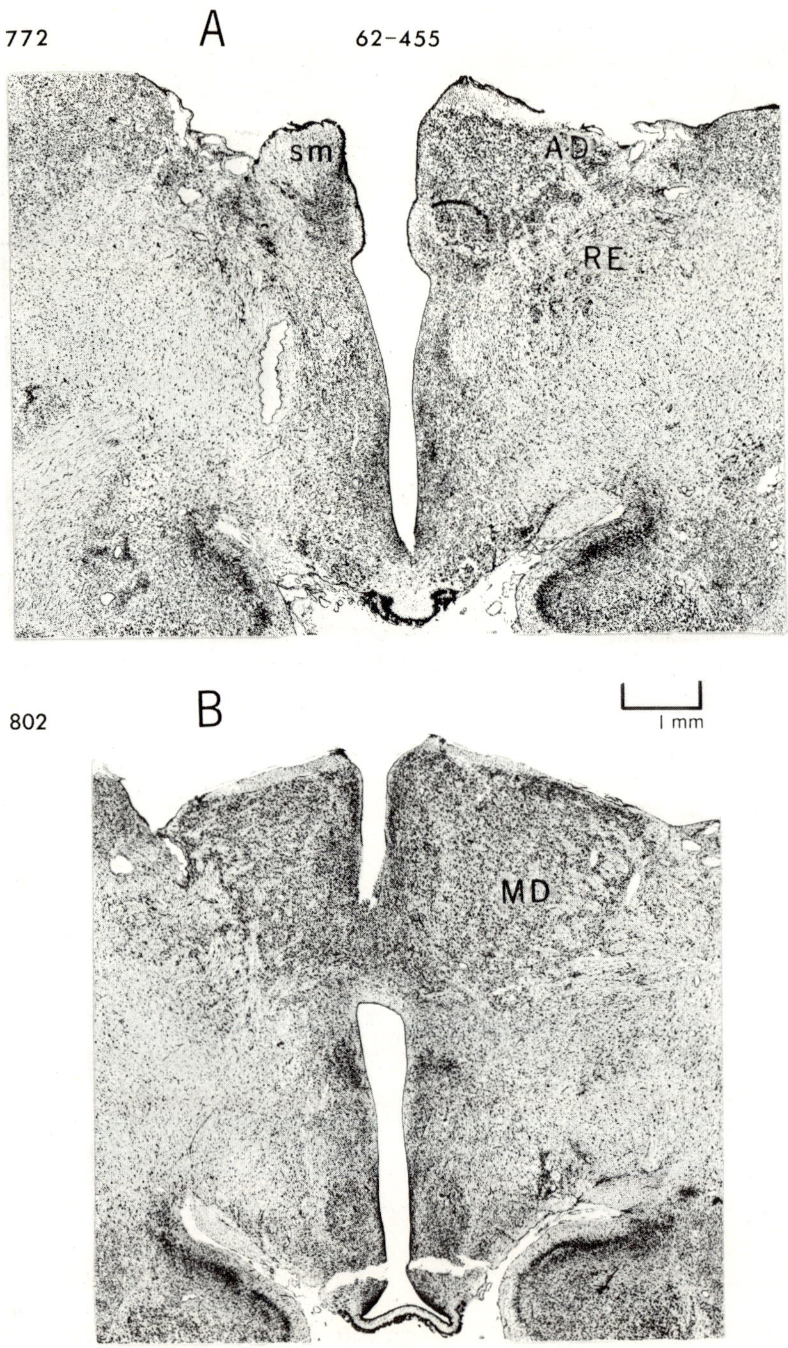
772
A
62-455
sm
AD
RE
802
B
1 mm
MD

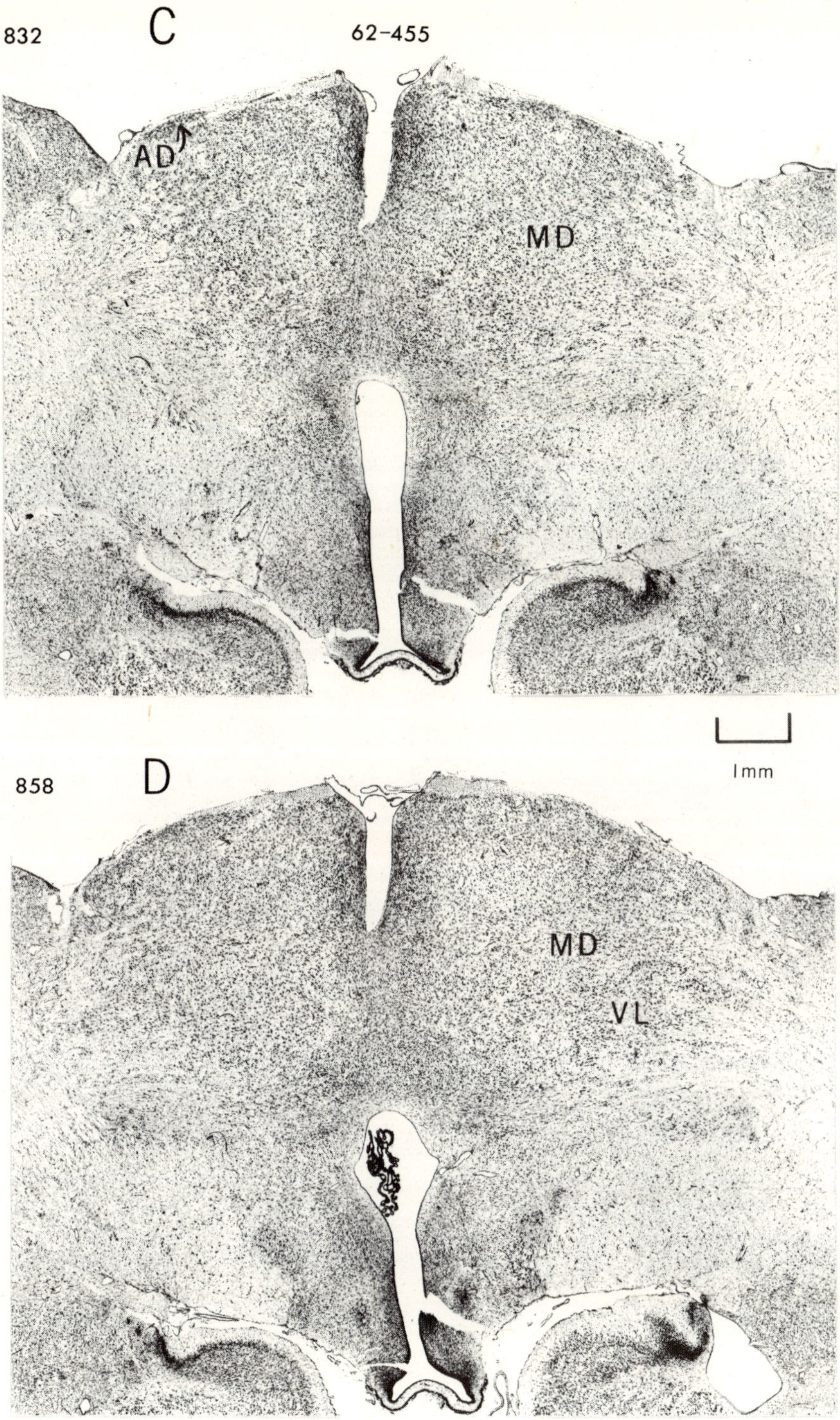
832
C
62-455
AD
MD
1mm
858
D
MD
VL

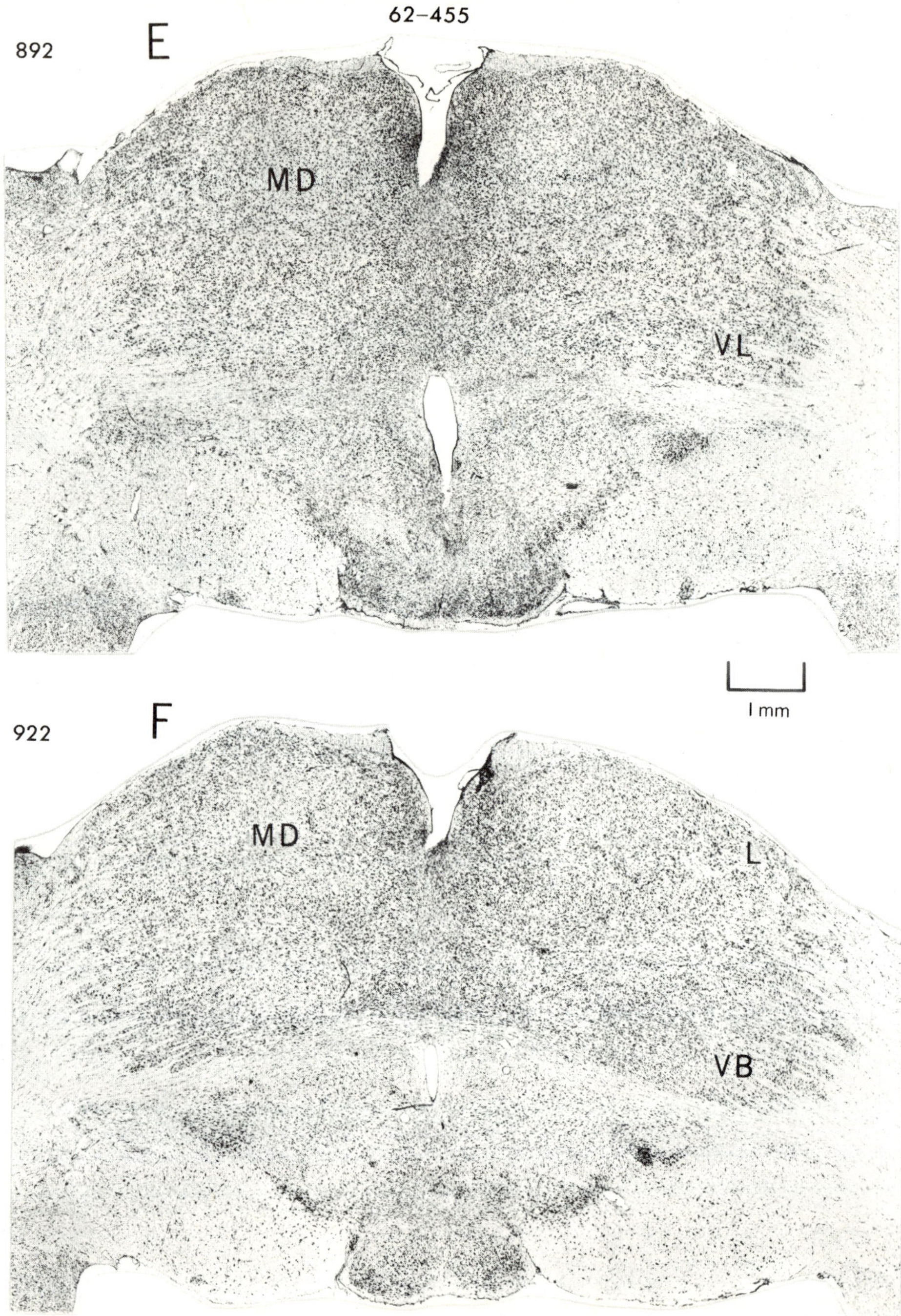
62–455
892
E
MD
VL
1 mm
922
F
MD
L
VB

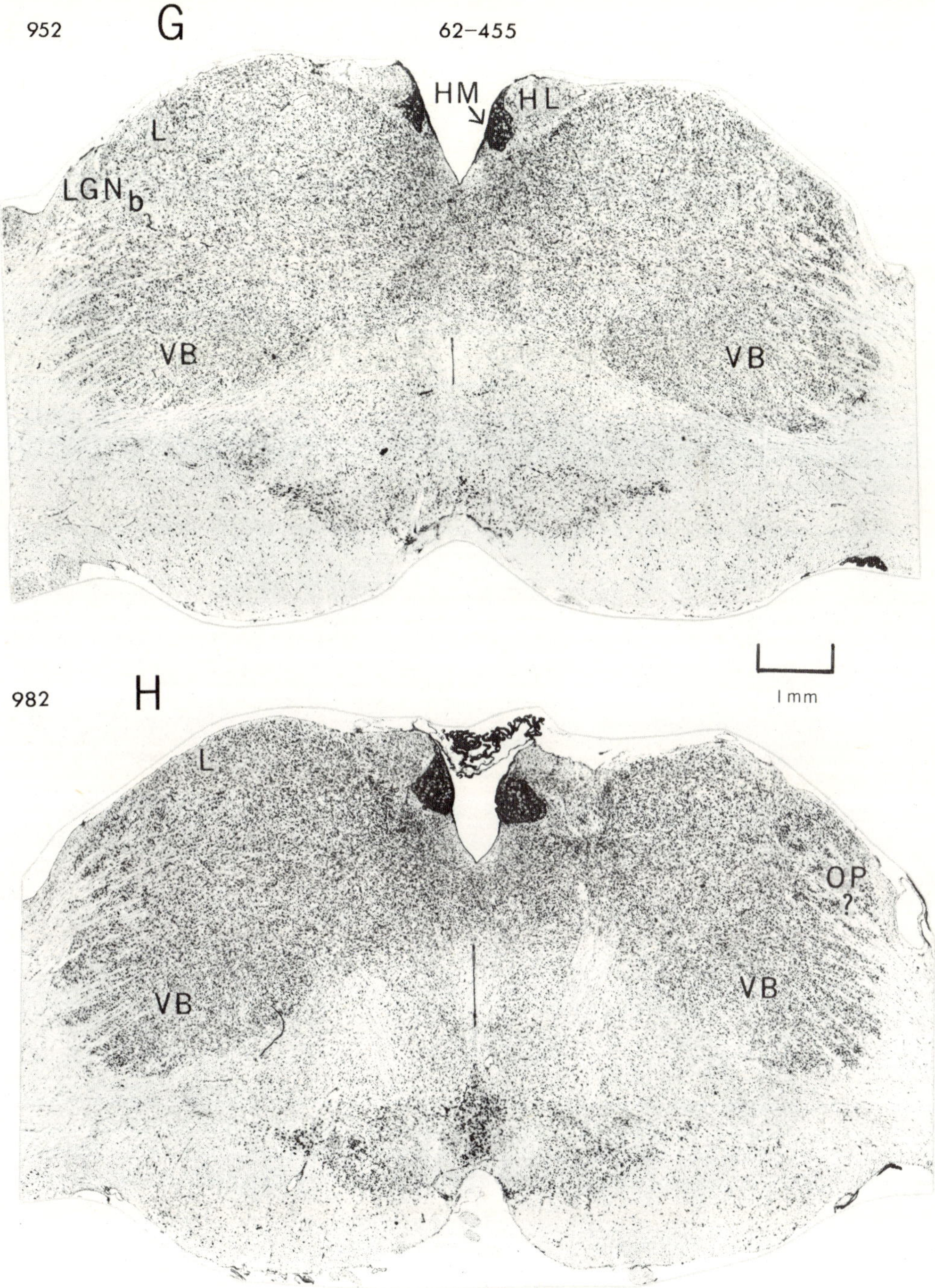
952
G
62–455
HM
HL
L
LGNb
VB
VB
1mm
982
H
L
OP
?
VB
VB

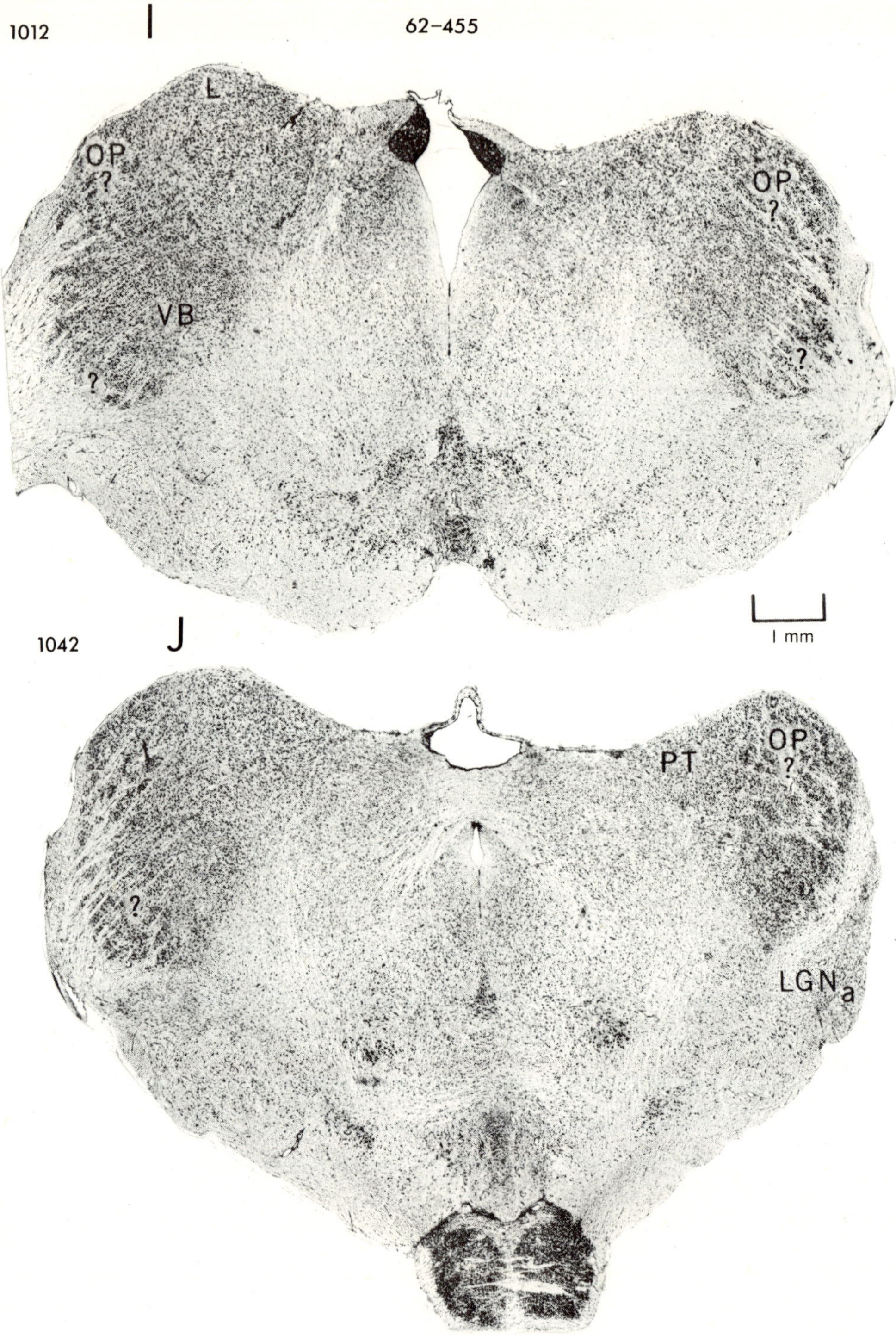
1012
I
62–455
L
OP
?
VB
?
OP
?
?
1 mm
1042
J
PT
OP
?
?
LGNa

1072 K 62–455

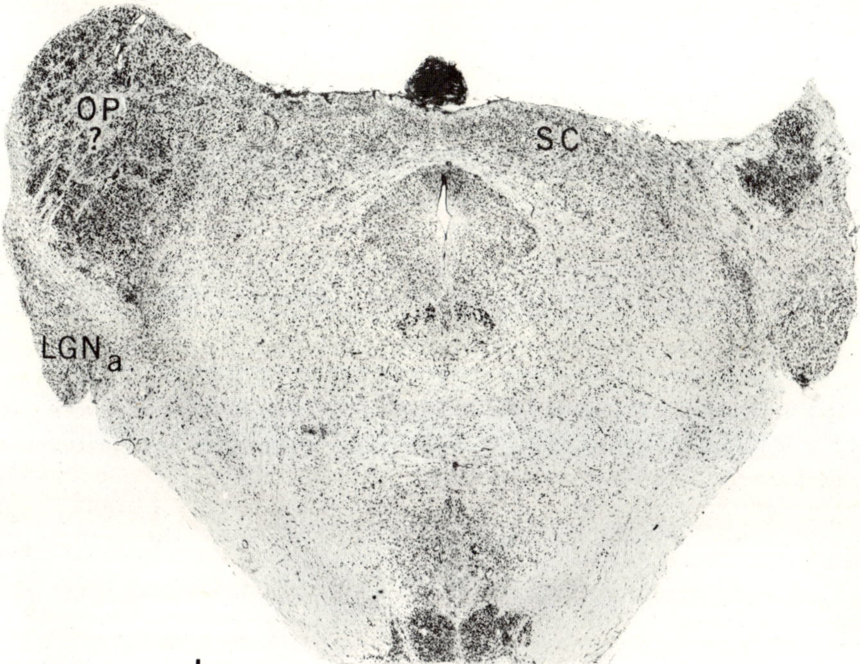

1102 L

1 mm

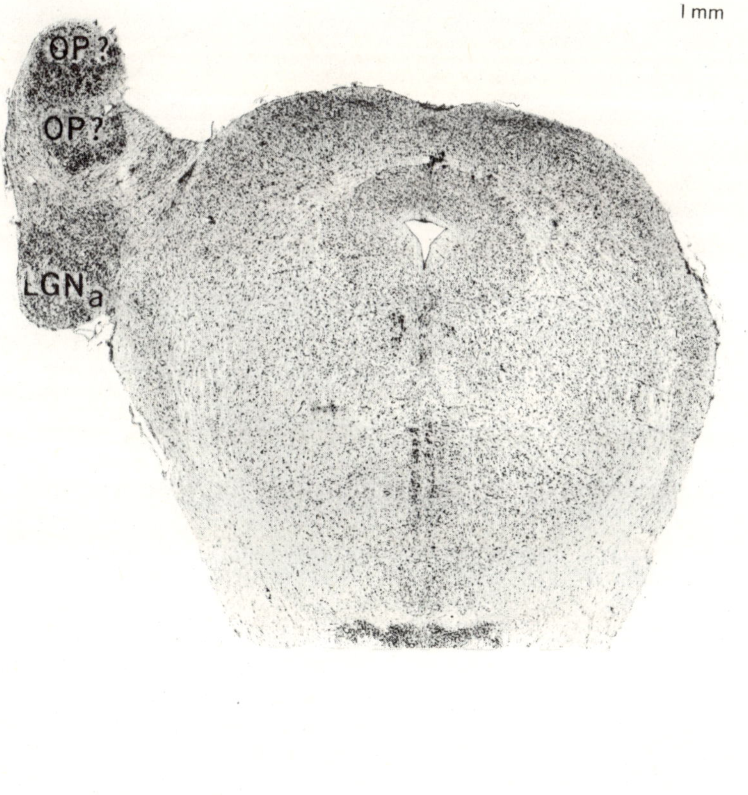

Killackey and Ebner, 1972, 1973; Lende, 1963*a,b,c,* 1969; Walsh and Ebner, 1970; see Section IV). However, the cortical motor and somatic sensory areas in echidna are separate and distinct (Lende, 1964), and our results show that the thalamic nuclear region (VL) that projects to the motor area is distinct from that (VB) projecting to somatic sensory cortex. Thus VL lies rostral to VB, as it does in other mammals with similar projections (Figs. 7D–F, 10B, and 11B). VL is relatively distinct as is apparent from the normal side in the animal in which motor cortex was ablated.

3. Mediodorsal Nuclear Region

The echidna's unusually expanded frontal cortex receives projections from a relatively large thalamic region situated in the midrostral half of the thalamus lateral to the more cell-dense midline nuclei (Figs. 7 and 9–14). In some mammals this region is occupied by an architecturally distinct mediodorsal nucleus (MD) bordered by several smaller nuclei (Akert, 1964; Bodian, 1936; Rose and Woolsey, 1947, 1949). However, in echidna the architectural boundaries are not very distinct. Instead, this thalamic region appears to consist of a relatively homogeneous mass of sparsely packed, medium-sized neurons.

Six lesions were made in different portions of the echidna's frontal cortex in order to determine the topographical organization of the thalamocortical projec-

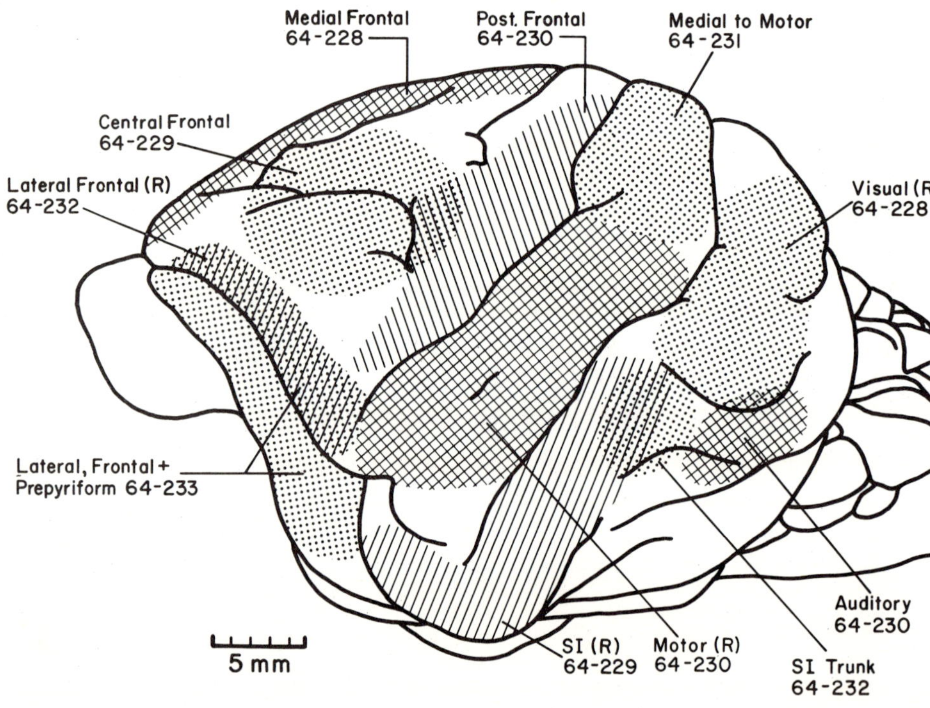

Figure 8. Locations of lesions of cerebral cortex of six echidnas indicated on left hemisphere of composite brain diagram. Animal numbers and side of each lesion (indicated by R if on right side) are indicated at margins of the drawing.

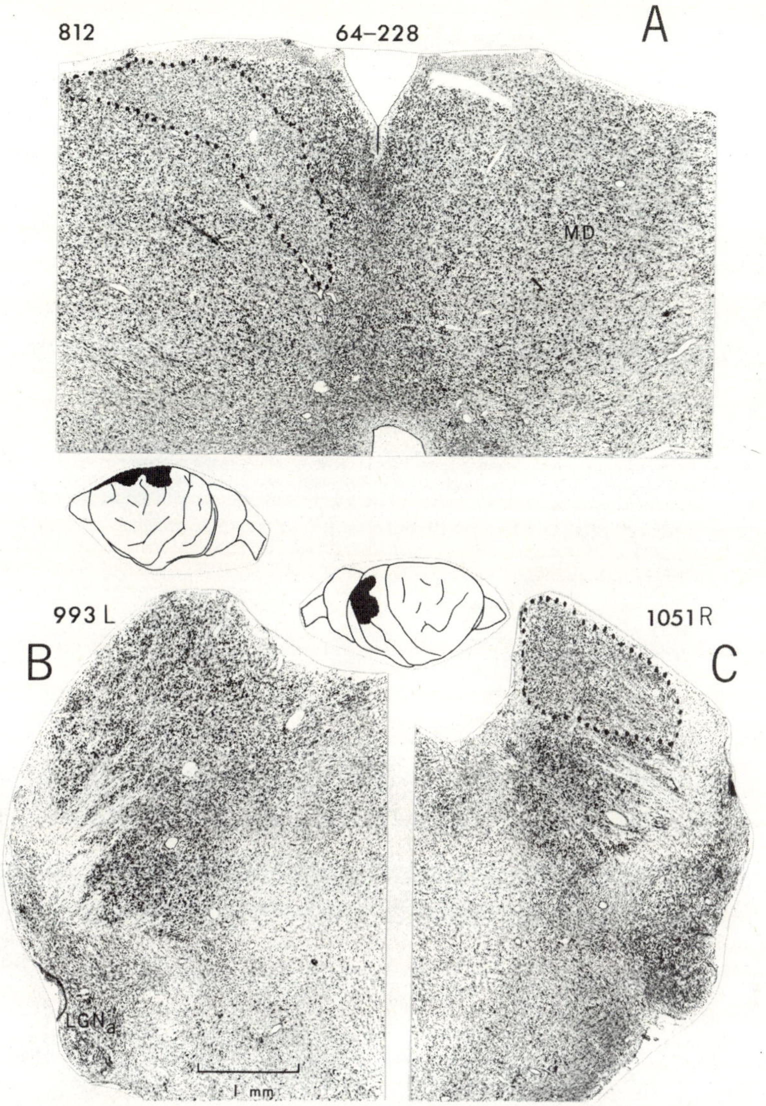

Figure 9. A: Thalamic degeneration (on left side) following ablation of left medial frontal cortex. This section is about at level D in the normal series of Fig. 7. Only the mediodorsal thalamic region is affected. Midline cortex is spared, and most, but not all, fibers to midline cortex are spared. This lesion is mostly confined to the cortical area intended. See Fig. 15D for summary diagrams of thalamic degeneration. BC: Thalamic degeneration following ablation of right "visual" cortex. Degeneration on right (C). Normal side on left (B). These sections are at about level K in the normal series of Fig. 7. Possible undercutting of fibers to cortex medial to visual area and of fibers from occipital pole. Sparing of SI. Possible invasion of auditory cortex. Thalamic degeneration involves the large nucleus (OP ?) in dorsocaudal aspect but also affects lateral thalamic neurons rostral to this large and dark-celled nuclear region (cf. Fig. 7J–L). Ventral nucleus (LGNa of Campbell and Hayhow, 1971) does not show clear-cut degeneration (?). See Fig. 15J,K for summary diagrams of thalamic degeneration. Echidna 64-228.

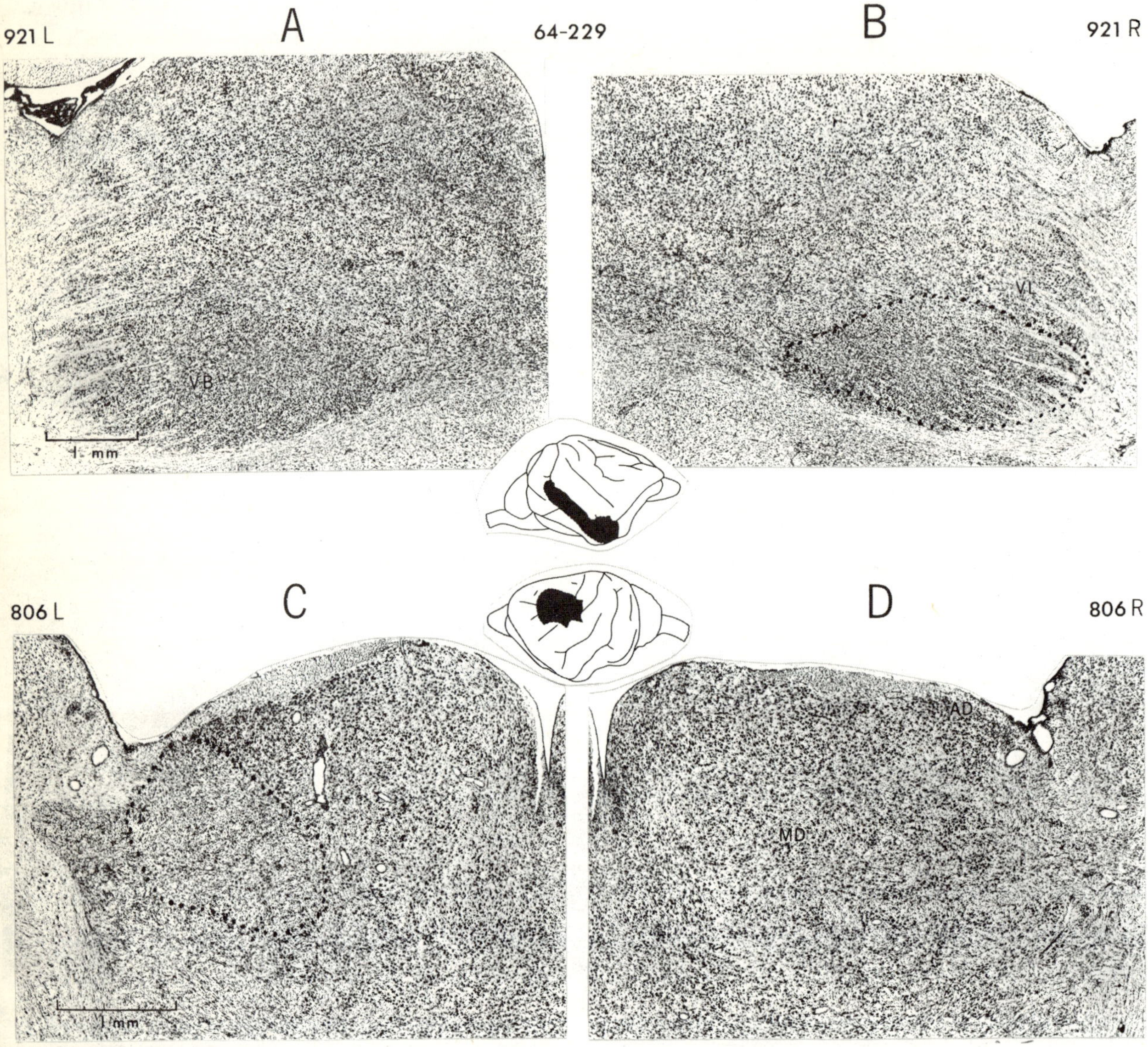

Figure 10. Thalamic degeneration (B) following ablation of right somatic sensory (SI) cortex. Normal side on left (A). These sections are about at level G in the normal series of Fig. 7. This lesion is nicely confined to the cortical area intended. See Fig. 15G for summary diagrams of thalamic degeneration. Thalamic degeneration (C) following ablation of left central frontal cortex. Normal side on right (D). These sections are at about level C in the normal series of Fig. 7. Possible slight undercutting of fibers to midline cortex. Caudate and hippocampus spared. This lesion is essentially confined to the region intended. See Fig. 15E for summary diagrams of thalamic degeneration. Echidna 64-229.

tions. The data reveal that adjacent frontal cortical regions receive inputs from adjacent dorsomedial thalamic regions (Fig. 15B–F,I), Of course, more than just an MD homologue may be involved in these cases, since the several different nuclei which border MD in other mammals are not distinguishable in our material. No attempt was made to place frontal cortical lesions within specific cytoarchitectural fields.

4. Cortex Medial to the Motor Area

The thalamic source of projections to the "silent" cortex medial to the motor area and caudal to the frontal cortex (Fig. 15A, horizontal series) is located at the dorsolateral margin of the thalamus dorsocaudal to the thalamic source (VL) of afferents to motor cortex (Fig. 14A,C). This may be the nucleus lateralis dorsalis.

5. Degeneration in Other Nuclei

The darkly staining large-celled nuclei (labeled OP? in Figs. 7H–L, 9B,C, and 14I) in the dorso-caudo-lateral thalamus is not a clear homologue, on the basis of our data with the lateral geniculate nucleus despite its appearance and location (cf. Kaas *et al.,* 1972). It is related to cortex somewhere on the occipital pole since it degenerates most completely (Fig. 9C) in cases with the larger occipital lesions (Fig. 15J,K).

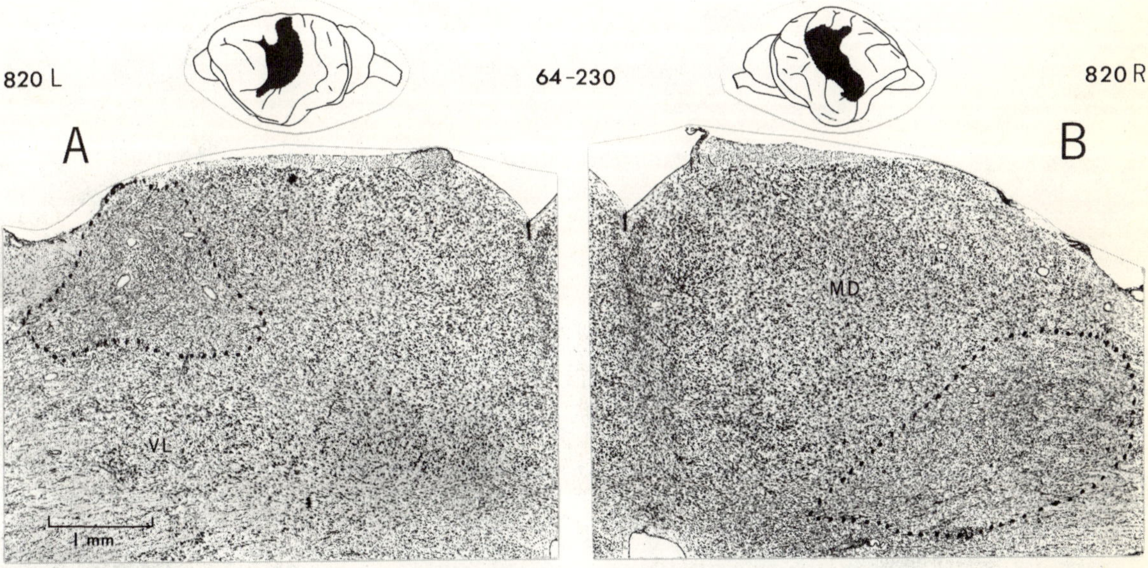

Figure 11. Thalamic degeneration following ablation of left posterior frontal (A) and right motor (B) cortex. This section is at about level E in the normal series of Fig. 7. The caudal frontal lesion (A) may undercut some fibers to motor cortex and to midline cortex and cortex medial to the motor area and possibly invades portion of tip of gyrus containing SI representation of the beak and tongue. Also, possible undercutting of visual cortex in depth. The lesion of motor cortex (B) possibly undercut some fibers to SI cortex in one location and definitely invaded fibers to visual cortex and the occipital pole. See Fig. 15H,I for summary diagrams of thalamic degeneration. The ablation of auditory cortex was minimal and clear retrograde degeneration was not seen. Echidna 64-230.

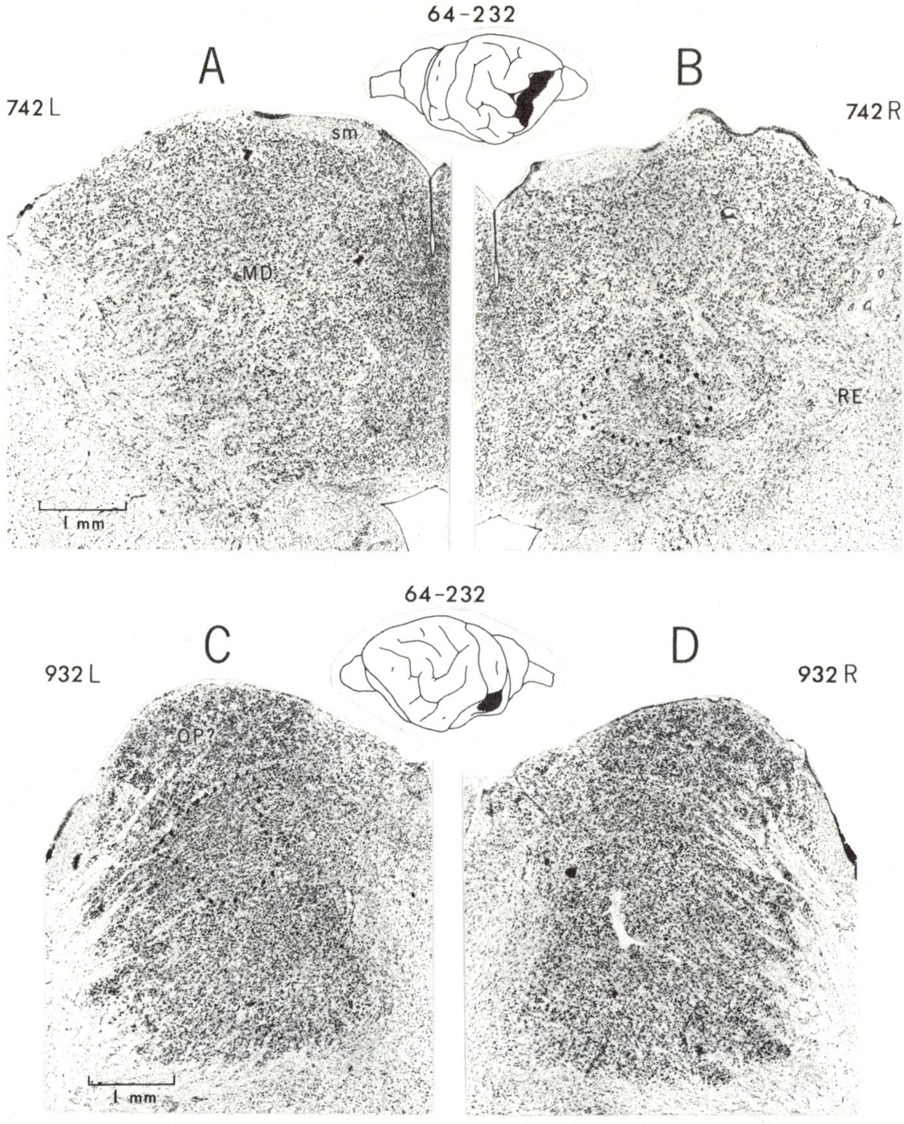

Figure 12. Thalamic degeneration (B) following ablation of right lateral frontal cortex. Normal side on left (A). These sections are at about level C in the normal series of Fig. 7. This cortical lesion is minimal and confined to the area intended. See Fig. 15F for summary diagrams of thalamic degeneration. C,D: Ablation of trunk region of left somatic sensory (SI) cortex. Degeneration on left (C). Normal side on right (D). These sections are at about levels J–K in the normal series of Fig. 7. Lesion is mainly confined to intended SI body region, but there is possible slight invasion of caudolateral aspect of visual gyrus or of cortex on occipital pole including the auditory area. The degenerated region in the thalamus appears too far dorsal and caudal to the major portion of Vb as identified on normal sections (Fig. 7F–I) or in the case with ablation of total SI (Fig. 10B). See Fig. 15L for summary diagrams of thalamic degeneration. Echidna 64-232. Coronal sections.

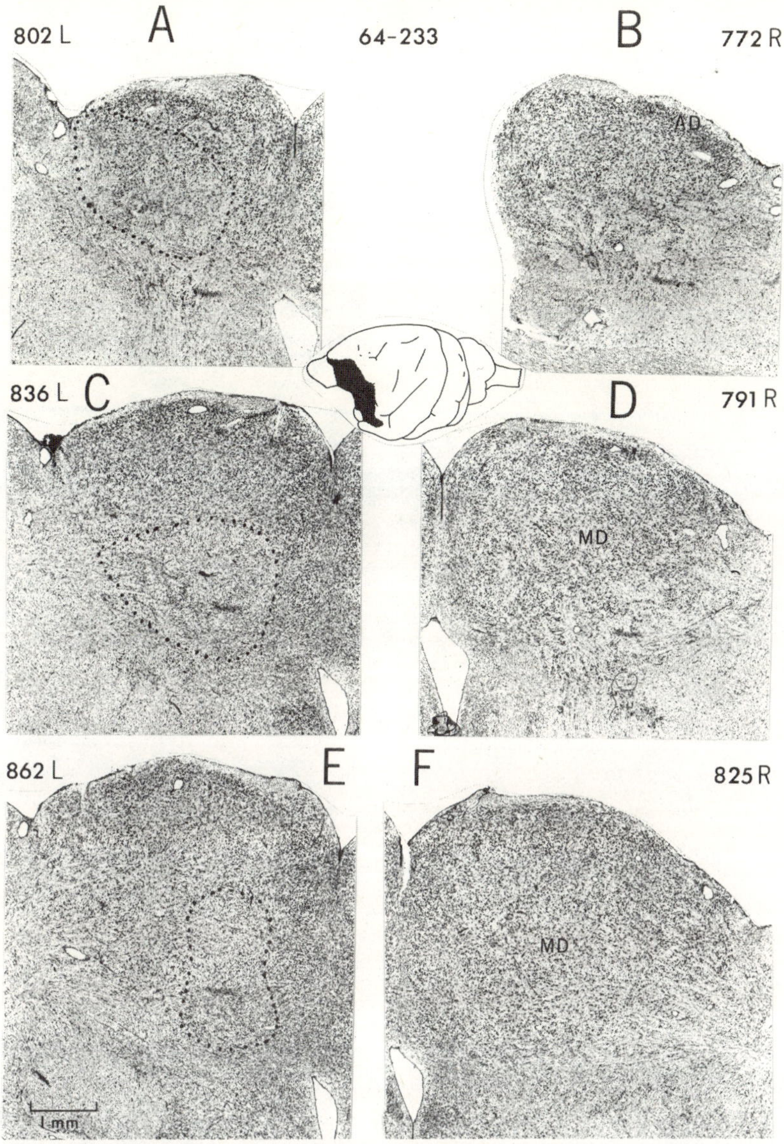

Figure 13. Thalamic degeneration (A,C,E) following ablation of left lateral frontal cortex plus left prepyriform cortex. Normal side on right (B,D,F). These three right and left pairs of sections are at about levels B–E in the normal series of Fig. 7. This lesion invaded the olfactory bulb dorsolaterally, destroyed rostrolateral aspects of prepyriform cortex, but spared medioventral and caudolateral portions of prepyriform cortex. Possible undercutting of fibers to medial frontal cortex. See Fig. 15C for summary diagrams of thalamic degeneration. Degeneration following lesion of right occipital pole is not shown, but this cortical lesion was the only one to produce clear degeneration of the large-celled nuclear groups (OP ?) in the caudolateral thalamus (Fig. 7I–L). Echidna 64-233. Coronal sections.

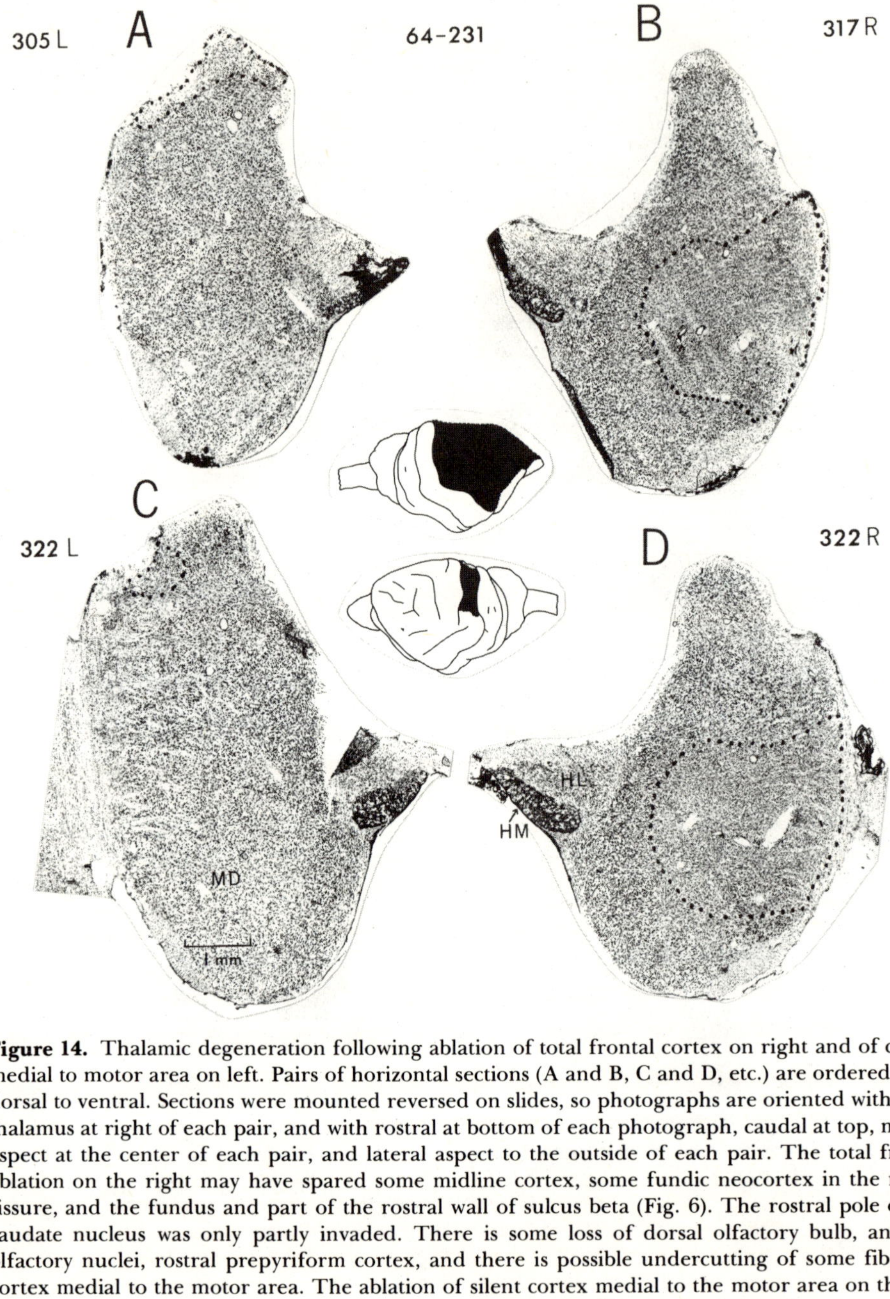

Figure 14. Thalamic degeneration following ablation of total frontal cortex on right and of cortex medial to motor area on left. Pairs of horizontal sections (A and B, C and D, etc.) are ordered from dorsal to ventral. Sections were mounted reversed on slides, so photographs are oriented with right thalamus at right of each pair, and with rostral at bottom of each photograph, caudal at top, medial aspect at the center of each pair, and lateral aspect to the outside of each pair. The total frontal ablation on the right may have spared some midline cortex, some fundic neocortex in the rhinal fissure, and the fundus and part of the rostral wall of sulcus beta (Fig. 6). The rostral pole of the caudate nucleus was only partly invaded. There is some loss of dorsal olfactory bulb, anterior olfactory nuclei, rostral prepyriform cortex, and there is possible undercutting of some fibers to cortex medial to the motor area. The ablation of silent cortex medial to the motor area on the left side was confined to the gyral crown as intended. Echidna 64-231. Horizontal sections.

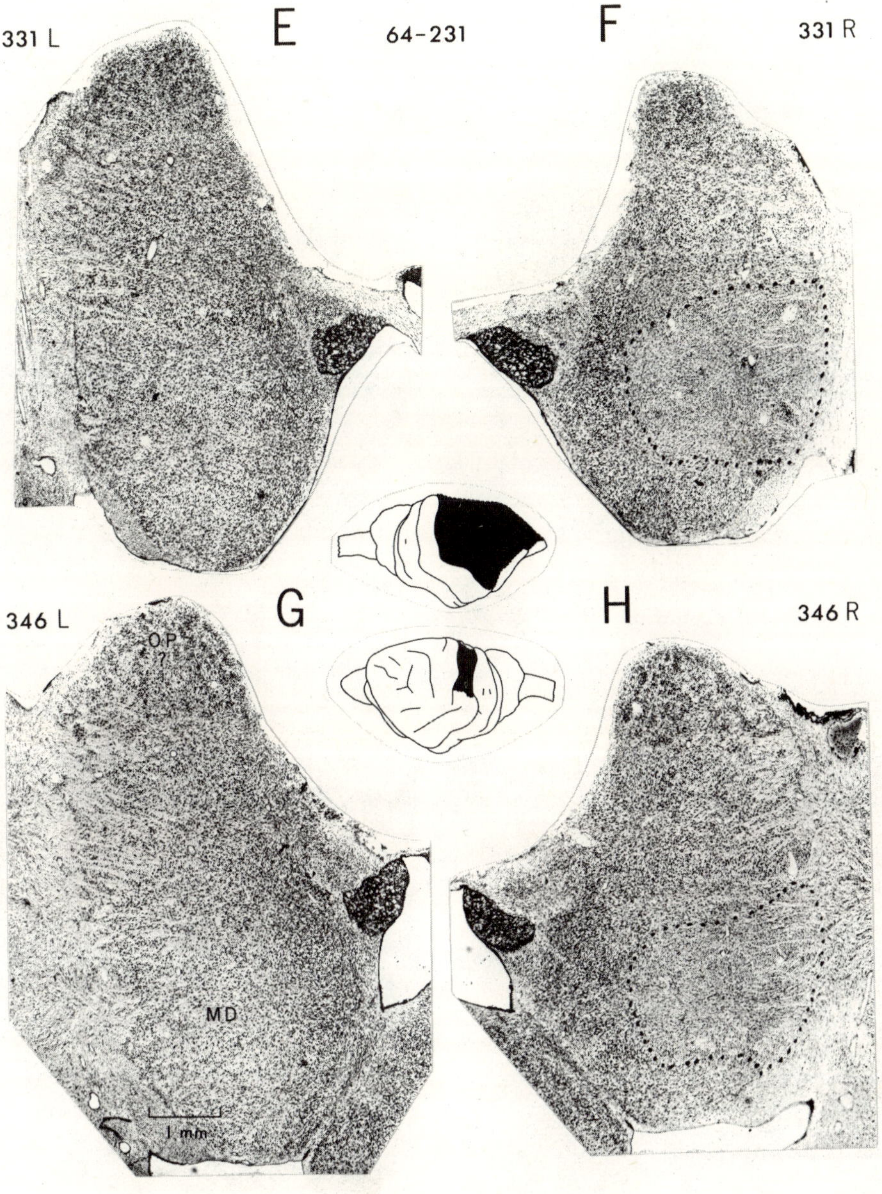

Figure 14. *(cont.)*

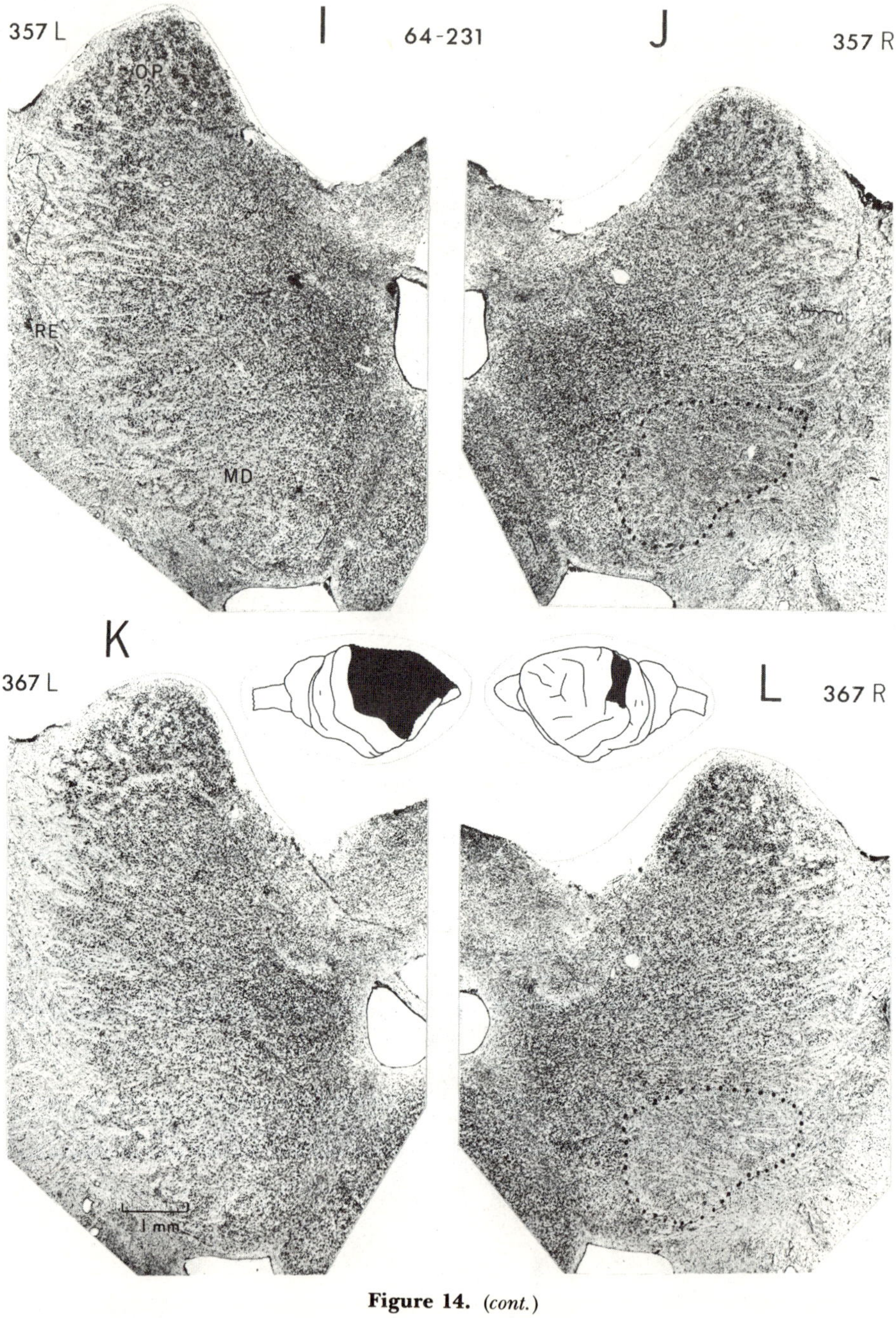

Figure 14. *(cont.)*

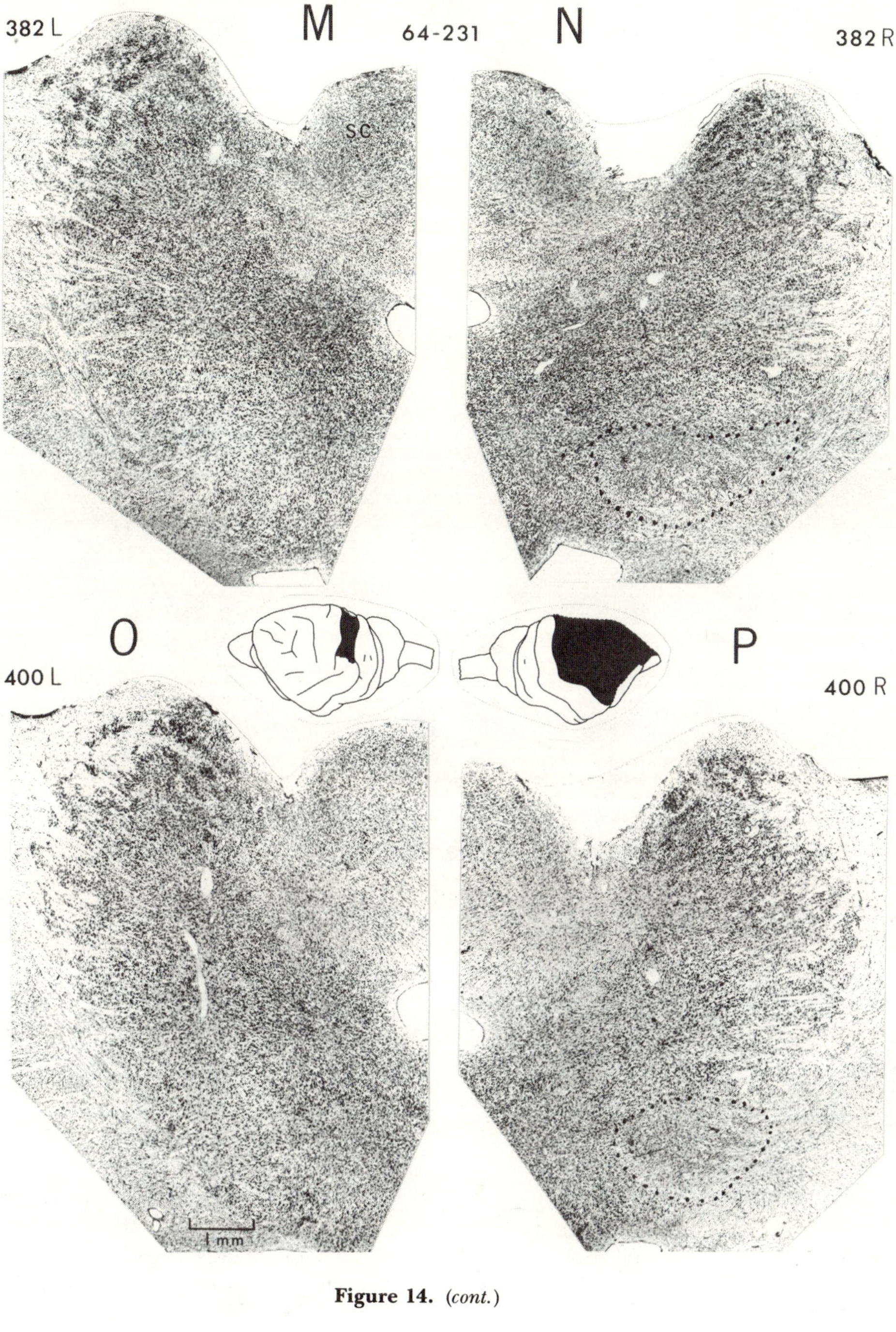

Figure 14. *(cont.)*

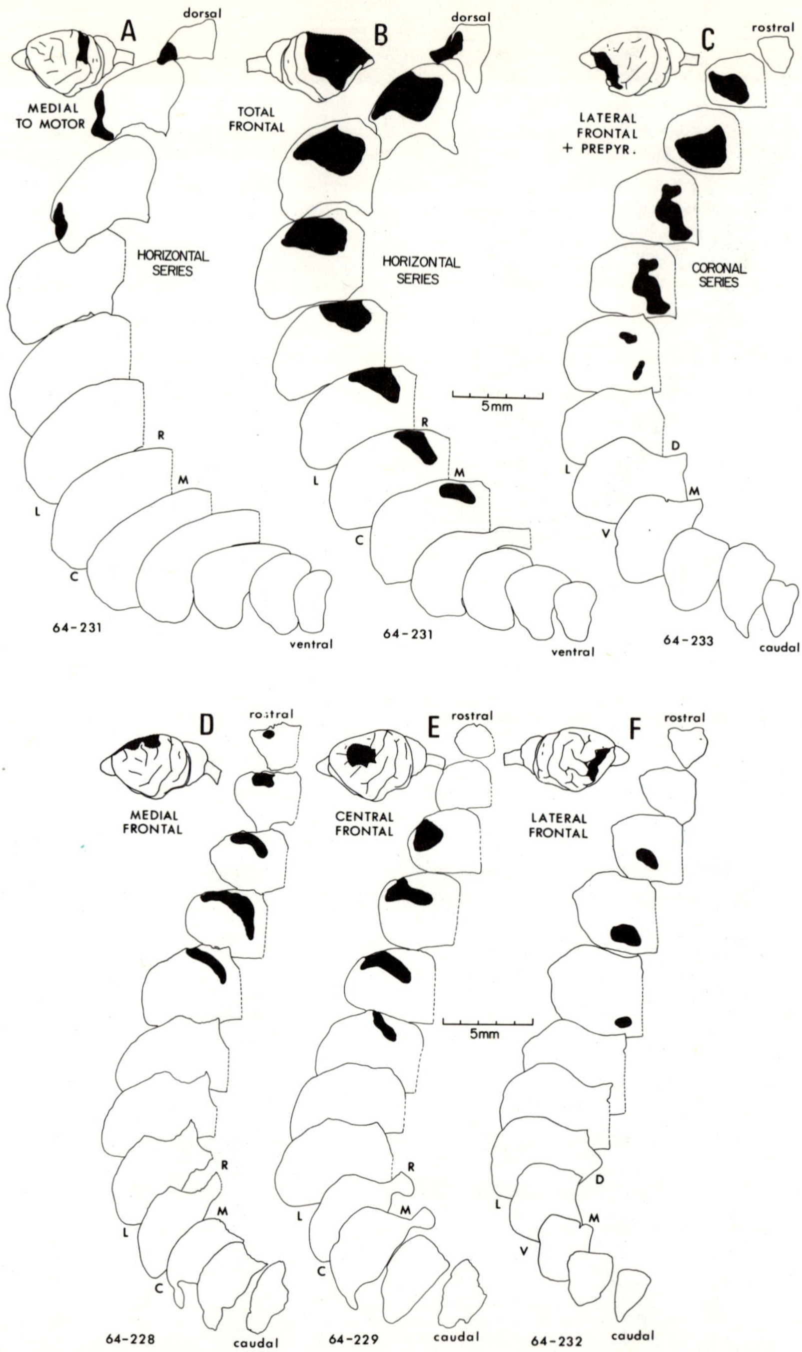

Figure 15. Summary reconstructions of thalamic degeneration on outline diagrams of 12 equally spaced sections through thalamus. Data are from 12 hemispheres of six animals. Degeneration is shown as black areas on thalamic diagrams (all cases reconstructed to appear as in left thalamus). Cortical lesions are indicated on inset brain diagrams. R, Rostral; C, caudal; M, medial; L, lateral; D, dorsal; V, ventral. A: Ablation of left cortex medial to motor area. Horizontal sections, with most dorsal section at top. B: Ablation of total frontal cortex on right. Horizontal sections, with most dorsal at top. C: Ablation of left lateral frontal and prepyriform cortex. This and all subsequent

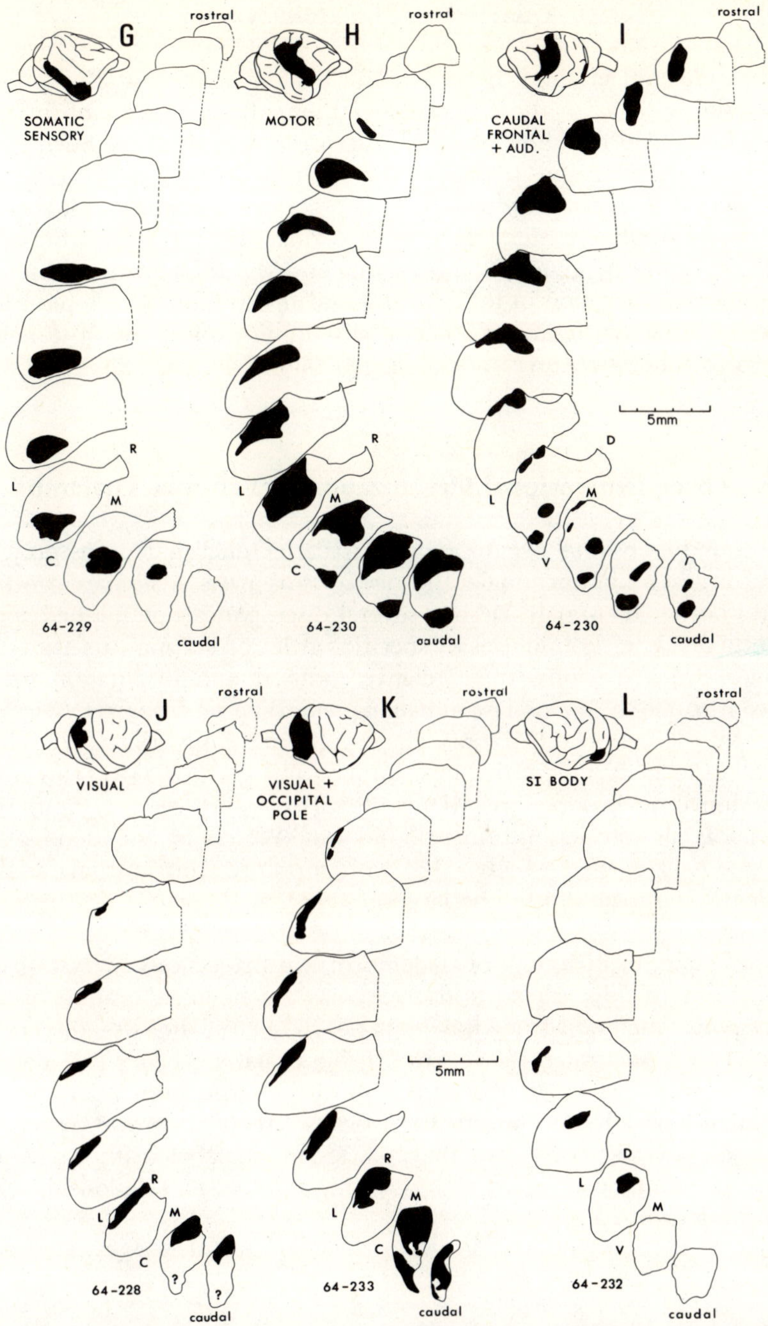

cases are coronal sections with most rostral sections at top. D: Ablation of medial frontal cortex. Coronal sections. E: Ablation of central frontal cortex. Coronal sections. F: Ablation of right lateral frontal cortex. Coronal sections. G: Ablation of right somatic sensory (SI) cortex. Coronal sections. H: Ablation of right motor cortex. Coronal sections. I: Ablation of left caudal frontal cortex. Coronal sections. J: Ablation of right visual cortex. Coronal sections. Question marks (?) on bottom sections indicate locations of likely but poorly defined degeneration. K: Ablation of right visual cortex and occipital pole. Coronal sections. L: Ablation of left cortex involving trunk (body) region of somatic sensory (SI) cortex. Coronal sections.

D. Unaffected Thalamic Nuclei

The reticular nucleus and the several nuclei lying adjacent to the ventricles, or those about the midline, or those near the caudomedial boundary of the thalamus with the midbrain did not show obvious retrograde degeneration. Such sparing of thalamic nuclei may be due in part to the fact that not all portions of cerebral neocortex were successfully destroyed in this series of animals. Thus there was some sparing of midline cortex, of occipital cortex, and possibly of buried cortex in the walls or depths of some of the fissures. However, the failure to observe clear-cut retrograde degeneration in the reticular and midline nuclei is typical for these structures and is likely due to presence of sustaining projections from neurons in these nuclei to other structures not damaged by our lesions (Rose and Woolsey, 1949).

E. Three-Dimensional Organization of Echidna Thalamus

The three-dimensional organization of thalamic nuclear regions projecting to cytoarchitecturally and functionally distinct cortical areas is similar in echidna to that found in other mammals. Despite several discrepancies mentioned above and some uncertainty as to boundaries of specific nuclei projecting to sensory, motor, and "silent" cortical regions, their relative location and orientation within the thalamus conform to the general mammalian plane. The ventrobasal (VB), ventrolateral (VL), and mediodorsal (MD) nuclear regions are easily identified. The visual nuclei (LGN_a and LGN_b) identified by Campbell and Hayhow (1971) are also clear. The mediodorsal nuclear region (MD) is identifiable and lies in a standard mammalian location, despite its indistinct boundaries. We could not identify auditory thalamus (medial geniculate body, MG) with certainty from our material. Of all these nuclei, MD appears to be the largest, with VB, VL, and LGN being successively smaller.

The principle of adjacency of thalamocortical projections was confirmed for echidna. Lesions of adjacent cortical areas resulted in degeneration of adjacent thalamic regions. Such adjacency was most clearly seen if the two adjacent cortical areas ablated were separated by a fissure. Projectional adjacency also was demonstrated for the four differently placed lesions of the large frontal cortex.

Greater precision in defining the specificity of thalamocortical projections will require more restricted cortical or thalamic lesions or labeled injections. For this study we were mainly concerned with assessing the overall relationships of thalamocortical projections.

IV. Discussion

It is an underlying concern of comparative vertebrate neurobiologists to understand what kinds of evolutionary changes have occurred in the nervous systems of the several vertebrate lineages. Neural circuits at all levels of the neuroaxis participate in behavioral and physiological adaptations to numerous specific perceived features of the environment. Since this is so, thorough understanding of all these sensory neural mechanisms is essential in gaining insight into the evolutionary courses and outcomes of brain evolution. As new information accumulates, it becomes clear that several kinds of reorganization of neural circuits occurred as evolutionary experiments among different vertebrate lines.

Comparisons of neural organization between reptiles and mammals are particularly important for understanding what circuit changes occurred in the evolution of mammals. Studies of the brains of living monotremes, marsupials, and "primitive" therian mammals by several investigators are concerned with the discovery of phyletic variations in neural circuitry. In this chapter we have reported on one set of circuits between thalamus and cerebral cortex in a monotreme. In this section we will briefly discuss our data in the light of findings of others obtained in other mammals, as well as review some of the problems and concepts that all these data generate.

A. Variations in Thalamocortical Circuit Connections among Vertebrates: The Search for Homologies

Comparisons between circuits in different animal types are most meaningful if homologous circuits are compared (Campbell, 1976). This is easiest if circuits are traced centrally (anatomically, biochemically, or physiologically) from the major sense organs since a stable pattern of organization of receptors was established early in vertebrate evolution. Consequently, homologous sensory circuits are more clearly distinguished in different taxa.

With respect to thalamocortical portions of sensory circuits, the problem of identifying comparative homologues is more difficult, requiring a series of studies that trace, in stepwise fashion, both their anatomical connections with the periphery and their physiological responsiveness to sensory stimuli. Among mammals, the locations of general features of homologous sensory nuclei of the thalamus have been identified in a variety of species (Bodian, 1936; Oswaldo-Cruz and Rocha-Miranda, 1968; Rose, 1942; Rose and Woolsey, 1947, 1949; cf. Welker, 1973, for review). Cortical sensory areas have been mapped out in several forms (Johnson, Chapter 14, this volume; Welker and Campos, 1963; Woolsey, 1952, 1964, 1971*a,b*). Although finer details of connectivity and function of thalamocortical circuit components remain to be discovered, or are currently being studied, homologous thalamocortical sensory connections (e.g., Rose and Woolsey, 1949) have been established for several mammals. Studies of some cortical and thalamic sensory subcircuits in several marsupials have revealed that these forms share with placental mammals a common plan of organization (Bodian, 1936, 1942; Johnson, Chapter 14, this volume; Lende, 1969; Oswaldo-Cruz and Rocha-Miranda, 1968; Pubols, 1968; Pubols *et al.,* 1976; Rose and Woolsey, 1947, 1949). However, the discovery by Lende that opossums do not have a motor area distinct from the SI somatic sensory area (Lende, 1963*a,c*, 1969; cf. Abbie, 1940) indicated an important variation in the common placental plan of sensory–motor organization (cf. Lende and Sadler, 1967). Ebner and his colleagues have verified other differences in these neural circuits in opossums (Benevento and Ebner, 1971; Ebner, 1969; Killackey and Ebner, 1972, 1973; Tobias and Ebner, 1973) and have further opened the door to the search for species differences in circuitry. Johnson (Chapter 14, this volume), Welker (1973), and others have emphasized the wide flexibility of somatic sensory circuits with respect to specific features of their differential enlargement and spatial pattern of organization. Both Pubols *et al.* (1976, for somatic sensory cortex) and Erickson *et al.* (1964, for thalamus) have revealed additional variations in organization of sensory nuclei. Contrary to what was expected, Lende's study of cortical sensory and motor areas in echidnas (1964) and the data presented in this chapter reveal that several thalamocortical relationships in this monotreme are more similar to those of most placental mammals than they are to those of the marsupials studied. The discovery of relatively voluminous thalamocortical connections to the echidna frontal cortex and the realization that olfactory inputs project to this thalamocortical subcircuit in several mammals (Benjamin and Jackson, 1974; Ferrer, 1969; Heimer, 1972; Jackson and Benjamin, 1974; Jackson *et al.*, 1977; Leonard, 1972; Powell *et al.*, 1965; Scott and Leonard, 1971) pointed up additional variations among mammals.

Campbell and Hayhow's (1971) discovery of an aberrant pattern of nuclear organization in the optic thalamus and its input from the eye in echidnas, and our rather uncertain data regarding thalamocortical connections to the echidna's physiologically defined visual cortex, suggest further novel circuits in this monotreme. Preliminary data from another monotreme, the platypus (Bohringer and Rowe, 1975), suggest similarities to echidna with respect to presence of a relatively large "frontal" region but differences with respect to organization within the somatic sensory cortex.

Comparative studies of sensory and other circuits are continuing for several mammalian groups. More exciting is the increased interest in identifying homologous and divergent sensory circuits within and between other vertebrate groups, and between reptiles and mammals. Such studies have accelerated in the last decade or so and have been the subject matter of several symposia (e.g., Petras and Noback, 1969; Masterton *et al.*, 1976*a,b*), including that which led to this volume.

B. Theoretical Concepts

Theories and hypotheses regarding principles of organization of neural circuits and of their evolution, diversity, complexity, and degree of specialization among vertebrates have become increasingly more testable. The validity of concepts such as a sensory–motor amalgam (Lende, 1963*a*, 1969), polymodal circuits (Erickson *et al.*, 1964; Lende, 1969), submodal differential circuits (Paul *et al.*, 1972; Powell and Mountcastle, 1959), and association circuits (Lende, 1969; Rose and Woolsey, 1949; Sanides, 1962) is being checked experimentally.

Our data on echidna do not warrant further conjecture on these issues. Much additional experimental work remains. The limited view of thalamocortical connections revealed both by the retrograde degeneration methods of this study and by macroelectrode evoked potential methods (Lende, 1964) must be extended and focused by other more specific anatomical and physiological circuit tracing methods in order to reach more precise and expanded conceptions of comparative differences in neural circuits and their evolutionary functional significance.

ACKNOWLEDGMENTS. Appreciation is expressed to JoAnn Ekleberry for preparation of the histological material, to Terry Stewart for photographic work, to Carol Dizack for the artwork, and to Jean Johnson for typing the manuscript. Supported by Grants NB 3249 and NS-06225.

V. References

Abbie, A. A., 1938, The excitable cortex in the monotremata, *Aust. J. Exp. Biol. Med. Sci.* **16:**143.

Abbie, A. A., 1940, The excitable cortex in *Perameles, Sarcophilus, Dasyurus, Trichosurus* and *Wallabia (Macropus), J. Comp. Neurol.* **72:**469.

Akert, K., 1964, Comparative anatomy of frontal cortex and thalamo-frontal connections, in: *The Frontal Granular Cortex and Behavior* (J. M. Warren and K. Akert, eds.), pp. 372–396, McGraw-Hill, New York.

Benevento, L. A., and Ebner, F. F., 1971, The contribution of the dorsal lateral geniculate nucleus to the total pattern of thalamic terminations in striate cortex of the Virginia opossum, *J. Comp. Neurol.* **143:**243.

Benjamin, R. M., and Jackson, J. C., 1974, Unit discharges in the mediodorsal nucleus of the squirrel monkey evoked by electrical stimulation of the olfactory bulb, *Brain Res.* **75:**181.

Bodian, D., 1936, Studies on the diencephalon of the Virginia opossum. Part I. The nuclear pattern in the adult, *J. Comp. Neurol.* **71:**259.

Bodian, D., 1942, Studies on the diencephalon of the Virginia opossum. Part III. The thalamo-cortical projection, *J. Comp. Neurol.* **77:**525.

Bohringer, R. C., and Rowe, M. J., 1975, Functional organization of the somatosensory cortex of the platypus (*Ornithorhynchus anatinus*), *Proc. Aust. Physiol. Pharm. Assoc.* **6:**27.

Campbell, C. B. G., 1976, Morphological homology and the nervous system, in: *Evolution, Brain and Behavior: Persistent Problems* R. B. Masterton, W. Hodos, and H. J. Jerison, eds.), Chap. 11, Erlbaum Associates, Hillsdale, N.J.

Campbell, C. B. G., and Hayhow, W. R., 1971, Primary optic pathways in the echidna *Tachyglossus aculeatus*: An experimental degeneration study, *J. Comp. Neurol.* **143:**119.

Ebner, F. F., 1969, A comparison of primitive forebrain organization in metatherian and eutherian mammals, *Ann. N.Y. Acad. Sci.* **167:**241.

Elliot-Smith, G., 1902, Descriptive and illustrated catalogue of the physiological series of comparative anatomy contained in the Museum of the Royal College of Surgeons of England, Vol. 2, 2nd ed., pp. 110–518, Taylor and Francis, London.

Erickson, R. P., Jane, J. A., Waite, R., and Diamond, I. T., 1964, Single neuron investigation of sensory thalamus of the opossum, *J. Neurophysiol.* **27:**1026.

Ferrer, N. G.. 1969, Efferent projections of the anterior olfactory nucleus, *J. Comp. Neurol.* **137:**309.

Gray, P. A., 1924, The cortical lamination pattern of the opossum, *Didelphis marsupialis virginiana, J. Comp. Neurol.* **37:**221.

Griffiths, M., 1968, *Echidnas,* Pergamon Press, Oxford.

Heimer, L., 1972, The olfactory connections of the diencephalon in the rat, *Brain Behav. Evol.* **6:**484.

Hopson, J. A., and Crompton, A. W., 1969, Origin of mammals, *Evol. Biol.* **3:**15.

Jackson, J. C., and Benjamin, R. M., 1974, Unit discharges in the mediodorsal nucleus of the rabbit evoked by electrical stimulation of the olfactory bulb, *Brain Res.* **75:**193.

Jackson, J. C., Golden, G. T., and Benjamin, R. M., 1977, The distribution of olfactory input in the opossum mediodorsal nucleus, *Brain Res.* **138:**229.

Jerison, H. J., 1973, *Evolution of the Brain and Intelligence,* Academic Press, New York.

Kass, J. H., Guillery, R. W., and Allman, J. M., 1972, Some principles of organization in the dorsal lateral geniculate nucleus, *Brain Behav. Evol.* **6:**253.

Killackey, H. P., and Ebner, F. F., 1972, Two different types of thalamocortical projections to a single cortical area in mammals, *Brain Behav. Evol.* **6:**141.

Killackey, H. P., and Ebner, F. F., 1973, Anatomical correlates of amalgamated sensory–motor cortex in opossum: The projection of three thalamic nuclei to a single cortical area, *Science* **179:**283.

Lende, R. A., 1963*a*, Cerebral cortex: A sensorimotor amalgam in the Marsupalia, *Science* **141:**730.

Lende, R. A., 1963*b*, Sensory representation in the cerebral cortex of the opossum (*Didelphis virginiana*), *J. Comp. Neurol.* **121:**395.

Lende, R. A., 1963*c*, Motor representation in the cerebral cortex of the opossum (*Didelphis virginiana*), *J. Comp. Neurol.* **121:**405.

Lende, R. A., 1964, Representation in the cerebral cortex of a primitive mammal; sensorimotor, visual and auditory fields in the echidna (*Tachyglossus aculeatus*), *J. Neurophysiol.* **27:**37.

Lende, R. A., 1969, A comparative approach to the neocortex: Localization in monotremes, marsupials and insectivores, *Ann. N.Y. Acad. Sci.* **167:**262.

Lende, R. A., and Sadler, K. M., 1967, Sensory and motor areas in neocortex of hedgehog (*Erinaceous*), *Brain Res.* **5:**390.

Leonard, C. M., 1972, The connections of the dorsomedial nuclei, *Brain Behav. Evol.* **6:**524.

Masterton, R. B., Bitterman, M. E., Campbell, C. B. G., and Hotton, N. (eds.), 1976*a*, *Evolution of Brain and Behavior in Vertebrates,* Erlbaum Associates, Hillsdale, N.J.

Masterton, R. B., Hodos, W., and Jerison, H. J. (eds.), 1976*b*, *Evolution, Brain and Behavior: Persistent Problems,* Erlbaum Associates, Hillsdale, N.J.

Oswaldo-Cruz, E., and Rocha-Miranda, C. E., 1968, *The Brain of the Opossum* (*Didelphis marsupialis*): *A Cytoarchitectonic Atlas in Stereotaxic Coordinates,* Instituto de Biofisica, Univ. Fed. do Rio de Janeiro.

Paul, R. L., Merzenich, M., and Goodman, H., 1972, Representation of slowly and rapidly adapting cutaneous mechanoreceptors of the hand in Brodmann's areas 3 and I of *Macaca mulatta, Brain Res.* **36:**229.

Petras, J. M., and Noback, C. R. (eds.), 1969, Comparative and evolutionary aspects of the vertebrate central nervous system, *Ann. N.Y. Acad. Sci.* **167:**1.

Powell, T. P. S., and Mountcastle, V. B., 1959, Some aspects of the functional organization of the cortex of the postcentral gyrus of the monkey: A correlation of findings obtained in a single unit analysis with cytoarchitecture, *Bull. Johns Hopkins Hosp.* **105:**133.

Powell, T. P. S., Cowan, W. M., and Raisman, G., 1965, The central olfactory connections, *J. Anat.* **99:**791.

Pubols, B. H., Jr., 1968, Retrograde degeneration study of somatic sensory thalamocortical connections in brain of Virginia opossum, *Brain Res.* **7:**232.

Pubols, B. H., Jr., Pubols, L. M., Di Pette, D. J., and Sheely, J. C., 1976, Opossum somatic sensory cortex: A microelectrode mapping study, *J. Comp. Neurol.* **165:**229.

Romer, A. S., 1968, *Notes and Comments on Vertebrate Paleontology,* University of Chicago Press, Chicago.

Rose, J. E., 1942, The ontogenetic development of the rabbit's diencephalon, *J. Comp. Neurol.* **77:**61.

Rose, J. E., and Woolsey, C. N., 1947, The orbitofrontal cortex and its connections with the mediodorsal nucleus in rabbit, sheep and cat, *Res. Publ. Assoc. Res. Nerv. Ment. Dis.* **27:**210.

Rose, J. E., and Woolsey, C. N., 1949, Organization of the mammalian thalamus and its relationship to the cerebral cortex, *Electroencephalogr. Clin. Neurophysiol.* **1:**391.

Sanides, F., 1962, Die Architektonic des meschlichen Stirnhirns: Zugleich eine Darstellung der Prinzipien seiner Gestaltung als Spiegel der Stammesgeschichtlichen Differenzierung der Grosshirn Rinde, *Gesamtgeb. Neurol. Psychiat.* **98:**1.

Scott, J. W., and Leonard, 1971, C. M., 1971, The olfactory connections of the lateral hypothalamus in the rat, mouse and hamster, *J. Comp. Neurol.* **141:**331.

Simpson, G. G., 1945, The principles of classification and a classification of mammals, *Bull. Am. Mus. Nat. Hist.* **85:**1.

Tobias, T. J., and Ebner, F. F., 1973, Thalamocortical projections from the mediodorsal nucleus in the Virginia opossum, *Brain Res.* **52:**79.

Van Valen, L., 1960, Therapsids as mammals, *Evolution* **14:**304.

Walsh, T. M., and Ebner, F. F., 1970, The cytoarchitecture of somatic sensory–motor cortex in the opossum (*Didelphis marsupialis virginiana*): A Golgi study, *J. Anat.* **107:**1.

Welker, W. I., 1973, Principles of organization of the ventrobasal complex in mammals, *Brain Behav. Evol.* **7:**253.

Welker, W. I., and Campos, G. B., 1963, Physiological significance of sulci in somatic sensory cerebral cortex in mammals of the family Procyonidae, *J. Comp. Neurol.* **120:**19.

Woolsey, C. N., 1952, Patterns of localization in sensory and motor areas of the cerebral cortex, in: *The Biology of Mental Health and Disease,* pp. 192–206, Hoeber, New York.

Woolsey, C. N., 1964, Cortical localization as defined by evoked potential and electrical stimulation studies, in: *Cerebral Localization and Organization* (G. Schaltenbrand and C. N. Woolsey, eds.), pp. 17–32, University of Wisconsin Press, Madison.

Woolsey, C. N., 1971*a*, Comparative studies on cortical representation of vision, *Vision Res.* **11:**365 (Suppl. 3).

Woolsey, C. N., 1971*b*, Tonotopic organization of the auditory cortex, in: *Physiology of the Auditory System* (M. B. Sachs, ed.), pp. 271–282, National Educational Consultants, Baltimore.

16

A Comparative Survey of Visual Cortex Organization in Mammals

JON H. KAAS

And at last came the monkey, and anybody could see that man was not far off now. And in truth that was so. The monkey went on developing for close upon five million years, and then turned into a man—to all appearances.

MARK TWAIN—*Letters from Earth*

I. Introduction

A large region of posterior neocortex in a number of species of mammals has been found to be responsive to visual stimuli. In some of these mammals more detailed studies have subdivided the responsive region into separate systematic maps or representations of visual space, and there are several reasons for thinking that these maps are important as functionally distinct subdivisions of the visual system. For instance, it appears that each systematic map is associated with a cortical region having a unique architectonic character and a distinctive pattern of connections with other visual structures. In addition, there is evidence that neurons in separate visual representations differ in the way they respond to visual stimuli. Finally, lesions of different visual maps have produced distinctively different behavior changes.

While it is generally agreed that visual representations constitute the functionally important subdivisions of visual cortex, it is not certain how many visual areas exist in any particular mammalian species, how or if mammalian species differ in numbers of visual areas, and what areas are homologous between species. This uncertainty stems from the lack of extensive comparative information and the incompleteness of even the most detailed of studies. Thus it is presently difficult to develop an overview that is satisfying. However, considerable mapping and anatomical data are now available for a few species of mammals, and partial data

JON H. KAAS • Department of Psychology, Vanderbilt University, Nashville, Tennessee 37240.

are available for a wide range of other mammals. It is now possible to broadly survey the available information, suggest a few homologies, point out the possibility of several specializations, and indicate mammals for which additional information would be extremely useful for further progress. The goal is to derive a general mammalian plan and to indicate the major variations of this plan. Such an overall perspective would allow better evaluation of the many types of studies that, at least initially, are performed on a limited number of species.

The format used here for considering the organization of visual cortex of different mammals is by major phylogenetic groups. A recent revision of phylogenetic classification of mammals by McKenna (1975) has provided a useful framework for discussing species differences and similarities, although the present conclusions are as yet too general to fully benefit from a detailed knowledge of the phylogenetic relationships.

In brief, McKenna (1975) divides the class Mammalia into two major subclasses, Prototheria, with only monotremes as the living representatives, and Theria, which later divided into the supercohort Marsupialia and the supercohort Eutheria. Marsupialia is divided into nine families with living representatives, and all other therian mammals are eutherian. The first division of eutherian mammals is into two cohorts, Edentata, including the living anteaters and armadillos, and Epitheria, including all other eutherian mammals. Epitheria divides into the superorder Leptictida, consisting of Macroscelidea (elephant shrews) and Lagomorpha (rabbits, hares, and pikas), and into the superorder Tokotheria, encompassing the remaining extant mammals. Tokotheria gives rise to four grand orders: (1) Insectivora, (2) Ferae (carnivores), (3) Archonta (primates, bats, tree shrews, and flying lemurs), and (4) Ungulata. The relationship of rodents to the subdivisions of Tokotheria is not certain, and therefore rodents are discussed separately as a fifth group. The order Pholidota (pangolins or scaly anteaters) is not closely related to other mammals, and the exact relationship is also uncertain. No investigations of visual cortex have been attempted in pangolins and they are not discussed further.

II. Survey of Extant Mammals

A. Monotremes

The most basic division of mammals is into the subclasses of Prototheria (monotremes) and Theria (all other mammals). The only surviving members of the prototherian radiation of mammals are the spiny anteaters, or echidnas, and the duck-billed platypuses. Monotremes diverged from therian mammals perhaps 150–170 million years ago, and they differ from therian mammals in that they lay eggs and have a single external opening for the excretory and reproductive systems (hence the name Monotremata). The cerebral hemispheres of echidnas and platypuses are quite different in external morphology; the neocortex of the platypus is smooth and relatively undeveloped, while the enormous development of the deeply fissured neocortex in echidna has long been a puzzle to neuroanatomists (Elliott Smith, 1902). It is unfortunate that our understanding of the brains of nontherian mammals must come from only these two surviving families, both with obvious and unusual specializations for rather restricted environmental niches. It is also unfortunate that very few studies using modern experimental methods have been attempted with monotremes. Because of these limitations, little is known about the visual cortex of monotremes. However, Lende (1964) identified a field of dorsomedial cortex in the occipital region of echidnas that is responsive to visual stimulation. Auditory and somatosensory fields were located just ventral and caudal, respectively, to the visual cortex. We expect that part or all of the visually responsive zone might be striate cortex or primary visual cortex (V I), since the retina projects to a thalamic nucleus that is the presumed homologue of the dorsal lateral geniculate nucleus (Campbell and Hayhow, 1972). Presently, however, there is no certain evidence in monotremes of striate cortex or any other visual areas as defined in other animals. Thus we are almost totally ignorant of the organization of the visual system of prototherian mammals.

B. Marsupials

Therian mammals separated into metatherian or pouched marsupial mammals and eutherian or placental mammals about 100 million years ago. The living marsupials are extremely diverse in body form and behavior, a result of long-term isolation and protection from eutherian competition in the Australian region. A number of marsupials appear to occupy behavioral niches very similar to those occupied by variously specialized eutherian mammals. Outside of the Australian region, marsupials have not been widely successful, and have been restricted to the "opossum" type. It would be of great interest to determine if the apparent convergences of behavior and body type of marsupial "mice," "cats," "wolves," "anteaters," "moles," "rabbits," etc., are reflected in similarities in brain structure with their placental counterparts, but such studies have not yet been attempted on a useful scale. Information about the visual systems of marsupials is extremely limited, and what is known is principally about the American opossum, *Didelphis*.

The American opossums, *Didelphis* and *Marmosa,* are not closely related to other (Australian) marsupials. The brain of *Didelphis* has been extensively studied, although we have only a partial understanding of the organization of the poorly developed visual system and visual cortex. The early cytoarchitectonic study of Gray (1924) distinguished a striate cortex and a "peristriate" belt. The striate cortex is clearly homologous to the striate cortex of eutherian mammals. It receives topologically organized projections from the dorsal lateral geniculate nucleus (Bodian, 1942; Diamond and Utley, 1963; Benevento and Ebner, 1971*b*) and contains a systematic and typical representation of the contralateral visual hemifield (Fig. 1; also see Sousa *et al.,* 1978). In comparison with that of other mammals, the representation is only slightly expanded in the portion corresponding to central or frontal vision, an observation compatible with the small eyes and poorly differentiated visual structures of the opossum.

Cortex lateral to striate cortex is also visually responsive in *Didelphis* (Lende, 1963*a*; Magalhães-Castro and Saraiva, 1971) and probably contains several subdivisions. Corticocortical connections (Benevento and Ebner, 1971*a*) suggest that the medial half of the "peristriate" cortex of Gray (1924) is a second representation of the visual field, i.e., V II or area 18. This medial half of the "peristriate" zone has been architectonically characterized by Benevento and Ebner (1971*a*), and it shares features, such as poorly developed lamination, with area 18 of many placental mammals. The medial margin of the "peristriate" band receives commissural connections from visual cortex of the opposite cerebral hemisphere, as it does in placental mammals, although the fibers course through the anterior commissure in the absence of a corpus callosum. These connections suggest a rerepresentation of the zero vertical meridian or the line of decussation of the retina in a second visual area. Indeed, some of our incomplete microelectrode mapping studies indicate the representation of the region of the zero vertical meridian along the medial margin of peristriate cortex of the opossum. Furthermore, the pattern of projections from striate cortex is congruent with the concept of a V II connected homotopically with V I. Each locus in the striate cortex projects to a locus in the medial "peristriate" belt, with the rostral part of striate cortex projecting to the rostral part of the belt and the caudal part of striate cortex projecting to the caudal part of the belt (Benevento and Ebner, 1971*a*). Thus there is electrophysiological, anatomical, and architectonic evidence for a second visual area, V II, in an Amer-

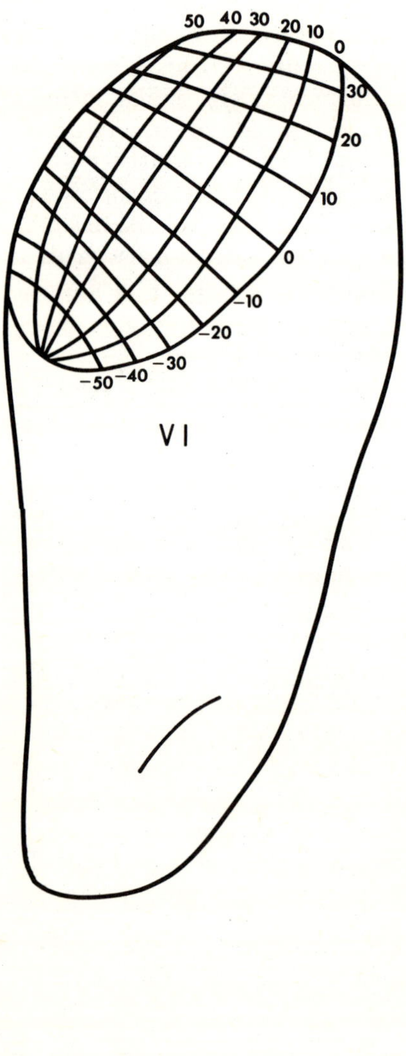

Figure 1. Dorsal view of the left cerebral hemisphere of an opossum (*Didelphis marsupialis-virginianus*). The visuotopic organization of striate cortex or primary visual cortex (V I) is shown in vertical meridians and horizontal parallels. The zero horizontal parallel corresponds to the horizontal midline of the eye, and the zero vertical meridian indicates the dividing line between the right and left visual hemifields and the line of decussation in the temporal retina. Cortex on the medial wall of the cerebral hemisphere represents more temporal parts of the hemifield. Note the relatively even representation of the hemifield with little expansion of frontal vision. Based on unpublished microelectrode mapping experiments of Kaas and Allman. For an example of the type of data used to construct such summaries, see Fig. 3.

ican opossum. However, the full extent, exact boundaries, and detailed visuotopic organization of this second visual area are not known.

Besides the projection pattern to the presumptive V II, the corticocortical efferents from V I also implicate a more lateral region of peristriate cortex and a caudal region of temporal cortex in visual functions (Fig. 2). Thus visual cortex of the opossum may contain a number of subdivisions, in addition to V I and V II, but it is uncertain what these subdivisions are, or if they correspond to any of the subdivisions identified in placental mammals.

Little is known about the organization of visual cortex in the Australian marsupials. The region of cortex responsive to visual stimulation has been shown in the wallaby (*Thylogale eugenii*) (Lende, 1963*b*), and it extends laterally beyond striate cortex to the border of the auditory region. Thus there is an expansive visual region but no evidence as to how it is subdivided. In the marsupial phalanger (*Trichosurus valpecula*) the interhemispheric connections of the lateral border region of striate cortex have been described (Heath and Jones, 1971), and the results are similar to those of the American opossum in that connections to the contralateral peristriate cortex just on the striate border suggest the presence of a second visual area, V II. A second focus of interhemispheric visual projections was found in the caudal portion of temporal cortex near the rhinal sulcus of the marsupial phalanger. Heath and Jones (1971) state that this projection zone "may represent the third visual area (V III or area 19) of the cat brain" or "the equivalent of the fourth or lateral suprasylvian visual area of the cat." It is not clear what is meant by "equivalent," but there is insufficient evidence to argue that the temporal projection zone is or is not homologous with any area of the cat brain.

C. Edentates

According to McKenna (1975), the first major offshoot of Eutheria was cohort Edentata, separating from the remaining eutherians (cohort Epitheria) perhaps in the early Cretaceous period. The extant edentates consist of a small number of species with pronounced specializations and restricted ecological distributions. Edentates are divided into three families: anteaters, tree sloths, and armadillos. While anteaters have no teeth, tree sloths and armadillos have cheek but not frontal teeth.

Little is known about the organization of visual cortex in edentates. However, the cortex of an armadillo has been divided into architectonic areas and regions

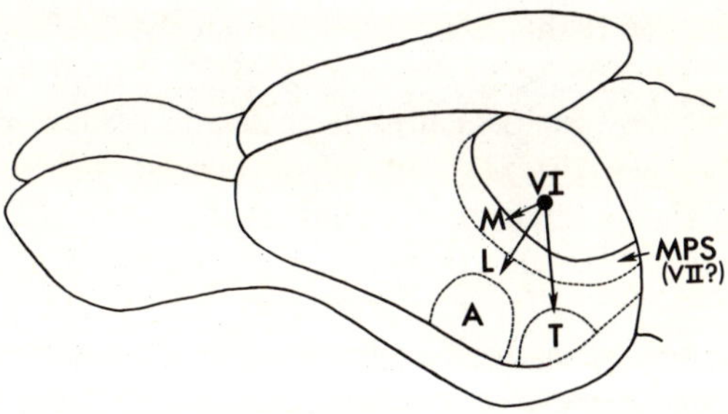

Figure 2. A dorsolateral view of an opossum (*Didelphis*) brain showing the location of primary visual cortex (V I), the medial peristriate band probably corresponding to the second visual area (V II), and projections from V I to medial peristriate cortex (M), lateral striate cortex (L), and temporal cortex (T). The projection pattern suggests the existence of at least three visual areas in addition to V I. A, Auditory region. Projections are based on Benevento and Ebner (1971*a*).

responsive to sensory stimulation (Royce *et al.,* 1975), and sensory areas have been shown in a sloth (Saraiva and Magalhães-Castro, 1975). The armadillo has a high rhinal fissure and an almost smooth neocortex. The small region responsive to visual stimuli is poorly differentiated architectonically, but it can be divided in myelin-stained brain sections into a large, densely stained medial area and a narrower, lightly stained lateral region. These two subdivisions of visual cortex may be the visual areas V I and V II (areas 17 and 18), but confirmation of this possibility awaits receptive field mapping. It is also possible that other visual areas exist in the temporal lobe, where some overlap of auditory and visual responses was noted. However, it is unlikely that other subdivisions of visual cortex exist rostral to the densely myelinated visual region since the immediately rostral cortex was found to be responsive to somatosensory stimulation.

The larger tree sloth brain has several fissures, one of which separates cortex responsive to visual stimuli from cortex responsive to auditory stimuli. The visually responsive area is located far more laterally than in most mammals, and it may be only part of the total area. It is uncertain if the responsive region represents V I, some other area, or several areas. The somatosensory cortex does not appear to immediately adjoin the visual region as in the armadillo.

D. Lagomorphs and Elephant Shrews

The next significant branch from the mainstream of eutherian mammals (ernotherian mammals) appears to have led to the present-day lagomorphs and macroscelidids (elephant shrews) (McKenna, 1975). This classification represents a significant change in presumed relationships since the elephant shrews have been generally considered to be insectivores, and at one time lagomorphs were thought to be rodents.

Lagomorphs are represented as rabbits, hares, and pikas. Only the visual system of the domestic rabbit has been studied in any detail. As early as 1950, primary (V I) and secondary (V II) visual areas were identified in the domestic rabbit by electrophysiological mapping methods (Thompson, *et al.,* 1950). The representation of the visual field in striate cortex, which is topographically connected to the dorsal lateral geniculate nucleus (Rose and Malis, 1965), is interesting in that a horizontal strip of retina with a high ganglion cell density relates to a disproportionately large segment of the total representation (Hughes, 1971; Thompson *et al.,* 1950). Our incomplete studies of the primary area in the cottontail rabbit (*Sylvilagus floridanus*) indicate that a horizontal strip of retina receives an expanded representation in this lagomorph also (Fig. 3), and it would be interesting to see if this feature is characteristic of lagomorphs in general.

The second visual area, V II, of the domestic rabbit appears to occupy a narrow strip of architectonically distinct cortex, area 18, just lateral to area 17 or striate cortex. As in V I of the rabbit, the representation of the horizontal strip of retina is disproportionately large (Hughes, 1971; Thompson *et al.,* 1950; Woolsey *et al.,* 1973). The basic organization of V II is like that of other mammals, with the 17/18 border corresponding to the zero vertical meridian, or line of decussation of the retina, with more temporal parts of the contralateral hemifield represented more laterally. However, the lateral border of V II is reached before the representation of the extreme temporal periphery occurs, and it appears that part of the representation is missing or displaced in a nontopographic manner toward the ends of the VII belt (Woolsey *et al.*, 1973). As in other mammals, V I projects in a point-to-point manner onto V II (Montero and Murphy, 1976), and callosal connections are along the boundary between V I and V II (Hughes and Wilson, 1969).

Besides the primary and secondary visual areas in the rabbit, there are both electrophysiological mapping and cortico-cortical connection evidence for at least two additional representations of the visual field in the cortex immediately lateral to V II (Woolsey *et al.*, 1973; Montero and Murphy, 1976; Towns *et al.*, 1977). Furthermore, a region of temporal cortex just caudal to auditory cortex is respon-

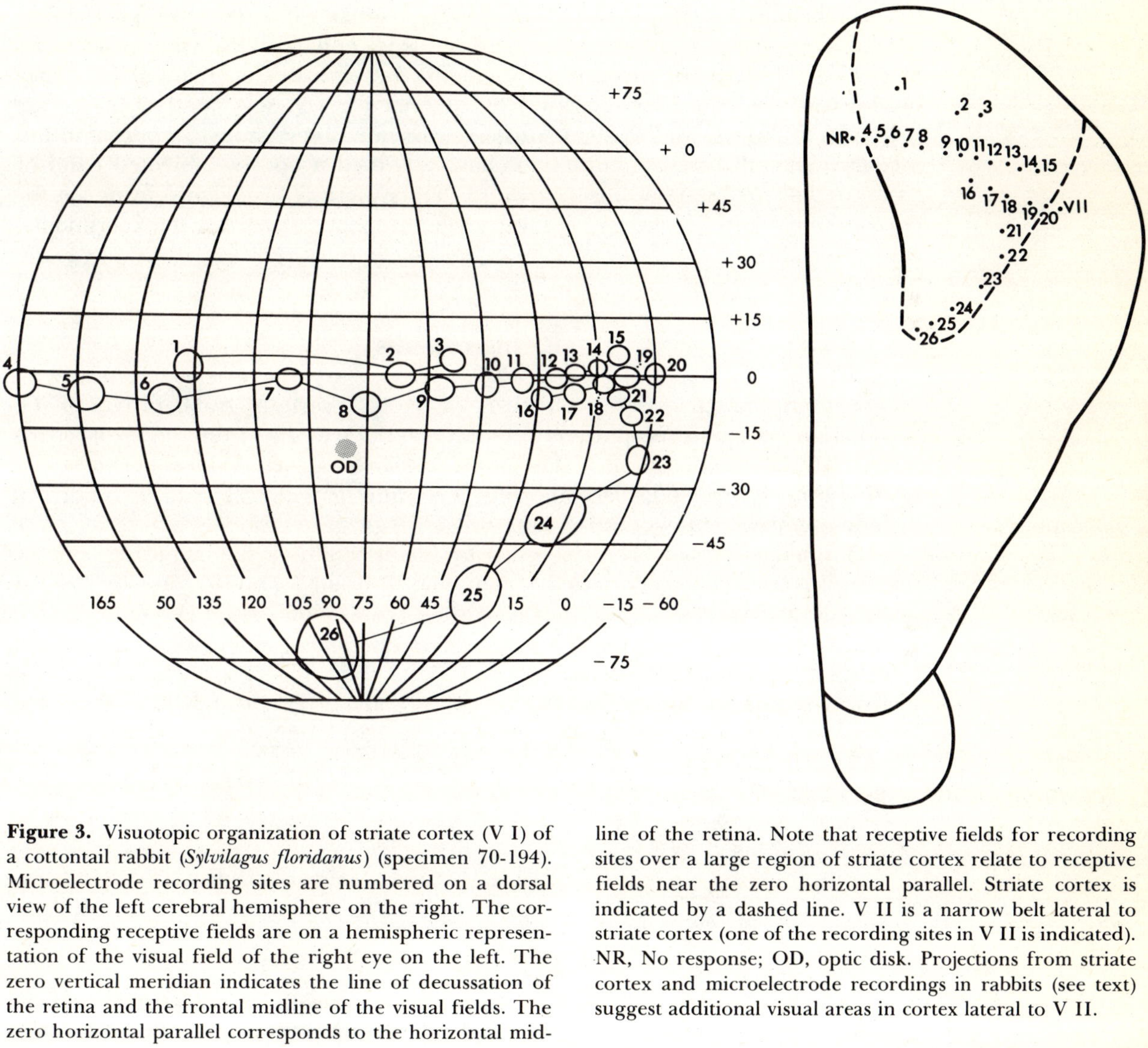

Figure 3. Visuotopic organization of striate cortex (V I) of a cottontail rabbit (*Sylvilagus floridanus*) (specimen 70-194). Microelectrode recording sites are numbered on a dorsal view of the left cerebral hemisphere on the right. The corresponding receptive fields are on a hemispheric representation of the visual field of the right eye on the left. The zero vertical meridian indicates the line of decussation of the retina and the frontal midline of the visual fields. The zero horizontal parallel corresponds to the horizontal midline of the retina. Note that receptive fields for recording sites over a large region of striate cortex relate to receptive fields near the zero horizontal parallel. Striate cortex is indicated by a dashed line. V II is a narrow belt lateral to striate cortex (one of the recording sites in V II is indicated). NR, No response; OD, optic disk. Projections from striate cortex and microelectrode recordings in rabbits (see text) suggest additional visual areas in cortex lateral to V II.

sive to visual stimuli (Chow *et al.,* 1977), and this region receives direct projections from striate cortex and the visual thalamus (Mathers *et al.,* 1977). Finally, the limbic cortex medial to striate cortex has been shown to receive a projection from striate cortex (Montero and Murphy, 1976), implicating part of the limbic system in visual functions.

In conclusion, the domestic rabbit has been shown to have complex visual system with a number of separate cortical representations of the visual field. Two of these, V I and V II, are undoubtedly homologous with V I and V II of other mammals. The homologies of the other visual areas remain uncertain, but the temporal visual area is similar in location and connections to a temporal visual area found in some other mammals.

Elephant shrews are the other surviving ernotherian mammals. Formerly, elephant shrews were grouped with tree shrews as a suborder of insectivores with a close relationship with primates. Now, it appears that, while tree shrews are closely related to primates, elephant shrews are not (McKenna, 1975). Aside from histological investigations of preserved specimens, the brains of elephant shrews have not been studied. Le Gros Clark (1928) described a well-developed striate cortex in elephant shrews, and this is consistent with our observations. In addition, immediately lateral to striate cortex, we have observed a poorly laminated band of tissue perhaps corresponding to area 18. Thus there is histological evidence for both primary and secondary visual areas in elephant shrews, but experimental evidence is lacking.

E. Insectivores

Surviving insectivores are members of one of the four grand orders of the tokotherian mammals recognized by McKenna (1975) as distinct in the fossil record by the late Cretaceous period. The "true insectivores" are divided by McKenna (1975) into two orders, erinaceomorphs, including hedgehogs, and soricomorphs, including tenrecs, shrews, and moles.

The hedgehog has been described by Elliott Smith (1902) as having "one of the simplest and most generalized of mammalian brains," and this opinion has led to considerable interest in the details of the organization of the hedgehog brain. Electrophysiological mapping studies have defined two systematic maps of the visual field in caudal neocortex, V I and V II (Fig. 4) (Kaas *et al.,* 1970). The primary visual area, V I, is coextensive with striate cortex, or area 17 (Kaas *et al.,*

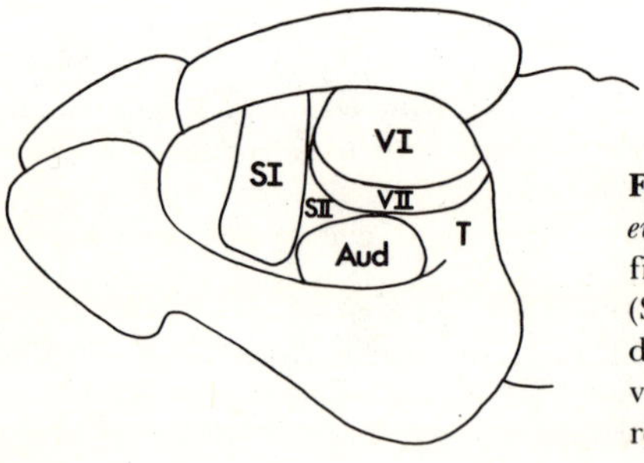

Figure 4. Cortical visual areas in the hedgehog (*Erinaceus europaeus*). The primary (V I) and secondary (V II) visual fields are indicated, as well as the locations of the primary (SI) and secondary (SII) somatosensory areas and the auditory field (Aud). Only two visual areas have been revealed, but it is possible that part or all of the temporal region (T) is involved in vision. Based on Kaas *et al.* (1970).

1970), and receives a retinotopically organized projection from the thalamic relay nucleus, the dorsal lateral geniculate nucleus (Gould *et al.*, 1978; Hall and Diamond, 1968). The second visual area, V II, also occupies a distinct architectonic field. Cortex immediately rostral to V I and V II is part of the primary somatosensory area, and auditory cortex and the second somatosensory cortex appear to adjoin much of the lateral and rostral parts of V II (Kaas *et al.*, 1970). The possibility for other visual areas in a small segment of temporal cortex exists, but there is no supportive electrophysiological evidence, and the cortical connections of V I appear to be only with V II and not with temporal cortex as in several other mammals (Gould and Ebner, 1978). Thus there is clear evidence for two subdivisions of visual cortex in hedgehogs, V I and V II, but evidence for other visual areas is lacking.

Little is known of the visual system of the morphologically more diverse soricomorphs. The Madagascar tenrecs have small poorly developed eyes and visual structures in the brain stem. Nothing is known about visual cortex. Vision is also poorly developed in shrews and moles. Unsuccessful attempts have been made to record visual responses from posterior neocortex in both anesthetized and unanesthetized moles (Allison and Twyver, 1970). Furthermore, the location of somatosensory cortex is very caudal, excluding the possibility of much visual cortex. In addition, the central visual pathway is poorly developed, and may not even include input to the dorsal lateral geniculate nucleus (Lund and Lund, 1966). Thus the central visual system in moles is degenerate, and visually responsive cortex may not even exist in some species.

F. Archonta

An important branch of the tokotheres appears to have led to the semiarboreal and arboreal tree shrews, bats, dermopterans, and primates (McKenna, 1975). All these separate lines, at least originally, were highly dependent on vision, and the extant forms (except for Microchiroptera) have well-developed visual systems.

1. Tupaiids

The tree shrews have many generalized and insectivorelike features and are regarded as primitive members of Archonta (McKenna, 1975; Romer, 1967). Tree shrews have a highly developed visual system characterized by a laminated lateral geniculate nucleus, a large and clearly laminated superior colliculus, and well-differentiated and distinct architectonic divisions of visual cortex. Some of these features may be a consequence of the taxonomic relationship between tree shrews and primates, as Le Gros Clark (1959) proposed. However, Campbell (1966) has correctly noted that many of the progressive features of the tupaiid visual system that are shared with primates are also widely found in other highly visual mammals, and therefore may have been independently acquired. One feature of the visual system that clearly distinguishes tree shrews from primates is that the superior colliculus of tree shrews has the generalized feature of receiving projections from all parts of the contralateral eye (Lane *et al.*, 1971; Kaas *et al.*, 1974) rather than from only the nasal retina as in primates.

Two visual areas, V I (Fig. 5) and V II, have been demonstrated by electrophysiological mapping methods in the tree shrew, and these representations correspond to the architectonic areas 17 and 18, respectively (Kaas *et al.,* 1972*b*). Temporal cortex lateral to area 18 in the temporal lobe responds to visual stimuli (Kaas *et al.,* 1972*b*), receives projections from the visual thalamus (Harting *et al.,* 1973), and is involved in visual behavior (Killackey *et al.,* 1971). Certainly it is reasonable to believe that this large temporal region of visual cortex contains functional subdivisions, but these subdivisions have not yet been demonstrated.

2. Bats

The Chiroptera include two suborders, Megachiroptera, or Old World fruit bats, and Microchiroptera, including all other bats with more varied behavioral and morphological adaptations. Megachiroptera have large eyes, while many Microchiroptera do not. The visual system is clearly regressive in some echolocating bats,

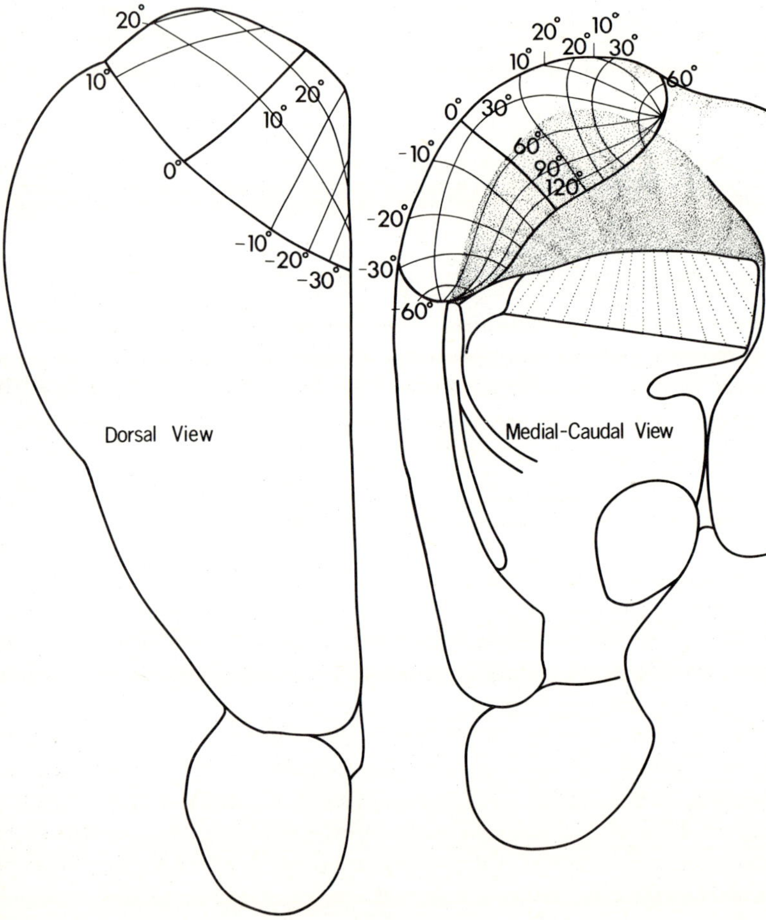

Figure 5. Visuotopic organization of striate cortex (V I) in the tree shrew (*Tupaia glis*). The coordinate system is as in Figs. 1 and 3. V I is bordered laterally by a narrow V II. In addition, large parts of temporal cortex respond to visual stimuli. Based on Kaas *et al.* (1972*b*).

where the occipital cortex is reduced so much in size that the brain stem is not completely covered. The retinal projections have been studied in an Old World fruit bat (Crowle, 1974); the dorsal lateral geniculate nucleus is well differentiated with clear lamination. In another Old World fruit bat, Brodmann (1909) described an area 17 bounded laterally by a narrow area 18; no Area 19 was noted. Thus there is architectonic evidence for V I and V II in Old World bats, but confirming experimental data are necessary, and there may be other visual areas.

3. Dermopterans (Gliding Lemurs)

The gliding lemurs are restricted to two species of gliding mammals of the Philippines and Southeast Asia. The eyes are large, the dorsal lateral geniculate nucleus is laminated (Kaas *et al.*, 1978), and a distinct striate cortex (area 17) can be identified (personal observation). Other subdivisions of visual cortex are unknown.

4. Primates

The primate order is divided into two suborders, the Stepsirhini and the Haplorhini. The Stepsirhini include lemurs, lorises, and galagos. The Haplorhini include three infraorders, tarsiers, platyrrhine (New World) monkeys, and catarrhine primates (Old World monkeys, apes, and humans).

In all the primates that have been studied, the primary area, striate cortex or area 17, is very distinct and easily identified. The representation of the visual field has been determined for striate cortex of a number of primates, and in each case a disproportionately large amount of tissue represents frontal vision at the center of gaze (for review, see Kaas, 1978). As in other mammals, V I is a topological representation of the contralateral visual hemifield.

A second visual area, V II, has been identified by electrophysiological mapping in galagos (Allman and Kaas, unpublished) and New World monkeys (Allman and Kaas, 1974; Cowey, 1964), and has been inferred from projection patterns from V I in Old World monkeys (Cragg, 1969; Zeki, 1974). The second visual area of the primates appears to "split" along much of the horizontal meridian so that V II forms a long belt around 90% or more of V I, with the outer boundary of V II being formed by the horizontal meridian. Since V II in primates is not completely topological, it has been referred to as a second-order transformation of the visual field (Allman and Kaas, 1974). The electrophysiological and projection studies show a close correspondence between V II and area 18 as defined in prosimians and New World monkeys. However, the experimental studies suggest that the belt usually designated as area 18 in Old World monkeys is too wide for V II and that "area 18" needs to be redefined in these primates.

A number of other visual areas have been found in a New World monkey, the owl monkey (Fig. 6). The details of organization of these areas have been reviewed elsewhere (Kaas, 1978; Allman and Kaas, 1976). Briefly, a small topological representation of the visual field in the temporal lobe has been called the middle temporal visual area (MT). MT is almost completely surrounded by a crescent-shaped representation, the dorsolateral crescent or DL. The dorsolateral crescent is split along the horizontal meridian, as is V II, and interconnects with MT. Other visual areas include the dorsomedial area, DM, a second-order transformation like DL and V II, the medial area, M, with a very reduced representation of central vision, and the posterior parietal area with visual input but undetermined organization. Cortex ventral to MT and DL in the owl monkey is responsive to visual stimuli, and this cortex is in the position of the inferotemporal (IT) cortex of rhesus monkeys.

MT has also been identified in the prosimian *Galago* by electrophysiological mapping methods (Allman *et al.,* 1973), and the existence of MT in Old World monkeys seems probable from studies of cortical connections. The other visual areas of the owl monkey have not yet been described for other primates. Thus it appears that at least three visual areas, V I, V II, and MT, are basic to all primates, but it is not yet certain if other areas found in the owl monkey are widespread in primates, or if primates vary in patterns of visual cortex organization.

G. Carnivores

The living representatives of the grand order Ferae are the present-day carnivores (McKenna, 1975). Pinnipeds, the seals and walruses, are often treated as a suborder of Carnivora, with the remaining carnivores consisting of seven families including cats, dogs, bears, skunks, raccoons, mongooses, and hyenas. The domestic cat has been extensively investigated, but little attention has been paid to other carnivores.

The two visual areas, V I and V II, were first described in the cat (Talbot, 1942; Talbot and Marshall, 1942), but detailed maps of the two areas have only recently become available (Woolsey, 1971; Tusa *et al.,* 1978, 1979). The primary visual area is coextensive with area 17. It contains a topographical representation of the contralateral visual hemifield, with a greatly expanded representation of the center of gaze. The second visual area forms a long, narrow band along the

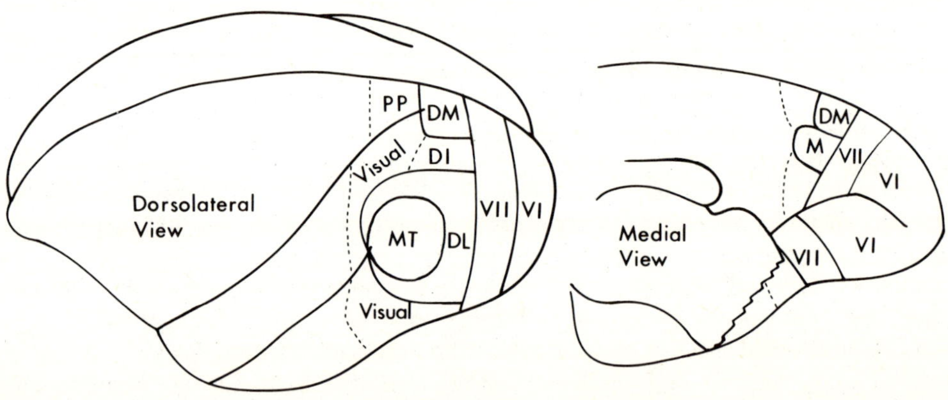

Figure 6. Some of the visual areas of the owl monkey (*Aotus trivirgatus*). The primary visual area (V I), secondary visual area (V II), dorsolateral area (DL), dorsomedial area (DM), medial area (M), and middle temporal area (MT) all contain systematic representations of the visual hemifield. The detailed organization of the posterior parietal region (PP), the dorso-intermediate region (DI), and other visually responsive zones has not yet been determined. Based on experiments of Allman and Kaas (1976 and others).

complete representation of the zero vertical meridian in V I. The band, V II or area 18, is split so that part of the outer (lateral) border of V II corresponds to the paracentral visual field, and the representation of the extreme temporal periphery appears to be missing. Furthermore, the representations of the upper and lower quadrants in V II are not symmetrical. More of the outer border of the upper quadrant of V II represents the horizontal meridian. Thus V II in the cat is a split or second-order transformation of the visual hemifield, with the complications of missing parts and asymmetry.

A third visual area, V III, has been described as forming the complete outer border of V II in cats (Tusa *et al.,* 1979); V III is roughly coextensive with area 19 of Sanides and Hoffman (1969).

In addition to V I, V II, and V III, a large region lateral to V III in the suprasylvian sulcus responds to visual stimuli (Spear and Baumann, 1975; Palmer *et al.,* 1978). Palmer *et al.* (1978) have divided the total region into six separate areas distinguished by differences in retinotopic organizations and in cortical and subcortical connections. The six areas form three mirror symmetrical pairs. The two anterior areas (anterior medial and anterior lateral) are topological (first-order) representations, but they appear to include only part of the hemifield.

The four caudal suprasylvian areas have an organization that has not been described for other areas or other mammals (Kaas, 1978). Each area systematically represents the horizontal dimension, but there is no systematic representation of the vertical dimension. Most receptive fields for neurons within one of these areas lie along or near the horizontal meridian. A particular recording site corresponds to a particular location along the horizontal meridian, but receptive fields "situated higher or lower in the visual field appear to be randomly scattered among the majority on the horizontal meridian." Palmer *et al.* (1978) characterize this type as a "line-to-surface" representation. The suprasylvian areas differ in internal organization, thalamic connections, and cytoarchitecture.

Finally, a small representation of at least part of the contralateral hemifield has been described for cortex bordering V I on the medial wall of the cerebral hemisphere in the splenial sulcus (Kalia and Whitteridge, 1973).

In addition to the domestic cat, parts of V I and V II have been mapped in the lion, where proportionately even more of these two visual areas is devoted to central vision (Kaas, Ladpli, and Hoffman, unpublished). In another carnivore, the mink (*Mustela vison*), the existence of V I and V II was established by electrophysiological mapping, but the detailed organization of these areas was not determined (Sanderson and Kaas, 1974).

In summary, there is evidence for V I and V II in at least three carnivores, and in the domestic cat a number of other visual areas have been established. It is not known if any of these additional visual areas have homologues in other mammals. The "line-to-surface" type of organization found in two of the cat visual areas has not been reported for any visual area of any other mammal.

H. Ungulates

The grand order Ungulata arose from cretaceous tokotheres according to McKenna (1975), and soon divided into four major groups (mirorders) of extant "ungulates": (1) the tubulidentates (aardvarks) and artiodactyls (even-toed hoofed mammals), (2) hyraxes and perissodactyls (odd-toed hoofed mammals), (3) elephants and the aquatic sea cows and manatees (Sirenia), and (4) cetaceans (whales).

The domestic sheep, an artiodactyl, is the only ungulate for which there are electrophysiological data bearing on the organization of visual cortex. Previously, Rose (1942) defined an area striata with "such a characteristic structure that there can scarcely be any doubt about it being equivalent to the area striata of other mammals." This opinion stands verified by the electrophysiological experiments of Clarke and Whitteridge (1976), which demonstrate a systematic map of the contralateral hemifield within the striate cortex of Rose (1942). Although the map has the general orientation and topological features of V I in other mammals, there are unusual features. First, the primary area has expanded representations of both frontal vision and a horizontal band of vision. These expanded representations correspond to a temporal area and a horizontal strip of high ganglion cell densities in the retina. The expanded representation of horizontal vision is similar to that found in rabbits. A further peculiarity is that the lateral part of what was judged to be V I was found to represent 10–15° of the ipsilateral visual hemifield. Immediately lateral to this unusual strip of cortex, the midline or zero vertical meridian was represented for a second time. Then a reverse order representation of the contralateral hemifield was found as mapping proceeded further laterally in the cortex. The general features of the retinotopic organization of the second area are clearly those of V II, but it is not yet known if V II in the sheep is either a complete or a topological representation of the contralateral hemifield. However, the receptive fields for the most lateral recording sites are only about 30° from the vertical meridian, suggesting that the representation is either incomplete, split in some way, or both. Finally, cortex lateral to V II also responded to visual stimuli in the sheep. This result clearly suggests the possibility of additional visual areas.

I. Rodents

The phylogenetic affinities of Rodentia are presently uncertain, although relationships to Ferae or primates have been suggested (McKenna, 1975). Thirty-five families of rodents are included in the highly successful order with a worldwide distribution. Rodentia includes members specialized for underground, terrestrial, arboreal, and semiaquatic life. Most of what is known of the visual system of rodents is based on laboratory rats. Important information is also available for gray squirrels, mice, and hamsters. In addition, visually responsive cortex has been identified in porcupines (Lende and Woolsey, 1956), guinea pigs (Zeigler, 1964; Campos and Welker, 1976), and capybaras (Campos and Welker, 1976).

The primary area, V I, of rats has been mapped by Adams and Forrester (1968) and by Montero *et al.* (1973*a*). In this rodent, V I has only a moderate expansion of the representation of frontal vision. For cortex lateral to V I, both groups of investigators have recordings that support the concept of a narrow V II, but the detailed organization and precise location of this second area are unknown. Additional mapping results, as well as the pattern of cortical projections from V I (Montero *et al.,* 1973*b*), indicate the presence of probably two additional visual areas lateral and rostral to V I. Further work is needed to identify and delimit these areas.

V I and V II have also been identified by electrophysiological mapping procedures in mice (Dräger, 1974; Wagor *et al.,* 1979), hamsters (Tiao and Blakemore, 1976), and gray squirrels (Hall *et al.,* 1971). In the mouse and hamster the representation of the visual field is relatively uniform in V I, while the more visual squirrel has proportionately more cortex devoted to frontal than temporal vision. In all these rodents, recordings across the width of the V II band fail to produce receptive fields in the extreme temporal periphery. As few as 15° of the frontal visual field is represented across the width of the central portion of V II in the squirrel, although the ends of the belt represent more temporal parts of the contralateral hemifield. It is not yet certain if some of the temporal periphery of the hemifield is missing from the representation in these rodents, or if it is displaced toward the ends of V II, producing a "split" or second-order transformation.

Cortex lateral to V II in the squirrel is responsive to visual stimuli, but the organizations, extents, and boundaries of other possible subdivisions of visual cortex are unknown. However, projections from striate cortex (Robson and Hall, 1977) to the densely myelinated posterior portion of the temporal cortex, Tp (Kaas *et al.,* 1972*a*), suggest the location of another visual area. A small visual representation has been reported in cortex immediately medial to V I in both the hamster (Tiao and Blakemore, 1976) and the mouse (Dräger, 1974; Wagor *et al.,* 1979). This visual area is similar in location and organization to the splenial visual area in the cat. As an added complication, there is evidence in the mouse (Wagor *et al.,* 1979) that this medial cortex might actually consist of two separate representations. Finally, there appears to be at least one visual representation in addition to V II in cortex lateral to V I in the mouse (Wagor *et al.*, 1979) and the rat (Montero *et al.,* 1973*b*).

In summary, two visual areas, V I and V II, have been demonstrated in rodents. As in other mammals, the second representation is not a simple first-order transformation (Allman and Kaas, 1974) as is V I, in that it is either incomplete or, more probably, "split." There is clear evidence for other visual areas, including a medial visual area, but these subdivisions need to be further defined.

III. Conclusions

Studies of the organization of visual cortex in mammals seldom reflect a comparative or phylogenetic point of view. Studies usually use mammals that are easily accessible or offer other practical advantages. While we can clearly benefit from an approach that is cognizant of phylogenetic taxonomy, the available results do allow several conclusions. First, a primary visual area, V I, has been identified by its distinctive visuotopic organization, architectonic structure, position, and pattern of connections in a wide range of mammals. It seems reasonable to conclude that, with the possible exceptions of monotremes (where further investigations are needed) and mammals such as moles, which are adapted to nonvisual environments, all mammals have a homologous primary visual area.

A second conclusion is that there are at least two distinct types of specializations of the visuotopic organization of V I in mammals, and that each of these specializations has occurred several times. In visually unspecialized or generalized mammals, such as hedgehogs (Fig. 7) and opossums (Fig. 1), the representation of the visual field is relatively uniform and there is only a slight expansion of the part of V I representing frontal vision. A common type of specialization is an increase in the proportion of V I devoted to frontal vision. Squirrels and tree shrews (Figs. 5 and 7) are two examples of mammals with such an increase. The expansion of frontal vision is even greater in primates and in cats. Another type of specialization of V I is the expansion of the amount of cortex that represents a broad horizontal strip of retina or visual field. This type of specialization might aid in the detection of predators as they appear at a distance on the midhorizontal plane from almost any direction. The cortical expansion of the region of midhorizontal vision has been reported for sheep and rabbits (Fig. 3), but it probably exists in many other mammals as well.

A third conclusion is that the second visual area, V II, is part of the basic mammalian plan of visual system organization (again with the possible exceptions of monotremes and moles). Although V II has been found in fewer mammals than V I, there is evidence for V II in a wide range of mammals, including marsupials, lagomorphs, insectivores, primates, tree shrews, carnivores, ungulates, and rodents. Since it is unlikely that V II arose independently in all these lines of descent, V II must have existed in a common ancestor. In all these mammals, V II appears to differ from V I in that the representation is either "split" or incomplete. V II shares an inner boundary with V I along the representation of the zero vertical meridian. The outer boundary of V II appears to relate to various parts of the paracentral visual field in different mammals. In primates this outer boundary of V II repre-

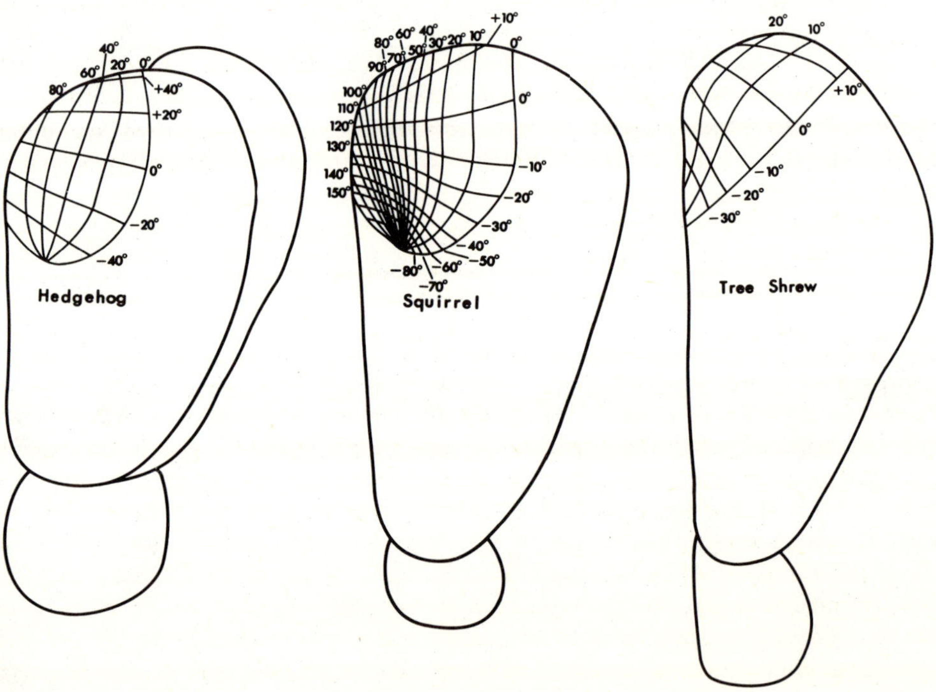

Figure 7. Distortion of the visual hemifield representation in V I of hedgehogs, squirrels, and tree shrews. Based on experiments by Kaas *et al.* (1970, 1972*a,b*) and Hall *et al.* (1971). Conventions as in Figs. 1, 3, and 5.

sents the zero horizontal meridian. In cats the representation of the upper and lower visual quadrants is organized differently in V II, with the horizontal meridian forming much of the outer boundary of V II in the representation of the upper but not the lower quadrant. In tree shrews and squirrels most of the outer boundary of V II corresponds to parts of the visual field only 15–20° from the zero vertical meridian, often at some distance from the zero horizontal. As more is known about the organization of V II in different mammals, it is likely that other interesting species differences will be revealed.

Because of insufficient evidence, it is yet uncertain if any other visual areas are basic to Mammalia. A small visual area has been described on the border of V I within the limbic cortex in cats and some rodents. It would be interesting to look for this visual area in other mammals. It is also possible that a visual area in the temporal lobe is common to many or all mammals. Many different mammals have been shown to have visual input from striate cortex and from the visual thalamus or pulvinar to the temporal lobe, and this region has been shown to represent systematically the visual field in some primates. A complication is that primates, cats, and probably many other mammals have more than one visual area in the temporal lobe, so that suggestions of homologies should be made with caution.

While visual areas V I, V II, and perhaps one or more others appear to be part of a basic mammalian plan of visual system organization, it is hard to avoid the conclusion that some of the additional visual areas found in visually advanced mammals such as monkeys and cats are specializations found in some lines of evolution and not in others. In some mammals apparently approximating the ancestral condition, the neocortex is small relative to the rest of the brain. In these mammals neocortex is largely occupied by V I, V II, and somatic, auditory, and motor areas, leaving very little room for other sensory areas. In hedgehogs, for example, the primary visual area, V I, borders the primary somatosensory area, SI (Fig. 4). In cats and monkeys the neocortex is greatly expanded, and the primary sensory areas, V I, SI, and AI, are widely separated. Between the primary areas, a number of visual areas have been defined. These observations strongly suggest that some of the visual areas of cats and monkeys are not homologous. A major goal of future experiments should be to determine what visual areas are unique to certain lines of descent.

The acquisition of new visual areas in any line of evolution would certainly be an outstanding accomplishment of mammalian evolution. By comparison, the specializations, differentiations, and expansions of common brain areas would be minor accomplishments since new areas have much more potential for altering and increasing behavioral capabilities. As Gregory (1935) pointed out, a major factor in evolution has been the duplication of existing body parts to create new ones. Over time, the "new" parts can diverge in function and thereby acquire new functions without interfering with the original functions which still can be maintained by the "old" parts.

As a final point, the survey presented here shows that we know very little about the organization of visual cortex for the living members of some of the major branches of mammalian evolution. Thus it is very important to gain some understanding of the organization of visual cortex in monotremes and edentates. In addition, a better understanding of the early stages of the evolution of the primate visual system might come from studies of dermopterans and Old World fruit bats.

Yet these mammals have been almost totally neglected in studies of the visual system. The phylogenetic revision presented by McKenna (1975) also suggests that elephant shrews and lagomorphs might share some common features of visual cortex organization. Studies of visual cortex in elephant shrews comparable to those already completed on rabbits might reveal similarities in cortical organization.

IV. References

Adams, A. D., and Forrester, J. M., 1968, The projection of the rat's visual field on the cerebral cortex, *Q. J. Exp. Physiol.* **53**:327.

Allison, T., and Twyver, H. V., 1970, Sensory representation in the neocortex of the mole, *Scalopus aquaticus, Exp. Neurol.* **27**:554.

Allman, J. M., and Kaas, J. H., 1974, The organization of the second visual area (VII) in the owl monkey: A second order transformation of the visual hemifield, *Brain Res.* **76**:247.

Allman, J. M., and Kaas, J. H., 1976, Representation of the visual field on the medial wall of occipital-parietal cortex in the owl monkey, *Science* **191**:572.

Allman, J. M., Kaas, J. H., and Lane, R. H., 1973, The middle temporal visual area (MT) in the bushbaby, *Galago senegalensis, Brain Res.* **57**:197.

Benevento, L. A., and Ebner, F. F., 1971*a*, The areas and layers of corticocortical terminations in the visual cortex of the virginia opossum, *J. Comp. Neurol.* **141**:157.

Benevento, L. A., and Ebner, F. F., 1971*b*, The contribution of the dorsal lateral geniculate nucleus to the total pattern of thalamic terminations in striate cortex of the virginia opossum, *J. Comp. Neurol.* **143**:243.

Bodian, D., 1942, Studies on the diencephalon of the virginia opossum. III. The thalamocortical projection, *J. Comp. Neurol.* **77**:259.

Brodmann, K., 1909, *Vergleichende Lokalisationslehre der Gosshirnrinde,* pp. 1–324, Verlag V. A. Barth, Leipzig.

Campbell, C. B. G., 1966, The relationships of the tree shrews: The evidence of the nervous system, *Evolution* **20**:276.

Campbell, C. B. G., and Hayhow, W. R., 1971, Primary optic pathways in the echidna, *Tachyglossus aculeatus:* An experimental degeneration study, *J. Comp. Neurol.* **143**:119.

Campbell, C. B. G., and Hayhow, W. R., 1972, Primary optic pathways in the duckbill platypus *Ornithorynchus anatinus:* An experimental degeneration study, *J. Comp. Neurol.* **145**:195.

Campos, G. B., and Welker, W. I., 1976, Comparisons between brains of a large and a small hystricomorph rodent: capybara, *Hydrochoesus* and guinea pig, *Cavia;* neocortical projection regions and measurements of brain subdivisions, *Brain Behav. Evol.* **13**:327.

Chow, K. L., Douville, A., Mascetti, G., and Grobstein, P., 1977, Receptive field characteristics of neurons in a visual area of the rabbit temporal cortex, *J. Comp. Neurol.* **171**:135.

Clarke, P. G. H., and Whitteridge, D., 1976, The cortical visual areas of the sheep, *J. Physiol.* **256**:497.

Cowey, A., 1964, Projection of the retina onto striate and prestriate cortex in the squirrel monkey, *Saimiri sciureus, J. Neurophysiol.* **27**:366.

Cragg, B. G., 1969, The topography of the afferent projections in the circumstriate visual cortex of the monkey studied by the Nauta method, *Vision Res.* **9**:733.

Crowle, P. K., 1974, Experimental investigation of retinofugal connections to the diencephalon and midbrain of Chiroptera, thesis, Indiana University.

Diamond, I. T., and Utley, J. D., 1963, Thalamic retrograde degeneration study of sensory cortex in opossum, *J. Comp. Neurol.* **120**:129.

Dräger, U. C., 1974, Receptive fields of single cells and topography in mouse visual cortex, *J. Comp. Neurol.* **160**:269.

Elliot Smith, G., 1902, Descriptive and illustrated catalogue of the physiological series of comparative anatomy, in: *R. C. Surg. Mus. Cat. Physiol. Ser.* **2**:133.

Gould, H. J., III, and Ford, F. E., 1978, Connections of the visual cortex in the hedgehog (*Paraechinus hypomelas*). II. Corticocortical projections, *J. Comp. Neurol.* **177**:473.

Gould, H. J., III, Hall, W. C., and Ebner, F. F., 1978, Connections of the visual system in the hedgehog (*Paraechinus hypomelas*). I. Thalamocortical projections, *J. Comp. Neurol.* **177:**445.

Gray, P. A., 1924, The cortical lamination pattern of the opossum, *Didelphys virginiana, J. Comp. Neurol.* **37:**221.

Gregory, W. K., 1935, Reduplication in evolution, *Q. Rev. Biol.* **10:**272.

Hall, W. C., and Diamond, I. T., 1968, Organization and function of the visual cortex in hedgehog. I. Cortical cytoarchitecture and thalamic retrograde degeneration, *Brain Behav. Evol.* **1:**181.

Hall, W. C., Kaas, J. H., Killackey, H., and Diamond, I. T., 1971, Cortical visual areas in the grey squirrel (*Sciurus carolinesis*): A correlation between cortical evoked potential maps and architectonic subdivisions, *J. Neurophysiol.* **34:**437.

Harting, J. K., Diamond, I. T., and Hall, W. C., 1973, Anterograde degeneration study of the cortical projections of the lateral geniculate and pulvinar nuclei in the tree shrew (*Tupaia glis*), *J. Comp. Neurol.* **150:**393.

Heath, C. J., and Jones, E. G., 1971, Interhemispheric pathways in the absence of a corpus callosum, *J. Anat.* **109:**253.

Hughes, A., 1971, Topographical relationships between the anatomy and physiology of the rabbit visual system, *Doc. Ophthalmol.* **30:**33.

Hughes, A., and Wilson, M. E., 1969, Callosal terminations along the boundary between visual areas I and II in the rabbit, *Brain Res.* **12:**19.

Kaas, J. H., 1978, Organization of visual cortex in primates, in: *Sensory Systems of Primates* (C. R. Noback, ed.), pp. 151–179, Plenum Press, New York.

Kaas, J. H., Hall, W. C., and Diamond, I. T., 1970, Cortical visual areas I and II in the hedgehog: Relation between evoked potential maps and architectonic subdivisions, *J. Neurophysiol.* **33:**595.

Kaas, J. H., Hall, W. C., and Diamond, I. T., 1972*a*, Visual cortex of the grey squirrel (*Sciurus carolinensis*): Architectonic subdivisions and connections from the visual thalamus, *J. Comp. Neurol.* **145:**273.

Kaas, J. H., Hall, W. C., Killackey, H., and Diamond, I. T., 1972*b*, Visual cortex of the tree shrew (*Tupaia glis):* Architectonic subdivisions and representations of the visual field, *Brain Res.* **42:**491.

Kaas, J. H., Harting, J. K., and Guillery, R. W., 1974, Representation of the complete retina in the contralateral superior colliculus of some mammals, *Brain Res.* **65:**343.

Kaas, J. H., Huerta, M. F., Weber, J. T., and Harting, J. K., 1978, Patterns of retinal terminations and laminar organizations of the lateral geniculate nucleus of primates, *J. Comp. Neurol.* **182:** 517.

Kalia, M., and Whitteridge, D., 1973, The visual areas in the splenial sulcus of the cat, *J. Physiol.* **232:**275.

Killackey, H., Snyder, M., and Diamond, I. T., 1971, Function of striate and temporal cortex in the tree shrew, *J. Comp. Physiol. Psychol.* **74:**1.

Lane, R. H., Allman, J. M., and Kaas, J. H., 1971, Representation of the visual field in the superior colliculus of the grey squirrel (*Sciurus carolinensis*) and the tree shrew (*Tupaia glis*), *Brain Res.* **26:**277.

Le Gros Clark, W. E., 1928, On the brain of *Macroscelididae, J. Anat.* **62:**245.

Le Gros Clark, W. E., 1959, *The Antecedents of Man,* Edinburgh University, Press, Edinburgh.

Lende, R. A., 1963*a*, Sensory representation in the cerebral cortex of the opossum (*Didelphis virginiana*), *J. Comp. Neurol.* **121:**395.

Lende, R. A., 1963*b*, Cerebral cortex: A sensorimotor amalgam in the Marsupialia, *Science* **141:**730.

Lende, R. A., 1964, Representation in the cerebral cortex of a primitive mammal, *J. Neurophysiol.* **27:**37.

Lende, R. A., and Woolsey, C. N., 1956, Sensory and motor localization in cerebral cortex of porcupine (*Erethizon dorsatus*), *J. Neurophysiol.* **19:**544.

Lund, R. D., and Lund, J. S., 1966, The central visual pathways and their functional significance in the mole (*Tala Europaea*), *J. Zool.* **149:**95.

Magalhães-Castro, B., and Saraiva, P. E. S., 1971, Sensory and motor representation in the cerebral cortex of the marsupial *Didelphis azarae azarae, Brain Res.* **34:**291.

Mathers, L. H., Douville, A., and Chow, K. L., 1977, Anatomical studies of a temporal visual area in the rabbit, *J. Comp. Neurol.* **171:**147.

McKenna, M. C., 1975, Toward a phylogenetic classification of the mammalia, in: *Phylogeny of the Primates* (W. P. Luckett and F. S. Szalay, eds.), pp. 21–46, Plenum Press, New York.

Montero, V. M., and Murphy, E. H., 1976, Cortico-cortical connections from the striate cortex in the rabbit, *Anat. Rec.* **184:**483.

Montero, V. M., Rojas, A., and Torrealba, F., 1973*a*, Retinotopic organization of striate and peristriate visual cortex in the albino rat, *Brain Res.* **53:**197.

Montero, V. M., Bravo, H., and Fernández, V., 1973*b*, Striate-peristriate cortico-cortical connections in the albino and gray rat, *Brain Res.* **53:**202.

Palmer, L. A., Rosenquist, A. C., and Tusa, R. J., 1978, The retinotopic organization of lateral suprasylvian visual areas in the cat, *J. Comp. Neurol.* **177:**237.

Robson, J. A., and Hall, W. C., 1977, The organization of the pulvinar in the grey squirrel (*Sciurus carolinensis*), *J. Comp. Neurol.* **173:**355.

Romer, A. S., 1967, Major steps in vertebrate evolution, *Science* **158:**1629.

Rose, J. E., 1942, A cytoarchitectural study of the sheep cortex, *J. Comp. Neurol.* **76:**1.

Rose, J. E., and Malis, L. I., 1965, Geniculostriate connections in the rabbit. II. Cytoarchitectonic structure of the striate region and of the dorsal lateral geniculate body; organization of the geniculo-striate projections, *J. Comp. Neurol.* **125:**121.

Royce, G. V., Martin, G. F., and Dom, R. M., 1975, Functional and cortical architecture in the nine-banded armadillo (*Dasypus novemcinctus mexicanus*), *J. Comp. Neurol.* **164:**495.

Sanderson, K. J., and Kaas, J. H., 1974, Thalamocortical interconnections of the visual system of the mink, *Brain Res.* **70:**139.

Sanides, F., and Hoffman, J., 1969, Cyto-and myeloarchitecture of the visual cortex of the cat and of the surrounding integration cortices, *J. Hirnforsch.* **11:**79.

Saraiva, P. E. S., and Magalhães-Castro, B., 1975, Sensory and motor representation in the cerebral cortex of the three-toed sloth (*Bradypus tridactylus*), *Brain Res.* **90:**181.

Sousa, A. P. B., Gattass, R., and Oswaldo-Cruz, E., 1978, The projection of the opossum's visual field on the cerebral cortex, *J. Comp. Neurol.* **177:**569.

Spear, P. D., and Baumann, T. P., 1975, Receptive-field characteristics of single neurons in lateral suprsylvian visual area of the cat, *J. Neurophysiol.* **38:**1403.

Talbot, S. A., 1942, A lateral location cat's visual cortex, *Fed. Proc.* **1:**84.

Talbot, S. A., and Marshall, W. H., 1942, Physiological studies on neural mechanisms of visual localization and discrimination, *Arch. Ophthalmol.* **27:**213.

Thompson, J. M., Woolsey, C. N., and Talbot, S. A., 1950, Visual areas I and II of cerebral cortex of rabbit, *J. Neurophysiol.* **13:**277.

Tiao, Y.-C., and Blakemore, C., 1976, Functional organization in the visual cortex of the golden hamster, *J. Comp. Neurol.* **168:**459.

Towns, L. C., Giolli, R. A., and Haste, D. A., 1977, Corticocortical fiber connections of the rabbit visual cortex: A fiber degeneration study, *J. Comp. Neurol.* **173:**537.

Tusa, R. J., Palmer, L. A., and Rosenquist, A. C., 1978, The retinotopic organization of area 17 (striate cortex) in the cat, *J. Comp. Neurol.* **177:**213.

Tusa, R. J., Rosenquist, A. C., and Palmer, L. A., 1979, Retinotopic organization of areas 18 and 19 in the cat, *J. Comp. Neurol.* **185:**657.

Wagor, E., Mangini, N. J., and Pearlman, A. L., 1979, Retinotopic organization of striate and extrastriate visual cortex in the mouse, *Mus musculus,* in preparation.

Woolsey, C. N., 1971, Comparative studies on cortical representation of vision, *Vision Res. Suppl.* **3:**365.

Woolsey, C. N., Sitthi-Amorn, C., Keesey, U. T., and Holub, R. A., 1973, Cortical visual areas of the rabbit, *Soc. Neurosci. Abstr.* **3:**180.

Zeigler, H. P., 1964, Cortical sensory and motor areas of the guinea pig (*Cavia porcellus*), *Arch. Ital. Biol.* **102:**587.

Zeki, S. M., 1974, The mosaic organization of the visual cortex in the monkey, in: *Essays on the Nervous System: A Festschrift for Professor J. F. Young* (R. Bellairs and E. G. Grey, eds.), Clarendon Press, Oxford.

Index